Veterinary Diseases: Identification, Treatment and Prevention

Veterinary Diseases: Identification, Treatment and Prevention

Editor: Shawn Kiser

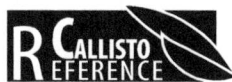

R CALLISTO
REFERENCE

www.callistoreference.com

Callisto Reference,
118-35 Queens Blvd., Suite 400,
Forest Hills, NY 11375, USA

Visit us on the World Wide Web at:
www.callistoreference.com

ISBN: 978-1-63239-846-8 (Hardback)

The publisher's policy is to use permanent paper from mills that operate a sustainable forestry policy. Furthermore, the publisher ensures that the text paper and cover boards used have met acceptable environmental accreditation standards.

Printed in the United States of America.

Cataloging-in-publication Data

Veterinary diseases : identification, treatment and Prevention / edited by Shawn Kiser.
    p. cm.
Includes bibliographical references and index.
ISBN 978-1-63239-846-8
1. Animals--Diseases. 2. Veterinary medicine--Diagnosis. 3. Veterinary therapeutics.
4. Animals--Diseases--Control. 5. Veterinary medicine. I. Kiser, Shawn.
SF745 .V48 2017
636.089--dc23

Table of Contents

Permissions

List of Contributors

Index

Preface

This book provides comprehensive insights into the field of veterinary diseases. It elucidates new techniques and their applications in a multidisciplinary approach. Veterinary diseases are the disorders found in animals. Some of the most common diseases in animals are aflatoxicosis, rabies, tick fever, tuberculosis, ringworm, etc. Laboratory tests are performed to diagnose the disease and then a treatment plan is formed to cure the same. This text provides significant information of this discipline to help develop a good understanding of veterinary diseases and related fields. Different approaches, evaluations, methodologies and advanced studies on diagnosis and treatment of veterinary diseases have been included in this book. It is a compilation of chapters that discussed the most vital concepts and emerging trends in this field. The readers would gain knowledge that would broaden their perspective about this subject. Students, researchers, experts and all associated with the field of veterinary medicine will benefit alike from this book.

The researches compiled throughout the book are authentic and of high quality, combining several disciplines and from very diverse regions from around the world. Drawing on the contributions of many researchers from diverse countries, the book's objective is to provide the readers with the latest achievements in the area of research. This book will surely be a source of knowledge to all interested and researching the field.

In the end, I would like to express my deep sense of gratitude to all the authors for meeting the set deadlines in completing and submitting their research chapters. I would also like to thank the publisher for the support offered to us throughout the course of the book. Finally, I extend my sincere thanks to my family for being a constant source of inspiration and encouragement.

Editor

A Comparison between Two Simulation Models for Spread of Foot-and-Mouth Disease

Tariq Halasa[1]*, Anette Boklund[1], Anders Stockmarr[1,2], Claes Enøe[1], Lasse E. Christiansen[2]

1 Section of Epidemiology, The National Veterinary Institutes, Technical University of Denmark, Copenhagen, Denmark, **2** Department of Applied Mathematics and Computer Science, Technical University of Denmark, Lyngby, Denmark

Abstract

Two widely used simulation models of foot-and-mouth disease (**FMD**) were used in order to compare the models' predictions in term of disease spread, consequence, and the ranking of the applied control strategies, and to discuss the effect of the way disease spread is modeled on the predicted outcomes of each model. The DTU-DADS (version 0.100), and ISP (version 2.001.11) were used to simulate a hypothetical spread of FMD in Denmark. Actual herd type, movements, and location data in the period 1st October 2006 and 30th September 2007 was used. The models simulated the spread of FMD using 3 different control scenarios: 1) A basic scenario representing EU and Danish control strategies, 2) pre-emptive depopulation of susceptible herds within a 500 meters radius around the detected herds, and 3) suppressive vaccination of susceptible herds within a 1,000 meters radius around the detected herds. Depopulation and vaccination started 14 days following the detection of the first infected herd. Five thousand index herds were selected randomly, of which there were 1,000 cattle herds located in high density cattle areas and 1,000 in low density cattle areas, 1,000 swine herds located in high density swine areas and 1,000 in low density swine areas, and 1,000 sheep herds. Generally, DTU-DADS predicted larger, longer duration and costlier epidemics than ISP, except when epidemics started in cattle herds located in high density cattle areas. ISP supported suppressive vaccination rather than pre-emptive depopulation, while DTU-DADS was indifferent to the alternative control strategies. Nonetheless, the absolute differences between control strategies were small making the choice of control strategy during an outbreak to be most likely based on practical reasons.

Editor: Yury E. Khudyakov, Centers for Disease Control and Prevention, United States of America

Funding: This study was financially supported by the Directorate for Food, Agriculture and Fisheries, Denmark (grant nr. 3304-FVFP-07-782-01). The funders had no role in study design, data collection and analysis, decision to publish, or preparation of the manuscript.

Competing Interests: The authors have declared that no competing interests exist.

* E-mail: tahbh@vet.dtu.dk

Introduction

Foot-and-mouth disease (**FMD**) is a highly contagious disease of ruminants and pigs that can cause large economic damage [1]. Several countries have imposed strict legislations and control strategies to eradicate FMD, such as the western European countries [2]. Despite of the successful eradication of FMD from these countries, some suffered severe outbreaks during the past 15 years, which indicates that FMD remains a constant threat to FMD-free countries. Following the 2001 UK outbreak, the EU has revised the regulations, in which the use of emergency vaccination was emphasized, and more emphasis on member states to show permanent awareness and preparedness to an FMD outbreak was enforced [3].

Simulation models are widely used to support veterinary authorities to setup contingency plans for FMD awareness and preparedness [1,4,5,6,7]. They are also used to study the potential spread of FMD and to evaluate potential control strategies to minimize the impact of the outbreak [7,8]. During the 2001 UK outbreak, simulation models were used to help the veterinary authorities control the spread of the outbreak [9,10]. Despite of the wide use of FMD simulation models, different models may substantially differ from each other due to different assumptions regarding the modeled processes. Moreover, models can differ in their flexibility to include changes to the models' basic structure,

their data requirement to run, and their ease of use. For example, the InterSpread Plus model (**ISP**) [11,12,13,14] has a user friendly interface, but it is not flexible, when it comes to including changes to the basic structure of the model. On the other hand, the Davis Animal Disease Simulation model (**DADS**) that has been further developed at the Technical University of Denmark to **DTU-DADS** [15,16] requires good programming skills, and hence is not user friendly. However, because it is possible to include changes to the model structure, this model is very flexible. In order to understand the simulated processes, the spread mechanisms and the results of the models, it is important to understand how the differences between models affect the results.

Because of the absence of outbreak data in some countries, and hence the difficulty to validate outcomes of an FMD simulation model, relative validity has been proposed [17,18]. This method suggests that two or more scenarios are defined and two or more independently developed models are used to simulate the spread of disease using these test scenarios [18]. Agreement among the different models in their prediction provides evidence that the developers of each model were consistent in their approach to simulate the spread of the disease [18]. The spread of FMD was compared using 3 simulation models; ISP, the North American Animal Disease Spread (NAADSM) and the Australian model (AusSpread) [18]. The authors found that the predicted outcomes were statistically significantly different between the different models. Nonetheless, the authors did not provide a detailed description of the effects of differences between models on the predicted outcomes of the models.

The objective of this paper is to simulate a hypothetical spread of FMD in Denmark using two widely used simulation models of FMD spread (DADS and ISP), in order to compare the models' predictions in term of disease spread, consequence, the ranking of the applied control strategies, and the effect of the way disease spread is modeled on the predicted outcomes of each model.

Materials and Methods

Data Description

Both simulation models used the same herd data, which contained information on all Danish cattle, swine, sheep and goats herds in the period from 1st October 2006 until 30th September 2007. For each herd, the herd data included the Danish Herd Identification System, referred to as CHR number, herd type, UTM geo-coordinates, number of animals, and number of off-farm animal movements per day. Herds were categorized into 3 categories; cattle, swine, and small ruminants (in this paper referred to as "sheep"). Cattle herds were categorized as dairy or non-dairy herds. Swine herds were categorized into 19 different types based on their production type and SPF (specific pathogen-free herd) status [19]. The number of animal movement was divided into animal movement from a herd to another and animal movement to the abattoir. For swine herds, animal movements were described as movements of either sows or weaners. When a farm included several animal species, each species was given a different ID and set as a different herd on the same location and with the same CHR number.

The input parameters of the models were based on Danish data, the literature and personal communication to experts [15]. Due to the large number of input parameters used in the models, we have described only parameters that influence the difference between the two models in this paper. All other parameters are described in a previous publication [15].

The Simulation Study

General framework. A hypothetical spread of FMD between herds in Denmark was simulated using two spatial simulation models; namely DTU-DADS (version 0.100), and ISP (version 2.001.11). The DADS model (version 0.05) was upgraded to DTU-DADS [15], to incorporate changes necessary to model FMD spread in Denmark. The simulation starts with the models loading the input data, and thereafter selecting the index herd, which is the first infected and detected herd in the epidemic. The index herd was randomly chosen for each herd type and when relevant for different animal densities. The index herds were 1,000 cattle herds located in high density cattle areas and 1,000 in low density cattle areas, 1,000 swine herds located in high density swine areas and 1,000 in low density swine areas, and 1,000 sheep herds. This was done to consider the variation between index herds, and for each index herd, the epidemic was simulated only once (= 1 iteration). The same index herds were used in both models and in all control scenarios to minimize variation between the models and scenarios.

Disease spread and dynamics. Spread of infection between herds was simulated through 7 spread mechanisms: 1) direct animal movement between herds; 2) abattoir trucks; 3) milk tankers; 4) veterinarians, artificial inseminators, and/or milk controllers (referred to as medium risk contacts); 5) visitors, feedstuff and/or rendering trucks (referred to as low risk contacts); 6) markets; and 7) local spread.

Based on actual animal movement data, a rate of animal movements per day was calculated for each herd. The individual daily movement rate was used as lambda in a Poisson distribution to represent the number of movements per day. Similarly, a rate of abattoir deliveries per day was calculated based on herds' actual data and used in a Poisson distribution to simulate the number of movements to the abattoir per day from the infectious herd. Thereafter, the number of herds visited by an abattoir truck on the way to the abattoir following visit to an infected herd was estimated from a Poisson distribution with a lambda depending on the herd type. For all milking herds, the average probability of having milk picked up was used as lambda in a Poisson

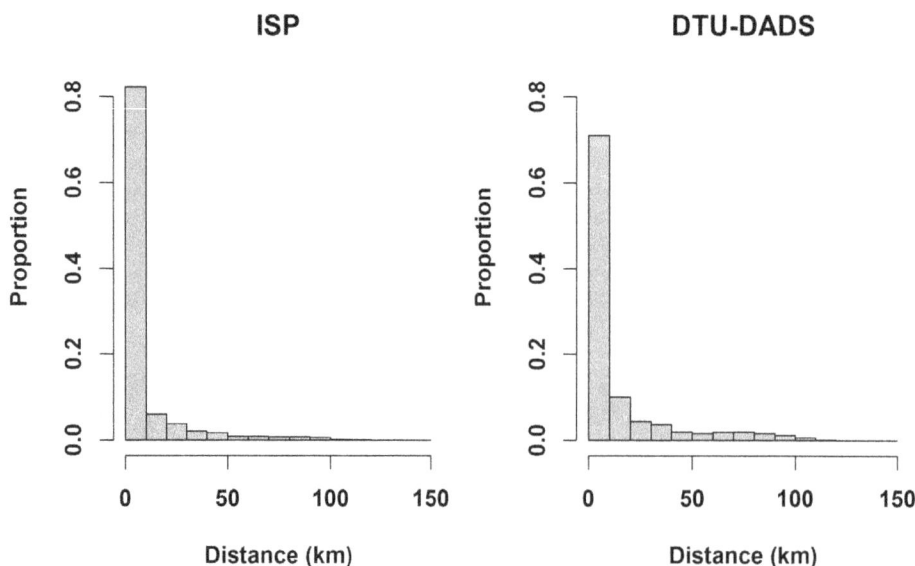

Figure 1. Distribution of distances (km) between infected herds and the source herd in two stochastic models simulating spread of FMD in Denmark (DTU-DADS (black) and ISP (gray)). Epidemics were initiated in cattle herds located in high density cattle area, using the basic control strategy(EU and Danish regulation of FMD control). Distances over 150 km were removed (<0.01% of distances).

Table 1. Epidemiological and economic results of a simulated FMD-epidemic in Denmark, using two simulation models: DTU-DADS and ISP.

Scenario and outcome parameter	Model - Median (5th and 95th percentiles)	
	DTU-DADS	ISP
High cattle		
Duration (days)	56**(16–142)	80 (5–255)
Infected	67**(13–245)	137 (3–696)
Depopulated	67**(13–245)	141 (3–718)
Total costs (€×10^6)	565**(402–946)	665 (399–1,137)
Area (km^2)	9,869*(567–28,687)	11,114 (0–35,178)
Low cattle		
Duration (days)	71 (19–179)	66 (2–226)
Infected	94 (15–371)	81 (2–521)
Depopulated	94 (15–371)	80 (1–539)
Total costs (€×10^6)	608**(416–1,061)	547 (363–1,101)
Area (km^2)	11,414**(339–36,207)	5,994 (0–32,588)
High swine		
Duration (days)	43**(8–130)	25 (2–180)
Infected	36**(5–195)	12 (1–313)
Depopulated	36**(5–195)	13 (1–322)
Total costs (€×10^6)	498**(376–869)	429 (341–961)
Area (km^2)	5,053**(11–27,254)	771 (0–22,680)
Sheep		
Duration (days)	38**(6–139)	9 (2–155)
Infected	29**(3–198)	4 (1–222)
Depopulated	29**(3–198)	4 (1–233)
Total costs (€×10^6)	476**(364–876)	410 (345–723)
Area (km^2)	3,881**(0–24,473)	1 (0–17,538)

refers to a **p-value <0.01, *refers to a **p-value <0.05,** and no sign refers to a **p-value ≥0.05.**
Basic control measures are simulated to control the epidemic. Epidemics are starting in cattle herds located in high and low density cattle areas, swine herds located in high density swine areas and in sheep herds, resulting in 5000 simulated epidemics. Results are given as medians (5–95%).

distribution describing contacts between herds by milk tankers. Likewise, medium and low risk contacts were simulated, but with different lambdas and risks of infection [15]. Once an infectious herd had a contact with a susceptible herd, the susceptible herd might become infected based on probabilities of infection per contact type [15]. It was assumed that all herds are equally susceptible, while the infectiousness was related to the proportion of infected animal within the herd. Because markets in Denmark are restricted to cattle only, an infection spreading from a market can initially affect only cattle herds [15]. Local spread was defined as infection of susceptible herds within a 3 km radius around the infected herd due to unexplained reasons, such as rodents, birds, flies and a limited airborne spread.

The disease was modelled to always start in one herd (the index case) and develop until the disease was detected, and hence the herd was depopulated. The period from a herd starts showing clinical signs and until detection was dependent on the herd type, e.g. cattle herds were detected faster than sheep herds, because some sheep do not show clinical signs. Moreover, herds within the protection and surveillance zones would have higher probability of detection, because of surveillance. Detection of the first infected farm was assumed to always be at day 21 following the start of the epidemic. This was based on experience from the UK [20,21] and

the Dutch 2001 FMD outbreaks [22]. In the simulations, the infection spread freely between herds during the first 21 days.

Basic control measures following detection of infection. After detection of the first infected herd, a set of default control strategies were applied representing the basic scenario. These included: 1) depopulation, cleaning and disinfection of detected herds; 2) a 3 days national stand still on animal movements in the country; 3) a 10 km radius zone (surveillance zone) around the detected herds; in which movements between herds and out of the zone were restricted and herds were surveyed one time before lifting the zone; 4) a 3 km radius zone (protection zone) around the detected herd, in which movements between herds and out of the zone were restricted, and herds are surveyed during the first week and a second time, 21 days later; 5) backward and forward tracing of contacts from and to detected herds. When a herd had received animals from a detected herd, the receiving herd was also depopulated and disinfected, while in case of other kind of contacts, the herd was surveyed. When a herd was subject to surveillance, the animals were inspected for clinical signs of FMD. In case of sheep herds, the animals were also sampled for serological analysis [15]. The daily animal depopulation capacity was set at 2,400 ruminants and 4,800 pigs [15]. Detected herds had higher priority for depopulation than traced herds. In case of

Empirical cumulative distribution

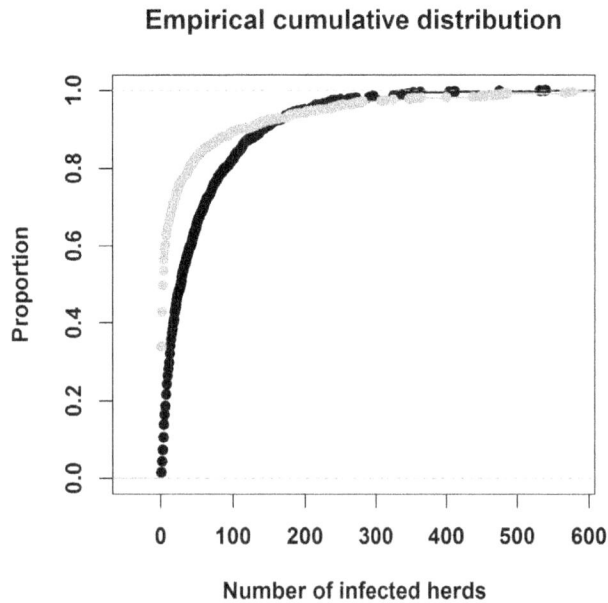

Figure 2. Empirical cumulative distribution of the number of infected herds predicted by the DTU-DADS (black) and ISP (gray), when the epidemic started in sheep herds and under the basic scenario, in which the EU and Danish regulation of FMD control were simulated.

several herds on the same farm, all herds on the farm were depopulated, when one herd was depopulated.

Simulated scenarios. Three spread scenarios were run in the models. The scenarios were: 1) the basic scenario, in which the EU and Danish control strategies were implemented as explained bellow, 2) pre-emptive depopulation, including the basic scenario plus depopulation of herds within 500 meters around detected herds, and 3) suppressive vaccination, including the basic scenario plus emergency vaccination of herds within 1,000 meters around detected herds. Vaccination and depopulation were initiated 14 days following the detection of the first infected herd.

When a susceptible herd was vaccinated, the herd was assumed to be susceptible for 4 days before the immunity would start to build up and reach its maximum potential at day 9 following vaccination. Vaccinated herds that became infected would be fully infectious, if they had been vaccinated ≤4 days before exposure to the virus, otherwise, the infectiousness reduced until day 9 following vaccination, where it was reduced by 90% [15]. The efficacy of the vaccine was obtained from a meta-analysis study on FMD vaccine efficacy [23].

The daily animal vaccination capacity was assumed to be 60,000 ruminants and 50,000 pigs [15]. Before vaccination, cattle and pig herds were clinically surveyed and sheep herds were serological surveyed. Thirty days following vaccination, the herds were surveyed again, before the vaccination zone was lifted.

Vaccinated herds were assumed to be depopulated after the end of the outbreak [5]. In this paper, only the effect of suppressive vaccination is presented. Results simulating the effect of protective vaccination are presented in a previous publication [15].

Differences between the Models

Despite that the models were setup to simulate the same spread scenarios, there are several dissimilarities between the models and it was not possible to make all simulations identical in the two models. These differences are:

When direct and indirect contact is modelled, a susceptible herd can become infected, based on a distance-based probability, a probability of contact between the different herd types, and a probability of disease transmission. In the DTU-DADS, these risks are multiplied and then a herd is selected from all herds within the country. In the ISP, the model will first select a distance band and then a herd will be selected within the band. Herds of the same type within a distance band will have similar probability of selection.

Disease spread within a herd in DTU-DADS is modeled stochastically. This means that disease spread within herds of the same type can be different. In ISP, herds of the same type would have similar patterns of within herd disease spread. This means that the infectiousness of a herd can be different between DTU-DADS and ISP, despite of similar herd characteristics and time of infection.

Several parameters are stochastic in the models. However, the way the stochasticity of these parameters is implemented can be different for some of the parameters. In DTU-DADS, risk of infection following low, medium or high risk contacts are stochastic across iterations. This means the risk for a specific herd would be the same during the iteration. Such parameters are stochastic per day in ISP, which means that the values differ between days within iteration for the same herd.

When modeling the number of contacts the truck makes on its way to the abattoir to deliver pigs and sheep, ISP uses the herds-specific abattoir lambda to determine whether a movement to the abattoir will occur at that day. Thereafter, it determines the number of herds that will be contacted on the way to the abattoir, based on a probability distribution function. In DTU-DADS, the herd-specific abattoir lambda is used in a Poisson distribution to determine the number of contacts a truck makes picking up pigs or sheep on its way to the abattoir.

In DTU-DADS all infected herds will eventually be detected. However, small herds might be infected and then recover without being detected in ISP.

Other differences do exist, but are not presented here, because of their minor impact on models' predictions, following investigation through sensitivity analysis [15].

Cost-benefit Analysis

The costs and losses due to the epidemics per control scenario were calculated as explained previously [15]. Briefly, the total costs of an epidemic were the sum of the direct and indirect costs. The direct costs consisted of surveillance, depopulation, cleaning and disinfection, empty stable, compensation, national standstill, and vaccination costs. The indirect costs included losses incurred from restrictions on exports to EU and non-EU countries. Total costs were calculated per iteration and their summaries were thereafter estimated.

Comparison between the Models

The predicted epidemiologic, total costs and epidemic area outputs of each scenario were compared between the two models. Epidemiologic predictors consisted of number of infected premises and the epidemic duration. The spatial spread (or epidemic area) was calculated by plotting the locations of the detected herds per iterations and constructing a minimum convex hull around the herds and then measuring the area of the resulting convex hull polygon. Predictions of each scenario of the two models were compared using the Wilcoxon Signed Rank Sum test in R 2.14.0 [24].

Table 2. Epidemiological and economic results of a simulated FMD-epidemic in Denmark, using two simulation models: DTU-DADS and ISP.

Scenario and outcome parameter	Model - Median (5th and 95th percentiles)	
	DTU-DADS	**ISP**
High cattle		
Duration (days)	46**(16–100)	66 (5–184)
Infected	59**(12–177)	109 (3–469)
Depopulated	84**(13–282)	175 (3–806)
Total costs (€×10^6)	533**(403–773)	614 (398–948)
Area (km^2)	9,372**(527–25,448)	9,779 (0–31,422)
Low cattle		
Duration (days)	51 (18–117)	52 (2–166)
Infected	71 (15–231)	59 (2–367)
Depopulated	104 (18–368)	93 (1–604)
Total costs (€×10^6)	543**(412–811)	510 (363–936)
Area (km^2)	9,672**(338–30,628)	4,608 (0–29,507)
High swine		
Duration (days)	37**(8–96)	23 (2–132)
Infected	31**(5–126)	11 (1–195)
Depopulated	43**(5–205)	16 (1–341)
Total costs (€×10^6)	480**(376–731)	422 (340–805)
Area (km^2)	4,386**(11–22,704)	642 (0–19,010)
Sheep		
Duration (days)	34**(6–100)	9 (2–133)
Infected	25**(3–130)	4 (1–157)
Depopulated	34**(3–210)	4 (1–285)
Total costs (€×10^6)	464**(364–716)	405 (345–681)
Area (km^2)	3,301**(0–19,842)	1 (0–13,396)

refers to a **p-value <0.01, *refers to a **p-value <0.05,** and no sign refers to a **p-value ≥0.05.**
Basic control measures **plus pre-emptive depopulation in 500 meters** are simulated to control the epidemic. Epidemics are starting in cattle herds located in high and low density cattle areas, swine herds located in high density swine areas and in sheep herds, resulting in 5000 simulated epidemics. Results are given as medians (5–95%).

Results

Basic Scenario

When epidemics were initiated in cattle herds located in high density cattle area, the proportion of disease spread through animal movements, indirect contacts and local spread predicted by DTU-DADS were, consecutively, 0.003%, 0.547% and 0.45%, while ISP prediction of disease spread through these mechanisms were, consecutively, 0.01%, 0.33% and 0.66%. Similar trends were observed when epidemics were initiated using the other index herd types. The distributions of distance between the infected herd and the source herd from both models are shown in Figure 1. It shows that DTU-DADS tends to have higher probability to spread the disease over long distances, while ISP tends to spread the disease over shorter distances, and hence cluster the spread in smaller areas than DTU-DADS. The 5th, 25th, 50th, 75th, 95th percentiles and maximum values of the predicted distances by DTU-DATS were, respectively, 0.00, 0.55, 1.92, 13.61, 72.44 and 163 km, while the predicted values by ISP were, respectively, 0.00, 0.53, 1.47, 3.49, 43.99 and 300 km.

DTU-DADS predicted larger epidemics of longer duration than the ISP, except from epidemics starting in cattle herds located in high density cattle areas. In these epidemics, ISP predicted larger

and longer duration epidemics (Table 1). There is a significant difference between the results of DTU-DADS and ISP in the basic scenarios, when the epidemic started in cattle herds located in high density cattle and swine herds located in high density swine areas and in sheep herds (Table 1). When the epidemic started in cattle herds located in low density cattle areas, the epidemiologic predictors (epidemic duration, number of infected and depopulated herds) show an insignificant difference between the models' results (Table 1). However, the differences in total costs and epidemic area between the 2 models were significant, in which DTU-DADS predicted wider spread and more costly epidemics. Generally, DTU-DADS seems to predict disease spread over larger areas than ISP (Table 1). This is not only when DTU-DADS predicted larger number of infected herds, but also when the difference in the predicted number of affected herds was not significantly different between the 2 models, as the case when epidemics started in cattle herds located in low density cattle area (Table 1). In this case, the predicted epidemic area by DTU-DADS was almost double the size of the predicted area by ISP (Table 1). Results from epidemics started in swine herds located in high and low density swine areas were very similar, and therefore

Table 3. Epidemiological and economic results of a simulated FMD-epidemic in Denmark, using two simulation models: DTU-DADS and ISP.

Scenario and outcome parameter	Model - Median (5ᵗʰ and 95ᵗʰ percentiles)	
	DTU-DADS	**ISP**
High cattle		
Duration (days)	47**(16–100)	59 (5–141)
Infected	60**(12–193)	93 (3–368)
Depopulated	60**(12–193)	96 (3–383)
Vaccinated	90**(3–350)	160 (0–711)
Total costs (€×10⁶)	535**(400–788)	573 (400–803)
Area (km²)	10,473 (549–25,236)	8,218 (0–28,349)
Low cattle		
Duration (days)	52*(19–103)	48 (2–137)
Infected	74**(15–232)	53 (2–287)
Depopulated	74**(15–232)	53 (1–303)
Vaccinated	117 (7–434)	84 (0–579)
Total costs (€×10⁶)	546**(410–799)	497 (365–820)
Area (km²)	11,683**(351–31,036)	4,136 (0–25,236)
High swine		
Duration (days)	37**(8–86)	23 (2–115)
Infected	31**(5–124)	11 (1–155)
Depopulated	31**(5–125)	12 (1–161)
Vaccinated	41**(0–253)	12 (0–357)
Total costs (€×10⁶)	479**(375–694)	421 (341–728)
Area (km²)	6,784**(10–21,497)	627 (0–17,225)
Sheep		
Duration (days)	35**(6–85)	9 (2–98)
Infected	26**(3–125)	4 (1–114)
Depopulated	26**(3–125)	4 (1–118)
Vaccinated	34**(0–251)	0 (0–270)
Total costs (€×10⁶)	469**(365–691)	404 (346–598)
Area (km²)	5,930**(0–19,977)	1 (0–10,664)

refers to a **p-value <0.01, *refers to a **p-value <0.05**, and no sign refers to a **p-value ≥0.05**.
Basic control measures **plus suppressive vaccination in 1000 meters** are simulated to control the epidemic. Epidemics are starting in cattle herds located in high and low density cattle areas, swine herds located in high density swine areas and in sheep herds, resulting in 5000 simulated epidemics. Results are given as medians (5–95%).

we chose to present only those started in swine herds located in high density swine areas.

ISP shows larger variability's and extreme situations than the DTU-DADS model as presented in the 5ᵗʰ and 95ᵗʰ percentiles of the predicted outcomes (Table 1). When the epidemic started in sheep herds, DTU-DADS showed significantly larger number of infected herds than the ISP (Table 1). However, ISP showed larger variability and more extreme epidemics than DTU-DADS (Figure 2).

Depopulation and Vaccination Scenarios

In the depopulation and vaccination scenarios (Tables 2 and 3), we generally observed similar trends in differences between DTU-DADS and ISP as those observed in the basic scenario. DTU-DADS showed significantly larger, wider spread and costlier epidemics than the ISP, except when the epidemic started in cattle herds located in high density cattle areas. When the epidemic

started in cattle herds located in low density cattle areas using vaccination 14 days following the detection of the first infected herd, the difference between the 2 models' prediction became significant (Table 3).

Generally, the models showed that zone depopulation or suppressive vaccination resulted in significantly shorter epidemics, fewer infected herds and cheaper epidemics than the basic scenario in both models (p-values <0.05). Using DTU-DADS, there was no significant difference in the costs of epidemics between depopulation in 500 meters and suppressive vaccination in 1 km control scenarios (p-values >0.05), regardless the index-herd type. However, using ISP, suppressive vaccination in 1 km was generally a cheaper choice than depopulation in 500 meters (p-value <0.05). Nonetheless, given the large variation, the difference in the absolute values is rather small.

Discussion

Generally, DTU-DADS showed significantly larger and longer duration of outbreaks than the ISP, when the epidemic started in swine herds located in high density swine areas and in sheep herds. The opposite was true when the epidemic started in cattle herds located in high density cattle areas. When epidemics started in cattle herds located in low density cattle areas, there was no significant difference in the predicted number of infected herds and epidemic duration between the 2 models, but DTU-DADS predicted larger epidemic area and costs than ISP. The tendency that DTU-DADS predicts larger epidemics and epidemic area than ISP could be explained by the way the newly infected herds are selected. In DTU-DADS, when an infected herd would infect other herds, the newly infected herds would be selected from all herds in the country based on distance and contact probabilities. In ISP, a distance band is drawn around the infected herd and then newly infected herds are selected from within the band. Herds of the same type would have similar probability of infection. In case no herds with positive probability of infection were found in the band, a new band will be selected with a maximum retries sat to 100 times in the current project. This means that in DTU-DADS, herds located close to and herds located far away from the infectious herd would be subjected to selection directly in one step. These herds would of course have different probabilities of selection, in which herds located far away would have lower probabilities than herds located close by. Nonetheless, the number of susceptible herds located far away is very large, which means that some might be selected more often compared to the way selection of new infected herds is carried out in ISP. This is because, in ISP such herds would have extremely small chance of selection, because the closer bands would most likely be selected. This means that DTU-DADS tend to spread the disease over longer distances and thus generally larger epidemics and epidemic area than ISP. This can be seen from Figure 1, which shows clearly that DTU-DADS have a higher chance to spread the disease over longer distances than ISP.

Furthermore, local spread dominated the different types of spread mechanisms in ISP (66%), while lower percentage (45%) of infection through local spread was predicted by DTU-DADS. This indicates as well that ISP tends to restrict outbreaks to a small area, while DTU-DADS would spread them out over longer distances, and hence larger areas. We speculate that the higher percentage of disease spread through local spread, and the short distance jumps of new infections through indirect contacts (e.g. low risk contact), combined with the presence of large number of susceptible herds in the area have resulted in larger epidemics size in ISP than DTU-DADS, when the index herd was cattle located in high density cattle area.

ISP tended to show larger variation and more extreme situations than the DTU-DADS (Table 1 and Figure 2). It is actually not completely clear why ISP creates larger variability and extreme situations than DTU-DADS. Nevertheless, the way disease spread is modelled might explain the larger variability predicted by ISP.

From this study, it was not possible to judge which way of modelling disease spread is the correct one. A way to get closer to the answer, would most likely be to compare models' output to actual outbreak data, and then use the method that best explain the data. Recent outbreak data is not available in Denmark, given that the last outbreak was in 1982 [25]. Furthermore, it is actually unknown whether the models would have similar trends, as observed in the current study, had this exercise been conducted on data from another region. This is because the structure of the

herds, the movement and contact patterns and intensity between herds in that region would also affect disease spread.

The models agreed that zone depopulation and suppressive vaccination are cheaper than the basic scenario. When depopulation and vaccination were compared, DTU-DADS was indifferent to the choices, while ISP estimated the costs, size and duration of suppressive vaccination to be smaller. This would indicate that the choice of control strategy might differ depending on the chosen model. However, from a practical point of view, the absolute differences were small, and given the large variation in the results, the final decision on strategy will most likely be based on other issues as well, such as practical, political, ethical and social effects of the epidemic. In this exercise, pre-emptive depopulation and suppressive vaccination were chosen to be implemented 14 day following the detection of the first infected herd. Following consultation with the National Veterinary Authorities, this timeframe seems reasonable before suppressive vaccination can be started. Despite that the two models did not fully agree on the chosen control strategy using this scenario, they have actually agreed that depopulation following the detection of 10 infected herds was the optimal scenario to control FMD spread in Denmark [15].

From a practical point of view, the advantage of DTU-DADS is that the structure of the model can be changed easily as soon as new data or knowledge arises, e.g. by adding new modules, because the source code is available. An important advantage, DTU-DADS runs on free software, but it demands personnel trained in programming. On the other hand, ISP is not free and cannot be extended to include changes to the structure of the model by the user. However, the model demands much less programming skills and training than DTU-DADS. ISP ran in few hours on personal computers, which is faster than the DTU-DADS that required one day for some scenarios in this study. Nonetheless, DTU-DADS can be run on a server, and hence can practically be very fast, because many scenarios can run at the same time. The cost-benefit analysis has been integrated within the DTU-DADS, which means that after the end of the model run, all necessary outputs can be obtained and only statistical analysis is still to be carried out. On the other hand, cost-benefit analysis on ISP outputs was carried out separately following the model run. Finally, DTU-DADS (in its current version) does not include elements of airborne spread, while ISP does. Important to mention, for the current exercise, spread of infection through airborne was not modelled, in order to keep the models as close to each other as possible. In a country where detailed herd, movement and contact data is available, ISP and DTU-DADS can both be useful, as they can represent the spread mechanism in details. This allows identifying risky contacts, which can be helpful to the veterinary authorities, while they are setting the preparedness and contingency plans.

The spread of FMD was compared using hypothetical data in 3 simulation models: ISP, North American Animal Disease Spread Model (NAADSM) and the Australian model (AusSpread) [17]. They found that the predicted number of infected premises and temporal and spatial spread predicted by the three models differed significantly, but the absolute differences were small and from a practical perspective would have resulted in a similar management decision being adopted. In a follow up study [18] and using actual population data, it was found that the predicted outcomes were also statistically significantly different between the different models, but the absolute results of ISP and AusSpread were clearly close compared to the results of the NAADSM, using standard EU control measures [18]. In the current study, the results also showed frequently a statistically significant difference in the predicted outcomes of the 2 models, with small absolute differences as well.

The current study provided insight into the differences between the models and discussed how those differences could have influenced models' predictions. Moreover, the current study estimated the financial impact of the epidemics, which is important, because significant epidemiological differences between the models could be financially indifferent or vice-versa. It is important to mention that efforts have been made to include the NAADSM in the comparison. Nonetheless, it was not possible to run the scenarios in the setup defined in the study using the available version of NAADSM when the study was performed, and thus the model was excluded. The restricted access to the source code of ISP has limited our capacity of investigating the effect of differences between the models on their predictions. Thus future research should have unlimited access to models' code, and should focus on investigating, which method of modeling disease spread between herds would best represent reality. This can be done either by comparing the predicted outputs to outbreak data, or to kernel models that are estimated based on outbreak data [8,9]. Furthermore, the larger variability that is predicted by ISP, compared to the DTU-DADS, should be further investigated.

Author Contributions

Conceived and designed the experiments: TH AB AS CE LEC. Performed the experiments: TH AB AS CE LEC. Analyzed the data: TH AB. Contributed reagents/materials/analysis tools: TH AB AS CE LEC. Wrote the paper: TH.

References

1. Pendell DL, Leatherman J, Schroeder TC, Alward GS (2007) The economic impact of foot-and-mouth disease outbreak: a regional analysis. J Agr App Econ 39: 19–33.
2. Cox SJ, Barnett PV (2009) Experimental evaluation of foot-and-mouth disease vaccines for emergency use in ruminants and pigs: a review. Vet Res 40: 13–43.
3. European Commission (2003) Council Directive 2003/85/EC on community measures for the control of foot-and-mouth disease repealing, Directive 85/511/EEC and amending directive 92/46/EEC. Official J Eur Union L306, 46, 22 November 2003.
4. Bates T, Thurmond MC, Carpenter TE (2003) Description of and epidemic simulation model for use in evaluating strategies to control an outbreak of foot-and-mouth disease. AJVR 64: 195–204.
5. Velthuis AGJ, Mourits MCM (2007) Effectiveness of movement prevention regulations to reduce the spread of foot-and-mouth disease in The Netherlands. Prev Vet Med 82: 262–281.
6. Tildesley MJ, Keeling MJ (2008) Foot-and-Mouth Disease - A Modelling Comparison between the UK and Denmark. Prev Vet Med 85: 107–124.
7. Martínez-López B, Perez AM, Sánchez-Vizcaíno JM (2010) A simulation model for the potential spread of foot-and-mouth disease in the Castile and Leon region of Spain. Prev Vet Med 96: 19–29.
8. Backer JA, Hagenaars TJ, Nodelijk G, van Roermund HJW (2012) Vaccination against foot-and-mouth disease I: Epidemiological consequences. Prev Vet Med107: 27–40.
9. Keeling MJ, Woolhouse MEJ, Shaw DJ, Mathews L, Chase-Topping M, et al. (2001) Dynamics of the 2001 UK foot and mouth disease epidemic: Stochastic dispersal in heterogeneous landscape. Science 294: 813–817.
10. Taylor N (2003) Review of the use of models in informing disease control policy development and adjustment. Defra, London, the UK.
11. Sanson RL (1993) The development of a decision support system for animal disease emergency. PhD Thesis, Massey University, Palmerston North, New Zealand.
12. Stern MW (2003) InterSpread Plus, User Guide. Massey University, New Zealand.
13. Stevenson M, Sanson RL, Stern M, O'Leary BD, Mackereth G, et al. (2005) InterSpread Plus: a spatial and stochastic simulation model of disease in animal populations. Technical paper for research project BER-60–2004. Biosecurity New Zealand, Wellington, New Zealand.
14. Stevenson MA, Sanson RL, Stern MW, O'Leary BD, Sujau M, et al. (2013) InterSpread Plus: A spatial and stochastic simulation model of disease in animal populations. Prev Vet Med 109: 10–24.
15. Boklund A, Halasa T, Christiansen LE, Enøe C (2013) Comparing control strategies against foot- and-mouth disease: Will vaccination be cost-effective in Denmark? Prev Vet Med 111: 206–219.
16. Halasa T, Willeberg P, Christiansen LE, Boklund A, AlKhamis M, et al. (2013) Decisions on control of foot-and-mouth disease informed using model predictions. Prev Vet Med 112: 194–202.
17. Dube C, Stevenson MA, Garner MG, Sanson RL, Carso BA, et al. (2007) A comparison of predictions made by three simulation models of foot-and-mouth disease. NZ Vet J 55: 280–288.
18. Sanson RL, Harvey N, Garner MG, Stevenson MA, Davis TM, et al. (2011) Foot and mouth disease model varification and 'relative validation' through a formal model comparison. Rev Sci Tech Off Int Epiz 30: 527–540.
19. Boklund A, Alban L, Toft N, Uttenthal Å (2009) Comparing the epidemiological and economic effects of control strategies against classical swine fever in Denmark. Prev Vet Med 90: 180–193.
20. Gibbens JC, Sharpe CE, Wilesmith JW, Mansley LM, Michalopoulou E, et al. (2001) Descriptive epidemiology of the 2001 foot-and-mouth disease epidemic in Great Britain: the first five months. Vet Rec 149: 729–743.
21. Gibbens JC, Wilesmith JW (2002) Temporal and geographical distribution of the cases of foot-and-mouth disease during the early weeks of the 2001 epidemic in Great Britain. Vet Rec 151: 407–412.
22. Pluimers FH, Akkerman AM, van der Wal P, Dekker A, Bianchi A (2002) Lessons from the foot and mouth disease outbreak in the Netherlands in 2001. Rev Sci Tech Off Int Epiz 21: 711–721.
23. Halasa T, Boklund A, Cox S, Enøe C (2011) Meta-analysis on the efficacy of foot-and-mouth disease emergency vaccination. Prev. Vet. Med. 98, 1–9.
24. R Development Core Team (2011) R: A language and environment for statistical computing. R Foundation for Statistical Computing, Vienna, Austria. ISBN 3-900051-07-0, URL http://www.R-project.org/.
25. Westergaard JM (1982) Report on the eradication of foot-and-mouth disease on the Island of Funen and Zealand, Denmark 1982. The Danish Veterinary Service, Frederiksgade 21, 1265 Copenhagen 21, Denmark.

2

Hand-Rearing, Release and Survival of African Penguin Chicks Abandoned Before Independence by Moulting Parents

Richard B. Sherley[1,2*¤], **Lauren J. Waller**[1,3], **Venessa Strauss**[4], **Deon Geldenhuys**[3], **Les G. Underhill**[1], **Nola J. Parsons**[4]

1 Animal Demography Unit and Marine Research Institute, University of Cape Town, Rondebosch, Western Cape, South Africa, 2 Bristol Zoological Society, Bristol Zoo Gardens, Bristol, United Kingdom, 3 CapeNature, Hermanus, Western Cape, South Africa, 4 Southern African Foundation for the Conservation of Coastal Birds, Bloubergrant, Western Cape, South Africa

Abstract

The African penguin *Spheniscus demersus* has an 'Endangered' conservation status and a decreasing population. Following abandonment, 841 African penguin chicks in 2006 and 481 in 2007 were admitted to SANCCOB (Southern African Foundation for the Conservation of Coastal Birds) for hand-rearing from colonies in the Western Cape, South Africa, after large numbers of breeding adults commenced moult with chicks still in the nest. Of those admitted, 91% and 73% respectively were released into the wild. There were veterinary concerns about avian malaria, airsacculitis and pneumonia, feather-loss and pododermatitis (bumblefoot). Post-release juvenile (0.32, s.e. = 0.08) and adult (0.76, s.e. = 0.10) survival rates were similar to African penguin chicks reared after oil spills and to recent survival rates recorded for naturally-reared birds. By December 2012, 12 birds had bred, six at their colony of origin, and the apparent recruitment rate was 0.11 (s.e. = 0.03). Hand-rearing of abandoned penguin chicks is recommended as a conservation tool to limit mortality and to bolster the population at specific colonies. The feasibility of conservation translocations for the creation of new colonies for this species using hand-reared chicks warrants investigation. Any such programme would be predicated on adequate disease surveillance programmes established to minimise the risk of disease introduction to wild birds.

Editor: William Hughes, University of Sussex, United Kingdom

Funding: The authors acknowledge financial support from our institutes, the SeaChange Programme of the National Research Foundation, the Earthwatch Institute, Dyer Island Conservation Trust, the Norway South Africa Fisheries Agreement (NORSA), IFAW and the Leiden Conservation Foundation. The funders had no role in study design, data collection and analysis, decision to publish, or preparation of the manuscript.

Competing Interests: The authors have declared that no competing interests exist.

* Email: richard.sherley@gmail.com

¤ Current address: Environment and Sustainability Institute, University of Exeter, Penryn, Cornwall, United Kingdom

Introduction

The conservation status of the world's seabirds is poor with c. 47% of species showing population declines and c. 28% occupying positions in the IUCN Red List's threatened categories [1]. In many cases, species face numerous threats, not all of which are well understood in form or function. This highlights the need for further research to improve seabird conservation [2], but also the importance of management actions that can reduce mortality and sustain populations in the short-term [1].

The African penguin *Spheniscus demersus* is 'Endangered' following a decrease in the global population of >70% between 2001 and 2013 [3,4]. Decreases in the Western Cape of South Africa (Figure 1) conform to an altered distribution of their main prey species, sardine *Sardinops sagax* and anchovy *Engraulis encrasicolus* [3,5]. Adult survival, juvenile survival and breeding productivity of African penguins have been influenced by the availability these two forage fish species [3,6–9] and competition with the local purse-seine fishery has been noted [3,10]. In

addition, growth rates and body condition of chicks at Robben Island decreased between 2004 and 2009 [11–13], while fledging periods increased concurrently in apparent response to a decline in the availability of sardine [8]. Spatial management of the fishery has been recommended [3,8–10] and the potential benefits of alternative approaches are being investigated [10,14].

Concurrently, conservation efforts are focused on strategies to increase breeding success, such as providing artificial nests [15], and to reduce mortality at breeding colonies, for example by rehabilitating oiled and injured adults [16] and their chicks abandoned as a result [16,17]. Chicks hand-reared after catastrophic oil spills had survival and recruitment rates analogous to naturally-reared cohorts [17,18] and reproduced successfully once they entered the breeding population [17]. On that basis, a number of African penguin chicks are hand-reared each year at the Southern African Foundation for the Conservation of Coastal Birds (SANCCOB), Cape Town. These chicks may be removed from the wild during the breeding season because they have been orphaned or abandoned by their parents following flooding of

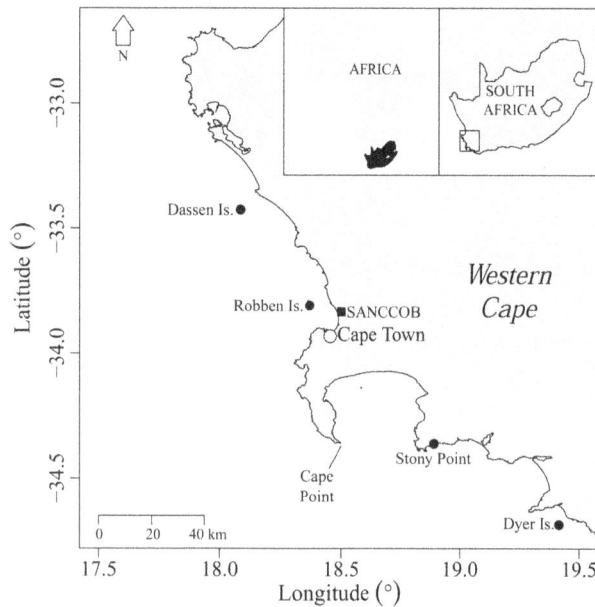

Figure 1. Map of the Western Cape, South Africa, showing the locations of the main African penguin breeding colonies (black circles) mention in the text and the location of SANCCOB (black square) in relation to Cape Town (white circle).

their nest site, building operations or the parents being removed for rehabilitation after being oiled [16]. In addition, at the end of the breeding season, some adults may enter moult with chicks still present in the nest [16]. African penguins usually make short foraging trips (<24 hours, [10]) and leave their chicks unattended when feeding conditions are poor (the post-guard phase) [19]. However, moulting penguins are without adequate waterproofing and must fast for c.21 days [20]; unfledged chicks would thus starve in the nest [21]. Here, we use the term 'abandoned' to indicate situations where chicks are no longer being provisioned prior to independence, rather than temporary abandonment that occurs naturally in penguins during the post-guard phase [22].

From 2001 to 2005, small numbers (24–99) of abandoned African penguin chicks were retrieved annually from Robben and Dyer Islands and sent to SANCCOB for hand-rearing (Table S1). However, in 2006 and 2007, large numbers (>400) of chicks were abandoned at Dyer Island between September and December, as their parents entered moult. This paper is a case study of the interventions made in 2006 and 2007 to hand-rear these chicks and considers the conservation merit of rearing penguin chicks abandoned prematurely by moulting parents.

Methods

In the Western Cape, penguins breed from February to September [23] and predominately moult between September and January, once chicks have fledged [24]. The penguin colonies at Dyer Island, Robben Island and Stony Point (Figure 1) were checked regularly for signs of abandoned chicks from the end of the breeding season. Abandoned chicks, identified by appearance and behaviour (apparently low mass relative to structural growth, "hollow" abdomens, lethargy, peck wounds on head and neck), were removed from all three sites and sent to SANCCOB to be hand-reared.

Chick removals from Dyer Island

At Dyer Island, most adults moult from October to December [24] and do so in in groups within the breeding colony (LJW pers. obs.). The colony was monitored for signs of abandoned chicks from September each year. In 2006, a large proportion of the breeding adults at Dyer Island commenced moult while chicks were still present in nests (Table S2). The managing authority was concerned about the impact that regular approaches into the colony to search for abandoned chicks would have on adult moulters, with birds showing signs of stress at a distance of 20–30 m. It was thus decided to remove chicks *en masse* in both 2006 and 2007 based on four considerations: (1) one operation would minimise disturbance to moulting adults; (2) the timing of moult is highly synchronised at Dyer Island [12], so the remaining chicks would likely be abandoned when parents ultimately commenced moult; (3) hand-reared chicks could potentially boost the breeding population in three to five years' time, depending on juvenile survival and recruitment processes [25,26]; (4) the poorer the condition of a chick when it reached the rehabilitation centre, the smaller the chances for successful rearing and release.

At Dyer Island, penguins form small, localised sub-colonies. Sub-colonies were slowly surrounded by 4–5 people to prevent adult birds, especially moulters, from moving off, while one person captured the chicks by hand. The chicks were sorted by size into indoor holding pens and gavaged 60 ml electrolyte solution after capture and again before removal to the mainland if kept overnight. The chicks were transported in aerated boxes by boat to the mainland (c. 0.5 hour) and then to SANCCOB by truck (c. 3 hours). In 2006, chicks were removed in large groups and were generally transported to SANCCOB the day after being removed from their nests. In 2007, daily capture numbers were smaller and chicks were transported to SANCCOB on the capture date.

Chick removals from Robben Island and Stony Point

At Robben Island, the colony was monitored from the end of October and at Stony Point the colony was monitored in November and December. Abandoned chicks were captured from nests by hand on an individual basis or in small groups. There were placed in aerated boxes and transported to SANCCOB the same day by truck (c. 2 hours) from Stony Point and by ferry (c. 0.5 hour) and truck (c. 0.5 hour) from Robben Island.

Hand-rearing procedures

On arrival at SANCCOB, chicks were grouped into stages of development based on their weight and the level of down present ([11,27], Appendix S1) and their condition was estimated by "habitus", scored from 1–4 (weak to strong; Appendix S1) [16].

Chicks were reared following guidelines based on Turner and Plutchak [28]. Chicks were given formula (liquidised fish and vitamin mixture), fluids and whole fish. Veterinary treatment requirements, changes in mass and waterproofing of feathers were evaluated on a weekly basis [16]. Blood samples (haematocrit, total serum protein and blood smears) to evaluate blood parasites, anaemia and systemic inflammatory response were taken weekly or fortnightly. Both flies and mosquitoes were abundant during the chick-rearing period; the netting surrounding the centre at the time was inadequate to exclude insects. Insecticides were used in the pens and applied locally to the birds' heads to help prevent flies and mosquitoes. Various fly traps and fly control products were also employed.

On live birds, conditions such as airsacculitis and pneumonia, avian pox, bumblefoot and feather-loss disorder were diagnosed based on clinical symptoms and lesions only. On birds that died, avian malaria was diagnosed on macroscopic pathology lesions together with positive blood and/or kidney impression smears [29]. Most other diagnoses were determined from macroscopic pathology lesions only. Fungal airsacculitis and pneumonia was differentiated from bacterial cases on the presence of fungal plaques and mats and was not specifically identified to species level. When birds died, the carcase was refrigerated immediately and post-mortem examination conducted on c. 85% of cases within four days. Histopathology and other tests were not routinely performed, except in cases where the cause of death could not otherwise be determined.

Release and resighting data

Juvenile penguins that met the criteria outlined by Parsons and Underhill [16] were released ashore at Dyer or Robben Islands or else at sea near to Robben Island. Movement of juvenile penguins is extensive [30] and breeding at non-natal colonies occurs [6,26]. It was thus not deemed vital to return chicks to their natal site. Of those released, 511 were marked with flipper bands from the 2006 cohort and 190 from the 2007 cohort (Table S3).

As part of routine monitoring carried out at African penguin colonies, searches were made for banded individuals and band numbers from throughout the species range (Namibia and South Africa) were reported to a central database (see [6]). The records from this database covering the period 1 January 2007 to 31 December 2012 were searched for resightings.

Ethics statement

Capture, transportation, rearing, diagnostic screening, care and release of the birds were carried out by SANCCOB on behalf of the Western Cape Nature Conservation Board (CapeNature) and the then Department of Environmental Affairs and Tourism (DEAT, now the Department of Environmental Affairs) under permits (Reference No. V1/1/5/1) issued by DEAT according to the Sea Birds and Seals Protection Act No. 46 of 1973 and the Marine Living Resources Act No. 18 of 1998. SANCCOB is a registered veterinary practice with the South African Veterinary Council (registration number FCO02/5650) and blood samples were taken by a state registered veterinarian to ensure that the birds were fit to be released and were not carrying any diseases that might be introduced to the wild population. Stainless steel flipper bands were applied under license from the South African Bird Ringing Unit (SAFRING) and according to the guidelines approved by the Banding Forum and the Animal Ethics Committee of the DEAT [31].

Statistical analyses

We estimated survival (φ), encounter (or resighting) (ρ), and recruitment (ψ) probabilities using multistate mark-recapture models (e.g. [32]). We considered three states; 'alive as a non-breeding individual', 'alive and confirmed breeding', and 'dead' and three events; 'not encountered', 'encountered as a non-breeding individual' and 'encountered as a breeder', which were conditional on the states (see Appendix S2). We implemented our multistate models in a hidden Markov models framework [33] using program E-SURGE v1.9.0 [34] and tested for goodness-of-fit using U-CARE v2.2.3, which indicated little evidence for overdispersion ($\hat{c} = 1.11$). Parameter estimates are given ± 1 standard error (s.e.), with 95% confidence intervals (95% CI) computed from the Hessian matrix.

We developed a set of candidate models that assumed survival probabilities to depend on age, encounter probabilities to be either constant or to vary with time, and recruitment probabilities to depend on age (years after release), time, or be constant across time. Due to sparse resighting data, we did not attempt to estimate time-dependent survival, or to estimate separate survival parameters for the two release cohorts. For the age effects on survival, we distinguished between juveniles (first year after release) and adults (all subsequent years; [6]). For recruitment probabilities, we modelled three age categories, $0-1$ years old, $1-2$ years old, and >2 years old as African penguins usually breed for the first time at 3 years of age or older [25]. Model selection was performed using the Akaike's Information Criterion adjusted for small sample size and overdispersion (QAICc, [35]).

Results

In total, 841 and 481 chicks were removed from the three colonies in 2006 and 2007 respectively (Table 1). At Dyer Island, 19 chicks were collected between 18 September and 15 October 2006, prior to the decision to remove chicks *en masse*. Between 16 and 21 October 2006, 668 chicks were captured at Dyer Island on three separate days and transported to SANCCOB. In 2007, the decision to remove all abandoned chicks from Dyer Island was taken on 27 October and 427 chicks were collected. An additional 201 chicks were admitted to SANCCOB from the other two colonies across the two years (Table 1).

Hand-rearing success

The abandoned chicks were generally underweight for their age [15] and many were not yet losing their down, indicating that they were at least 20 days from fledging [18]. In 2006 and 2007 respectively, 6% and 20% of chicks from Dyer Island were small to medium downy chicks, for Stony Point the corresponding values were 6% and 2%, while none of the birds from Robben Island were small to medium downy chicks.

The chicks were reared in 2006 for a mean of 44 days (range: 11–127 days) for those that were released and 36 days (range: 0–88 days) for those that died. In 2007 rearing lasted a mean of 48 days (range: 15–130 days) for those released and 50 days (0–158 days) for those that died (Table 2 and 3). In both years, chicks that died had a lower habitus on admission than those that were released (2006: $\chi^2 = 76.0$, p<0.001; 2007: $\chi^2 = 19.2$, p<0.001; Table 2).

In 2006 and 2007, 114 chicks (14%) and 112 chicks (23%) respectively were found to be positive for avian malaria *Plasmodium* spp. (Table S4). Positive birds were treated according to a set of basic treatment protocols (Appendix S1). Those that were released took 20% longer in 2006 and 95% longer in 2007 than all chicks to reach the conditions for release. Malaria was diagnosed as the cause of death for 36% of deaths in 2006 and 59% in 2007 (Table 3).

The second main cause of death was bacterial airsacculitis and pneumonia (Table 3), which can spread from the lungs to infect other organs. No specific aetiological diagnosis was made. Fungal airsacculitis and pneumonia caused 7% of deaths in 2006 and 2% in 2007 (Table 3). Birds diagnosed as "chesty" (laboured breathing, crackly lung noises on auscultation and coughing) were treated with a course of systemic antibiotics (Appendix S1) and nebulised in an enclosed box with a disinfectant. Attempts were made to isolate "chesty" birds, although there was a lack of space when there were large numbers of birds in the facility. Antifungal treatment was also given if there was no response to the antibacterial treatment (Appendix S1).

One bird was euthanized due to blindness caused by avian pox (Table 3). Lesions occurred around the eyes, the ceres, the beak, inside the mouth and occasionally on the feet of the chicks that contracted the disease [36]. The pox lesions were debrided and treated locally with antibiotic eye cream. When swelling occurred

Table 1. Numbers of African penguin chicks admitted to and released from SANCCOB by colony in 2006 and 2007.

Year	Colony	Admissions	Releases	Release rate	Mean ± SD duration
2006	Robben Island	113	90	80%	35±21
	Dyer Island	694	647	93%	45±16
	Stony Point	34	29	85%	42±18
2007	Robben Island	7	3	43%	25±8
	Dyer Island	427	324	76%	48±22
	Stony Point	47	24	51%	47±25
Total		**1322**	**1117**	**84%**	**45±19**

The mean ± standard deviation (SD) duration (in days) of stay in rehabilitation for the released birds is also shown.

around the eyes, the penguins were also treated with systemic antibiotics and anti-inflammatories (Appendix S1). The lesions usually healed after three weeks; in severe cases, scarring caused a smaller eye opening.

In both years, a number of chicks also contracted pododermatitis (bumblefoot; Table 3). Lesions were treated with topical antibiotics and severe cases were also treated with systemic antibiotics and anti-inflammatories (Appendix S1). In 2007, bandages were applied as cushioning to provide some relief to the birds when standing. One bird was euthanased each year due to bumblefoot (Table 3). A feather-loss disorder also occurred in both years, delaying hand-rearing significantly, but did not cause any mortality. These results are discussed in detail by Kane et al. [37].

Release, survival and recruitment rates

In 2006, 766 hand-reared penguins were released (91% of admissions) and in 2007, 351 chicks were released (73% of admissions, Table S3). Of those released with flipper bands, 92 (13%) were resighted by 31 December 2012. Twelve individuals were confirmed as breeding, all from the 2006 cohort, and 22 others were resighted at breeding age. Of the breeding birds, six were at Dyer Island, three were at Robben Island, two at Stony Point and one at Dassen Island (Table S5). They all originated from Dyer Island (Table S5).

Model selection on the resighting data favoured the model with a constant recruitment probability and time-dependent encounter rates (Model 2, Table 4). Apparent survival was 0.32 ± 0.08 (95% CI: 0.18–0.49) in the first year after release (juvenile survival) and 0.76 ± 0.10 (0.51–0.90) in subsequent years (adult survival). Encounter rates were low initially at 0.01 ± 0.01 (0.00–0.06) in 2007 and 0.06 ± 0.02 (0.03–0.12) in 2008, but increased to 0.31 ± 0.11 (0.14–0.55) in 2011, before falling back in 2012

(Figure 2). The recruitment probability was 0.11 ± 0.03 (0.06–0.19) and there was no support for a change in this parameter over time or within the age structure we identified (Table 4).

Discussion

The use of hand- or captive-reared chicks to reinforce or restore threatened bird populations is now relatively widespread [38]. The approach has been used successfully in combination with translocation in the conservation of at least 11 seabird species worldwide [39–42]. However, efforts to restore or reinforce penguin populations appear to be scarce [42], even though the Spheniscidae may represent good candidates species. All members of the family exhibit apparent post-fledging independence, they generally have low levels of parental attendance following the guard stage, and they can be easily hand-fed [43]. Although prolonged hand-feeding of nestlings can reduce fledging success in some seabirds [44], this does not occur with African penguins and, because hand-reared chicks are as fit as naturally-reared chicks [17,27], the species has been considered a promising candidate for reinforcement and conservation translocation [17].

Our results confirm that the success of hand-rearing African penguin chicks after oiling incidents extends to chicks abandoned by moulting parents. Survival in the first year after release (0.32 ± 0.08) was within the range of estimates for chicks hand-reared after oil spills (0.20–0.42, [17,45]) and apparent adult survival (0.76 ± 0.10) was also similar to estimates for chicks hand-reared after the 1994 (0.79, [45]) and 2000 oil spills [17]. In addition, juvenile survival compared well to a previous estimate from naturally-reared birds at Robben and Dassen Island from 1987 to 1994 (0.35, [45]) and was towards the upper end of estimates for both juvenile (0.06–0.52) and adult (0.46–0.77) survival at these colonies during our study period [3,6].

Table 2. The habitus of African penguin chicks admitted to SANCCOB in 2006 and 2007.

Habitus	2006			2007		
	Admissions	Releases	Mean ± SD duration	Admissions	Releases	Mean ± SD duration
1	29	16	58±16	25	11	59±11
2	140	113	53±21	173	116	57±25
3–4	672	637	42±15	283	224	43±20
Total	**841**	**766**	**44±17**	**481**	**351**	**48±22**

Habitus is scored from 1–4, with one being weak and four being strong (Appendix S1, [16]). The mean ± standard deviation (SD) duration (in days) of stay in rehabilitation is also shown for those birds that were released.

Table 3. Causes of death of abandoned African penguin chicks admitted to SANCCOB in 2006 and 2007.

Cause of death	2006			2007		
	N	Deaths	Mean ± SD duration	N	Deaths	Mean ± SD duration
Abscess on heart	1	1.3%	(28)	–	–	–
Airsacculitis and pneumonia	16	21.3%	41±32	23	17.6%	41±31
Fungal airsacculitis and pneumonia	5	6.6%	31±15	3	2.3%	34±24
Multiple organ infection	8	10.5%	33±29	1	0.8%	(52)
Pododermatitis (Bumblefoot)	1	1.3%	(84)	1	0.8%	(46)
Enteritis	–	–	–	3	2.3%	59±28
Blind	1	1.3%	(47)	–	–	–
Nervous symptoms	2	2.6%	48±52	–	–	–
Avian malaria	27	35.5%	48±26	77	59.2%	58±28
Weak, emaciated chick	11	14.7%	7±5	11	8.5%	10±9
Tubed down trachea	2	2.6%	10±6	1	0.8%	(96)
Died during transport	–	–	–	7	5.4%	47±3
Undetermined	1	1.3%	(8)	3	2.3%	54±34
Total	75		36±29	130		50±30

The mean ± standard deviation (SD) duration (in days) in rehabilitation for individuals in each cause of death category is also shown. Where only one individual died in any category, the duration of stay (days) for that individual in given in parentheses.

Despite a decreasing breeding population in the Western Cape and poor feeding conditions between 2005 and 2010 [3], an estimated 11% of the hand-reared chicks subsequently recruited into the breeding population. Survival rates measured in this study suggest that around 14% would have survived to breeding age (4 years old [25]). Half of those individuals confirmed as breeding returned to their natal colony, suggesting that this action ultimately acted to reinforce the breeding population at the source colonies [17]. However, removing and hand-rearing African penguin chicks is expensive, labour intensive, and has potential implications for the source populations. Collection of penguin chicks can cause disturbance to moulting adults or other breeding seabirds if not carefully managed. In addition rearing of chicks in captivity exposes them to diseases which could potentially be introduced to wild

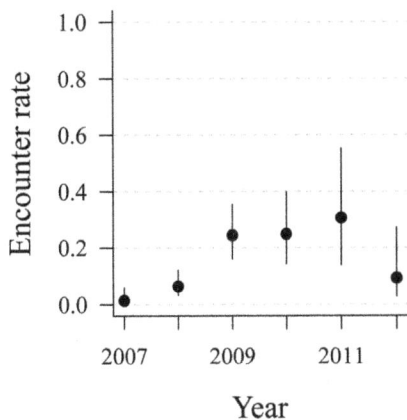

Figure 2. Time-dependent encounter (or resighting) probabilities for banded, hand-reared African penguins released by SANCCOB in 2006 and 2007. Resightings were made over the period 2007 to 2012. Encounter probabilities are based on model 2, Table 4. Error bars show the 95% confidence intervals.

populations and fledglings may be returned to an environment which cannot support them if prey availability is poor.

Role of prey availability in chick abandonment

Long-lived birds can alter their reproductive performance according to their body condition and the needs of their offspring [46], choosing not to breed or to abandon a breeding attempt in order to safeguard their own survival [5]. In contrast, moult is obligatory in penguins [24]. It must be undertaken annually and, once initiated, cannot be abandoned prematurely [47,48]. Thus, the acquisition of insufficient reserves prior to moult compromises survival [21] and the need to exploit a predictable food source during summer – not the fledging of chicks – appears to determine the timing of moult in African penguins [24,49].

In the Western Cape, moult coincides with the availability of high energy prey [24] while the breeding season is synchronised to the availability of fish in the vicinity of the colonies in winter [50]. During good years, African penguins can successfully rear two broods in a season, but chick growth rates show high plasticity in response to variable feeding conditions [8,11]. The duration of the fledging period varies as a function of both the local foraging conditions and the energy that parents can afford to invest in chick provisioning [8,48]. Thus, we hypothesise that the date of egg-laying in the nests which produced the abandoned chicks was early enough to produce fledglings in most years but, in 2006 and 2007, the chicks exhibited such slow growth that they were still nestlings at a point when their parents could no longer delay the initiation of moult. Very slow growth rates were observed at Dyer Island in subsequent years [11] and an increase in fledging periods, similar to that observed at Robben Island [8], may well have occurred. Prey availability in the Western Cape was relatively poor in both 2006 and 2007 [3], such that abandonments could have been mediated either by poor food availability close to the colonies during chick-rearing, poor availability of adult fish during the preceding pre-breeding period, or a combination of the two [8].

African penguins exhibit some natal philopatry [26] and half of the birds breeding in this study returned to their natal site. This

Table 4. Model selection results for mark-recapture modelling of hand-reared African penguins released by SANCCOB in 2006 and 2007.

Model No.	Model structure	K	Deviance	QAICc	ΔQAICc	w
2	$\varphi(a)\rho(t)\psi(c)$	11	1000.05	1022.37	0	0.82
1	$\varphi(a)\rho(t)\psi(a)$	14	996.87	1025.38	3.01	0.18
3	$\varphi(a)\rho(t)\psi(t)$	20	993.12	1034.15	11.78	0.00
5	$\varphi(a)\rho(c)\psi(c)$	6	1054.41	1066.51	44.15	0.00
4	$\varphi(a)\rho(c)\psi(a)$	9	1051.24	1069.45	47.09	0.00
6	$\varphi(a)\rho(c)\psi(t)$	15	1047.49	1078.07	55.70	0.00

The model components were survival (φ), encounter (ρ) and recruitment (ψ), the rate of transition from a non-breeder to a breeding individual. Survival probabilities were assumed to depend on age (a), encounter probabilities to be either constant (c) or to vary with time (t), and recruitment probabilities to depend on age (years after release), time, or be constant across time. K is the number of estimated parameters in each model, QAICc is Akaike's information criterion (AIC) adjusted for overdispersion and sample size, ΔQAICc is the difference in QAICc between each model and the best model and w denotes the Akaike weights (relative support given to each model).

was despite evidence that juvenile African penguins may emigrate to non-natal colonies if the food environment is heterogeneous [3,5], and apparently poor conditions for breeding penguins at Dyer Island in recent years [12,51] However, if the poor prey availability persists, their subsequent survival and reproductive success would be compromised relative to birds at colonies where conditions are more favourable [3,6,8]. As the situation for African penguin has continued to deteriorate on the West Coast [3,6], plans have been developed to use conservation translocations to establish new breeding colonies in areas of higher prey availability along the South African coast [52].

Our results suggest abandoned chicks as an obvious source of birds for such an endeavour, but the split in recruitment to natal and non-natal sites in birds from Dyer Island suggests that natal imprinting in African penguins occurs before fledging. Nevertheless, translocated individuals will undertake some prospecting behaviour to evaluate the quality of their new habitat, relative to that available to the rest of the meta-population [53]. As such, return rates to translocation sites might well be higher if those sites can be placed in areas perceived to be of high habitat quality or prey availability [53]. The current approach of rearing chicks at SANCCOB to release back at existing colonies (natal and non-natal) provides an opportunity to better understand the dispersal and recruitment process of African penguins [17]. In future, consideration should to be given to whether more could be gained by employing alternative strategies to maximise the conservation benefit of translocations. Rearing birds *in situ* at future release sites has yielded high success rates in chick translocation projects with Procellariiformes [42]. However, this approach comes with additional logistical and financial costs, as well as different risks of disease introduction and environmental impacts. In addition, it may not be necessary for all seabird species, as little penguins *Eudyptula minor* have been successfully translocated by simply keeping them overnight at a release site in artificial nest boxes (N. Carlile, pers. comm.).

Veterinary concerns

The hand-reared chicks were susceptible to various conditions, in part due to being in captivity (pododermatitis), at high-density (airsacculitis and pneumonia, avian pox) and being exposed to vectors transmitting disease (avian pox, avian malaria).

Pododermatitis can be avoided through the use of varied substrate levels and textures and by having birds regularly walk through disinfectant baths; however, these techniques are gener-

ally incompatible with the logistics of large-scale captive rearing. The condition generally improved once the birds were swimming and spending less time standing and does not pose a risk to wild populations.

The severity of avian pox varies between species [36,54] and the symptoms seen in African penguins are mild to moderate, although mortality of Magellanic penguin S. *magellanicus* chicks has occurred [55]. Prevention of the disease involves control of the vector, isolating heavily infected birds and thorough disinfection of pens, equipment and clothing [36]. It is unlikely to pose a risk to wild populations after release as the lesions resolved over time, although outbreaks can occur in the wild dependent on vector occurrence.

Infections of avian malaria are an ongoing concern at SANCCOB [16]. Avian malaria is present at a low prevalence in wild African penguins [56,57] although the possibility exists of spreading a pathogenic species from rehabilitated birds into the wild population [29]. This risk is reinforced by the identification of potential vectors on some of the offshore islands (SANCCOB unpubl. data). The incidence of avian malaria at the facility has been dramatically reduced since the erection of new shade cloth netting in 2008 (SANCCOB unpubl. data).

Fungal airsacculitis and pneumonia (most likely to be caused by Aspergillus sp.) occasionally causes deaths in wild African penguin chicks (SANCCOB unpubl. data) and is likely to be more widespread than reported. This is not a condition in released birds that poses a threat to the wild population due to the ubiquitous nature of the organism where infections generally occur secondarily to an immunosuppressive event [54].

While it is possible that releasing large numbers of hand-reared birds into the wild introduced disease into the population [17,29,58–60] this seems unlikely as surveillance of the colonies is near-continuous and there were no mass mortalities of African penguins during the study period. Sub-clinical diseases remain a possibility [58–60], although the comparable subsequent breeding success of hand-reared and naturally-reared African penguins [17] makes this unlikely too. All birds undergo basic disease screening and veterinary evaluation before release in order to reduce any disease introduction risk. A programme of ongoing disease surveillance throughout the breeding range is also recommended to minimise this risk.

Finally, one missing element in the strategy for chick removal in this study was quantitative criteria to decide whether individual chicks were in sufficiently poor condition to conclude that they had been abandoned. The development and use of a body condition index for African penguin chicks [13] provides the opportunity to relate chick condition at admission to survival and to generate adaptive decision rules about the need for chick removal, and its timing in future.

Conclusions

Hand-rearing of African penguin chicks is a valuable conservation tool in light of the declining population. Continued monitoring of body condition in penguin chicks should be a priority in the management of colonies to ensure the timely collection of abandoned chicks. Further research on the relationship between these abandonment events and variations in prey availability at different temporal and spatial scales is warranted and a programme of disease surveillance is recommended to help limit any possibility of disease outbreak. Finally, additional research on how the dispersal of fledging African penguins relates to prey availability could pave the way for successful conservation translocations to establish new colonies in favourable breeding localities for this 'Endangered' species.

Supporting Information

Appendix S1 Additional information on the chick-rearing methods and results: (a) the system used to classify chicks by stage of development, (b) the system used to classify chicks by Habitus, (c) the basic treatment protocols used during hand-rearing.

Appendix S2 The state-transition and observation matrices for the multistate models.

Appendix S3 Data on the African penguin chicks admitted to SANCCOB in 2006 and 2007.

Table S1 Numbers of African penguin chicks admitted to SANCCOB from 2001 to 2005.

Table S2 Numbers of African penguin chicks removed in 2006 and 2007, compared to the number of breeding pairs at Dyer Island, Robben Island and Stony Point.

Table S3 Numbers of abandoned African penguin chicks released according to area of origin and area of release, with number of banded individuals.

Table S4 Numbers of African penguin chicks which were positive for avian malaria.

Table S5 Additional information on the 12 hand-reared chicks observed breeding by December 2012.

Acknowledgments

The staff of CapeNature, Robben Island Museum (RIM), the City of Cape Town's (CCT) Environmental Resource Management Department, Overstrand Municipality and SANCCOB captured and removed chicks. The Dyer Island Conservation Trust, K. de Kock and RIM provided boat transport. Staff and volunteers of SANCCOB, CapeNature, CCT and the International Fund for Animal Welfare (IFAW) oil spill response team helped rear the chicks. Flipper bands were supplied by the Department of Environmental Affairs (DEA) and the Bristol Zoological Society (BZS). Banding information was administered by the South African Bird Ringing Unit (SAFRING) at the Animal Demography Unit (ADU). This study contributes to the African Penguin Chick Bolstering Project, a partnership between SANCCOB, BZS, ADU, DEA (Oceans and Coasts), CapeNature, RIM, BirdLife South Africa and IFAW. We thank Nicholas Carlile and Ralph Vanstreels for helpful comments on an earlier version of the manuscript.

Author Contributions

Conceived and designed the experiments: RBS LJW VS DG LGU NJP. Analyzed the data: RBS NJP. Wrote the paper: RBS NJP. Contributed substantially to revisions: RBS NJP LGU. Contributed to data collection: RBS LJW VS DG LGU NJP.

References

1. Croxall JP, Butchart SHM, Lascelles B, Stattersfield AJ, Sullivan B, et al. (2012) Seabird conservation status, threats and priority actions: a global assessment. Bird Conserv Int 22: 1–34. doi:10.1017/S0959270912000020.

2. Lewison R, Oro D, Godley B, Underhill L, Bearhop S, et al. (2012) Research priorities for seabirds: improving conservation and management in the 21st century. Endanger Species Res 17: 93–121. doi:10.3354/esr00419.

3. Crawford RJM, Altwegg R, Barham BJ, Barham PJ, Durant JM, et al. (2011) Collapse of South Africa's penguins in the early 21st century. Afr J Mar Sci 33: 139–156. doi:10.2989/1814232X.2011.572377.

4. Crawford RJM, Makhado AB, Waller LJ, Whittington PA (2014) Winners and losers – response to recent environmental change by South African seabirds that compete with purse-seine fisheries for food. Ostrich: doi: 10.2989/00306525.2014.955141. doi:10.2989/00306525.2014.955141.

5. Crawford RJM, Underhill LG, Coetzee JC, Fairweather T, Shannon LJ, et al. (2008) Influences of the abundance and distribution of prey on African penguins Spheniscus demersus off western South Africa. Afr J Mar Sci 30: 167–175. doi:10.2989/AJMS.2008.30.1.17.467.

6. Sherley RB, Abadi F, Ludynia K, Barham BJ, Clark AE, et al. (2014) Age-specific survival and movement among major African Penguin Spheniscus demersus colonies. Ibis 156: 716–728. doi:10.1111/ibi.12189.

7. Duffy DC, Wilson RP, Ricklefs RE, Broni SC, Veldhuis H (1987) Penguins and purse seiners: competition or coexistence? Natl Geogr Res 3: 480–488.

8. Sherley RB, Underhill LG, Barham BJ, Barham PJ, Coetzee JC, et al. (2013) Influence of local and regional prey availability on breeding performance of African penguins Spheniscus demersus. Mar Ecol Prog Ser 473: 291–301. doi:10.3354/meps10070.

9. Durant JM, Crawford RJM, Wolfaardt AC, Agenbag K, Visagie J, et al. (2010) Influence of feeding conditions on breeding of African penguins – importance of adequate local food supplies. Mar Ecol Prog Ser 420: 263–271. doi:10.3354/meps08857.

10. Pichegru L, Ryan PG, Eeden R Van, Reid T, Grémillet D, et al. (2012) Industrial fishing, no-take zones and endangered penguins. Biol Conserv 156: 117–125. doi:10.1016/j.biocon.2011.12.013.

11. Sherley RB (2010) Factors influencing the demography of Endangered seabirds at Robben Island, South Africa. PhD thesis. Bristol: University of Bristol. 237 p.

12. Waller LJ (2011) The African penguin Spheniscus demersus: conservation and management issues. PhD thesis. Cape Town: University of Cape Town. 290 p.

13. Lubbe A, Underhill LG, Waller LJ, Veen J (2014) A condition index for African penguin Spheniscus demersus chicks. Afr J Mar Sci 36: 143–154. doi:10.2989/1814232X.2014.915232.

14. Robinson WML (2013) Modelling the impact of the South African small pelagic fishery on African penguin dynamics. PhD thesis, University of Cape Town, Cape Town. 221 p.

15. Sherley RB, Barham BJ, Barham PJ, Leshoro TM, Underhill LG (2012) Artificial nests enhance the breeding productivity of African Penguins (Spheniscus demersus) on Robben Island, South Africa. Emu 97: 97–106. doi:10.1071/MU11055.

16. Parsons NJ, Underhill LG (2005) Oiled and injured African penguins Spheniscus demersus and other seabirds admitted for rehabilitation in the Western Cape, South Africa, 2001 and 2002. Afr J Mar Sci 27: 289–296. doi:10.2989/18142320509504087.

17. Barham PJ, Underhill LG, Crawford RJM, Altwegg R, Leshoro MT, et al. (2008) The efficacy of hand-rearing penguin chicks: evidence from African Penguins (Spheniscus demersus) orphaned in the Treasure oil spill in 2000. Bird Conserv Int 18: 144–152. doi:10.1017/S0959270908000142.

18. Underhill LG, Bartlett PA, Baumann L, Crawford RJM, Dyer BM, et al. (1999) Mortality and survival of African penguins *Spheniscus demersus* involved in the *Apollo Sea* oil spill: an evaluation of rehabilitation efforts. Ibis 141: 29–37.

19. Seddon PJ, van Heezik YM (1993) Behaviour of the jackass penguin chick. Ostrich 64: 8–12. doi:10.1080/00306525.1993.9634188.

20. Cooper J (1978) Moult of the black-footed penguin *Spheniscus demersus*. Int Zoo Yearb 18: 22–27. doi:10.1111/j.1748-1090.1978.tb00211.x.

21. Kemper J, Roux J-P, Underhill LG (2008) Effect of age and breeding status on molt phenology of adult African penguins (*Spheniscus demersus*) in Namibia. Auk 125: 809–819. doi:10.1525/auk.2008.06262.

22. Wilson D (2009) Causes and benefits of chick aggregations in penguins. Auk 126: 688–693. doi:10.1525/auk.2009.9709b.

23. Crawford RJM, Williams AJ, Hofmeyr JH, Klages NTW, Randall RM, et al. (1995) Trends of African penguin *Spheniscus demersus* populations in the 20th century. S Afr J Mar Sci 16: 101–118. doi:10.2989/025776195784156403.

24. Crawford RJM, Hemming M, Kemper J, Klages NTW, Randall R, et al. (2006) Molt of the African penguin, *Spheniscus demersus* in relation to its breeding season and food availability. Acta Zool Sin 52 (Supp.): 444–447.

25. Whittington PA, Klages NTW, Crawford RJM, Wolfaardt AC, Kemper J (2005) Age at first breeding of the African penguin. Ostrich 76: 14–20. doi:10.2989/00306520509485468.

26. Whittington PA, Randall RM, Crawford RJM, Wolfaardt AC, Klages NTW, et al. (2005) Patterns of immigration to and emigration from breeding colonies by African penguins. Afr J Mar Sci 27: 205–213. doi:10.2989/18142320509504079.

27. Barham PJ, Underhill LG, Crawford RJM, Leshoro TM (2007) Differences in breeding success between African penguins (*Spheniscus demersus*) that were and were not oiled in the MV *Treasure* oil-spill in 2000. Emu 107: 7–13. doi:10.1071/MU06028.

28. Turner WA, Plutchak L (1998) SeaWorld California penguin hand-rearing guidelines. Penguin Conserv 11: 2–9.

29. Grim KC, van der Merwe E, Sullivan M, Parsons N, McCutchan TF, et al. (2003) *Plasmodium juxtanucleare* associated with mortality in black-footed penguins (*Spheniscus demersus*) admitted to a rehabilitation center. J Zoo Wildl Med 34: 250–255. doi:10.1638/02-070.

30. Sherley RB, Ludynia K, Lamont T, Roux J-P, Crawford RJM, et al. (2013) The initial journey of an endangered penguin: implications for seabird conservation. Endanger Species Res 21: 89–95. doi:10.3354/esr00510.

31. Petersen SL, Branch GM, Crawford RJM, Cooper J, Underhill LG (2005) The future for flipper banding African penguins: discussion recommendations and guidelines. Mar Ornithol 33: E1–E4.

32. Lebreton J-D, Nichols JD, Barker RJ, Pradel R, Spendelow JA (2009) Modeling individual animal histories with multistate capture–recapture models. In: Caswell H, editor. Advances in Ecological Research. Burlington: Academic Press, Vol. 41. 87–173. doi:10.1016/S0065-2504(09)00403-6.

33. Gimenez O, Lebreton J-D, Gaillard J-M, Choquet R, Pradel R (2012) Estimating demographic parameters using hidden process dynamic models. Theor Popul Biol 82: 307–316. doi:10.1016/j.tpb.2012.02.001.

34. Choquet R, Rouan L, Pradel R (2009) Program E-Surge: A software application for fitting multievent models. In: Thomson DL, Cooch EG, Conroy MJ, editors. Modeling Demographic Processes In Marked Populations. Boston: Springer US. 845–865. doi:10.1007/978-0-387-78151-8.

35. Burnham KP, Anderson DR (2002) Model selection and multimodel inference: a practical information-theoretic approach. 2nd ed. New York: Springer.

36. Hansen W (1999) Avian pox. In: Friend M, Franson JC, editors. Field manual of wildlife diseases: general field procedures and diseases of birds. Washington DC: United States Geological Survey, Biological Resources Division. 163–169.

37. Kane OJ, Smith JR, Boersma PD, Parsons NJ, Strauss V, et al. (2010) Feather-loss disorder in African and Magellanic penguins. Waterbirds 33: 415–421. doi:10.1675/063.033.0321.

38. Jones CG, Merton DV (2012) A tale of two islands: the rescue and recovery of Endemic birds in New Zealand and Mauritius. In: Ewen J, Armstrong D, Parker K, Seddon P, editors. Reintroduction Biology: Integrating Science and Management. Chichester, UK: Wiley-Blackwell. 33–72.

39. Miskelly CM, Taylor GA, Gummer H, Williams R (2009) Translocations of eight species of burrow-nesting seabirds (genera *Pterodroma*, *Pelecanoides*,

40. Deguchi T, Jacobs J, Harada T, Perriman L, Watanabe Y, et al. (2011) Translocation and hand-rearing techniques for establishing a colony of threatened albatross. Bird Conserv Int 22: 66–81. doi:10.1017/S0959270911000438.

41. Carlile N, Priddel D, Madeiros J (2012) Establishment of a new, secure colony of Endangered Bermuda Petrel *Pterodroma cahow* by translocation of near-fledged nestlings. Bird Conserv Int 22: 46–58. doi:10.1017/S0959270911000372.

42. Jones HP, Kress SW (2012) A review of the world's active seabird restoration projects. J Wildl Manage 76: 2–9. doi:10.1002/jwmg.240.

43. Gummer H (2003) Chick translocation as a method of establishing new surface-nesting seabird colonies: a review. DOC Science Internal Series 150. Department of Conservation, Wellington. Available: http://csl.doc.govt.nz/documents/science-and-technical/dsis150.pdf.

44. Miskelly CM, Taylor GA (2004) Establishment of a colony of common diving petrels (*Pelecanoides urinatrix*) by chick transfers and acoustic attraction. Emu 104: 205–211. doi:10.1071/MU03062.

45. Whittington PA (2002) Survival and movements of African penguins, especially after oiling. PhD thesis. Cape Town: University of Cape Town. 296 p.

46. Erikstad KE, Fauchald P, Tveraa T, Steen H (1998) On the cost of reproduction in long-lived birds: the influence of environmental variability. Ecology 79: 1781–1788. doi:10.2307/176796.

47. Payne R (1972) Mechanisms and control of molt. In: Farner DC, King JR, editors. Avian Biology Vol. 2. New York and London: Academic Press. 103–155.

48. Randall RM (1989) Jackass penguins. In: Payne AIL, Crawford RJM, van Dalsen AP, editors. Oceans of Life of Southern Africa. Cape Town: Vlaeberg. 244–256.

49. Wolfaardt AC, Underhill LG, Crawford RJM (2009) Comparison of moult phenology of African penguins *Spheniscus demersus* at Robben and Dassen Islands. Afr J Mar Sci 31: 19–29. doi:10.2989/AJMS.2009.31.1.2.773.

50. Crawford RJM, Barham PJ, Underhill LG, Shannon LJ, Coetzee JC, et al. (2006) The influence of food availability on breeding success of African penguins *Spheniscus demersus* at Robben Island, South Africa. Biol Conserv 132: 119–125. doi:10.1016/j.biocon.2006.03.019.

51. Ludynia K, Waller LJ, Sherley RB, Abadi F, Galada Y, et al. (2014) Processes influencing the population dynamics and conservation of African penguins on Dyer Island, South Africa. Afr J Mar Sci 36: 253–267. doi:10.2989/1814232X.2014.929027.

52. Schwitzer C, Simpson N, Roestorf M, Sherley RB (2013) The African Penguin Chick Bolstering Project: a One Plan approach to integrated species conservation. WAZA Mag 14: 23–26.

53. Oro D, Martínez-Abraín A, Villuendas E, Sarzo B, Mínguez E, et al. (2011) Lessons from a failed translocation program with a seabird species: Determinants of success and conservation value. Biol Conserv 144: 851–858. doi:10.1016/j.biocon.2010.11.018.

54. Ritchie B, Harrison G, Harrison L (1994) Avian medicine: principles and application. Lake Worth, Florida: Wingers Publishing Inc.

55. Kane OJ, Uhart MM, Rago V, Pereda AJ, Smith JR, et al. (2012) Avian pox in Magellanic penguins (*Spheniscus magellanicus*). J Wildl Dis 48: 790–794. doi:10.7589/0090-3558-48.3.790.

56. Brossy J-J (1992) Malaria in wild and captive jackass penguins *Spheniscus demersus* along the southern African Coast. Ostrich 63: 10–12.

57. Graczyk TK, Cranfield MR, Brossy JJ, Cockrem JF, Jouventin P, et al. (1995) Detection of avian Malaria infections in wild and captive penguins. J Helminthol Soc Washingt 62: 135–141.

58. Peirce MA (1989) The significance of avian haematozoa in conservation strategies. In: Cooper JE, editor. Diseases and Threatened Birds. Cambridge: ICBP Technical Publication No. 10, Vol. 10. 69–76.

59. Brossy J-J, Plös AL, Blackbeard JM, Kline A (1999) Diseases acquired by captive penguins; what happens when they are released into the wild? Mar Ornithol 27: 185–186.

60. Jones HI, Shellam GR (1999) Blood parasites in penguins, and their potential impact on conservation. Mar Ornithol 27: 181–184.

Pachyptila and *Puffinus*: Family Procellariidae). Biol Conserv 142: 1965–1980. doi:10.1016/j.biocon.2009.03.027.

3

Emerging Infectious Diseases in Free-Ranging Wildlife– Australian Zoo Based Wildlife Hospitals Contribute to National Surveillance

Keren Cox-Witton[1]*, Andrea Reiss[2], Rupert Woods[1], Victoria Grillo[1], Rupert T. Baker[3], David J. Blyde[4], Wayne Boardman[5¤], Stephen Cutter[6], Claude Lacasse[7], Helen McCracken[8], Michael Pyne[9], Ian Smith[5], Simone Vitali[10], Larry Vogelnest[11], Dion Wedd[6], Martin Phillips[2], Chris Bunn[12], Lyndel Post[12]

1 Australian Wildlife Health Network, Mosman, New South Wales, Australia, 2 Zoo and Aquarium Association Australasia, Mosman, New South Wales, Australia, 3 Healesville Sanctuary, Zoos Victoria, Healesville, Victoria, Australia, 4 Sea World, Gold Coast, Queensland, Australia, 5 Adelaide Zoo, Zoos South Australia, Adelaide, South Australia, Australia, 6 Territory Wildlife Park, Berry Springs, Northern Territory, Australia, 7 Australia Zoo Wildlife Hospital, Beerwah, Queensland, Australia, 8 Melbourne Zoo, Zoos Victoria, Parkville, Victoria, Australia, 9 Currumbin Wildlife Sanctuary, Currumbin, Queensland, Australia, 10 Perth Zoo, South Perth, Western Australia, Australia, 11 Taronga Zoo, Taronga Conservation Society Australia, Mosman, New South Wales, Australia, 12 Australian Government Department of Agriculture, Canberra, Australian Capital Territory, Australia

Abstract

Emerging infectious diseases are increasingly originating from wildlife. Many of these diseases have significant impacts on human health, domestic animal health, and biodiversity. Surveillance is the key to early detection of emerging diseases. A zoo based wildlife disease surveillance program developed in Australia incorporates disease information from free-ranging wildlife into the existing national wildlife health information system. This program uses a collaborative approach and provides a strong model for a disease surveillance program for free-ranging wildlife that enhances the national capacity for early detection of emerging diseases.

Editor: Patrick C Y. Woo, The University of Hong Kong, Hong Kong

Funding: The zoo based wildlife disease surveillance program described in this paper was funded by the Australian Government Department of Agriculture and the Australian Centre of Excellence for Risk Analysis. The funders had no role in study design, data collection and analysis, decision to publish, or preparation of the manuscript.

* E-mail: kcox-witton@wildlifehealthaustralia.com.au

¤ Current address: School of Animal and Veterinary Sciences, The University of Adelaide, Adelaide, South Australia, Australia

Introduction

Emerging infectious diseases are increasingly originating from wildlife, due in part to increasing urbanisation, globalised trade, habitat loss and other environmental changes. This is a real trend that cannot be fully explained by an increase in detection through improved surveillance, recognition, diagnosis or reporting [1], [2], [3], [4], [5]. Many of these diseases have significant impacts on human health, domestic animal health, wildlife health and biodiversity.

Zoonoses represent a rising threat to global health [5], [6]. Recent examples of emerging infectious diseases in humans with a wildlife origin include severe acute respiratory syndrome (SARS), Nipah virus and Ebola virus. Wildlife can act as a source and reservoir of diseases of domestic livestock such as bovine tuberculosis and avian influenza, and can result in significant economic losses [7], [8], [9]. Emerging diseases may also directly threaten wildlife health and biodiversity, as demonstrated in recent years by the emergence of white nose syndrome, Tasmanian devil facial tumour disease (DFTD) and chytridiomycosis [10], [11], [12], [13]. In Australia a number of diseases have emerged over the last 15 years with confirmed or suspected involvement of

wildlife. Many of these diseases have had significant impacts on biodiversity, human health and domestic animal health, including chytrid fungus, DFTD, Australian bat lyssavirus (ABLV), Menangle virus, Japanese encephalitis and Hendra virus [14], [15], [16].

With the growing understanding of the importance of wildlife as a source or reservoir of emerging diseases, there is increased recognition of the need for disease surveillance in free-ranging wildlife. There are however inherent difficulties in conducting effective wildlife disease surveillance. Many wildlife disease events go unrecognised due to remote locations and a lack of obviously ill individuals or carcasses. Further challenges include a lack of validated diagnostic tests and laboratory capacity for the investigation of wildlife diseases, under-developed surveillance networks, difficulties in determining key parameters such as prevalence for diseases in wildlife populations, and lack of accurate ecological data on population size and density [17], [18]. Collection and validation of wildlife disease data can be challenging due to lack of funding, the 'anecdotal' nature of some reports, and the need to integrate data from disparate sources [16].

Utilising existing systems to establish a coordinated approach is an effective and efficient mechanism to overcome some of these difficulties, where they relate to reporting and data collection. This approach can be strengthened by a functional network that facilitates communication and information flow between those engaged at all levels in surveillance, diagnosis and management of wildlife disease. Surveillance information collected in this way may contribute to the early detection of new or emerging diseases [16], [19]. This paper describes a zoo based wildlife disease surveillance program, as an example of how such a system can assist in managing some of the issues associated with disease surveillance in free-ranging wildlife.

In Australia, the national animal health system is supported by a co-ordinated general wildlife health surveillance system. The primary responsibility for gathering animal health data, including wildlife disease data, rests with state and territory government agencies [20]. The Australian Wildlife Health Network (AWHN) is a national network of government and private stakeholders with an interest in wildlife health that receives core funding from the Australian Government Department of Agriculture. The AWHN is charged with collation and management of national wildlife surveillance data, and works within a 'One Health' framework by encouraging collaboration on wildlife health issues and investigations across human health, animal health and environmental sectors [21]. The AWHN manages wildlife health data through a national web-based database known as eWHIS (the 'electronic Wildlife Health Information System'). A key component of the wildlife health surveillance system are the 'wildlife coordinators', with a government representative in each of Australia's states and territories. Wildlife coordinators manage wildlife disease investigations in their jurisdiction and report data into eWHIS. State, territory and commonwealth agriculture, environment and human health agencies, universities, private veterinary practices and zoos all contribute to Australia's coordinated wildlife health surveillance system. The zoo based wildlife disease surveillance program was developed to formally incorporate disease information from free-ranging wildlife presented to Australian zoos into this existing national wildlife health information system.

Zoos are well suited to participation in surveillance efforts, as many zoos conduct active disease surveillance of collection animals as part of their routine preventative medicine programs, maintain serum and tissue banks and detailed medical records, and have staff with technical expertise in wildlife health [22], [23], [24]. The Zoo Animal Health Network in the USA, for example, is a collaborative program with the United States Department of Agriculture that is involved in early disease detection and outbreak response programs [25], [26], [27], [28]. The value of zoos for surveillance was demonstrated in 1999 when investigation of wild bird mortalities by veterinarians at New York City's Bronx Zoo led to the diagnosis of the first known occurrence of West Nile virus (WNV) in the western hemisphere, a disease with significant human and animal health impacts [22], [23].

Typically, however, zoo surveillance has largely focused on captive animals within zoo collections. In Australia, wildlife hospitals operated by the major zoos also treat a significant caseload of free-ranging and rehabilitation wildlife. A survey in 2008 found that 15 Australian zoos treated over 14,000 wildlife cases each year in their wildlife hospitals [29] and admissions to these hospitals appear to be increasing over time. As well as providing expertise in veterinary care, these hospitals have strong links to a network of wildlife rehabilitation, conservation, research and welfare organisations in their region.

The zoo based wildlife disease surveillance program was developed in recognition of the strong capacity and potential for wildlife hospitals at Australian zoos to contribute to national and international wildlife disease surveillance. The program aimed to integrate zoo based wildlife hospitals into Australia's animal health surveillance system. This paper describes the program and reviews the outcomes in the context of wildlife diseases that impact on human health, livestock health, trade and biodiversity.

Materials and Methods

Planning

In 2009 the Zoo Animal Health Reference Group [30] held a workshop to identify the role that Australian zoos could play in biosecurity, and surveillance was identified as a key area where a contribution could be made. A zoo based wildlife disease surveillance program was proposed and a collaborative project was subsequently developed between the AWHN and the Zoo and Aquarium Association Australasia (ZAA). The ZAA, with over 80 institutional members, is the peak body representing the zoo and aquarium industry in Australia and New Zealand. The AWHN and the ZAA worked with the Zoo Animal Health Reference Group and the senior veterinarians from the participating zoos to develop the scope and methodology for a pilot project to evaluate the potential of a zoo based surveillance program. The aim of the pilot project was to trial the integration of free-ranging wildlife disease information from zoo based wildlife hospitals into the national wildlife health information system. An additional objective was to strengthen and improve communication and the flow of information between zoo veterinarians and relevant government agencies.

Six major Australian zoos were selected to participate in the pilot project, each with a well-established and resourced on-site veterinary hospital treating free-ranging and rehabilitation wildlife and a permanent staff of experienced zoo and wildlife veterinarians. The six participating zoos are located in five Australian states: Adelaide Zoo in South Australia, Australia Zoo Wildlife Hospital in Queensland, Healesville Sanctuary and Melbourne Zoo in Victoria, Perth Zoo in Western Australia and Taronga Zoo in New South Wales (Figure 1). A formal survey of these zoos was conducted to gather baseline information and assist in planning for the pilot project. Data were collected on the number and taxonomic breakdown of wildlife cases seen by each of the zoo veterinary hospitals over a 12-month period during 2009 to 2010 (Table 1).

Operation

The pilot project commenced in November 2010 and finished in October 2011. During this time an agreed data set was collected from free-ranging and rehabilitation wildlife cases seen by the participating zoo veterinary hospitals. The scope of the pilot project did not include data from zoo collection animals and focused on the reporting of existing work, rather than expansion of disease investigations. Reporting into the national wildlife health information system in the pilot project was limited to selected disease event categories (Table 2), which had previously been established as a high priority for wildlife surveillance in Australia and aligned with data being reported from other sources. These categories are designed to collect wildlife disease information of potential importance to human health, livestock health, trade and biodiversity. While the priority for data collection was positive results, reporting of negative results was also encouraged, particularly where a specific disease was excluded that is a locally, nationally, or internationally notifiable or reportable disease. The 'interesting or unusual' category was designed to capture unusual events or findings that could indicate an emerging disease, syndrome or trend. Examples of disease events that could be reported in this category are significant clusters or patterns of disease, unexpected morbidities or mortalities, toxicity events,

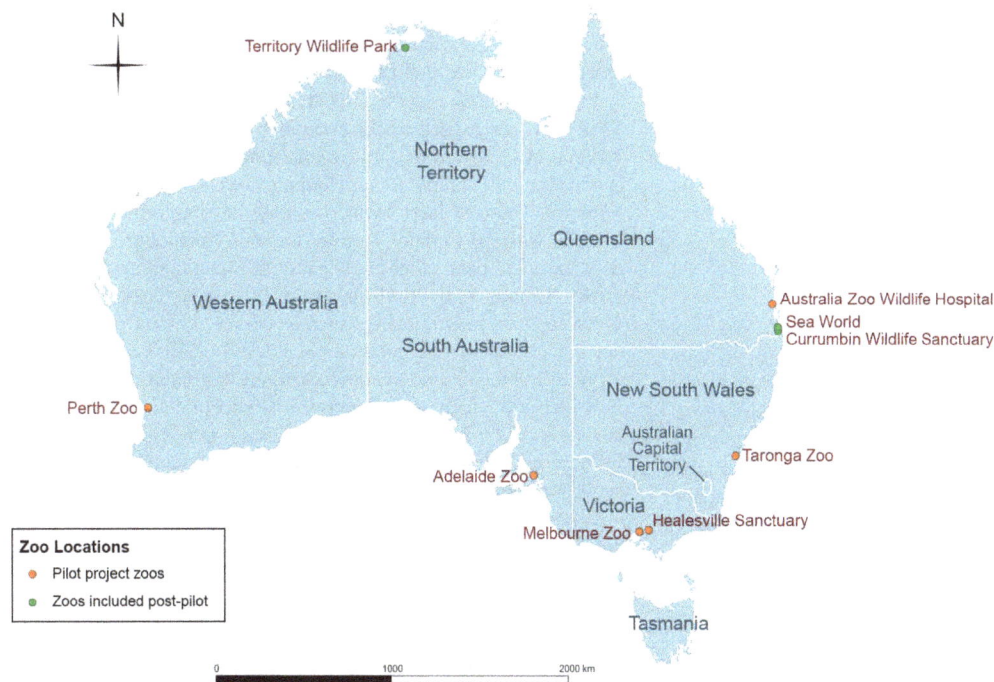

Figure 1. Geographic location of the zoos participating in the surveillance program.

marine wildlife strandings, and cases with possible linkages to international events or drivers. Cases for reporting were not confined to those where a necropsy or laboratory test had been conducted. Participants were encouraged to report a range of cases using different diagnostic tools, including where the diagnosis was based solely on clinical examination.

Cases were reported into the national wildlife health surveillance system via a web-enabled database, the 'electronic Wildlife Health Information System' (eWHIS). After initial training sessions provided by the AWHN, the zoo veterinarians entered data directly into the eWHIS database on a monthly basis for the duration of the pilot project, with ongoing training and support provided as needed. Fields captured included: event dates, event location, event type (e.g. individual, outbreak, monitoring), event category (see Table 2), species, number (affected and dead), state of captivity, presenting syndrome, diagnosis (one or multiple),

Table 2. Categories for selection of wildlife disease events for reporting into eWHIS.

Category
World Organisation for Animal Health (OIE) Listed diseases
Bat viral diseases
Mass mortalities
Arboviral diseases
Salmonella cases
'Interesting or unusual' cases

Table 1. Indicative numbers of free-ranging wildlife cases seen by veterinary hospitals at six major Australian zoos over a 12 month period during 2008/2009.

	Native species*				Feral species*	
ZOO	Mammals	Birds	Reptiles	Amphibia	All taxa	TOTAL
Australia Zoo Wildlife Hospital	2,579 (38%)	2,835 (42%)	1,126 (17%)	49 (0.7%)	197 (3%)	6,786
Healesville Sanctuary	567 (37%)	851 (56%)	95 (6%)	14 (0.9%)	*	1,527
Taronga Zoo	276 (39%)	341 (48%)	92 (13%)	5 (0.7%)	*	714
Perth Zoo	75 (12%)	328 (53%)	188 (31%)	8 (1%)	15 (2%)	614
Melbourne Zoo	135 (37%)	135 (37%)	76 (21%)	23 (6%)	*	369
Adelaide Zoo	85 (39%)	100 (46%)	8 (4%)	2 (0.9%)	18 (8%)	213
TOTAL	3,717 (36%)	4,590 (45%)	1,585 (16%)	101 (1%)	230 (2%)	10,229

*Data from three zoos did not differentiate feral from native species; for these zoos, feral animal cases are included with native species numbers.

laboratory test details and confidentiality level. The data entered into eWHIS were reviewed and moderated by the AWHN.

Participating zoo veterinarians were given the opportunity to discuss interesting disease events and operational aspects of the pilot project at regular teleconferences. All zoo participants were encouraged to engage with their state or territory agriculture agency via the wildlife coordinator, however this did not replace or bypass the legislated reporting of notifiable animal diseases through appropriate channels.

Evaluation

An independent review was conducted at the end of the pilot project by an internationally-recognised consulting company with expertise and experience in epidemiology and wildlife disease surveillance. Their evaluation of the project included an assessment of the value of the surveillance data and the potential for the project to deliver benefits to stakeholders, including the Australian commonwealth, state and territory governments. The sustainability of the system was also assessed. The evaluation process included an online stakeholder survey, interviews with the project coordinators and analysis of collected data.

Results

The preliminary survey indicated that the six zoos treated over 10,000 wildlife cases in a year (Table 1). All six selected zoos agreed to participate in the pilot project and the zoo veterinarians commenced entering data directly into the eWHIS database from November 2010. Sixteen zoo veterinarians participated for some or all of the pilot project period. A total of 211 events that occurred during the 12-month pilot project were reported into eWHIS by the participating zoos. This represented almost a third of all cases submitted to eWHIS during that period from all sources including state and territory departments of agriculture and human health, university researchers and private veterinary practitioners. A small subset of the cases presented to the zoo veterinary hospitals met the agreed criteria for data entry into eWHIS (Table 2). This subset was between 1 and 8% of all cases for individual zoos and approximately 2% for the six zoos overall. Examples of disease events reported for each of the categories are provided in Table 3.

A wide range of wildlife species was represented by the data collected during the pilot project. Accurate taxonomic identification of the animals under investigation was possible due to the expertise of the participating zoo veterinarians. The 211 disease events reported for the period from November 2010 to October 2011 covered 52 different species from 31 families and included birds (12 orders), turtles, marsupials, monotremes, marine mammals and bats (Table 4). The pilot project increased the overall species coverage of the data collected in eWHIS, with 18 species (9 bird, 7 mammal and 2 reptile species) reported through the pilot project that were not reported from other sources during the same period. A number of events reported through the pilot project came from geographic areas not represented by other sources.

The project captured data on diseases with potential human health implications, including confirmed or highly suspicious cases of salmonellosis, avian chlamydiosis (*Chlamydophila psittaci*), Australian bat lyssavirus in bats, mycobacteriosis (unspeciated) in a koala (*Phascolarctos cinereus*), and cryptosporidiosis in a hand-raised macropod. The cases of salmonellosis occurred in a variety of birds, marsupials and reptiles, and typing of these isolates contributed to the National Enteric Pathogens Surveillance Scheme [31]. Multiple cases of neurological signs in tawny

frogmouths (*Podargus strigoides*) in urban areas of Sydney were of interest as this species has been suggested as a sentinel for the emerging zoonosis angiostrongylosis [32], [33].

Of the records entered in eWHIS through the pilot project, 73% were categorised by the submitter as 'interesting or unusual', a grouping designed to capture information on possible emerging syndromes and trends. As an example, 14 cases of neoplasia were reported. Cancers have been recognised as emerging diseases of wildlife with potentially serious impacts, including Tasmanian devil facial tumour disease [11] and fibropapillomatosis of green turtles (*Chelonia mydas*) [34]. Additionally, cancer clusters in wildlife due to environmental causes such as chemical contamination can act as sentinels for risk to human health [35], [36]. Cases were also reported of recognised syndromes where the cause has not been fully identified, such as non-suppurative encephalitis in corvids and paralysis in rainbow lorikeets (*Trichoglossus haematodus*). This information could contribute to a better understanding of syndromes with unknown aetiology.

Cases in threatened species were reported, including the endangered Carnaby's black-cockatoo (*Calyptorhynchus latirostris*) and loggerhead turtle (*Caretta caretta*) and a number of vulnerable species (Table 5) [37], some of which were not represented in data captured from other sources for the same period. Data were collected on cases of psittacine circoviral (beak and feather) disease, which is listed as a key threatening process in endangered psittacine species under the *Environment Protection and Biodiversity Conservation (EPBC) Act 1999* [38]. Also reported was a diabetes syndrome affecting koalas in care that could impact on the rehabilitation success of koalas in Queensland, a species now listed as vulnerable under the *EPBC Act 1999* [37]. The first two confirmed clinical cases of chlamydiosis in koalas in South Australia were reported to the AWHN through the pilot project [39]. The South Australian koala population was thought to be free of *Chlamydia* [40], so these reports may be an indicator of an emerging disease in the South Australian koala population.

The project provided a framework for improved data capture for monitoring programs. For example, the AWHN holds responsibility for collating, moderating and maintaining a national dataset of bats tested for ABLV, and the pilot project resulted in the capture of more detailed information on the history and clinical signs of bats for this dataset.

The project framework assisted the management of a disease outbreak in 2011. A strain of avian paramyxovirus 1 (APMV1) not previously reported in Australia was detected in hobby pigeons in the Melbourne area in Victoria, and the virus was subsequently detected in free-living feral rock doves (*Columba livia*) and a spotted turtle dove (*Streptopelia chinensis*), and in a native collared sparrow hawk (*Accipiter cirrocephalus*) [41], [42]. The project provided a mechanism to update zoo veterinarians about the outbreak, highlighted the possible involvement of native pigeons and raptors, and most likely resulted in increased submission of free-ranging sick and dead birds to the Victorian Department of Primary Industries for testing. A number of notifications of other disease events and outbreaks of relevance to wildlife were disseminated through the project, including a cluster of Hendra virus cases in horses in New South Wales and Queensland [43], and neurological disease in horses due to arboviruses in New South Wales [44] in 2011.

Information reported into eWHIS by the participants contributed to Australia's reports to the World Organisation for Animal Health (OIE). Australia, as a contributor to the OIE, regularly reports on the country's animal health status, which is important to ensure that Australia's health status for animals and animal products is well recognised internationally [45].

Table 3. Examples of disease events captured for each reporting category (see Table 2).

Reporting Category	Examples
OIE Listed diseases*	• Avian chlamydiosis (*Chlamydophila psittaci*)
	• Botulism
	• Psittacine circoviral (beak and feather) disease
	• Toxoplasmosis
	• Trichomoniasis
Bat viral diseases	• Australian bat lyssavirus
Mass mortalities	• Six Carnaby's black-cockatoos (*Calyptorhynchus latirostris*) found dead in a similar location over a two-week period
	• Twenty-one rainbow lorikeets (*Trichoglossus haematodus*) and scaly-breasted lorikeets (*Trichoglossus chlorolepidotus*) with neurological signs over a period of a month
Arboviral diseases	• None reported
Salmonella cases	Salmonella cultured from:
	• Green turtle (*Chelonia mydas*) – corneal abscess
	• Australian Raven (*Corvus coronoides*) with neurological signs – muscle
	• Two hand-raised eastern grey kangaroos (*Macropus giganteus giganteus*) with diarrhoea and anorexia – faeces
	• Hand-raised koala (*Phascolarctos cinereus*) joey with neurological signs and septicaemia - caecum, blood and liver
'Interesting or unusual' cases	• Fourteen cases of neoplasia in a variety of species including yellow-bellied glider (*Petaurus australis*), New Zealand fur seal (*Arctocephalus forsteri*), koala (*Phascolarctos cinereus*), wedge-tailed eagle (*Aquila audax*), laughing kookaburra (*Dacelo novaeguineae*)
	• Australian fur seal (*Arctocephalus pusillus doriferus*) with acute suppurative meningitis; heavy growth of *Arcanobacterium*
	• Multisystemic lymphoproliferative disease in a wedge-tailed eagle (*Aquila audax*)
	• Green turtle (*Chelonia mydas*) with fibropapillomatous lesions on flippers
	• Australian raven (*Corvus coronoides*) with non-suppurative encephalitis; flavivirus, avian influenza and Newcastle disease excluded

*Includes 'non-listed' pathogens and agents of wildlife [49].

Evaluation

The independent review found that the pilot project increased the volume of cases and expanded the sources of data being entered into the national database [46]. According to the review, the project resulted in increased geographic and taxonomic coverage of the wildlife population, with data collected from additional 'catchment' areas and an increased species distribution, as well as a wider range of presenting syndromes and reporting reasons. The review concluded from these outcomes that the pilot project enhanced the capacity of the national wildlife health information system for early detection of disease and improved the sensitivity for demonstration of freedom from disease.

The survey of zoo participants found that most considered their institution had benefited from the pilot project. Participants

Table 4. Cases* for November 2010– October 2011 reported through the pilot project, by taxonomic group.

Taxonomic group	
A. ALL CASES	No. of cases (%)
Birds	109 (52%)
Mammals	79 (37%)
Reptiles	23 (11%)
Total	211
B. MAMMALS	No. of cases (% of mammal cases)
Non-macropod marsupial	34 (43%)
Bat+	28 (35%)
Macropod	10 (13%)
Marine mammal	4 (5%)
Monotreme	2 (3%)
Other mammal	1 (1%)
Total	79

*A case may involve single or multiple animals.
+The majority of bat cases were submitted for exclusion testing for Australian bat lyssavirus (ABLV).

Table 5. Threatened species for which data was captured through the pilot project.

Species	EPBC Act Listing Status
Carnaby's black-cockatoo (*Calyptorhynchus latirostris*)	Endangered
Loggerhead turtle (*Caretta caretta*)	Endangered
Chuditch or Western quoll (*Dasyurus geoffroii*)	Vulnerable
Flatback turtle (*Natator depressus*)	Vulnerable
Green turtle (*Chelonia mydas*)	Vulnerable
Grey-headed flying fox (*Pteropus poliocephalus*)	Vulnerable
Hawksbill turtle (*Eretmochelys imbricata*)	Vulnerable
Koala (*Phascolarctos cinereus*)*	Vulnerable
Quokka (*Setonix brachyurus*)	Vulnerable
Sub-Antarctic fur seal (*Arctocephalus tropicalis*)	Vulnerable

*The koala (combined populations of Queensland, New South Wales and the Australian Capital Territory) was listed as vulnerable in May 2012.

reported that the project provided additional focus for the zoos to investigate wildlife diseases; resulted in better recognition of their contribution to wildlife health; and improved collaboration, connection and communication with other institutions and organisations. It also contributed to a better understanding of the wider context of wildlife disease events, and assisted in identifying patterns in these events by providing a forum to share information on similar syndromes from different locations. The majority of participants agreed that participation in the project increased their awareness and understanding of diseases of national concern. The review identified some limitations of the program, including the clustering of cases around major population centres, and the collection of only a small proportion of the total caseload of the participating zoo wildlife hospitals.

The reviewers concluded that there was value in the project to both the stakeholders and the participants, and that it was sustainable. They recommended the program be continued and expanded to include more zoos in order to increase the coverage and volume of data collected and to build on the improved capacity for early detection of wildlife disease. Factors recommended for consideration in the selection of additional zoos included geographic location and the 'catchment' area of wildlife covered by the zoo, veterinary presence, caseload, nature of cases, and availability of resources for data entry.

Outcomes

Based on the success of the pilot project and the recommendations of the independent review, the zoo based wildlife disease surveillance program has continued. Each of the participating zoos has remained with the program, which has expanded to incorporate three additional zoos with the aim of increasing both the geographic and species range. These zoos are Currumbin Wildlife Sanctuary and Sea World in Queensland, and Territory Wildlife Park in the Northern Territory (Figure 1). This brings the total number of free-ranging wildlife cases seen by the nine participating zoos to around 17,000 cases each year. A total of 25 zoo wildlife hospital staff have directly participated in the program since its inception.

Discussion

Animal health surveillance is the key to early detection and management of emerging diseases. The need to include free-ranging wildlife populations in animal health surveillance programs is increasingly recognised in Australia and globally [1], [5], [14], however effective disease surveillance in free-ranging wildlife populations presents many challenges. In Australia, as in many countries, there is an established system for investigating wildlife disease events and reporting them into the national system, however a considerable number of wildlife cases are inevitably seen outside of this system. A significant caseload of free-ranging wildlife is presented for treatment to Australian zoo based veterinary hospitals by members of the public, wildlife carers and park rangers, or are referred by state and territory government agencies, and the cost of providing this service is mostly covered by the zoos' operating budgets [29].

Australian zoo based hospitals are recognised as one of the chief sources of information on wildlife health and are well placed to participate in wildlife disease surveillance as these zoos have veterinary staff with expertise in wildlife health, are well organised and represented by their peak body, the Zoo and Aquarium Association, and have an existing framework of communication and collaboration. Zoos also have strong linkages with a broad network of wildlife rehabilitators, wildlife researchers, conservation organisations and environmental officers in their districts. For these reasons, the existing framework for the national reporting of wildlife disease information was expanded to include zoo veterinarians working with free-ranging wildlife. A pilot project demonstrated that a zoo based surveillance program was able to capture useful information on disease in free-ranging wildlife that might otherwise not have been reported into the national system, or was reported earlier than would otherwise have occurred. The program has the ability to capture valuable information on diseases of humans and domestic animals originating from wildlife, diseases in threatened species and recognised syndromes of unknown aetiology.

Some limitations of the zoo surveillance pilot project were identified by the independent review and the authors. Geographic coverage of cases reported through the project was, as expected, clustered around the physical locations of the participating zoos, which are primarily in or near the major population centres in coastal areas of Australia. This reflects the inherent bias of general surveillance systems. Although primarily in coastal locations, the zoos are situated in a variety of geographic and climatic zones, and in both urban and rural settings. This source of surveillance information does not stand alone, but complements other sources of data. The program also allows clear identification of geographic areas where general surveillance is of lower intensity, which is valuable for planning and assessment of risk.

As described, the scope of the project resulted in the collection of only a small proportion of the total caseload of the zoo wildlife hospitals into the eWHIS database (1–8%). The majority of cases presenting to zoo wildlife hospitals involve orphaned animals and cases involving dog, cat or vehicular trauma. Most of these do not align with the categories for reporting, which are selected on the basis of nationally-agreed priorities for wildlife disease surveillance in Australia. Nonetheless a large volume of potentially valuable data is not captured through the program, and this aspect of data collection will be further investigated by the authors. There may also be cases that meet the selection criteria but are not being reported into eWHIS, as the decision on what to report rests with the submitter, however the AWHN provides training and ongoing guidance on case selection to minimise the loss of eligible data.

This program focuses on wildlife hospitals at zoos, however the caseload varies significantly between participating institutions and in some instances there are other organisations in the same region with a higher caseload, such as private veterinary clinics, and not-for-profit wildlife hospitals and rehabilitation centres, which are not yet formally integrated into the surveillance system. This program may be used as a model in future to integrate other types of organisations into the national wildlife health surveillance system.

The Australian zoo based wildlife disease surveillance program provides a model for an effective, low cost system that utilises existing capacity and routine activities to contribute to national and international surveillance efforts. The program generates information with the potential to assist earlier detection of emerging diseases and trends, as well as strengthening networks, improving communication and information flow, and building capacity in wildlife health professionals. These elements form the basis of a successful surveillance program. This program acknowledges the value of data where a range of diagnostic tools, including clinical assessment has been used. As a model, it demonstrates that meaningful surveillance can be conducted in a variety of circumstances, including those where laboratory capacity and financial resources are limited.

There is a recognition that successful surveillance relies on communication between stakeholders, including private practitioners and public officers [47]. There is a need for greater integration and linkage of animal - both wild and domestic - and human pathogen surveillance systems at the international and national level [48]. The need for a systematic approach to communication between the human and animal disease surveillance systems in Australia has been outlined [19]. A 'One Health' approach can result in increased interaction between professionals working in the veterinary, medical, wildlife and environmental spheres [14]. In an evaluation of the WNV surveillance program in the USA, an association was found between submission of samples by zoos for WNV testing and the level of communication between the zoos and the public health agency [24]. The authors concluded that a greater awareness of the importance of surveillance by zoos could result in better collaboration and

detection of possible human health threats from animal disease events.

The AWHN maintains a 'first alert' framework based on a national network of wildlife health professionals that can be used to coordinate and disseminate information in an emergency or a significant disease event. This network receives regular notifications of disease alerts, requests for information and samples, and publication of significant articles, guidelines and policy documents. The pilot project demonstrated the potential of the program to widen this network and raise the level of awareness of emerging diseases and diseases of potential national importance. The collaborative framework of the program also encourages discussion on new and interesting events and patterns of disease across multiple locations, and facilitates sharing of samples for testing and research.

The program has resulted in improved communication and flow of information, and strengthened relationships between the zoo industry and government agencies, in particular the state and territory departments of agriculture. Linking with zoos provides an avenue for information gathering and dissemination, and an opportunity to utilise the expertise and resources within their extensive networks. The program has the potential to build the capacity of zoos to play a rapid and effective role in a disease emergency by integrating zoo veterinarians into the national biosecurity surveillance network.

Conclusion

The science of understanding emerging infectious diseases with wildlife as part of their ecology has gained much attention over recent years, but it is often difficult to conduct meaningful surveillance in this area. The Australian zoo based wildlife disease surveillance program uses a collaborative approach involving government and the zoo industry, with a focus on collecting and reporting of wildlife disease events with potential impact on human health, livestock health and biodiversity. It provides a strong model for a disease surveillance program for free-ranging wildlife that could be adapted and utilised in other contexts. There is potential for expansion of the program to groups outside of zoo hospitals such as private veterinary practitioners from 'sentinel' hospitals with a high wildlife caseload, veterinary hospitals run by animal welfare organisations and universities involved in clinical wildlife work and research. Integration of these groups into the national wildlife health surveillance system has the potential to assist in the early detection of emerging diseases in Australia's free-ranging wildlife population.

Acknowledgments

Australia's states and territories, the zoos mentioned in the paper and the Zoo and Aquarium Association Australasia provided significant in-kind resources to enable the work to proceed. We thank Angus Cameron and Jenny Hutchison from AusVet Animal Health Services for their independent review of the pilot project, Susan Hester from ACERA for her interest and support, and the state and territory wildlife coordinators for their support and participation. We acknowledge the contribution of Helen Crabb, Bonnie McMeekin, Cree Monaghan, Tim Portas, Kimberley Vinette Herrin and Sam Young to the planning of the project. A particular thank you to the participating zoo veterinarians and staff, without whom the program could not run: Paul Eden, Sarah Frith, Leesa Haynes, Peter Holz, Robert Johnson, Trine Kruse, Anna Le Souef, Jenna McKenzie, David McLelland, Phillipa Mason, Jade Patterson, Karen Payne, Franciscus Scheelings, Tania Theuma, Gabrielle Tobias and Rebecca Vaughan-Higgins.

Author Contributions

Conceived and designed the experiments: KCW AR RW VG RTB DJB WB SC CL HMcC M. Pyne IS SV LV DW M. Phillips CB LP. Performed the experiments: KCW AR RW VG RTB DJB WB SC CL HMcC M. Pyne IS SV LV DW. Analyzed the data: KCW AR. Wrote the paper: KCW AR.

References

1. Kruse H, Kirkemo AM, Handeland K (2004) Wildlife as source of zoonotic infections. Emerg Infect Dis 10: 2067–2072.
2. Daszak P, Cunningham AA, Hyatt AD (2001) Anthropogenic environmental change and the emergence of infectious diseases in wildlife. Acta Trop 78: 103–116.
3. Daszak P, Cunningham AA, Hyatt AD (2000) Emerging infectious diseases of wildlife – threats to biodiversity and human health. Science 287: 443–449.
4. Cook RA, Karesh WB (2008) Chapter 6 - Emerging Diseases at the Interface of People, Domestic Animals, and Wildlife. In: Fowler ME, Miller RE, editors. Zoo and Wild Animal Medicine (Sixth Edition). Saint Louis: W.B. Saunders. pp. 55–65.
5. Jones KE, Patel NG, Levy MA, Storeygard A, Balk D, et al. (2008) Global trends in emerging infectious diseases. Nature 451: 990–993.
6. McFarlane R, Sleigh A, McMichael T (2012) Synanthropy of wild mammals as a determinant of emerging infectious diseases in the Asian-Australasian region. Ecohealth 9: 24–35.
7. O'Neil BD, Pharo HJ (1995) The control of bovine tuberculosis in New Zealand. N Z Vet J 43: 249–255.
8. Nolan A, Wilesmith JW (1994) Tuberculosis in badgers (Meles meles). Vet Microbiol 40: 179–191.
9. Alexander DJ (2007) An overview of the epidemiology of avian influenza. Vaccine 25: 5637–5644.
10. Frick WF, Pollock JF, Hicks AC, Langwig KE, Reynolds DS, et al. (2010) An emerging disease causes regional population collapse of a common North American bat species. Science 329: 679–682.
11. McCallum H (2008) Tasmanian devil facial tumour disease: lessons for conservation biology. Trends Ecol Evol 23: 631–637.
12. Skerratt L, Berger L, Speare R, Cashins S, McDonald K, et al. (2007) Spread of chytridiomycosis has caused the rapid global decline and extinction of frogs. EcoHealth 4: 125–134.
13. Berger L, Speare R, Daszak P, Green DE, Cunningham AA, et al. (1998) Chytridiomycosis causes amphibian mortality associated with population declines in the rain forests of Australia and Central America. Proceedings of the National Academy of Sciences 95: 9031–9036.
14. Black PF, Murray JG, Nunn MJ (2008) Managing animal disease risk in Australia: the impact of climate change. Rev Sci Tech 27: 563–580.
15. Bunn C, Woods R (2005) Emerging wildlife diseases – impact on trade, human health and the environment. Microbiology Australia 26: 53–55.
16. Prowse SJ, Perkins N, Field H (2009) Strategies for enhancing Australia's capacity to respond to emerging infectious diseases. Vet Ital 45: 67–78.
17. Sleeman J, Brand C, Wright S (2012) Strategies for wildlife disease surveillance. In: Aguirre A, Ostfeld R, Daszak P, editors. New Directions in Conservation Medicine. New York, NY: Oxford University Press. pp. 539–551.
18. Mathews F (2009) Zoonoses in wildlife integrating ecology into management. Adv Parasitol 68: 185–209.
19. Murray KA, Skerratt LF, Speare R, Ritchie S, Smout F, et al. (2012) Cooling off health security hot spots: getting on top of it down under. Environ Int 48: 56–64.
20. Animal Health Australia (2013) Animal Health in Australia 2012. Canberra, Australia.
21. Australian Wildlife Health Network (2014) About AWHN. Available: http://wildlifehealthaustralia.com.au/AboutUs.aspx. Accessed 2014 Mar 10.
22. McNamara T (2007) The role of zoos in biosurveillance. International Zoo Yearbook 41: 12–15.
23. Ludwig GV, Calle PP, Mangiafico JA, Raphael BL, Danner DK, et al. (2002) An outbreak of West Nile virus in a New York City captive wildlife population. Am J Trop Med Hyg 67: 67–75.
24. Pultorak E, Nadler Y, Travis D, Glaser A, McNamara T, et al. (2011) Zoological institution participation in a West Nile Virus surveillance system: implications for public health. Public Health 125: 592–599.
25. McNamara T, Travis D, Nadler Y (2011) A bird in hand: the power of zoo sentinels. Ecohealth 7: S21–22.
26. Watanabe M (2003) Zoos act as sentinels for infectious diseases. BioScience 53: 792.
27. Zoo Animal Health Network (2012) Flu At The Zoo Tabletop Exercise. Available: http://www.zooanimalhealthnetwork.org/FluAtTheZoo.aspx. Accessed 2013 Nov 20.
28. USDA/AZA Avian Influenza Surveillance System for Zoological Institutions (2012) Available: http://www.zooanimalhealthnetwork.org/ai/Home.aspx.Accessed 2013 Nov 20.
29. Beri V, Tranent A, Abelson P (2010) The economic and social contribution of the zoological industry in Australia. International Zoo Yearbook 44: 192–200.
30. Australian Wildlife Health Network (nd) Zoo Animal Health Reference Group. Available: http://wildlifehealthaustralia.com.au/ProgramsProjects/ZooAnimalHealthReferenceGroup.aspx. Accessed 2014 Mar 10.
31. Powling J (2012) Quarterly Statistics – Surveillance Activities – Salmonella Surveillance. Animal Health Surveillance Quarterly Report 17: 27.
32. Spratt D (2005) Neuroangiostrongyliasis: disease in wildlife and humans. Microbiology Australia 26: 63–64.
33. Ma G, Dennis M, Rose K, Spratt D, Spielman D (2013) Tawny frogmouths and brushtail possums as sentinels for Angiostrongylus cantonensis, the rat lungworm. Vet Parasitol 192: 158–165.
34. Herbst LH, Klein PA (1995) Green turtle fibropapillomatosis: challenges to assessing the role of environmental cofactors. Environ Health Perspect 103 Suppl 4: 27–30.
35. McAloose D, Newton AL (2009) Wildlife cancer: a conservation perspective. Nat Rev Cancer 9: 517–526.
36. Newman SJ, Smith SA (2006) Marine mammal neoplasia: a review. Vet Pathol 43: 865–880.
37. Australian Government Department of the Environment (2009) EPBC Act List of Threatened Fauna. Available: http://www.environment.gov.au/cgi-bin/sprat/public/publicthreatenedlist.pl?wanted = fauna. Accessed 2013 Nov 20.
38. Australian Government Department of the Environment (2009) Listed Key Threatening Processes. Available: http://www.environment.gov.au/cgi-bin/sprat/public/publicgetkeythreats.pl. Accessed 2013 Nov 20.
39. Funnell O, Johnson L, Woolford L, Boardman W, Polkinghorne A, et al. (2013) Conjunctivitis Associated with Chlamydia pecorum in Three Koalas (Phascolarctos cinereus) in the Mount Lofty Ranges, South Australia. Journal of Wildlife Diseases 49: 1066–1069.
40. Australian Government Department of the Environment (2013) Species Profile and Threats Database 2012: Phascolarctos cinereus (combined populations of Qld, NSW and the ACT) – Koala (combined populations of Queensland, New South Wales and the Australian Capital Territory). Available: http://www.environment.gov.au/cgi-bin/sprat/public/publicspecies.pl?taxon_id = 85104. Accessed 2013 Nov 20.
41. Paskin R (2011) Avian paramyxovirus in pigeons. Animal Health Surveillance Quarterly Report 16: 3–5.
42. Grillo T, Post L (2012) Australian Wildlife Health Network. Animal Health Surveillance Quarterly Report 17: 6–8.
43. Field H, Crameri G, Kung NY, Wang LF (2012) Ecological aspects of Hendra virus. Curr Top Microbiol Immunol 359: 11–23.
44. Arthur R (2011) State and Territory Reports – New South Wales. Animal Health Surveillance Quarterly Report 16: 10–13.
45. Australian Government Department of Agriculture (2011) Australia and the World Organization for Animal Health. Available: http://www.daff.gov.au/animal-plant-health/animal/oie. Accessed 2013 Nov 20.
46. Cameron A, Hutchison J (2011) Review of the Zoo Based Wildlife Disease Surveillance Pilot Project. Unpublished report to the Australian Wildlife Health Network.
47. Halliday J, Daborn C, Auty H, Mtema Z, Lembo T, et al. (2012) Bringing together emerging and endemic zoonoses surveillance: shared challenges and a common solution. Philos Trans R Soc Lond B Biol Sci 367: 2872–2880.
48. Kuiken T, Leighton FA, Fouchier RA, LeDuc JW, Peiris JS, et al. (2005) Public health. Pathogen surveillance in animals. Science 309: 1680–1681.
49. World Organisation for Animal Health (OIE) (2012) Report of the Meeting of the OIE Working Group on Wildlife Diseases, Paris, 12–15 November 2012. Available: http://www.oie.int/fileadmin/Home/eng/Internationa_Standard_Setting/docs/pdf/WGWildlife/A_WGW_Nov2012.pdf. Accessed 2013 Nov 20.

4

Suboptimal Herd Performance Amplifies the Spread of Infectious Disease in the Cattle Industry

M. Carolyn Gates*, Mark E. J. Woolhouse

Epidemiology Group, Centre for Immunity, Infection and Evolution, School of Biological Sciences, University of Edinburgh, Ashworth Laboratories, Edinburgh, Scotland, United Kingdom

Abstract

Farms that purchase replacement breeding cattle are at increased risk of introducing many economically important diseases. The objectives of this analysis were to determine whether the total number of replacement breeding cattle purchased by individual farms could be reduced by improving herd performance and to quantify the effects of such reductions on the industry-level transmission dynamics of infectious cattle diseases. Detailed information on the performance and contact patterns of British cattle herds was extracted from the national cattle movement database as a case example. Approximately 69% of beef herds and 59% of dairy herds with an average of at least 20 recorded calvings per year purchased at least one replacement breeding animal. Results from zero-inflated negative binomial regression models revealed that herds with high average ages at first calving, prolonged calving intervals, abnormally high or low culling rates, and high calf mortality rates were generally more likely to be open herds and to purchase greater numbers of replacement breeding cattle. If all herds achieved the same level of performance as the top 20% of herds, the total number of replacement beef and dairy cattle purchased could be reduced by an estimated 34% and 51%, respectively. Although these purchases accounted for only 13% of between-herd contacts in the industry trade network, they were found to have a disproportionately strong influence on disease transmission dynamics. These findings suggest that targeting extension services at herds with suboptimal performance may be an effective strategy for controlling endemic cattle diseases while simultaneously improving industry productivity.

Editor: Hiroshi Nishiura, The University of Tokyo, Japan

Funding: This work was undertaken through the Centre of Expertise on Animal Disease Outbreaks (EPIC) supported by the Scottish Government and has made use of the resources provided by the Edinburgh Compute and Data Facility (ECDF). MCG was supported by the Principal's Career Development Scholarship and Scottish Overseas Research Student Award Scheme through the University of Edinburgh. The funders had no role in study design, data collection and analysis, decision to publish, or preparation of the manuscript.

Competing Interests: The authors have declared that no competing interests exist.

* E-mail: CarolynGatesVMD@gmail.com

Introduction

Beef and dairy herds require a constant supply of replacement breeding cattle to maintain or increase herd size. A key decision facing producers is whether to raise heifers internally for replacement or to purchase replacement breeding cattle directly from outside sources at the risk of introducing many economically important diseases [1–5]. The optimal strategy for any given herd depends on a number of complex factors including land and labour availability, cash flow needs, market prices, and future business goals [6–10]. Heifers require intensive management and nutritional support to reach an appropriate physical maturity by the target age at first breeding [11] and for farms that cannot provide this cost-effectively, there can be significant financial advantages to breeding calves with desirable growth and carcass characteristics for fattening instead [12,13]. Due to the long production cycle of cattle, farms that are undergoing rapid expansion to capture favourable market prices may also choose to purchase replacement cattle rather than rely on internal growth [14].

In some cases, however, the decision to purchase replacement cattle is directly influenced by herd reproductive performance. Farms that cull excessive numbers of animals for infertility, poor

production, and other health related issues have an increased demand for replacement breeding cattle [15], while farms with high calf mortality rates, delayed ages at first calving, and prolonged calving intervals may not have an adequate supply of heifers to meet replacement needs [16,17]. As well as losing significant profit through reduced productivity [17,18], these farms are potentially increasing their risk of disease introductions by purchasing greater numbers of replacement breeding cattle than would be needed if they were achieving industry standards for performance. Since the movements of replacement breeding cattle form part of a larger contact network, herds that purchase large numbers of animals to compensate for poor performance may also be contributing to the industry-level transmission dynamics of many infectious cattle diseases.

Although there have been many recent studies characterizing the frequency of between-herd cattle movements and the basic structure of cattle movement networks in countries with electronic movement recording systems [19–26], little is currently known about the underlying causes or epidemiological consequences of trade in replacement breeding cattle. In this analysis, data from the national cattle movement database in Great Britain was used as a case example to determine the relationship between key herd performance indicators (average age at first calving, interval between successive calvings, culling rates, and calf mortality rates) and the number of replacement breeding cattle purchased by beef and dairy herds. Simple disease simulation models were then used to study the effects of removing replacement breeding cattle movements from the contact network on the transmission dynamics of different endemic pathogens. Findings from both analyses were used to emphasize that the management decisions of individual herds can have a substantial impact on the epidemiology of infectious disease at the industry level.

Materials and Methods

Cattle movement data

Farmers across the European Union have been required to report the births, deaths, and movements of individual cattle to the government under Council Regulation (EC) No 820/97 as part of efforts to restore consumer confidence in the safety of livestock following the bovine spongiform encephalopathy (BSE) crisis in 1996. In Great Britain, these records have been stored electronically in the Cattle Tracing System (CTS) database operated by the British Cattle Movement Service (BCMS) since January 2001 [27,28]. Demographic information on the sex, breed classification (beef, dairy, or dual purpose breed), date of birth, birth location, date of death, death location, and identity of calves that survived parturition is also available for each animal and may be used to generate key performance indicators for cattle breeding herds [29]. Movements on or off livestock locations are recorded with information on the departure location, destination location, movement date, and movement type (birth, death, or movement). By linking the demographic information with the movement records, it is possible to infer the animal's production purpose at the time of movement.

The subsequent analyses used data from 01 January 2004 through 31 December 2006 to characterize the performance of British cattle farms and to reconstruct the network of cattle movements between them. Data were extracted from the CTS database using the Python programming language. For the purpose of this analysis, a farm was defined as any location with a unique county-parish-holding (CPH) number that was classified as an agricultural holding or landless keeper (farmer raising cattle on rented land). The primary reason for selecting this time period was to ensure that sufficient pre- and post-movement data was available to classify animals into production groups. It was assumed that animals intended for human consumption would be slaughtered by 30 months of age to comply with bovine spongiform encephalopathy (BSE) regulations [30] and that animals intended for breeding would deliver their first calf by 48 months of age. At the time of this analysis, CTS data was only available through April 2010.

Herd performance indicators

There were a total of 8,415,283 recorded calvings on 67,868 farm locations in Great Britain from January 2004 through December 2006. This analysis focused on the subset of 34,289 farms with an average of at least 20 beef and/or 20 dairy cattle births per year. This included 18,951 exclusively beef farms, 14,737 exclusively dairy farms, and 601 mixed production farms. Altogether these herds accounted for 89.6% of the total number of calvings in Great Britain. The main reasons for restricting the sample were to eliminate small scale operations where cattle breeding was unlikely to be the primary source of farm income [31] and to eliminate farms that may have been in the process of entering or exiting the cattle industry. Beef herds and dairy herds

managed on mixed production farms were treated as separate units in the remaining analyses.

For each calving event, the following information was recorded: calving farm, calving date, dam date of birth, dam breed classification, date and location of any previous or subsequent calvings, date of the next recorded movement off the calving farm, calf breed classification, calf sex, and calf date and location of death. The average number of calvings per year was used as an estimate of breeding herd size. The basic calving event records were aggregated by farm to generate the following performance indicators: average age at first calving, calving interval, culling rate, and calf mortality rate. The methodology used to calculate these indicators has been published in other studies [29,32].

The average age at first calving was calculated as the difference between the age at calving and date of birth in months for all heifers that calved on the farm during the specified time period. A heifer was defined as an animal between 19 and 48 months of age with no previously recorded calving dates in the CTS database. The purpose for placing restrictions on age was to eliminate potential outliers that may have been caused by data entry errors or animals that may have delivered an unrecorded stillborn calf at an appropriate age. The calving interval was calculated as the number of months between successive calving dates for the subset of dams that delivered another calf within 730 days. It was assumed that in most production herds, any animals that failed to deliver a calf within 24 months would be culled from the herd and outlying values were most likely attributable to data entry errors or unrecorded births. The culling rate was calculated as the percentage of calvings where the dam was subsequently slaughtered or sold within 500 days of calving. The calf mortality rate was calculated as the percentage of all calves born during the specified time period that died on an agricultural holding within 365 days of birth. It was assumed that calves slaughtered at an abattoir were intended for the veal production market and therefore excluded from the mortality calculations. The performance indicators were averaged over the 3 year study time period.

Network reconstruction

There were a total of 7,917,890 individual movements between cattle farms in the period from 01 January 2004 through 31 December 2006. The cattle movement network was reconstructed by aggregating the individual movement records into batch movement records such that all cattle moving from farm A to farm B on the same date were considered a single batch movement. This resulted in a network with 2,695,402 batch movements between 90,478 unique farm locations (including breeding herds, fattening herds, and hobby farms). Similar to previous studies, movements that occurred through a livestock market were treated as a single direct movement from the original departure herd to the final destination herd after sale [20,33]. Approximately 1% of individual movement records were discarded due to missing or inaccurate information.

For the purpose of this analysis, a replacement breeding heifer was defined as an animal that was born on a different location than the destination farm and subsequently calved on the destination farm, while a replacement breeding cow was defined as an animal that previously calved on a different location than the destination farm and subsequently calved on the destination farm. These definitions were used to distinguish true cattle sales from temporary movements between seasonal grazing pastures, movements between locations operated by the same cattle business, and movements through farms acting as livestock dealers. All batch movements that contained at least one replacement breeding female were subsequently classified as replacement breeding cattle movements. The remaining movements included store calves, fattening cattle, breeding bulls, and replacement heifers that were culled before breeding. The average number of replacement breeding cattle purchased by the study farms each year was also recorded.

Descriptive statistics

Basic descriptive statistics on the performance of beef and dairy herds were provided as frequency distributions. For illustrative purposes, the industry standards for performance were also indicated on the plots. In general, it is held that the average age at first calving should be less than 24 months, the average calving interval less than 365 days, the average culling rate for beef herds between 15 and 20%, the average culling rate for dairy herds between 25 and 35%, and the average calf mortality rate less than 5% [7,34–36].

Impact of herd performance on replacement breeding cattle trade

Zero-inflated negative binomial (ZINB) regression models were used to explore the relationship between herd performance and the purchase of replacement breeding cattle. Data for beef herds and dairy herds were analysed separately due to inherent difference in management practices. The logistic component of the ZINB model provided insight on factors influencing the odds of herds remaining closed over the three year study period, while the negative binomial component provided insight on factors influencing the expected count of replacement cattle purchased over the three year study period. Prior to analysis, a logarithmic transformation (base 10) was applied to herd size, and the performance variables (age at first calving, calving, interval, culling rate, and calf mortality rate) were divided into categories by quintile. For culling rate, the reference category was set as the middle quintile and for the remaining variables, the reference category was set as the top quintile.

As the purpose of the analysis was to explore the relationship between performance indicators and replacement breeding cattle trade rather than to generate the most parsimonious model, all variables were retained in both the logistic and negative binomial components of the final multivariate models. The Vuong test statistic was used to confirm the choice of a zero-inflated model over standard negative binomial regression. The odds ratios (ORs) and 95% confidence intervals were reported for the logistic components of the models, while the coefficients and standard errors (SEs) were reported for the negative binomial components of the models. All statistical analyses were performed in R [37].

The equations from the final ZINB regression models were then used to predict the effects of improving herd performance on the total number of replacement breeding cattle purchased by beef and dairy herds. As a baseline for comparison, we first used the empirically observed values for the performance indicators in the model equations to estimate the total number of replacement breeding cattle purchased. Then, each of independent variables (with the exception of herd size) was set to a target value and the new predicted values for the total number of replacement breeding cattle purchased were calculated. For age at first calving, calving interval, and calf mortality variables, the target values were set as the top quintile for performance. For culling rate, the target values were set as the middle quintile for performance. These quintiles were used as the target performance levels based on observations that the majority of British beef and dairy were failing to achieve industry standards for performance in practice. The objective was to provide a more realistic estimate for how much performance could be improved. Each variable was tested alone and in combination. The results were expressed as the percentage reduction in the total number of purchased replacement breeding cattle compared to the baseline value.

Impact of replacement breeding cattle trade on disease transmission dynamics

The effect of removing replacement breeding cattle movements from the contact network on disease transmission dynamics was evaluated with a simple Susceptible-Infectious-Susceptible (SIS) simulation model. At the beginning of each simulation, disease was seeded on 10,000 farms at random on 01 January 2004. Each affected farm was assigned an infectious period drawn at random from an exponential distribution with a half-life, h [2]. The model was then updated in time steps of one day. If an infected farm moved a batch of cattle to a susceptible farm, there was a fixed probability, p, that the destination farm would also become infected. The probability was not weighted according to the number of cattle moved. Farms that reached the end of their infectious period reverted back to a susceptible state. To ensure adequate time for the system to reach steady state equilibrium, the simulation was allowed to run for a total of 50 years by recycling the 3 year movement data set. Endemic prevalence was measured as the average number of farms infected on any given day over the last 3 years of the simulation. The simulation code was implemented in the C programming language.

In the first set of simulation scenarios, h was set at 1,095 days and p was set at 0.05 to approximate the transmission dynamics of a pathogen similar to bovine viral diarrhoea virus [2]. A targeted removal approach was used to assess the relative importance of replacement breeding cattle movements to network transmission dynamics [38]. At the beginning of each simulation, a proportion of replacement breeding cattle movements were removed from the network data set at random. The simulation was then run on the reduced movement network to monitor changes in the predicted endemic prevalence. A total of 10,000 simulations were performed with the proportion to be removed drawn at random from a uniform distribution bounded at 0 and 1 representing no removal and complete removal, respectively. Based on performance curves, this number of simulations was adequate to capture the variation in model outcomes. As a benchmark for comparison, another 10,000 simulations were performed where equivalent numbers of movements (including replacement breeding cattle movements and all other types of movements) were removed from the network at random. The results from both simulation sets were plotted as the percent of total network movements removed against the percent change in endemic prevalence using the maximum recorded value for endemic prevalence amongst the simulations as the baseline value.

In the second set of simulation scenarios, the proportion of replacement breeding cattle movements removed from the network was fixed at 1, but the values for h and p were varied in each replicate to determine whether the observed effects were consistent across for broader range of endemic pathogens. At the beginning of each simulation, the value for h was drawn from a uniform distribution ranging from 90 days to 1,825 days and the value for p was drawn from a uniform distribution ranging from 0.01 to 0.25. These parameter ranges were chosen based on how the simulated diseases behaved on the networks. Pathogens with farm infectious periods below 90 days were generally unable to persist. When the farm infectious period was increased above 1,825 days or the transmission probability was increased above 0.25, the network saturated and there was very little change in the endemic prevalence. A total of 100,000 simulations were performed. Similar to the first scenario, another 100,000 simulations were performed removing the equivalent number of movements (including replacement breeding cattle movements and all other types of movements) at random for comparison. The results were again expressed as the additional percentage change in endemic prevalence relative to the baseline simulations with random elimination of cattle movements.

Results

Descriptive statistics

Data on the performance of 19,552 beef herds and 15,338 dairy herds in Great Britain with an average of at least 20 calvings per year were derived from records stored in the national Cattle Tracing System (CTS) database between January 2004 and December 2006. The average size of beef herds in the sample was 56 breeding cattle (median: 41, range: 20 to 1,520) and the average size of dairy herds was 91 breeding cattle (median: 76, range: 20 to 1,241). As highlighted in Figure 1, there were a substantial number of herds performing below industry targets for average age at first calving, calving interval, culling rates, and calf mortality rates. An estimated 69% of beef herds and 59% of dairy herds purchased at least one replacement breeding animal over the three year period. The average number of replacement breeding cattle purchased by open beef herds in a given year was 6 (median: 2, range: 1 to 422), while the average number of replacement breeding cattle purchased by open dairy herds in a given year was 9 (median: 2, range: 1 to 847).

Impact of herd performance on replacement breeding cattle trade

Zero-inflated negative binomial (ZINB) regression models were constructed to explore the relationship between herd performance and the total number of replacement breeding cattle purchased by beef and dairy herds (Tables 1 and 2, respectively). The Vuong tests for beef (V = 11.36, p<0.001) and dairy (V = 11.43, p<0.001) herds had high positive values indicating that the zero-inflated models fit the data better than standard negative binomial regression.

In the logistic component of the models, the odds of a beef or dairy herd being closed decreased significantly as the calf mortality rate increased. Beef herds with average ages at first calving in the second and third quintiles (29.6 to 31.8 months and 31.9 to 33.8 months, respectively) were significantly less likely to be closed than herds in the top quintile (<29.6 months), while herds in the bottom quintile (>35.9 months) were significantly more likely to be closed. Similar trends with the average age at first calving were observed for dairy herds. Herds of both production types with culling rates above or below the industry target range were also significantly more likely to be closed. The average calving interval was not significantly associated with being a closed dairy herd. However, beef herds with calving intervals above the first quintile (>378 days) were generally less likely to be closed, although there was no clear trend as the calving interval increased. Herd size had no significant effect on the odds of either a beef or dairy herd being closed.

In the negative binomial component of the models, the total number of replacement breeding cattle purchased by beef and dairy herds generally increased with herd size, culling rate, and calf mortality rate. For dairy herds, there was also an increase in the number of replacement breeding cattle purchased as the average age at first calving increased. This trend was not observed for beef herds. For herds of both production types, having a calving interval in the bottom quintile (>412 days for beef and

>444 days for dairy) was significantly associated with purchasing greater numbers of replacement breeding cattle.

The ZINB models were then used to predict the effects of altering herd performance on the total number of replacement breeding cattle purchased by the study herds (Figure 2). Setting all the reproductive performance variables for each herds to the top quintile reduced the number of replacement breeding cattle purchased by 34.4% for beef and 50.8% for dairy.

Impact of replacement breeding cattle trade on disease transmission dynamics

The simulation models revealed that replacement breeding cattle movements had a disproportionately strong influence on network transmission dynamics. At a transmission probability of 0.05 and infectious period half-life of 1,095 days, removal of all replacement breeding cattle movements (13.3% of all between-herd movements) from the network resulted in an approximately 45.8% reduction in endemic prevalence (Figure 3). Removal of the equivalent number of movements at random decreased endemic prevalence by only 19%. The effects of removing replacement breeding cattle movements compared to removing movements at random were more pronounced for diseases with low transmission probabilities and short infectious periods (Figure 4).

Discussion

Although many studies have used records from the CTS database to investigate the spread of disease through cattle movement networks [20,33,39,40], this is the first to our knowledge that establishes a direct relationship between the management practices of individual herds and the theoretical risk of infectious disease transmission. The most significant finding in the present study was that herds with poor performance were not only losing profitability, but also contributing to the persistence of endemic diseases at the industry level by purchasing excess numbers of replacement breeding cattle. The wide variation in performance between herds suggests that there is significant potential to reduce the number of replacement breeding cattle purchased and therefore the number of potentially infectious contacts by improving herd management. As a disease control strategy, this approach may be particularly effective because of the disproportionately strong influence that replacement trade has on the industry-level transmission dynamics of many important livestock pathogens

Data limitations

There are several limitations in using the CTS database to calculate herd performance indicators that must be considered when interpreting the study findings. First, a breeding herd was defined as any location with a unique CPH number that had at least one recorded beef or dairy calving. Larger farm businesses may house cattle on several locations [41] and with the available data, it was not possible for us to determine which of these locations were linked. Therefore, some of the animals classified as replacement breeding cattle or culled cattle may have been transfers within the same farm business rather than transfers of ownership. We also assumed that dairy breeding cattle housed on the same location as beef breeding cattle were separate production units. However, these dairy cattle may have been strictly used to produce crossbreed calves for the beef production unit [42]. Second, farmers are not required to register the births of stillborn calves or calves that died within several hours of birth. The may lead to underestimation of calf mortality rates and breeding herd size as well as overestimation of the average age at first calving and

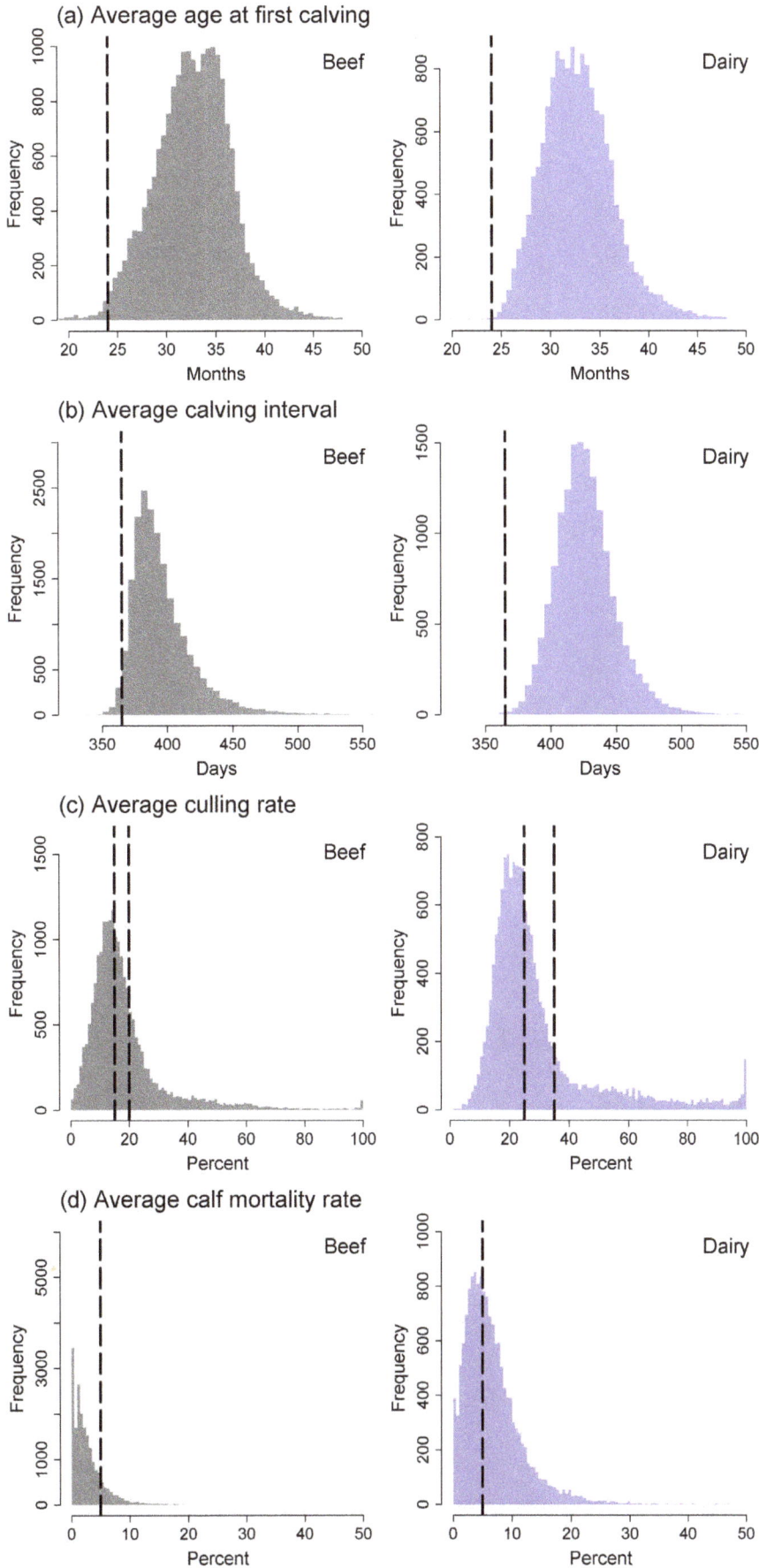

(a) Average age at first calving

(b) Average calving interval

(c) Average culling rate

(d) Average calf mortality rate

Figure 1. Descriptive statistics on the performance of beef and dairy herds in Great Britain. Frequency distributions of the (a) average age at first calving, (b) average calving interval, (c) average culling rate, and (d) average calf mortality rate amongst 24,093 beef herds and 14,754 dairy herds in Great Britain with at least 20 breeding dams per year between January 2004 and December 2006. The vertical dashed lines indicate the industry target values for performance.

calving intervals. Finally, records in the CTS database are not free from error and a small proportion of calving records were discarded due to missing or biologically implausible data.

Impact of herd performance on replacement breeding cattle trade

Descriptive statistics revealed that the majority of beef and dairy herds in Great Britain were calving heifers at significantly older ages than the recommended 24 months [11]. However, the relationship between average age at first calving and the risk of purchasing replacement breeding cattle was complex. Compared to herds ranked in the top 20% for performance, those in second quintile were significantly more likely to be open, while those in the bottom quintile were significantly more likely to be closed. Part of this trend may related to the difficulty in ensuring that heifers have reached an appropriate physical maturity by the start of the breeding season or the target age at first calving for the herd. Heifers that are bred too young have a greater risk of calving complications [43], which can effect subsequent fertility and performance [44]. Consequently, farmers may choose to retain

heifers for breeding in subsequent autumn or spring calving seasons [45], which would increase the average age at first calving, but reduce the need to purchase animals from outside sources. For dairy herds, the total number of replacement breeding cattle purchased increased with the average age at first calving. Based on unpublished data, this may be confounded by the fact that purchased replacement dairy heifers were also significantly older at the time of calving than home-raised heifers.

The average calving intervals observed in the study herds were also significantly greater than the recommended 365 days [42,46], which suggests that many cattle breeding herds in Great Britain are experiencing problems with fertility. Delays between successive calvings should in theory limit the number of replacement heifers an animal produces over its lifespan leading to an increased risk of purchasing replacement cattle as well as an increased number of cattle purchased. However, contrary to expectations, the average calving interval had little appreciable effect on replacement breeding cattle trade. One possible explanation is that calving intervals may be artificially low in herds that are culling excessive animals for poor fertility [47,48]. For example, beef herds that

Table 1. Zero-inflated negative binomial regression model for beef herds.

Predictor	Levels	(a) logistic			(b) negative binomial		
		OR	95% CI	p-value	Coef	SE	p-value
$\log_{10}$(herd size)	–	0.85	0.67–1.09	0.201	2.12	0.037	<0.001
Average age at first calving (months)	<29.5	Ref	-	-	Ref	-	-
	29.6 to 31.8	0.47	0.37–0.59	<0.001	0.063	0.030	0.038
	31.9 to 33.8	0.45	0.36–0.56	<0.001	0.082	0.030	0.006
	33.9 to 35.8	0.89	0.74–1.06	0.194	−0.012	0.031	0.695
	>35.9	1.33	1.13–1.58	0.001	−0.126	0.033	<0.001
Calving interval (days)	<378	Ref	-	-	Ref	-	-
	379 to 386	0.78	0.64–0.95	0.012	−0.005	0.031	0.881
	387 to 396	0.76	0.63–0.93	0.007	0.001	0.031	0.992
	397 to 411	0.73	0.59–0.89	0.002	−0.009	0.031	0.776
	>412	1.16	0.97–1.40	0.102	0.091	0.032	0.005
Culling rate (%)[a]	<9.8	2.10	1.67–2.63	<0.001	−0.059	0.030	0.066
	9.9 to 13.5	1.55	1.23–1.96	<0.001	−0.043	0.030	0.153
	13.6 to 17.2	Ref	-	-	Ref	-	-
	17.3 to 23.4	1.24	0.98–1.57	0.071	0.164	0.030	<0.001
	>23.5	1.95	1.57–2.42	<0.001	0.667	0.032	<0.001
Calf mortality rate (%)[b]	<0.68	Ref	-	-	Ref	-	-
	0.69 to 1.52	0.88	0.72–1.07	0.199	0.067	0.032	0.038
	1.53 to 2.59	0.90	0.74–1.09	0.265	0.105	0.032	0.001
	2.60 to 4.29	0.80	0.66–0.98	0.033	0.121	0.032	<0.001
	>4.30	0.78	0.64–0.95	0.014	0.345	0.031	<0.001

The (a) logistic and (b) negative binomial components of the zero-inflated negative binomial regression model predicting the likelihood of being a closed herd and the number of replacement breeding cattle purchased by beef herds, respectively. (OR = odds ratio, CI = confidence interval, Coef = coefficient, SE = standard error) Voung test V = 11.36, p<0.001
[a]The culling rate was calculated as the percentage of calvings where the dam was subsequently slaughtered or sold within 500 days of calving.
[b]The calf mortality rate was calculated as the percentage of all calves born during the specified time period that died on an agricultural holding within 365 days of birth.

Table 2. Zero-inflated negative binomial regression model for dairyherds.

Predictor	Levels	(a) logistic			(b) negative binomial		
		OR	95% CI	p-value	Coef	SE	p-value
$\log_{10}$(herd size)	–	0.90	0.73–1.11	0.333	1.707	0.051	<0.001
Average age at first calving (months)	<29.8	Ref	-	-	Ref	-	-
	29.9 to 31.7	0.62	0.52–0.74	<0.001	0.043	0.043	0.317
	31.8 to 33.5	0.81	0.69–0.95	0.012	0.172	0.044	<0.001
	33.6 to 35.6	0.93	0.80–1.09	0.398	0.167	0.045	<0.001
	>35.7	1.03	0.88–1.21	0.674	0.341	0.045	<0.001
Calving interval (days)	<408	Ref	-	-	Ref	-	-
	409 to 420	0.89	0.76–1.04	0.143	0.043	0.045	0.330
	421 to 429	0.89	0.75–1.04	0.138	0.005	0.045	0.907
	430 to 443	0.90	0.77–1.06	0.197	0.040	0.045	0.374
	>444	0.92	0.78–1.08	0.301	0.150	0.045	0.001
Culling rate (%)[a]	17.5	1.74	1.48–2.05	<0.001	−0.273	0.046	<0.001
	17.6 to 21.8	1.19	1.01–1.40	0.043	−0.199	0.043	<0.001
	21.9 to 26.4	Ref	-	-	Ref	-	-
	26.5 to 35.9	0.78	0.66–0.94	0.007	0.273	0.041	<0.001
	>36.0	1.41	1.20–1.66	<0.001	0.462	0.044	<0.001
Calf mortality rate (%)[b]	<2.86	Ref	-	-	Ref	-	-
	2.87 to 4.69	0.87	0.75–1.02	0.078	−0.029	0.047	0.538
	4.70 to 6.74	0.78	0.67–0.91	0.001	0.104	0.047	0.025
	6.75 to 9.80	0.59	0.50–0.69	<0.001	0.244	0.046	<0.001
	> 9.81	0.46	0.54–0.54	<0.001	0.376	0.046	<0.001

The (a) logistic and (b) negative binomial components of the zero-inflated negative binomial regression model predicting the likelihood of being a closed herd and the number of replacement breeding cattle purchased by dairy herds, respectively. (OR = odds ratio, CI = confidence interval, Coef = coefficient, SE = standard error) Voung test V = 11.43, p<0.001
[a]The culling rate was calculated as the percentage of calvings where the dam was subsequently slaughtered or sold within 500 days of calving.
[b]The calf mortality rate was calculated as the percentage of all calves born during the specified time period that died on an agricultural holding within 365 days of birth.

practice seasonal calving are under significant pressure to cull animals that fail to conceive within the narrow breeding window [32]. The results for dairy herds may also be confounded by the presence of high producing dairy herds that intentionally delay rebreeding in certain high yielding cows to increase farm profitability [49,50]. Future studies should explore the interaction between the different performance variables in greater detail.

The risk of purchasing at least one replacement breeding animal was less in herds with culling rates that were above or below the industry target ranges. It is possible that some of the herds with low culling rates were compensating for an inadequate supply of replacement heifers by retaining a greater percentage of mature breeding cattle, while some of the herds with high culling rates were in the process of exiting the cattle industry. A small number of herds in England and Wales may have also been subject to movement restrictions and increased culling as part of bovine tuberculosis control efforts [51]. Even though the risk of disease introductions is theoretically lower, herds that cull too few animals are losing opportunities to improve herd genetics and perfor- mance, while herds that cull too many animals are losing profitability through the costs of raising extra replacement heifers to maintain herd size [9,52]. The negative binomial portion of the ZINB models predicted that number of replacement breeding cattle increased with herd culling rates, which supports the hypothesis that herds with high culling rates have an increased demand for replacement cattle.

For herds of both production types, the total number of replacement breeding cattle purchased increased with the calf mortality rate. The magnitude of these results must be interpreted with some caution as the extent and effects of under-reporting the deaths of male calves are not well known [53]. Calf mortality has a direct impact on the supply of replacement heifers and it has been recommended that death losses should not exceed 5% [36]. The majority of beef herds were well below this threshold, which may explain why the risk of being a closed herd decreased only marginally as the calf mortality rate increased. In contrast, almost 60% of dairy herds had a mortality rate greater than 5%. This may be partly attributed to the fact that male dairy calves have a lower economic value and generally do not receive the same standard of care as replacement heifers [54]. Furthermore, dairy calves are separated from their dams shortly after birth and factors such as colostrum intake, housing conditions, nutritional manage- ment, and infectious disease control become even more critical in preventing calf deaths [55–57].

Impact of replacement breeding cattle trade on disease transmission dynamics

In a recent review, Carslake and colleagues emphasized the importance of finding disease control interventions that are effective against a wide range of endemic diseases to reduce trade-off in resource allocation [58]. Our ZINB models predicted that if all herds were able to achieve the same level of performance

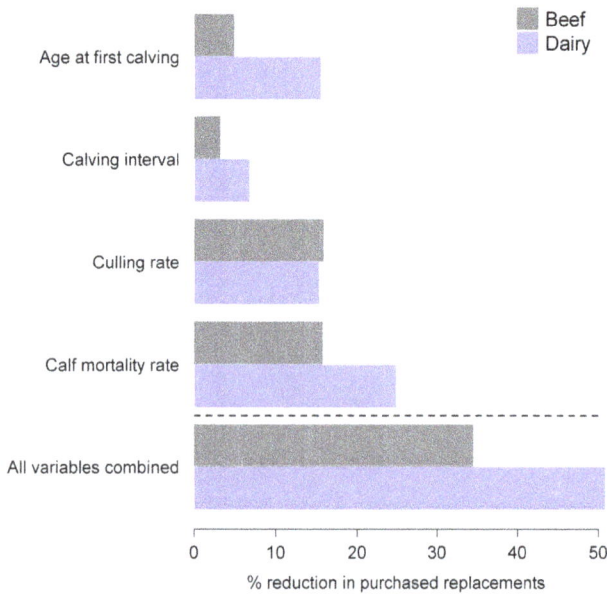

Figure 2. Estimated reduction in the number of purchased replacement breeding cattle with improved herd management. The horizontal bars show the percentage reduction in the total number of replacement breeding cattle purchased by the study herds when the values for age at first calving, calving interval, and calf mortality variables, the target value were set as the top quintiles and the values for culling rates were set at the middle quintile in the ZINB models. Each variable was tested alone and in combination.

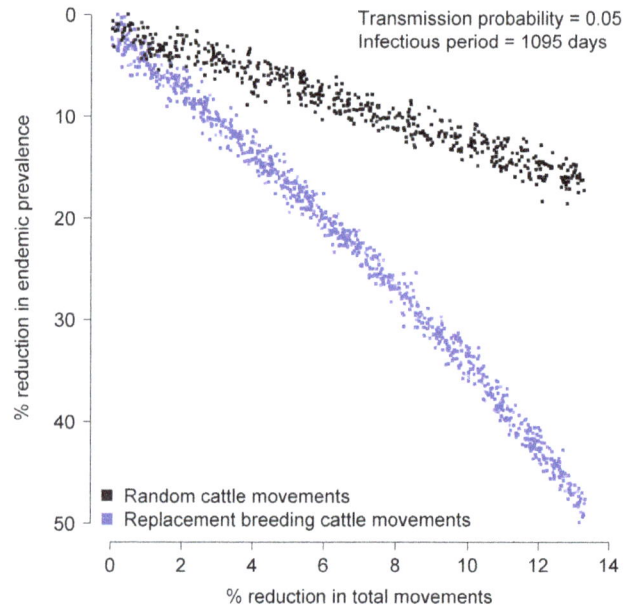

Figure 3. Estimated reduction in the endemic prevalence of BVDV following removal of replacement breeding cattle movements. The proportion of movements removed from the network was varied randomly between 0 and 13.3% at the beginning of each simulation. The black dots indicate the results from removing movements from the network at random. The blue dots indicate the results for the targeted removal of replacement breeding cattle movements. A total of 10,000 replicates were performed for each removal strategy. The transmission probability was set at 0.05 and the infectious period half-life was set at 1,095 days to simulate BVDV.

as the top 20%, the number of replacement breeding cattle purchased by beef and dairy herds could be reduced by a third and a half, respectively. Given that even herds in the top 20% were still operating below industry targets for performance, these may be conservative estimates for the potential reduction in replacement breeding cattle movements and subsequent risk of introducing multiple directly transmissible diseases to the herd. The primary advantage of this approach is that improving herd performance has readily demonstrable effects on farm profitability without relying on disease specific interventions. There is still, however, the challenge of providing appropriate incentives and education to encourage farmers to change their management practices.

Poor performance has traditionally been considered a herd level problem and therefore free from national regulation. However, as the results from our simulation model show, the practice of purchasing replacement breeding cattle has a disproportionately strong influence on the risk of disease spreading to other farms in the network. This may be related to the market structure of the British livestock industry since herds that purchase replacement breeding cattle must often source animals from multiple herds, which increases the number of inward contacts. These farms may also be selling larger numbers of cattle for fattening, which increases the number of outward contacts. Both factors are important determinants of network centrality. Even if these movements cannot be prevented through improved herd management, it may possible to apply disease specific biosecurity measures such as quarantine, vaccination, or diagnostic testing to effectively remove them from the contact network [21,59,60]. However, these measures may be more effective against some pathogens than others. Our results also showed that the magnitude of the observed effect increased as both the farm infectious period and movement transmission probability were decreased. This is

likely to be because diseases with short infectious periods and low transmission probabilities have difficulty persisting in cattle populations to begin with and therefore minor changes in the network structure are enough to push these diseases towards extinction. Other researchers have similarly shown that the

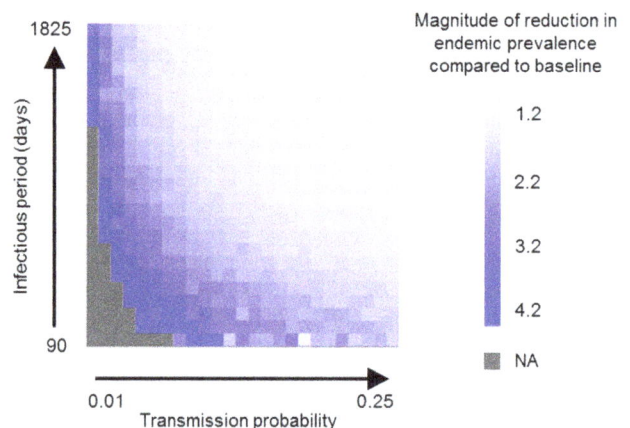

Figure 4. Effects of altering the transmission probability and infectious period half-life on simulation model results. The values shown are the predicted endemic prevalence when all replacement breeding cattle movements were removed from the network divided by the predicted endemic prevalence when an equivalent number of movements (including all movement types) were removed from the network at random. Grey squares indicate parameter combinations where disease was unable to persist on the network.

structural and temporal features of cattle movement networks matter less for diseases that spread over long time periods [61] or have a higher probability of spreading through batch movements [33].

Study limitations

Although we found many significant associations between herd performance and the purchase of replacement breeding cattle in the ZINB models, the interpretation of the study findings is complicated by the fact that poor performance can be both a cause and effect of purchasing replacement breeding cattle. For example, Thomsen and others [62] found that culling rates were significantly higher in Danish dairy herds with a large proportion of purchased cows. It was suggested that herds with excessively high culling rates may not have an adequate supply of heifers to meet replacement needs thereby necessitating the purchase of replacement breeding cattle from outside sources. However, herds that purchase replacement breeding cattle are at increased risk of introducing diseases like bovine viral diarrhoea virus (BVDV) and bovine herpesvirus type I (BHV I), which can in turn lead to increased culling through their effects on fertility and abortion [63–66]. Similarly, high calf mortality rates may limit the availability of replacement heifers, but may also be linked to the presence of infectious diseases introduced through animal movements [67,68].

Another striking feature of our results was the number of herds operating below industry standards for animal performance. The potential causes of poor performance in British beef and dairy herds have been discussed at length in a previous publication [29] and are likely farm specific and multifactorial. This leads to the question of how much farmers can reasonably be expected to improve herd performance in the field. Our models assumed that all herds would be capable of achieving the same level of performance as the top 20% of herds in the field, which in many cases was still below the industry targets for performance. Further

research is needed to determine whether this leads to an underestimation or overestimation of the effect size observed in the ZINB models.

The simulation study used a simplistic disease transmission model that considered all farms to be homogenous production units regardless of their size or demographic structure and all movements to carry the same risk of transmitting disease regardless of the number or production type of cattle moved. While these assumptions may be appropriate for highly infectious epidemic diseases that spread rapidly and indiscriminately between herds, endemic pathogens often have unique epidemiological features that can modify transmission risk [58]. For example, factors such as age, gender, and production type can influence the probability of purchased cattle being infected as well as their probability of being commingled directly with susceptible production groups in the receiving herd [69]. The rate of disease clearance from infected herds can also be influenced by size and other management practices [70,71]. We also assumed that no disease transmission occurred between animals in close contact at livestock markets, which again may change the industry level transmission dynamics. Therefore, the absolute values predicted by the model should be interpreted with caution, but the general trend that replacement breeding cattle movements have a greater importance to disease transmission should still be robust.

Acknowledgments

The authors gratefully acknowledge the RADAR team of DEFRA for their assistance with the CTS extracts.

Author Contributions

Conceived and designed the experiments: MCG MEJW. Performed the experiments: MCG. Analyzed the data: MCG. Wrote the paper: MCG MEJW.

References

1. Garcia Alvarez R, Webb C, Holmes M (2011) A novel field-based approach to validate the use of network models for disease spread between dairy herds. Epidemiol Infect 139: 1863–1874.
2. Tinsley M, Lewis FI, Brülisauer F (2012) Network modeling of BVD transmission. Vet Res 43.
3. Gilbert M, Mitchell A, Bourn D, Mawdsley J, Clifton-Hadley R, et al. (2005) Cattle movements and bovine tuberculosis in Great Britain. Nature Letters 435: 491–496.
4. Woodbine KA, Schukken YH, Green LE, Ramirez-Villaescusa A, Mason S, et al. (2009) Seroprevalence and epidemiological characteristics of Mycobacterium avium subsp. paratuberculosis on 114 cattle farms in south west England. Prev Vet Med 89: 102–109.
5. Woodbine KA, Medley GF, Moore SJ, Ramirez-Villaescusa AM, Mason S, et al. (2009) A four year longitudinal sero-epidemiological study of bovine herpesvirus type-1 (BHV-1) in adult cattle in 107 unvaccinated herds in south west England. BMC Vet Res 5: 5.
6. Gartner JA (1981) Replacement policy in dairy herds on farms where heifers compete with the cows for Grassland—part 1: Model construction and validation. Agr Sys 7: 289–318.
7. Groenendaal H, Galligan DT, Mulder HA (2004) An economic spreadsheet model to determine optimal breeding and replacement decisions for dairy cattle. J Dairy Sci 87: 2146–2157.
8. Van Arendonk JAM (1985) Studies on the replacement policies in dairy cattle. II. Optimum policy and influence of changes in production and prices. Livest Prod Sci 13: 101–121.
9. Heikkilä AM, Nousiainen JI, Jauhiainen L (2008) Optimal replacement policy and economic value of dairy cows with diverse health status and production capacity. J Dairy Sci 91: 2342–2352.
10. Vargas B, Herrero M, van Arendonk JAM (2001) Interactions between optimal replacement policies and feeding strategies in dairy herds. Livest Prod Sci 69: 17–31.
11. Le Cozler Y, Lollivier V, Lacasse P, Disenhaus C (2008) Rearing strategy and optimizing first-calving targets in dairy heifers: a review. Animal 2: 1393–1404.
12. Dal Zotto R, Penasa M, De Marchi M, Cassandro M, Lopez-Villalobos N, et al. (2009) Use of crossbreeding with beef bulls in dairy herds: effect on age, body weight, price, and market value of calves sold at livestock auctions. J Anim Sci 87: 3053–3059.
13. Roughsedge T, Amer PR, Simm G (2003) A bioeconomic model for the evaluation of breeds and mating systems in beef production enterprises. Anim Sci 77: 403–416.
14. Aadland D (2004) Cattle cycles, heterogeneous expectations, and the age distribution of capital. J Econ Dyn Control 28: 1977–2002.
15. Hadley GL, Wolf CA, Harsh SB (2006) Dairy cattle culling patterns, explanations, and implications. J Dairy Sci 89: 2286–2296.
16. Bascom SS, Young AJ (1998) A summary of the reasons why farmers cull cows. J Dairy Sci 81: 2299–2305.
17. Gröhn YT, Rajala-Schultz PJ (2000) Epidemiology of reproductive performance in dairy cows. Anim Reprod Sci 60–61: 605–614.
18. Britt JH (1985) Enhanced reproduction and its economic implications. J Dairy Sci 68: 1585–1592.
19. Bigras-Poulin M, Thompson RA, Chriel M, Mortensen S, Greiner M (2006) Network analysis of Danish cattle industry trade patterns as an evaluation of risk potential for disease spread. Prev Vet Met 76: 11–39.
20. Volkova VV, Howey R, Savill NJ, Woolhouse MEJ (2010) Potential for transmission of infections in networks of cattle farms. Epidemics 2: 116–122.
21. Natale F, Giovannini A, Savini L, Palma D, Possenti L, et al. (2009) Network analysis of Italian cattle trade patterns and evaluation of risks for potential disease spread. Prev Vet Met 92: 341–350.
22. Robinson S, Christley R (2006) Identifying temporal variation in reported births, deaths and movements of cattle in Britain. BMC Vet Res 2: 11.
23. Robinson SE, Christley RM (2007) Exploring the role of auction markets in cattle movements within Great Britain. Prev Vet Met 81: 21–37.
24. Vernon MC (2011) Demographics of cattle movements in the United Kingdom. BMC Vet Res 7.
25. Aznar MN, Stevenson MA, Zarich L, León EA (2011) Analysis of cattle movements in Argentina, 2005. Prev Vet Met 98: 119–127.

26. Baptista FM, Nunes T (2007) Spatial analysis of cattle movement patterns in Portugal. Vet Ital 43: 611–619.

27. Mitchell A, Bourn D, Mawdsley J, Wint W, Clifton-Hadley R, et al. (2005) Characteristics of cattle movements in Britain-an analysis of records from the Cattle Tracing System. Anim Sci 80: 265–273.

28. Green DM, Kao RR (2007) Data quality of the Cattle Tracing System in Great Britain. Vet Rec 161: 439–443.

29. Gates MC (2013) Evaluating the reproductive performance of British beef and dairy herds using national cattle movement records. Vet Rec 173: 499.

30. Department for Environment, Food, and Rural Affairs (2010) Bovine Spongiform Encephalopathy: Chronology of Events. Available: http://www.archive.defra.gov.uk/foodfarm/farmanimal/diseases/atoz/bse/publications/documents/chronol.pdf. Accessed 2014 Feb 19.

31. Ezanno P, Fourichon C, Beaudeau F, Seegers H (2006) Between-herd movements of cattle as a tool for evaluating the risk of introducing infected animals. Anim Res 55: 189–208.

32. Gates MC, Humphry RW, Gunn GJ (2013) Associations between bovine viral diarrhoea virus (BVDV) seropositivity and performance indicators in beef suckler and dairy herds. Vet J 198: 631–637.

33. Vernon MC, Keeling MJ (2009) Representing the UK's cattle herd as static and dynamic networks. P Roy Soc B Biol Sci 276: 469–476.

34. Berry DP, Cromie AR (2009) Associations between age at first calving and subsequent performance in Irish spring calving Holstein-Fresian dairy cows. Livest Sci 123: 44–54.

35. Haworth GM, Tranter WP, Chuck JN, Cheng Z, Wathes DC (2008) Relationships between age at first calving and first lactation milk yield, and lifetime productivity and longevity in dairy cows. Vet Rec 162: 643–647.

36. Youngquist RS, Threllfall W (1997) Current therapy in large animal theriogenology. Philadelphia: WB Saunders Company. 898p.

37. R-Development-Core-Team (2010) R: A language and environment for statistical computing. R Foundation for Statistical Computing.

38. Rautureau S, Dufour B, Durand B (2010) Vulnerability of animal trade networks to the spread of infectious diseases: a methodological approach applied to evaluation and emergency control strategies in cattle, France, 2005. Transbound Emerg Dis 58: 110–120.

39. Kao RR, Danon L, Green DM, Kiss IZ (2006) Demographic structure and pathogen dynamics on the network of livestock movements in Great Britain. P Roy Soc B Biol Sci 273: 1999–2007.

40. Robinson SE, Everett MG, Christley RM (2007) Recent network evolution increases the potential for large epidemics in the British cattle population. J Roy Soc Interface 4: 669–674.

41. Madders B (2006) Review of livestock movement controls. London. pp. 36. Available: http://archive.defra.gov.uk/foodfarm/farmanimal/movements/documents/livestock_movement_controls-review.pdf. Accessed 2014 Feb 19.

42. Amer PW, Simm G, Keane MG, Diskin MG, Wickham BW (2001) Breeding objectives for beef cattle in Ireland. Livest Prod Sci 67: 223–239.

43. Funston RN, Deutscher GH (2004) Comparison of target breeding weight and breeding date for replacement beef heifers and effects on subsequent reproduction and calf performance. J Anim Sci 82: 3094–3099.

44. Ettema JF, Santos JEP (2004) Impact of age at calving on lactation, reproduction, health, and income in first-parity Holsteins on commercial farms. J Dairy Sci 87: 2730–2742.

45. Hickson RE, Lopez-Villalobos N, Kenyon PR, Ridler BJ, Morris ST (2010) Profitability of calving heifers at 2 compared with 3 years of age and the effect of incidence of assistance at parturition on profitability. Anim Prod Sci 50: 354–358.

46. Veerkamp RF, Dillon P, Kelly E, Cromie AR, Groen AF (2002) Dairy cattle breeding objectives combining yield, survival and calving interval for pasture-based systems in Ireland under different milk quota scenarios. Livest Prod Sci 76: 137–151.

47. Bourdon R, Brinks J (1983) Calving date versus calving interval as a reproductive measure in beef cattle. J Anim Sci 57: 1412–1417.

48. MacGregor RG, Casey NH (1999) Evaluation of calving interval and calving date as measures of reproductive performance in a beef herd. Livest Prod Sci 57: 181–191.

49. Arbel R, Bigun Y, Ezra E, Sturman H, Hojman D (2001) The effect of extended calving intervals in high lactating cows on milk production and profitability. J Dairy Sci 84: 600–608.

50. Borman JM, Macmillan KL, Fahey J (2004) The potential for extended lactations in Victorian dairying: a review. Aust J Exp Agr 44: 507–519.

51. Abernethy DA, Upton P, Higgins IM, McGrath G, Goodchild AV, et al. (2013) Bovine tuberculosis trends in the UK and the Republic of Ireland, 1995–2010. Vet Rec 172: 312.

52. Korver S, Renkema JA (1979) Economic evaluation of replacement rates in dairy herds II. Selection of cows during the first lactation. Livest Prod Sci 6: 29–37.

53. Ortiz-Pelaez A, Pritchard DG, Pfeiffer DU, Jones E, Honeyman P, et al. (2008) Calf mortality as a welfare indicator on British cattle farms. Vet J 176: 177–181.

54. Lombard JE, Garry FB, Tomlinson SM, Garber LP (2007) Impacts of dystocia on health and survival of dairy calves. J Dairy Sci 90: 1751–1760.

55. Wathes DC, Brickell JS, Bourne NE, Swali A, Cheng Z (2008) Factors influencing heifer survival and fertility on commercial dairy farms. Animal 2: 1135–1143.

56. Brickell JS, McGowan MM, Pfeiffer DU, Wathes DC (2009) Mortality in Holstein-Friesian calves and replacement heifers, in relation to body weight and IGF-1 concentration, in 19 farms in England. Animal 3: 1175–1182.

57. Svensson C, Lundborg K, Emanuelson U, Olsson S-O (2003) Morbidity in Swedish dairy calves from birth to 90 days of age and individual calf-level risk factors for infectious diseases. Prev Vet Med 58: 179–197.

58. Carslake D, Grant W, Green LE, Cave J, Greaves J, et al. (2011) Endemic cattle diseases: comparative epidemiology and governance. PhilosT Roy Soc B 366: 1975–1986.

59. Rautureau S, Dufour B, Durand B (2012) Structural vulnerability of the French swine industry trade network to the spread of infectious disease. Animal 6: 1152–1162.

60. Natale F, Savini L, Giovannini A, Calistri P, Candeloro L, et al. (2011) Evaluation of risk and vulnerability using a disease flow centrality measure in dynamic cattle trade networks. Prev Vet Med 98: 111–118.

61. Kao RR, Green DM, Johnson J, Kiss IZ (2007) Disease dynamics over very different time-scales: foot-and-mouth disease and scrapie on the network of livestock movements in the UK. J Roy Soc Interface 4: 907–916.

62. Thomsen PT, Kjeldsen AM, Sørensen JT, Houe H, Ersbøll AK (2006) Herd-level risk factors for the mortality of cows in Danish dairy herds. Vet Rec 158: 622–626.

63. Rüfenacht J, Schaller P, Audigé L, Knutti B, Küpfer U, et al. (2001) The effect of infection with bovine viral diarrhea virus on the fertility of Swiss dairy cattle. Theriogenology 56: 199–210.

64. Valle PS, Wayne Martin S, Skjerve E (2001) Time to first calving and calving interval in bovine virus diarrhoea virus (BVDV) sero-converted dairy herds in Norway. Prev Vet Med 51: 17–36.

65. van Schaik G, Dijkhuizen AA, Huirne RBM, Schukken YH, Nielen M, et al. (1998) Risk factors for existence of Bovine Herpes Virus 1 antibodies on nonvaccinating Dutch dairy farms. Prev Vet Med 34: 125–136.

66. Tiwari A, VanLeeuwen JA, Dohoo IR, Stryhn H, Keefe GP, et al. (2005) Effects of seropositivity for bovine leukemia virus, bovine viral diarrhoea virus, Mycobacterium avium subspecies paratuberculosis, and Neospora caninum on culling in dairy cattle in four Canadian provinces. Vet Microbiol 109: 147–158.

67. Raboisson D, Delor F, Cahuzac E, Gendre C, Sans P, et al. (2013) Perinatal, neonatal, and rearing period mortality of dairy calves and replacement heifers in France. J Dairy Sci 96: 2913–2924.

68. Ersbøll AK, Rugbjerg H, Stryhn H (2003) Increased mortality among calves in Danish cattle herds during bovine virus diarrhoea infection. Acta Vet Scand 44: 49.

69. Ezanno P, Fourichon C, Seegers H (2008) Influence of herd structure and type of virus introduction on the spread of bovine viral diarrhoea virus (BVDV) within a dairy herd. Vet Res 39.

70. Brooks-Pollock E, Keeling M (2009) Herd size and bovine tuberculosis persistence in cattle farms in Great Britain. Prev Vet Med 92: 360–365.

71. Ståhl K, Lindberg A, Rivera H, Ortiz C, Moreno-López J (2008) Self-clearance from BVDV infections—A frequent finding in dairy herds in an endemically infected region in Peru. Prev Vet Med 83: 285–296.

5

Stability, Bifurcation and Chaos Analysis of Vector-Borne Disease Model with Application to Rift Valley Fever

Sansao A. Pedro[1,2,4]*, **Shirley Abelman**[1], **Frank T. Ndjomatchoua**[2,5], **Rosemary Sang**[3], **Henri E. Z. Tonnang**[2]

1 School of Computational and Applied Mathematics, University of the Witwatersrand, Johannesburg, South Africa, **2** Modelling, International Center of Insect Physiology and Ecology, Nairobi, Kenya, **3** Human Health, International Center of Insect Physiology and Ecology, Nairobi, Kenya, **4** Departamento de Matemática e Informática, Universidade Eduardo Mondlane, Maputo, Mozambique, **5** Departement de Physique, Universite de Yaoundé I, Yaoundé, Cameroun

Abstract

This paper investigates a RVF epidemic model by qualitative analysis and numerical simulations. Qualitative analysis have been used to explore the stability dynamics of the equilibrium points while visualization techniques such as bifurcation diagrams, Poincaré maps, maxima return maps and largest Lyapunov exponents are numerically computed to confirm further complexity of these dynamics induced by the seasonal forcing on the mosquitoes oviposition rates. The obtained results show that ordinary differential equation models with external forcing can have rich dynamic behaviour, ranging from bifurcation to strange attractors which may explain the observed fluctuations found in RVF empiric outbreak data, as well as the non deterministic nature of RVF inter-epidemic activities. Furthermore, the coexistence of the endemic equilibrium is subjected to existence of certain number of infected *Aedes* mosquitoes, suggesting that *Aedes* have potential to initiate RVF epidemics through transovarial transmission and to sustain low levels of the disease during post epidemic periods. Therefore we argue that locations that may serve as RVF virus reservoirs should be eliminated or kept under control to prevent multi-periodic outbreaks and consequent chains of infections. The epidemiological significance of this study is: (1) low levels of birth rate (in both *Aedes* and *Culex*) can trigger unpredictable outbreaks; (2) *Aedes* mosquitoes are more likely capable of inducing unpredictable behaviour compared to the *Culex*; (3) higher oviposition rates on mosquitoes do not in general imply manifestation of irregular behaviour on the dynamics of the disease. Finally, our model with external seasonal forcing on vector oviposition rates is able to mimic the linear increase in livestock seroprevalence during inter-epidemic period showing a constant exposure and presence of active transmission foci. This suggests that RVF outbreaks partly build upon RVF inter-epidemic activities. Therefore, active RVF surveillance in livestock is recommended.

Editor: Rick Edward Paul, Institut Pasteur, France

Funding: The lead author (SAP) received a personal PhD scholarship from German Academy Exchange Service (DAAD) under International Center of Insect Physiology and Ecology (ICIPE) ARPPIS programme. The funder had no role in study design and analysis, decision to publish or preparation of the manuscript.

Competing Interests: The authors have declared that no competing interests exist.

* Email: spedro@icipe.org

Introduction

Rift Valley fever (RVF) virus, a member of the genus phlebovirus and family Bunyaviridae, which has been isolated from at least 40 mosquito species in the field [1], infects both wild and domestic animals and humans. The RVF epizootics and epidemics are closely linked to the occurrence of the warm phase of the El Nino/Southern Oscillation (ENSO) phenomenon [2]. This phenomenon is characterized by elevated Indian Ocean temperatures which lead to heavy rainfall and flooding of habitats suitable for the production of immature *Aedes* and *Culex* mosquitoes that serve as the primary RVF virus (RVFV) vectors in East Africa [3,4]. Studies have shown that the life cycle of RVFV has distinct endemic and epidemic cycles. During the endemic cycle the virus persists during dry season/inter-epizootic periods through vertical transmission in *Aedes* mosquito eggs [3]. *Aedes* eggs need to be dry for several days before they can mature. After maturing, they hatch during the next flooding event large enough to cover them with water [5,6]. The eggs have high desiccation resistance and can survive dry conditions in a dormant form for months to years. At the beginning of the rainy season, *Aedes* mosquitoes quickly multiply into large numbers before declining due to the need for dry conditions for egg maturation [9]. There can be a second peak in mosquito densities at the end of the rainy season if there is a gap in rainfall for several days [5]. When these mosquitoes lay their eggs in flooded areas (including dambos), transovarially infected adults may emerge and transmit RVFV to nearby domestic animals, including sheep, goats, cattle, and camels. High viremias in these animals may then lead to the infection of secondary arthropod vector species including various *Culex* species [7].

Epizootic/epidemic cycles are driven by the subsequent elevation of various *Culex* mosquito populations, which serve as excellent secondary vectors if immature mosquito habitats remain flooded for a long enough period [4]. Their eggs require water to mature and hatch and the mosquitoes survive the dry season in adult form and during the rainy season, the population of *Culex* mosquitoes reaches a maximum towards the end of the season [9]. The propagation of these secondary vectors may spread the virus to additional infection in animal and human, causing an outbreak.

The disease is known to occur in outbreaks that come in cycles of 5–15 years in the Eastern Africa region and the Horn of Africa [10].

We observe that RVF outbreaks are highly linked to seasonal variations on rainfall, which is in turn reflected through seasonal fluctuations in mosquito population densities. *Aedes* eggs require water to hatch and dry condition for maturation, and at the beginning of the rainy season quickly grow to large numbers while *Culex* eggs require water to mature and hatch, and survive dry season in adult form and during the rainy season reach maximum numbers towards the end of the season. Thus, fluctuations in both seasons (wet and dry) favour the complex dynamics of both mosquito species. Hence the complexity observed on the dynamics of RVF virus transmission and maintenance.

The interplay between the internal nonlinear dynamic of ecological systems and various external factors that affect them, makes understanding of population fluctuation a unique problem [11].

Mathematical models have been developed in order to provide a better understanding of the nature and dynamics of the transmission and persistence of the disease, as well as predict outbreaks and simulate the impact of control strategies [9,12,17,18]. Most of these models considered constant mosquito oviposition rates, ignoring effects of seasonal fluctuations in the mosquito population size. Furthermore, some have ignored the effects of vertical transmission and secondary vectors [18] and some only considered *Aedes* species [9]. Temperature, rainfall and humidity have great influence in all stages of mosquito development from the emergence and viability of eggs, to the size and longevity of adults [19,20]. Recently, Mpeshe et al. [21] modified their previous study [18] to include vertical transmission in *Aedes* species and climate-driven parameters. These models provide important insights but do not investigate the stability dynamics and attractors structures of the model when there are external forces in the density of vector populations.

The most common manifestation of external forcing is through seasonality including both natural (e.g. the occurrence of the warm phase of the El Nino/Southern oscillation phenomenon) and induced (e.g human deforestation or human pollution).

Studies for understanding dynamical consequences of regular and stochastic external forcing are still ongoing but poorly understood [22–25]. To the best of our knowledge, no systematic investigation of stability and attractor structures of a realistic RVF model comprising two populations of mosquitoes (*Aedes* and *Culex*) and one livestock host population with two infected classes (asymptomatic and symptomatic) and seasonal variation on mosquito oviposition rates has been carried out.

Based on the model proposed by Gaff et al. [12], we investigate a two vector and one host epidemic model, to capture the dynamical behaviour of both the disease free and endemic equilibria, the effects of seasonality on mosquito oviposition rates (b_1,b_3), parametrized by δ_1, δ_3 and effects of asymptomatic class in livestock (parametrized by $1-\theta_2$). We prove existence and global stability of both the disease-free and the endemic equilibria in the absence of secondary vectors ($I_3=0$), as well as the existence and local stability of both disease free and endemic equilibrium points of the overall model. We then investigate the structures of model attractors through bifurcation analysis, taking as bifurcation parameters δ_1 and δ_3 the strengths of seasonality of mosquito oviposition rates. The bifurcation diagrams with simultaneous variation of seasonal forcing on the oviposition rates of the two mosquito species reveal the complexity induced by their interactions. The understanding of possible state space scenarios through bifurcation analysis is helpful for understanding RVF

epidemiological data with its seasonality aspects. To obtain robust analysis we then compute the largest Lyapunov exponents, Poincaré maps and maxima return maps.

The section methods gives a detailed description of the model and its parameters. In section results the model is used to study the dynamic behaviour of the disease stability and bifurcation analysis. Simulations are performed to investigate model dependence on initial condition and attractors structures of the model applying an external forcing on mosquito's oviposition rates.

Methods

Gaff et al. [12] proposed a one host and two vectors population model for RVF with vertical transmission in *Aedes* vectors to study the transmission of RVF and the impact of vertical transmission on the persistence of the disease. Chitnis et al. [9] analysed a RVF model with vertical transmission for *Aedes* mosquitoes and included asymptomatic class for livestock and removed one population of mosquitoes.

The model presented in this paper adopts a similar structure as in Gaff et al. [12]. We introduce an asymptomatic class for livestock [9], because for many species of livestock, RVF virus infection are frequently subclinical [26,27]. As the main purpose of this study is to study the dynamic behaviour of the disease, influenced by changes in climate and oscillation of rainfall, we include seasonal variation in the oviposition rates of both *Aedes* and *Culex* mosquitoes.

We divide the livestock population into four classes: susceptible, S_2, asymptomatic, A_2, infectious, I_2, and recovered (immune), R_2. Livestock enter the susceptible class through birth (at a constant rate). Birth rates are important because after an outbreak, herd immunity can reach 80% and the proportion of susceptible livestock must be renewed through birth or movement before another outbreak can occur [28]. When an infectious mosquito bites a susceptible animal, there is a finite probability that the animal becomes infected. Since the duration of the latent period in cattle is small relative to their life span, we do not model the exposed stage. Many adult cattle do not exhibit clinical signs apart from abortion of foetuses [6,26], thus, include an asymptomatic class for infectious animals that transmit the virus at a lower rate than those with acute clinical symptoms. After being successfully infected by an infectious *Aedes* and/or *Culex* mosquito, livestock move from the susceptible class S_2 to either the infected symptomatic I_2 or asymptomatic A_2 class. After some time, the symptomatic and asymptomatic livestock recover and move to the recovered class, R_2. The recovered livestock have immunity to the disease for life. Cattle leave the population through a per capita natural death rate and through a per capita disease-induced death rate only for symptomatic livestock. The size of the livestock population is given by $N_2 = S_2 + A_2 + I_2 + R_2$.

We divide the *Aedes* and *Culex* mosquitoes population into three classes: susceptible, S_a, exposed, E_a, and infectious, I_a. The subscripts $a=1$ and $a=3$ represent *Aedes* and *Culex* mosquitoes, respectively. Female mosquitoes (we do not include male mosquitoes in our model because only female mosquitoes bite animals for blood meals) enter the susceptible class through birth. The virus enters a susceptible mosquito, S_a, with finite probability, when the mosquito bites an infectious animal and the mosquito moves to the exposed class, E_a. After some period of time, depending on the ambient temperature and humidity [29], the mosquito moves from the exposed class to the infectious class, I_a. To reflect the vertical transmission in the *Aedes* species, compartments for uninfected P_1 and infected U_1 eggs are included. As the *Culex* species cannot transmit RVF vertically, only uninfected eggs P_3 are included. Mosquitoes once infected remain infectious during their lifespan. Mosquitoes leave the population through a per capita natural death rate. The size of each adult mosquito population is $N_1 = S_1 + E_1 + I_1$ for adult *Aedes* mosquitoes and $N_3 = S_3 + E_3 + I_3$ for adult *Culex* mosquitoes. The three populations are modelled with carrying capacity K_1, K_2, K_3, for *Aedes*, livestock and *Culex* respectively. While in [12], the total number of mosquito bites on cattle depends on the number of mosquitoes, in our model, the total number of bites varies with both the cattle and mosquito population sizes. This allows a more realistic modelling of situations where there is a high ratio of mosquitoes to cattle, and where cattle availability to mosquitoes is reduced through control interventions [9].

0.1 Mathematical Model

The state variables in Table 1 and parameters in Table 2 for the RVF model (Figure 1) satisfy the following system of equations:

Aedes

$$\dot{P}_1(t) = b_1(N_1 - q_1 I_1) - \theta_1 P_1,$$
$$\dot{U}_1(t) = b_1 q_1 I_1 - \theta_1 U_1,$$
$$\dot{S}_1(t) = \theta_1 P_1 - \frac{\sigma_1 \sigma_2 \beta_{12}}{\sigma_1 N_1 + \sigma_2 N_2} I_2 S_1 - \frac{\sigma_1 \sigma_2 \tilde{\beta}_{12}}{\sigma_1 N_1 + \sigma_2 N_2} A_2 S_1 - d_1 \frac{S_1 N_1}{K_1},$$
$$\dot{E}_1(t) = \frac{\sigma_1 \sigma_2 \beta_{12}}{\sigma_1 N_1 + \sigma_2 N_2} I_2 S_1 + \frac{\sigma_1 \sigma_2 \tilde{\beta}_{12}}{\sigma_1 N_1 + \sigma_2 N_2} A_2 S_1$$
$$\qquad - \gamma_1 E_1 - d_1 \frac{E_1 N_1}{K_1},$$
$$\dot{I}_1(t) = \gamma_1 E_1 + \theta_1 U_1 - d_1 \frac{I_1 N_1}{K_1},$$

(1)

Livestock

$$\dot{S}_2(t) = b_2 N_2 - \frac{\sigma_1 \sigma_2 \beta_{21}}{\sigma_1 N_1 + \sigma_2 N_2} I_1 S_2 - \frac{\sigma_3 \sigma_2 \beta_{23}}{\sigma_3 N_3 + \sigma_2 N_2} I_3 S_2 - d_2 \frac{S_2 N_2}{K_2},$$
$$\dot{A}_2(t) = (1 - \theta_2) \frac{\sigma_1 \sigma_2 \beta_{21}}{\sigma_1 N_1 + \sigma_2 N_2} I_1 S_2 + (1 - \theta_2) \frac{\sigma_3 \sigma_2 \beta_{23}}{\sigma_3 N_3 + \sigma_2 N_2} I_3 S_2 -$$
$$\qquad \tilde{\varepsilon}_2 A_2 - d_2 \frac{A_2 N_2}{K_2},$$
$$\dot{I}_2(t) = \theta_2 \frac{\sigma_1 \sigma_2 \beta_{21}}{\sigma_1 N_1 + \sigma_2 N_2} I_1 S_2 + \theta_2 \frac{\sigma_3 \sigma_2 \beta_{23}}{\sigma_3 N_3 + \sigma_2 N_2} I_3 S_2 - \epsilon_2 I_2 -$$
$$\qquad d_2 \frac{I_2 N_2}{K_2} - m_2 I_2,$$
$$\dot{R}_2(t) = \tilde{\varepsilon}_2 A_2 + \varepsilon_2 I_2 - d_2 \frac{R_2 N_2}{K_2},$$

(2)

Culex

$$\dot{P}_3(t) = b_3 N_3 - \theta_3 P_3,$$
$$\dot{S}_3(t) = \theta_3 P_3 - \frac{\sigma_3 \sigma_2 \beta_{32}}{\sigma_3 N_3 + \sigma_2 N_2} I_2 S_3 - \frac{\sigma_3 \sigma_2 \tilde{\beta}_{32}}{\sigma_3 N_3 + \sigma_2 N_2} A_2 S_3 - d_3 \frac{S_3 N_3}{K_3},$$
$$\dot{E}_3(t) = \frac{\sigma_3 \sigma_2 \beta_{32}}{\sigma_3 N_3 + \sigma_2 N_2} I_2 S_3 + \frac{\sigma_3 \sigma_2 \tilde{\beta}_{32}}{\sigma_3 N_3 + \sigma_2 N_2} A_2 S_3 - \gamma_3 E_3 - d_3 \frac{E_3 N_3}{K_3},$$
$$\dot{I}_3(t) = \gamma_3 E_3 - d_3 \frac{I_3 N_3}{K_3},$$

(3)

where from the model flowchart in Fig.1, μ_h for $h = 1, 2, 3$ represents the natural death rate given by $d_h \frac{X_h N_h}{K_h}$, X_h representing each compartment of every species in the model, with

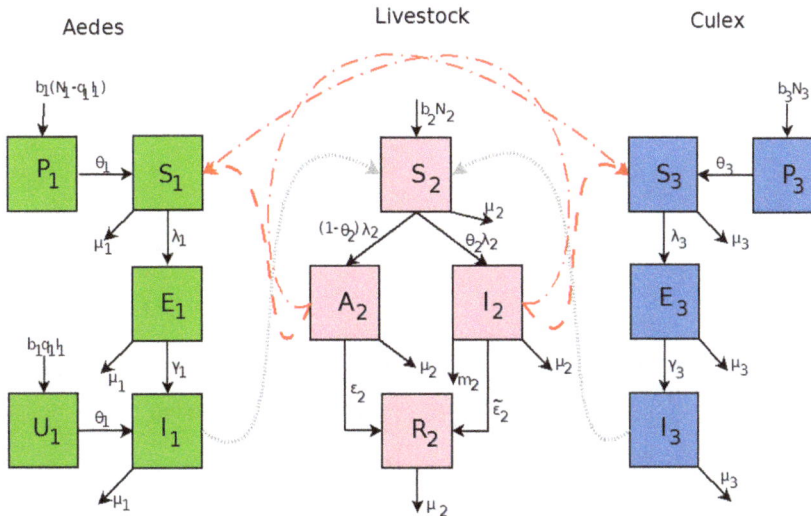

Figure 1. Flow diagram of RVFV transmission with each species, namely, *Aedes* mosquitoes, *Culex* mosquitoes and livestock (the solid lines represent the transition between compartments and the dash lines represent the transmission between different species).

Table 1. State variables for the model system (1,2,3).

Variable	Description
P_1	Number of uninfected *Aedes* mosquito eggs
Q_1	Number of infected *Aedes* mosquito eggs
S_1	Number of susceptible *Aedes* mosquitoes
E_1	Number of exposed *Aedes* mosquitoes
I_1	Number of infected *Aedes* mosquitoes
S_2	Number of susceptible livestock
E_2	Number of exposed livestock
A_2	Number of asymptomatic livestock
I_2	Number of infected livestock
P_3	Number of uninfected *Culex* mosquito eggs
S_3	Number of susceptible *Culex* mosquitoes
E_3	Number of exposed *Culex* mosquitoes
I_3	Number of infected *Culex* mosquitoes

$$\frac{dN_1}{dt} = b_1 N_1 - \frac{d_1}{K_1}(N_1)^2,$$
$$\frac{dN_2}{dt} = b_2 N_2 - \frac{d_2}{K_2}(N_2)^2 - m_2 I_2, \qquad (4)$$
$$\frac{dN_3}{dt} = b_3 N_3 - \frac{d_3}{K_3}(N_3)^2.$$

Following the approach in [9], σ_a, where $a=1$ for *Aedes* and $a=3$ for *Culex* is the rate at which a mosquito would like to bite livestock (related to the gonotrophic cycle length), and σ_2 is the maximum number of bites that an animal can support per unit time (through physical availability and any intervention measures on livestock taken by humans). Then, $\sigma_a N_a$ is the total number of bites that the mosquitoes would like to achieve per unit time and $\sigma_2 N_2$ is the availability of livestock. Thus, the total number of mosquito-livestock contacts is half the harmonic mean of $\sigma_a N_a$ and $\sigma_2 N_2$,

$$\bar{b} = \bar{b}(N_2, N_a) = \frac{\sigma_a N_a \sigma_2 N_2}{\sigma_a N_a + \sigma_2 N_2} = \frac{\sigma_a \sigma_2}{\sigma_a(N_a/N_2) + \sigma_2} N_a.$$

In addition to having the correct limits at zero and infinity, this form also meets the necessary criteria that $\bar{b} \leq min(\sigma_a N_a, \sigma_2 N_2)$ where $\bar{b}$ is the total number of bites per unit time. The total number of mosquito-livestock contacts depends on the populations of both species. We define $\bar{b}_2 = \bar{b}_2(N_2, N_a) = \bar{b}(N_2, N_a)/N_2$ as the number of bites per livestock per unit time, and $\bar{b}_a = \bar{b}_a(N_2, N_a) = \bar{b}(N_2, N_a)/N_a$ as the number of bites per mosquito per unit time.

We defined the force of infection from mosquitoes to livestock, $\lambda_2^a(t)$, as the product of the number of mosquito bites that one animal has per unit time, b_2, the probability of disease transmission from the mosquito to the animal, β_{2a}, and the probability that the mosquito is infectious, I_a/N_a. We define the

force of infection from livestock to mosquitoes, $\lambda_a^2(t)$, as the force of infection from infectious (symptomatic and asymptomatic) livestock. This is expressed as the number of livestock bites one mosquito has per unit time, $\bar{b}_a$; the probability of disease transmission from an infected (asymptomatic) animal to the mosquito, $\beta_{a2}(\tilde{\beta}_{a2})$; and the probability that the animal is infectious, $I_2/N_2(A_2/N_2)$. Therefore the forces of infection are given by:

$$\lambda_1^2 = \frac{\sigma_1 \sigma_2 N_2}{\sigma_1 N_1 + \sigma_2 N_2}(\beta_{12}\frac{I_2}{N_2} + \tilde{\beta}_{12}\frac{A_2}{N_2}) = \frac{\sigma_1 \sigma_2 \beta_{12} I_2}{\sigma_1 N_1 + \sigma_2 N_2} + \frac{\sigma_1 \sigma_2 \tilde{\beta}_{12} A_2}{\sigma_1 N_1 + \sigma_2 N_2},$$
$$\lambda_2^1 = \frac{\sigma_1 \sigma_2 N_1}{\sigma_1 N_1 + \sigma_2 N_2}\beta_{21}\frac{I_1}{N_1} = \frac{\sigma_1 \sigma_2 \beta_{21} I_1}{\sigma_1 N_1 + \sigma_2 N_2},$$
$$\lambda_2^3 = \frac{\sigma_3 \sigma_2 N_3}{\sigma_3 N_3 + \sigma_2 N_2}\beta_{23}\frac{I_3}{N_3} = \frac{\sigma_3 \sigma_2 \beta_{23} I_3}{\sigma_3 N_3 + \sigma_2 N_2},$$
$$\lambda_3^2 = \frac{\sigma_3 \sigma_2 N_2}{\sigma_3 N_3 + \sigma_2 N_2}(\beta_{32}\frac{I_2}{N_2} + \tilde{\beta}_{32}\frac{A_2}{N_2}) = \frac{\sigma_3 \sigma_2 \beta_{32} I_2}{\sigma_3 N_3 + \sigma_2 N_2} + \frac{\sigma_3 \sigma_2 \tilde{\beta}_{32} A_2}{\sigma_3 N_3 + \sigma_2 N_2},$$

The model system (1,2,3) is biologically relevant (solutions are positive) in the set

$$\Omega = \left\{ \begin{array}{l} (P_1, U_1, S_1, E_1, I_1, S_2, A_2, I_2, R_2, P_3, S_3, E_3, I_3) \in \mathbb{R}_+^{13} : P_1, U_1, \\ S_1, E_1, I_1, S_2, A_2, I_2, R_2, P_3, S_3, \\ E_3, I_3 \geq 0, N_1 \leq \frac{b_1 K_1}{d_1}, N_2 \leq \frac{b_2 K_2}{d_2}, N_3 \leq \frac{b_3 K_3}{d_3}, P_1 + U_1 \leq \frac{b_1 N_1}{\theta_1}, \\ P_3 \leq \frac{b_3 N_3}{\theta_3} \end{array} \right. \qquad (5)$$

Lemma 1. *The model system (1,2,3) is well-posed in Ω which is invariant and attracting.*

Proof 1. *When $S_i = 0$ for $i = 1, 2, 3$ then $\frac{dS_1}{dt} = \theta_1 P_1, \frac{dS_2}{dt} = b_2 N_2, \frac{dS_3}{dt} = \theta_3 P_3$ that is $\frac{dS_i}{dt} \geq 0$ for $i = 1, 2, 3$ for $t \geq 0$.*

Similarly, when $E_i = 0, I_i = 0, P_1 = U_1 = P_3 = A_2 = R_2 = 0$ for $i = 1, 2, 3$ we have $\frac{dE_i}{dt} \geq 0, \frac{dI_i}{dt} \geq 0, \frac{dP_1}{dt} \geq 0, \frac{dU_1}{dt} \geq 0, \frac{dP_3}{dt} \geq 0, \frac{dA_2}{dt} \geq 0, \frac{dI_2}{dt} \geq 0.$ If $S_i + E_i + I_i \geq 0$ for $i = 1, 2, 3$ and $S_2 + A_2 + I_2 + R_2 \geq 0$ we have $\frac{dN_i}{dt} = b_i N_i - d_i \frac{N_i^2}{K_i} \Leftrightarrow N_i(t) = \frac{b_i K_i}{d_i + N_i(0)e^{-b_i t}}$ for $i = 1, 3$ and we show that for $t \rightarrow \infty$ $N_i \leq \frac{b_i K_i}{d_i}$ for $i = 1, 3$.

Similarly, if $P_1 + U_1 \geq 0$ we can show that $\dot{P}_1 + \dot{U}_1 \leq \frac{b_1 N_1}{\theta_1}$ and $\dot{P}_3 \leq \frac{b_3 N_3}{\theta_3}$ for $t \geq 0$. Thus, the solution remain in the feasible region Ω if it starts in this region.

Results

0.2 Basic Reproduction Number

For epidemiology models, a quantity, R_0 is derived to assess the stability of the disease free equilibrium [12]. R_0 represents the the number of individuals infected by a single infected individual during his or her entire infectious period, in a population which is entirely susceptible [30]. When $R_0 < 1$, if a disease is introduced, there are insufficient new cases per case, and the disease cannot invade the population. When $R_0 > 1$, the disease may become endemic; the greater R_0 is above 1, the less likely stochastic fade out of the disease can occur. To compute this threshold we use the next generation operator approach, as described by Diekmann et al. [31] and van den Driessche and Watmough [32] as well as to describe the conditions for which the disease-free equilibrium points lose stability.

Since the model incorporates both vertical and horizontal transmission, R_0 for the system is the sum of the R_0 values for each mode of transmission determined separately [33],

$$R_0 = R_{0,V} + R_{0,H}.$$

To compute each component of R_0, the model equations in vector form are the difference between the rate of new infection in compartment i, F_i and the rate of transfer between compartment i and all other compartments due to other processes, V_i [32], (see Appendix S1). Then, R_0 is given by

$$R_0 = \frac{b_1 q_1}{2\mu_1} + \frac{1}{2}\sqrt{R_{0,V}^2 + 4R_{0,H}^2} \qquad (6)$$

where $R_{0,V} = \dfrac{b_1 q_1}{\mu_1}$ and

$$R_{0,H} = \sqrt{\frac{(l_3^0)^2 \beta_{23}\gamma_3 N_2^0 N_3^0}{\mu_3(\gamma_3 + \mu_3)}\left[\frac{(1-\theta_2)\tilde{\beta}_{32}}{\tilde{\varepsilon}_2 + \mu_2} + \frac{\theta_2\beta_{32}}{\varepsilon_2 + m_2 + \mu_2}\right] + \frac{(l_1^0)^2 \beta_{21}\gamma_1 N_1^0 N_2^0}{\mu_1(\gamma_1 + \mu_1)}\left[\frac{(1-\theta_2)\tilde{\beta}_{12}}{\tilde{\varepsilon}_2 + \mu_2} + \frac{\theta_2\beta_{12}}{\varepsilon_2 + m_2 + \mu_2}\right]}. \qquad (7)$$

0.3 Basic Reproduction Number for periodic environment

In periodic environment, the basic reproduction number is the generalization of the R_0 in non periodic environment. It is known as the transmissibility number $\bar{R}_0$, which is defined as the average number of secondary cases arising from the introduction of a single infectious individual into a completely susceptible population at a random time of the year [34]. Thus, $\bar{R}_0$ is defined through the spectral radius of a linear integral operator on a space of periodic functions, given by the integral operator G_j (see Appendix S1),

$$\begin{aligned} G_j =\ & \frac{b_1 q_1}{\mu_1 + 2\pi ji} \cdot \frac{\theta_1}{\theta_1 + 2\pi ji} + \frac{\gamma_1}{\gamma_1 + \mu_1 + 2\pi ji} \cdot \frac{(l_1^0)^2 \beta_{21} S_2^0 S_1^0}{\mu_1 + 2\pi ji} \\ & \left[\frac{(1-\theta_2)\tilde{\beta}_{12}}{\tilde{\varepsilon}_2 + \mu_2 + 2\pi ji} + \frac{\theta_2\beta_{12}}{\varepsilon_2 + m_2 + \mu_2 + 2\pi ji}\right] \\ & + \frac{\gamma_3}{\gamma_3 + \mu_3 + 2\pi ji} \cdot \frac{(l_3^0)^2 \beta_{23} S_3^0 S_2^0}{\mu_3 + 2\pi ji}\left[\frac{(1-\theta_2)\tilde{\beta}_{32}}{\tilde{\varepsilon}_2 + \mu_2 + 2\pi ji} + \frac{\theta_2\beta_{32}}{\varepsilon_2 + m_2 + \mu_2 + 2\pi ji}\right]. \end{aligned} \qquad (8)$$

As proposed by Bacaer [36], the transmissibility number $\bar{R}_0$ is given by

$$\bar{R}_0 = G_0 + \frac{\delta_i^2}{2} Re\left(\frac{G_0 G_1}{G_0 - G_1}\right) \qquad (9)$$

where $Re(.)$ is the real part of $(.)$. G_0 is the basic reproduction number for the non-seasonal model, obtained when $\delta_i = 0$.

The size of $\bar{R}_0$ is reduced compared to R_0 when oviposition rates are constant, and this makes it slightly difficult for the virus to invade the population with such fluctuations on the transmission rates [36].

From G_0 the following sub-reproduction numbers $R_{21}, R_{12}, R_{23}, R_{32}$ can be obtained: R_{21} is the number of new infections in livestock from one infected $Aedes$ mosquito and is given by

$$R_{21} = \frac{\gamma_1}{\gamma_1 + b_1} \times \frac{\beta_{21} l_1^0 N_2^0}{b_1},$$

representing the product of the probability that the $Aedes$ mosquito survives the exposed stage $\dfrac{\gamma_1}{\gamma_1 + b_1}$, the number of bites on livestock per mosquito $l_1^0 N_2^0$, the probability of transmission per bite β_{21}, and the infectious lifespan of $Aedes$ mosquito $1/b_1$.

R_{12} is the number of new infections in $Aedes$ mosquitoes from one infected (asymptomatic or symptomatic) animal, and is given by the weighted sum of new infections resulting from asymptomatic and symptomatic livestock

$$R_{12} = l_1^0 N_1^0\left(\frac{(1-\theta_2)\tilde{\beta}_{12}}{\tilde{\varepsilon}_2 + b_2} + \frac{\theta_2\beta_{12}}{\varepsilon_2 + b_2 + m_2}\right).$$

This is the product of the number of bites an animal receives $l_1^0 N_1^0$, the probability of transmission per bite ($\tilde{\beta}_{12}$ for an asymptomatic animal and β_{12} for symptomatic animal), and the duration of the infective period ($\dfrac{1}{\tilde{\varepsilon}_2 + b_2}$ for an asymptomatic animal and $\dfrac{1}{\varepsilon_2 + b_2 + m_2}$ for symptomatic animal) weighted by the probability that an animal either becomes asymptomatic or symptomatic upon infection.

R_{23} is the number of new infections in livestock from one infected $Culex$ mosquito and is given by

$$R_{23} = \frac{\gamma_3}{\gamma_3 + b_3} \times \frac{\beta_{23} l_3^0 N_2^0}{b_3}.$$

This is the product of the probability that the $Culex$ mosquito survives the exposed stage $\dfrac{\gamma_3}{\gamma_3 + b_3}$, the number of bites on livestock per mosquito $l_3^0 N_2^0$, the probability of transmission per bite β_{23}, and the infectious lifespan of $Culex$ mosquito $1/b_3$.

R_{32} is the number of new infections in $Culex$ mosquitoes from an infected (asymptomatic or symptomatic) animal and is given by the weighted sum of new infections resulting from asymptomatic and symptomatic livestock

$$R_{32} = l_3^0 N_3^0\left(\frac{(1-\theta_2)\tilde{\beta}_{32}}{\tilde{\varepsilon}_2 + b_2} + \frac{\theta_2\beta_{32}}{\varepsilon_2 + b_2 + m_2}\right).$$

This is the product of the number of bites one animal receives $l_3^0 N_3^0$, the probability of transmission per bite ($\tilde{\beta}_{32}$ for an asymptomatic animal and β_{32} for symptomatic animal), and the duration of the infective period ($\frac{1}{\tilde{\varepsilon}_2 + b_2}$ for an asymptomatic animal and $\frac{1}{\varepsilon_2 + b_2 + m_2}$ for symptomatic animal) weighted by the probability that an animal either becomes asymptomatic or symptomatic upon infection.

If $q_1 > 0$, R_0 increases because vertical transmission directly increases the number of infectious mosquitoes and indirectly increases the transmission from livestock to mosquitoes and back to livestock.

0.4 Stability analysis

The computation of the equilibria for model system $(1,2,3)$ yields, respectively: the disease-free equilibrium (DFE),

$$
\begin{aligned}
X^0 &= (P_1^0, U_1^0, S_1^0, E_1^0, I_1^0, S_2^0, A_2^0, I_2^0, R_2^0, P_3^0, S_3^0, E_3^0, I_3^0) \\
&= (\tfrac{b_1 N_1}{\theta_1}, 0, \tfrac{b_1 K_1}{d_1}, 0, 0, \tfrac{b_2 K_2}{d_2}, 0, 0, 0, \tfrac{b_3 N_3}{\theta_3}, \tfrac{b_3 K_3}{d_3}, 0, 0)
\end{aligned} \tag{10}
$$

and the endemic equilibrium (EE)

$$
X^* = (P_1^*, U_1^*, S_1^*, E_1^*, I_1^*, S_2^*, A_2^*, I_2^*, R_2^*, P_3^*, S_3^*, E_3^*, I_3^*)
$$

where

$$
P_1^* = \frac{b_1 N_1 - b_1 q_1 I_1^*}{\theta_1} \qquad U_1^* = \frac{b_1 q_1 I_1^*}{\theta_1} \tag{11}
$$

$$
S_1^* = \frac{b_1 N_1 - b_1 q_1 I_1^*}{g_1 I_2^* + g_2 A_2^* + \mu_1} \qquad E_1^* = \frac{\mu_1 - b_1 q_1}{\gamma_1} I_1^* \tag{12}
$$

$$
I_1^* = \frac{g_1 I_2^* + g_2 A_2^*}{g_1 I_2^* + g_2 A_2^* + \mu_1} \times \frac{b_1 N_1 - b_1 q_1 I_1^*}{(\gamma_1 + \mu_1) g_7} \tag{13}
$$

$$
S_2^* = \frac{b_2 N_2}{g_3 I_1^* + g_4 I_3^* + \mu_2} \tag{14}
$$

$$
A_2^* = \frac{g_3 I_1^* + g_4 I_3^*}{g_3 I_1^* + g_4 I_3^* + \mu_2} \times \frac{1}{g_8} \qquad I_2^* = \frac{g_3 I_1^* + g_4 I_3^*}{g_3 I_1^* + g_4 I_3^* + \mu_2} \times \frac{1}{g_9} \tag{15}
$$

$$
R_2^* = \frac{\tilde{\varepsilon}_2 A_2^* + \varepsilon_2 I_2^*}{\mu_2} \qquad P_3^* = \frac{b_3 N_3}{\theta_3} \tag{16}
$$

$$
S_3^* = \frac{b_3 N_3}{g_5 I_2^* + g_6 A_2^* + \mu_3} \quad E_3^* = \frac{\mu_3}{\gamma_3} I_3^* \quad I_3^* = \frac{g_5 I_2^* + g_6 A_2^*}{g_5 I_2^* + g_6 A_2^* + \mu_3} \times \frac{1}{l_4}, \tag{17}
$$

$$
g_1 = \frac{\sigma_1 \sigma_2 \beta_{12}}{\sigma_1 N_1 + \sigma_2 N_2}, \quad g_2 = \frac{\sigma_1 \sigma_2 \tilde{\beta}_{12}}{\sigma_1 N_1 + \sigma_2 N_2}, \quad g_3 = \frac{\sigma_1 \sigma_2 \beta_{21}}{\sigma_1 N_1 + \sigma_2 N_2},
$$

$$
g_4 = \frac{\sigma_3 \sigma_2 \beta_{23}}{\sigma_3 N_3 + \sigma_2 N_2}, \quad g_5 = \frac{\sigma_3 \sigma_2 \beta_{32}}{\sigma_3 N_3 + \sigma_2 N_2}, \quad g_6 = \frac{\sigma_3 \sigma_2 \tilde{\beta}_{32}}{\sigma_3 N_3 + \sigma_2 N_2},
$$

$$
g_7 = \frac{\mu_1 - b_1 q_1}{\gamma_1}, \quad g_8 = \frac{\tilde{\varepsilon}_2 + \mu_2}{(1 - \theta_2) b_2 N_2}, \quad g_9 = \frac{\varepsilon_2 + m_2 + \mu_2}{\theta_2 b_2 N_2},
$$

$$
l_4 = \frac{\mu_3 (\gamma_3 + \mu_3)}{\gamma_3 b_3 N_3}, \quad l_5 = (\gamma_1 + \mu_1) g_7.
$$

Substituting equations (15) into equation (13) we obtain

$$
b_1 N_1 g_3 l_6 I_1^* + b_1 N_1 g_4 l_6 I_3^* - \mu_1 \mu_2 l_5 I_1^* = g_3 l_7 (I_1^*)^2 + g_4 l_7 I_1^* I_3^* \tag{18}
$$

where $l_6 = \dfrac{g_1 g_8 + g_2 g_9}{g_8 g_9}, l_7 = b_1 q_1 l_6 + l_5 l_6 + \mu_1 l_5$.

In solving for the equilibria, we omit the expression containing R_2 because it can be determined when S_2, A_2 and I_2 are known. We then determine analytically the conditions under which these equilibria are stable or unstable. The following result holds without proof to avoid repetition:

Lemma 2. *The resulting model is biologically relevant (solutions are positive) in the set*

$$
\Omega^1 = \{(P_1, U_1, S_1, E_1, I_1, S_2, A_2, I_2, P_3, S_3, E_3, I_3) \ \mathbb{R}_+^{112} :
$$

$$
P_1, U_1, S_1, E_1, I_1, S_2, A_2, I_2, P_3, S_3, E_3, I_3 \geq 0, N_1 \leq \frac{b_1 K_1}{d_1}, \tag{19}
$$

$$
N_2 \leq \frac{b_2 K_2}{d_2}, N_3 \leq \frac{b_3 K_3}{d_3}, P_1 + U_1 \leq \frac{b_1 N_1}{\theta_1}, P_3 \leq \frac{b_3 N_3}{\theta_3}\}
$$

The model system $(1,2,3)$ being nonlinear, stability analysis will be carried out via linearisation. The Jacobian matrix of system $(1,2,3)$ at an arbitrary equilibrium is

$$
J = \begin{bmatrix}
-\theta_1 & 0 & 0 & 0 & -b_1 q_1 & 0 & 0 & 0 & 0 & 0 & 0 & 0 \\
0 & -\theta_1 & 0 & 0 & b_1 q_1 & 0 & 0 & 0 & 0 & 0 & 0 \\
\theta_1 & 0 & -a_1 - \mu_1 & 0 & 0 & 0 & -a_2 & -a_3 & 0 & 0 & 0 \\
0 & 0 & a_1 & -a_{14} & 0 & 0 & a_2 & a_3 & 0 & 0 & 0 \\
0 & \theta_1 & 0 & \gamma_1 & -\mu_1 & 0 & 0 & 0 & 0 & 0 & 0 \\
0 & 0 & 0 & 0 & -a_4 & -a_5 - \mu_2 & 0 & 0 & 0 & 0 & -a_9 \\
0 & 0 & 0 & 0 & (1-\theta_2)a_4 & (1-\theta_2)a_5 & -a_6 & 0 & 0 & 0 & (1-\theta_2)a_9 \\
0 & 0 & 0 & 0 & \theta_2 a_4 & \theta_2 a_5 & 0 & -a_7 & 0 & 0 & \theta_2 a_9 \\
0 & 0 & 0 & 0 & 0 & 0 & 0 & 0 & -\theta_3 & 0 & 0 \\
0 & 0 & 0 & 0 & 0 & 0 & -a_{10} & -a_{11} & \theta_3 & -a_{12} - \mu_3 & 0 \\
0 & 0 & 0 & 0 & 0 & 0 & a_{10} & a_{11} & 0 & a_{12} & -a_{13} & 0 \\
0 & 0 & 0 & 0 & 0 & 0 & 0 & 0 & 0 & \gamma_3 & -\mu_3
\end{bmatrix} \tag{20}
$$

where $a_1 = g_1 I_2 + g_2 A_2, a_2 = g_2 S_1, a_3 = g_1 S_1, a_4 = g_3 S_2, a_5 = g_3 I_1 + g_4 I_3, a_6 = \tilde{\varepsilon}_2 + \mu_2, a_7 = \varepsilon_2 + m_2 + \mu_2, a_9 = g_4 S_2, a_{10} = g_6 S_3, a_{11} = g_5 S_3, a_{12} = g_5 I_2 + g_6 A_2, a_{13} = \gamma_3 - \mu_3, a_{14} = \gamma_1 + \mu_1$.

Evaluating J at the disease-free equilibrium and using basic properties of matrix algebra, it is evident from the characteristic polynomial of J that the following eigenvalues $\lambda_1 = -\mu_1, \lambda_2 = -\theta_1, \lambda_3 = -\mu_2, \lambda_4 = -\theta_3, \lambda_5 = -\mu_3$ have negative real part and the remaining reduced matrix is

$$
J_1 = \begin{pmatrix}
-\theta_1 & 0 & b_1 q_1 & 0 & 0 & 0 & 0 \\
0 & -(\gamma_1 + \mu_1) & 0 & g_2 S_1^0 & g_1 S_1^0 & 0 & 0 \\
\theta_1 & \gamma_1 & -\mu_1 & 0 & 0 & 0 & 0 \\
0 & 0 & (1-\theta_2)g_3 S_2^0 & -(\tilde{\varepsilon}_2 + \mu_2) & 0 & 0 & (1-\theta_2)g_4 S_2^0 \\
0 & 0 & \theta_2 g_3 S_2^0 & 0 & -(\tilde{\varepsilon}_2 + m_2 + \mu_2) & 0 & \theta_2 g_4 S_2^0 \\
0 & 0 & 0 & g_6 S_3^0 & g_5 S_3^0 & -(\gamma_3 + \mu_3) & 0 \\
0 & 0 & 0 & 0 & 0 & \gamma_3 & -\mu_3
\end{pmatrix} \tag{21}
$$

The stability of a disease-free equilibria should be established from the eigenvalues of the reduced Jacobian matrix (21). To simplify the computations, we perform the following operations on matrix (21): first we add the first row to the third one and take the resultant as the new third row; second we multiply the second row by $\gamma_1/(\gamma_1+\mu_1)$ and add it to the new third row, then take the resultant as the new third row and at last we multiply the sixth row by $\gamma_3/(\gamma_3+\mu_3)$ and add it to the last row and maintaining the rest as it is, we obtain the following matrix

$$J_2 = \begin{pmatrix} -\theta_1 & 0 & b_1q_1 & 0 & 0 & & \\ 0 & -(\gamma_1+\mu_1) & 0 & g_2S_1^0 & g_1S_1^0 & 0 & 0 \\ 0 & 0 & b_1q_1-\mu_1 & \dfrac{\gamma_1g_2S_1^0}{\gamma_1+\mu_1} & \dfrac{\gamma_1g_1S_1^0}{\gamma_1+\mu_1} & 0 & 0 \\ 0 & 0 & (1-\theta_2)g_3S_2^0 & -(\tilde{\varepsilon}_2+\mu_2) & 0 & 0 & (1-\theta_2)g_4S_2^0 \\ 0 & 0 & \theta_2g_3S_2^0 & 0 & -(\tilde{\varepsilon}_2+m_2+\mu_2) & 0 & \theta_2g_4S_2^0 \\ 0 & 0 & 0 & g_6S_3^0 & g_5S_3^0 & -(\gamma_3+\mu_3) & 0 \\ 0 & 0 & 0 & \dfrac{\gamma_3g_6S_3^0}{\gamma_3+\mu_3} & \dfrac{\gamma_3g_5S_3^0}{\gamma_3+\mu_3} & 0 & -\mu_3 \end{pmatrix} \tag{22}$$

From the basic properties of matrix algebra, it is evident from the characteristic polynomial of J_2 that the following eigenvalues $\lambda_1 = -\theta_1, \lambda_2 = -(\gamma_1+\mu_1)$ and $\lambda_3 = -(\gamma_3+\mu_3)$ have negative real part and the remaining reduced matrix is

$$\tilde{J}(X^0) = \begin{pmatrix} b_1q_1-\mu_1 & \dfrac{\gamma_1g_2S_1^0}{\gamma_1+\mu_1} & \dfrac{\gamma_1g_1S_1^0}{\gamma_1+\mu_1} & 0 \\ (1-\theta_2)g_3S_2^0 & -(\tilde{\varepsilon}_2+\mu_2) & 0 & (1-\theta_2)g_4S_2^0 \\ \theta_2g_3S_2^0 & 0 & -(\tilde{\varepsilon}_2+m_2+\mu_2) & \theta_2g_4S_2^0 \\ 0 & \dfrac{\gamma_3g_6S_3^0}{\gamma_3+\mu_3} & \dfrac{\gamma_3g_5S_3^0}{\gamma_3+\mu_3} & -\mu_3 \end{pmatrix} \tag{23}$$

0.5 Stability analysis of the model (1,2,3) without *Culex* species

In the absence of *Culex* species, $I_3^* = 0$, equation (18) can be written as

$$g_3l_7(I_1^*)^2 - (b_1N_1g_3l_6 - \mu_1\mu_2l_5)I_1^* = 0. \tag{24}$$

Equation (24) has two possible solutions $I_1^* = 0$ or $I_1^* \neq 0$. The case $I_1^* = 0$ implies an existence of a disease-free equilibria and the case $I_1^* \neq 0$ implies an existence of an endemic equilibria. Let us now derive conditions under which positive endemic equilibria exist. For $I_1^* \neq 0$, we get

I_1^* is epidemiologically meaningful, that is, $I_1^* > 0$ if and only if

$$b_1N_1\gamma_1g_3[\theta_2b_2N_2g_1(\tilde{\varepsilon}_2+\mu_2) + (1-\theta_2)b_2N_2g_2(\varepsilon_2+m_2+\mu_2)$$
$$> \mu_1\mu_2(\gamma_1+\mu_1)(\mu_1-b_1q_1)(\tilde{\varepsilon}_2+\mu_2)(\varepsilon_2+m_2+\mu_2)$$

which can be written in the form

$$\frac{b_1b_2}{\mu_1\mu_2(1-\frac{b_1q_1}{\mu_1})} \times \frac{g_3\gamma_1N_2}{\mu_1(\gamma_1+\mu_1)} \times \left[\frac{(1-\theta_2)g_2N_1}{\tilde{\varepsilon}_2+\mu_2} + \frac{\theta_2g_1N_1}{\varepsilon_2+m_2+\mu_2}\right] > 1$$

where $R_0^1 = \dfrac{g_3\gamma_3N_2}{\mu_1(\gamma_1+\mu_1)} \times \left[\dfrac{(1-\theta_2)g_2N_1}{\tilde{\varepsilon}_2+\mu_2} + \dfrac{\theta_2g_1N_1}{\varepsilon_2+m_2+\mu_2}\right]$ is the basic reproductive number for the model without *Culex* species and $R_{21} = \dfrac{g_3\gamma_3N_2}{\mu_1(\gamma_1+\mu_1)}$ represents the number of new infections in livestock from one infected *Aedes* mosquito and $R_{12} = \dfrac{(1-\theta_2)g_2N_1}{\tilde{\varepsilon}_2+\mu_2} + \dfrac{\theta_2g_1N_1}{\varepsilon_2+m_2+\mu_2}$ represent the number of new infections in *Aedes* mosquitoes from one infected (asymptomatic or symptomatic) animal and $R_{0,V} = \dfrac{b_1q_1}{\mu_1}$ represents the vertical transmission reproductive number. Therefore, $I_1^* > 0$ if and only if $R_{0,V} < 1$ and $R_0^1 > 1$. Thus, the following result holds:

Theorem 1. *The RVF model (1,2,3) without Culex species has exactly one disease-free equilibrium point (DFE),* $X_1^0 = (P_1^0, U_1^0, S_1^0, E_1^0, I_1^0, S_2^0, A_2^0, I_2^0, R_2^0) = (\frac{b_1N_1}{\theta_1}, 0, \frac{b_1K_1}{d_1}, 0, 0, \frac{b_2K_2}{d_2}, 0, 0, 0)$ *for* $R_0^1 \leq 1$ *and exactly one endemic equilibrium point (EE),* $X_1^* = (P_1^*, U_1^*, S_1^*, E_1^*, I_1^*, S_2^*, A_2^*, I_2^*, R_2^*)$ *whenever* $R_0^1 > 1$.

The result in Theorem 1 indicates the impossibility of backward bifurcation in the RVF model system (1,2,3) without *Culex* species since it has no endemic equilibrium when $R_0^1 < 1$. This explains that the model (1,2,3) without *Culex* species has a globally asymptotically stable disease-free equilibrium whenever $R_0^1 \leq 1$.

In its simplest form, backward bifurcation in epidemic models usually implies the existence of two subcritical endemic equilibria when the basic reproductive number for $R_0^1 < 1$, and a unique supercritical endemic equilibrium for $R_0^1 > 1$ [37]. Thus, a unique

$$I_1^* = \frac{b_1N_1\gamma_1g_3(g_1\dfrac{\tilde{\varepsilon}_2+\mu_2}{(1-\theta_2)b_2N_2} + g_2\dfrac{\varepsilon_2+m_2+\mu_2}{\theta_2b_2N_2}) - \mu_1\mu_2(\gamma_1+\mu_1)(\mu_1-b_1q_1)\dfrac{(\tilde{\varepsilon}_2+\mu_2)(\varepsilon_2+m_2+\mu_2)}{(1-\theta_2)\theta_2b_2b_2N_2N_2}}{g_3[b_1q_1\gamma_1(g_1g_8+g_2g_9) + (\gamma_1+\mu_1)(\mu_1-b_1q_1)(g_1g_8+g_2g_9) + \mu_1(\gamma_1+\mu_1)(\mu_1-b_1q_1)g_8g_9]}, \tag{25}$$

positive endemic equilibrium exists only when $R_0^1 > 1$. We note that the increase in complexity of an epidemic model (by adding more infected classes, for example) can lead to backward bifurcation and even more complicated phenomena associated with endemic equilibria [37]. However, increase in complexity of the proposed RVF model does not appear to give rise to more complex behaviour with regard to endemic equilibria.

0.5.1 Local stability of DFE, X_1^0. In the absence of secondary vector (*Culex* species) that serve as RVF outbreak amplifiers the Jacobian matrix $\tilde{J}(X^0)$ in (23) reduces to

$$J(X_1^0) = \begin{pmatrix} b_1 q_1 - \mu_1 & \frac{\gamma_1 g_2 S_1^0}{\gamma_1 + \mu_1} & \frac{\gamma_1 g_1 S_1^0}{\gamma_1 + \mu_1} \\ (1-\theta_2)g_3 S_2^0 & -(\tilde{\varepsilon}_2 + \mu_2) & 0 \\ \theta_2 g_3 S_2^0 & 0 & -(\varepsilon_2 + m_2 + \mu_2) \end{pmatrix} \quad (26)$$

The characteristic equation corresponding to the above Jacobian matrix is

$$\lambda^3 + A\lambda^2 + B\lambda + C = 0 \quad (27)$$

where $\quad A = \varepsilon_2 + m_2 + \mu_2 + \tilde{\varepsilon}_2 + \mu_2 + \mu_1\left(1 - \frac{b_1 q_1}{\mu_1}\right), \quad B =$
$- \theta_2 g_3 S_2^0 \frac{\gamma_1 g_1 S_1^0}{\gamma_1 + \mu_1} - (1-\theta_2) g_3 S_2^0 \frac{\gamma_1 g_2 S_1^0}{\gamma_1 + \mu_1} + (\varepsilon_2 + m_2 + \mu_2)(\tilde{\varepsilon}_2 + \mu_2) + (\varepsilon_2 + m_2 + \mu_2)(\mu_1 - b_1 q_1) + (\tilde{\varepsilon}_2 + \mu_2)(\mu_1 + b_1 q_1),$

$C = -\theta_2 g_3 S_2^0 \frac{\gamma_1 g_1 S_1^0}{\gamma_1 + \mu_1}(\tilde{\varepsilon}_2 + \mu_2) - (1-\theta_2)g_3 S_2^0 \frac{\gamma_1 g_2 S_1^0}{\gamma_1 + \mu_1}(\varepsilon_2 + m_2 + \mu_2) + (\tilde{\varepsilon}_2 + \mu_2)(\varepsilon_2 + m_2 + \mu_2)(\mu_1 - b_1 q_1).$

Here $A > 0$ for $\frac{b_1 q_1}{\mu_1} < 1$, $B > 0 \wedge C > 0$ for $\frac{b_1 q_1}{\mu_1} < 1 \wedge R_0^1 < 1$. Thus the equation (27) has no root which is positive or zero (Descartes' rule of sign). The equation (27) will only have negative roots or complex roots with negative real part if $AB - C > 0$ (according to Routh-Hurwitz criteria), that is, $\frac{b_1 q_1}{\mu_1} < 1 \wedge R_0^1 < 1$. Thus, the system (1,2,3) without *Culex* species is stable about the interior equilibrium X_1^0 and the following result holds:

Theorem 2. *For $R_0^1 < 1$ the model system (1,2,3) without Culex mosquitoes has a unique DFE point which is locally asymptotically stable in Ω^1.*

0.5.2 Global asymptotic stability of DFE, X_1^0. To ensure that the disease elimination is independent of the initial sizes of the populations, we need to show that the disease-free equilibrium X_1^* is globally asymptotically stable (GAS). This is established using the approach proposed in Castillo-Chavez et al. [38]. There are two conditions that if met guarantee the global asymptotic stability of the disease-free state. First, system (1,2,3) without *Culex* mosquitoes must be written in the form:

$$\frac{dX}{dt} = F(x,Z), \\ \frac{dZ}{dt} = G(X,Z), \, G(x,0) = 0 \quad (28)$$

where $X \in R^m$ denotes (its components) the number of uninfected individuals and $Z \in R^n$ denotes (its components) the number of infected individuals including latent and infectious. $U^0 = (x^0, 0)$ denotes the disease-free equilibrium of this system.

(H1) For $\frac{dX}{dt} = F(X,0)$, X^0 is globally asymptotic stable

(H2) $G(X,Z) = AZ - \hat{G}(X,Z)$, $\hat{G}(X,Z) \geq 0$ for $(X,Z) \in \Omega^1$ where $A = D_Z G(X^0, 0)$ (see [31] for more details) is an M-matrix (the off diagonal elements of A are nonnegative) and Ω^1 is the region where the model makes biological sense.

If the system (28) satisfies the above two conditions then the following Theorem holds.

Theorem 3. *The fixed point $U^0 = (x^0, 0)$ is globally asymptotic stable equilibrium of system (28) provided that $R_0^1 < 1$ (locally asymptotic stable) and that assumptions (H1) and (H2) are satisfied.*

Proof 2. *Rewriting the model system (1,2,3) without Culex mosquitoes in the form of equation (28) then $X = (P_1, S_1, S_2, R_2)$, $Z = (U_1, E_1, I_1, A_2, I_2)^T$ and $F(X,0) = (b_1 N_1 - \theta_1 P_1, \theta_1 P_1 - \mu_1 S_1, b_2 N_2 - \mu_2 S_2, 0)$, then*

$$A = D_Z G(X^0, 0) = \begin{pmatrix} -\theta_1 & 0 & b_1 q_1 & 0 & 0 \\ 0 & -(\gamma_1 + \mu_1) & 0 & \frac{\sigma_1 \sigma_2 \tilde{\beta}_{12}}{\sigma_1 N_1 + \sigma_2 N_2}S_1^0 & \frac{\sigma_1 \sigma_2 \beta_{12}}{\sigma_1 N_1 + \sigma_2 N_2}S_1^0 \\ \theta_1 & \gamma_1 & -\mu_1 & 0 & 0 \\ 0 & 0 & (1-\theta_2)\frac{\sigma_1 \sigma_2 \beta_{21}}{\sigma_1 N_1 + \sigma_2 N_2}S_2^0 & -(\tilde{\varepsilon}_2 + \mu_2) & 0 \\ 0 & 0 & \theta_2 \frac{\sigma_1 \sigma_2 \beta_{21}}{\sigma_1 N_1 + \sigma_2 N_2}S_2^0 & 0 & -(\varepsilon_2 + m_2 + \mu_2) \end{pmatrix} \quad (29)$$

and $\hat{G}(X,Z) = AZ - G(X,Z) =$

$$= \begin{pmatrix} -\theta_1 & 0 & b_1 q_1 & 0 & 0 \\ 0 & -(\gamma_1 + \mu_1) & 0 & \frac{\sigma_1 \sigma_2 \tilde{\beta}_{12}}{\sigma_1 N_1 + \sigma_2 N_2}S_1^0 & \frac{\sigma_1 \sigma_2 \beta_{12}}{\sigma_1 N_1 + \sigma_2 N_2}S_1^0 \\ \theta_1 & \gamma_1 & -\mu_1 & 0 & 0 \\ 0 & 0 & (1-\theta_2)\frac{\sigma_1 \sigma_2 \beta_{21}}{\sigma_1 N_1 + \sigma_2 N_2}S_2^0 & -(\tilde{\varepsilon}_2 + \mu_2) & 0 \\ 0 & 0 & \theta_2 \frac{\sigma_1 \sigma_2 \beta_{21}}{\sigma_1 N_1 + \sigma_2 N_2}S_2^0 & 0 & -(\varepsilon_2 + m_2 + \mu_2) \end{pmatrix} \begin{pmatrix} U_1 \\ E_1 \\ I_1 \\ A_2 \\ I_2 \end{pmatrix} -$$

$$- \begin{pmatrix} b_1 q_1 I_1 - \theta_1 U_1 \\ \frac{\sigma_1 \sigma_2 \beta_{12}}{\sigma_1 N_1 + \sigma_2 N_2}S_1 I_2 + \frac{\sigma_1 \sigma_2 \tilde{\beta}_{12}}{\sigma_1 N_1 + \sigma_2 N_2}S_1 A_2 - (\gamma_1 + \mu_1)E_1 \\ \gamma_1 E_1 + \theta_1 U_1 - \mu_1 I_1 \\ (1-\theta_2)\frac{\sigma_1 \sigma_2 \beta_{21}}{\sigma_1 N_1 + \sigma_2 N_2}S_2 I_1 - (\tilde{\varepsilon}_2 + \mu_2)A_2 \\ \theta_2 \frac{\sigma_1 \sigma_2 \beta_{21}}{\sigma_1 N_1 + \sigma_2 N_2}S_2 I_1 - (\varepsilon_2 + m_2 + \mu_2)I_2 \end{pmatrix} =$$

$$\begin{pmatrix} 0 \\ \frac{\sigma_1 \sigma_2}{\sigma_1 N_1 + \sigma_2 N_2}(\beta_{12}I_2 + \tilde{\beta}_{12}A_2)(S_1^0 - S_1) \\ 0 \\ (1-\theta_2)\frac{\sigma_1 \sigma_2 \beta_{21}}{\sigma_1 N_1 + \sigma_2 N_2}(S_2^0 - S_2) \\ \theta_2 \frac{\sigma_1 \sigma_2 \beta_{21}}{\sigma_1 N_1 + \sigma_2 N_2}(S_2^0 - S_2) \end{pmatrix}$$

Since $0 \leq S_1 \leq K_1$ and $0 \leq S_2 \leq K_2$ it is clear that $\hat{G}(X,Z) \geq 0$. Then $X^0 = (b_1 N_1 - \theta_1 P_1, \theta_1 P_1 - \mu_1 S_1, b_2 N_2 - \mu_2 S_2, 0)$ is globally asymptotic stable equilibrium of $\frac{dX}{dt} = F(X,0)$. Hence, by the above Theorem, U^0 which represents the disease-free equilibrium X_1^0 is globally asymptotic stable.

0.5.3 Global asymptotic stability of EE, X_1^*. Since the DFE is locally stable when $R_0^1 < 1$ (this will suggest local stability of the EE for the reverse condition [32]), we only investigate the global stability of the endemic equilibrium.

Theorem 4. *For $R_0^1 > 1$, the model system (1,2,3) without Culex mosquitoes has unique positive EE point X_1^*, such that*

$$\frac{E_1^*}{E_1} \leq \frac{F_1^* S_1^* E_1}{F_1 S_1 E_1^*} \leq 1 \ for \ 0 < E_1 < E_1^*,$$

$$\frac{S_2^*}{S_2} \geq \frac{I_1^* S_2}{I_1 S_2} \geq 1 \ for \ 0 < S_2 < S_2^* \wedge 0 < I_1 < I_1^* \ and$$

$$\frac{S_1^*}{S_1} \leq \frac{P_1 S_1^* G_1^*}{P_1^* S_1 G_1} \leq 1 \ for \ 0 < S_1^* < S_1 \wedge 0 < P_1 < P_1^*$$

Then, X_1^* is globally asymptotic stable in $\overset{\circ}{\Omega}{}^1 \subset \Omega^1$.

Proof 3. *Global stability of the EE is explored via the construction of a suitable Lyapunov function. Let us consider the following function:*

$$
\begin{aligned}
&V(P_1, U_1, S_1, E_1, I_1, S_2, A_2, I_2) \\
&= e_1(P_1 - P_1^* \ln P_1) + e_2(U_1 - U_1^* \ln U_1) + e_3(S_1 - S_1^* \ln S_1) \\
&+ e_4(E_1 - E_1^* \ln E_1) + e_5(I_1 - I_1^* \ln I_1) + e_6(S_2 - S_2^* \ln S_2) \\
&+ e_7(A_2 - A_2^* \ln A_2) + e_8(I_2 - I_2^* \ln I_2),
\end{aligned}
\tag{30}
$$

where $e_i > 0$ for $i = 1, 2, \cdots, 8$ with $e_7 = \dfrac{1}{I_1^* S_2^*}, e_8 = \dfrac{1 - \theta_2}{\theta_2} \dfrac{1}{I_1^* S_2^*}$. e_2 and e_5 are chosen very small such $e_2 X^* < \delta$, $e_5 X^* < \delta$ for $\delta \in (0,1)$.

V (> 0 in $\overset{\circ}{\Omega}{}^1$) is a Lyapunov function (Korobeinikov [39]). The time derivative of V is

$$
\begin{aligned}
\dot{V} &= e_1(1 - \frac{P_1^*}{P_1})\dot{P}_1 + e_2(1 - \frac{U_1^*}{U_1})\dot{U}_1 + e_3(1 - \frac{S_1^*}{S_1})\dot{S}_1 \\
&+ e_4(1 - \frac{E_1^*}{E_1})\dot{E}_1 + e_5(1 - \frac{I_1^*}{I_1})\dot{I}_1 + e_6(1 - \frac{S_2^*}{S_2})\dot{S}_2 \\
&+ e_7(1 - \frac{A_2^*}{A_2})\dot{A}_2 + e_8(1 - \frac{I_2^*}{I_2})\dot{I}_2 \\
&= e_1(1 - \frac{P_1^*}{P_1})[b_1(N_1 - q_1 I_1) - \theta_1 P_1] \\
&+ e_2(1 - \frac{U_1^*}{U_1})[b_1 q_1 I_1 - \theta_1 U_1] \\
&+ e_3(1 - \frac{S_1^*}{S_1})[\theta_1 P_1 - g_1 I_2 S_1 - g_2 A_2 S_1 - \mu_1 S_1] \\
&+ e_4(1 - \frac{E_1^*}{E_1})[g_1 I_2 S_1 + g_2 A_2 S_1 - (\gamma_1 + \mu_1)E_1] \\
&+ e_5(1 - \frac{I_1^*}{I_1})[\gamma_1 E_1 + \theta_1 U_1 - \mu_1 I_1] \\
&+ e_6(1 - \frac{S_2^*}{S_2})(b_2 N_2 - g_3 I_1 S_2 - \mu_2 S_2) \\
&+ e_7(1 - \frac{A_2^*}{A_2})[(1 - \theta_2) g_3 I_1 S_2 - (\tilde{\varepsilon}_2 + \mu_2)A_2] \\
&+ e_8(1 - \frac{I_2^*}{I_2})[\theta_2 g_3 I_1 S_2 - (\varepsilon_2 + m_2 + \mu_2)I_2].
\end{aligned}
\tag{31}
$$

At X_1^*, we have $b_1 N_1 = b_1 q_1 I_1^* + \theta_1 P_1^*$, $b_1 q_1 = \dfrac{\theta_1 U_1^*}{I_1^*}$, $\theta_1 = \dfrac{g_1 I_2^* S_1^* + g_2 A_2^* S_1^* + \mu_1 S_1^*}{P_1^*}$, $\gamma_1 + \mu_1 = \dfrac{g_1 I_2^* S_1^* + g_2 A_2^* S_1^*}{E_1^*}$, $\mu_1 = \dfrac{\gamma_1 E_1^* + \theta_1 U_1^*}{I_1^*}$, $b_2 N_2 = g_3 I_1^* S_2^* + \mu_2 S_2^*$, $\tilde{\varepsilon}_2 + \mu_2 = \dfrac{(1 - \theta_2) g_3 I_1^* S_2^*}{A_2^*}$, $\varepsilon_2 + m_2 + \mu_2 = \dfrac{\theta_2 g_3 I_1^* S_2^*}{I_2^*}$.

Let $F_1 = g_1 I_2 + g_2 A_2$, $F_1^* = g_1 I_2^* + g_2 A_2^*$, $G_1 = g_1 I_2 + g_2 A_2 + \mu_1$, $G_1^* = g_1 I_2^* + g_2 A_2^* + \mu_1$, $H_1 = \gamma_1 E_1 + \theta_1 U_1$, $H_1^* = \gamma_1 E_1^* + \theta_1 U_1^*$. Then, $\dot{V}$ can now be written as

$$
\begin{aligned}
\dot{V} &= e_1(1 - \frac{P_1^*}{P_1})(b_1 q_1 I_1^* + \theta_1 P_1^* - b_1 q_1 I_1 - \theta_1 P_1) \\
&+ e_2(1 - \frac{U_1^*}{U_1})(\frac{\theta_1 U_1^*}{I_1^*} - \theta_1 U_1) + e_3(1 - \frac{S_1^*}{S_1})(\frac{P_1 G_1^* S_1^*}{P_1^*} - G_1 S_1) \\
&+ e_4(1 - \frac{E_1^*}{E_1})(F_1 S_1 - \frac{F_1^* S_1^* E_1}{E_1^*}) + e_5(1 - \frac{I_1^*}{I_1})(H_1 - \frac{H_1^* I_1}{I_1^*}) \\
&+ e_6(1 - \frac{S_2^*}{S_2})[(g_3 I_1^* + \mu_2)S_2^* - (g_3 I_1 + \mu_2)S_2] \\
&+ e_7(1 - \frac{A_2^*}{A_2})[(1 - \theta_2)g_3 I_1 S_2 - \frac{(1 - \theta_2)g_3 I_1^* S_2^* A_2}{A_2^*}] \\
&+ e_8(1 - \frac{I_2^*}{I_2})[\theta_2 g_3 I_1 S_2 - \frac{\theta_2 g_3 I_1^* S_2^* I_2}{I_2^*}].
\end{aligned}
\tag{32}
$$

Further simplification yields

$$
\begin{aligned}
\dot{V} &= -e_1(1 - \frac{P_1^*}{P_1})^2 \theta_1 P_1 - e_6(1 - \frac{S_2^*}{S_2})^2 \mu_2 S_2 \\
&+ F(P_1, U_1, S_1, E_1, I_1, S_2, A_2, I_2)
\end{aligned}
\tag{33}
$$

where

$$
\begin{aligned}
F &= e_1 b_1 q_1 (1 - \frac{P_1^*}{P_1})(\frac{I_1^*}{I_1} - 1)I_1 \\
&+ e_2 \theta_2 (1 - \frac{U_1^*}{U_1})(\frac{U_1^* I_1}{U_1 I_1^*} - 1)U_1 \\
&+ e_3(1 - \frac{S_1^*}{S_1})(\frac{P_1 S_1^* G_1^*}{P_1^* S_1 G_1} - 1)S_1 G_1 \\
&+ e_4(1 - \frac{E_1^*}{E_1})(1 - \frac{F_1^* S_1^* E_1}{F_1 S_1 E_1^*})S_1 F_1 \\
&+ e_5(1 - \frac{I_1^*}{I_1})(1 - \frac{H_1^* I_1}{H_1 I_1^*})H_1 \\
&+ e_6 g_3 (1 - \frac{S_2^*}{S_2})(\frac{I_1^* S_2^*}{I_1 S_2} - 1)I_1 S_2 \\
&+ e_7(1 - \theta_2)g_3(1 - \frac{A_2^*}{A_2})(1 - \frac{I_1^* S_2^* A_2}{I_1 S_2 A_2^*})I_1 S_2 \\
&+ e_8 \theta_2 g_3 (1 - \frac{I_2^*}{I_2})(1 - \frac{I_1^* S_2^* I_2}{I_1 S_2 I_2^*})I_1 S_2.
\end{aligned}
\tag{34}
$$

Recalling that $U_1^* = \frac{b_1 q_1}{\theta_1} I_1^*$, $e_7 = \frac{1}{I_1^* S_2^*}$ *and* $e_8 = \frac{1-\theta_2}{\theta_2} \frac{1}{I_1^* S_2^*}$ *we obtain,*

$$e_2\theta_2(1-\frac{U_1^*}{U_1})(\frac{U_1^* I_1}{U_1 I_1^*}-1)U_1$$
$$= e_2\theta_2 U_1^*(1-\frac{U_1}{U_1^*}-\frac{U_1^* I_1}{U_1 I_1^*})+e_2\theta_2\frac{b_1 q_1}{\theta_1}I_1, \quad (35)$$

$$e_5(1-\frac{I_1^*}{I_1})(1-\frac{H_1^* I_1}{H_1 I_1^*})H_1 = e_5 H_1(1-\frac{I_1^*}{I_1}-\frac{H_1^* I_1}{H_1 I_1^*})+e_5 H_1^*, \quad (36)$$

and $\quad e_7(1-\theta_2)g_3(1-\frac{A_2^*}{A_2})(1-\frac{I_1^* S_2^* A_2}{I_1 S_2 A_2^*})I_1 S_2 + e_8\theta_2 g_3(1-\frac{I_2^*}{I_2})$
$(1-\frac{I_1^* S_2^* I_2}{I_1 S_2 I_2^*})I_1 S_2 = (1-\theta_2)g_3\frac{I_1 S_2}{I_1^* S_2^*}(2-\frac{A_2^*}{A_2}-\frac{I_1^* S_2^* A_2}{I_1 S_2 A_2^*}-\frac{I_2^*}{I_2}-$
$\frac{I_1^* S_2^* I_2}{I_1 S_2 I_2^*})+2(1-\theta_2)g_3.$

By theorems hypothesis,

$$e_1 b_1 q_1(1-\frac{P_1^*}{P_1})(\frac{I_1^*}{I_1}-1)I_1 \leq 0,$$

$$e_3(1-\frac{S_1^*}{S_1})(\frac{P_1 S_1^* G_1}{P_1^* S_1 G_1}-1)S_1 G_1 \leq 0,$$

$$e_4(1-\frac{E_1^*}{E_1})(1-\frac{F_1^* S_1^* E_1}{F_1 S_1 E_1^*})S_1 F_1,$$

$$e_6 g_3(1-\frac{S_2^*}{S_2})(\frac{I_1^* S_2^*}{I_1 S_2}-1)I_1 S_2 \leq 0,$$

where strict equalities holds only when,

$$P_1 = P_1^*, I_1 = I_1^*, S_1 = S_1^*, E_1 = E_1^* \text{ and } S_2 = S_2^*$$

Furthermore,

$$\frac{U_1}{U_1^*}+\frac{U_1^* I_1}{U_1 I_1^*} \geq 2,$$

$$\frac{I_1^*}{I_1}+\frac{H_1^* I_1}{H_1 I_1^*} \geq 2,$$

$$\frac{A_2^*}{A_2}+\frac{I_1^* S_2^* A_2}{I_1 S_2 A_2^*}+\frac{I_2^*}{I_2}+\frac{I_1^* S_2^* I_2}{I_1 S_2 I_2^*} \geq 4,$$

for all $I_1, S_2, A_2, I_2 \geq 0$, *because the arithmetic mean is greater than or equal to the geometric mean. Thus,* $F \leq 0$ *for* $P_1, U_1, S_1, E_1, I_1, S_2, A_2, I_2 > 0$. *Hence,* $\dot{V} \leq 0$ *for all* $P_1, U_1, S_1, E_1, I_1, S_2, A_2, I_2 > 0$ *and is equal to zero for* $P_1 = P_1^*, U_1 = U_1^*, S_1 = S_1^*, E_1 = E_1^*, I_1 = I_1^*, S_2 = S_2^*, A_2 = A_2^*, I_2 = I_2^*$

and X_1^* *is the only equilibrium state of the system on this plane.*

Therefore, the largest compact invariant set in Ω^1 *such that* $\dot{V} \leq 0$ *is the singleton* X_1^* *which is the endemic equilibrium point. LaSalle's invariant principle [40] guarantees that* X_1^* *is globally asymptotically stable (GAS) in* $\overset{\circ}{\Omega}^1$, *the interior of* Ω^1.

0.6 Stability analysis of the overall model (1,2,3)

The overall model system (1,2,3) describes the epidemiological and ecological complexity involved on RVF dynamics. Theorem 2 in van den Driesche and Watmough [32] states that the local stability of the disease-free equilibrium of the model can be determined by its basic reproduction number, R_0. However, in host-vector models where multiple transmission cycle are observed to occur as in the case of our model (vertical transmission, host to *Aedes* infection, *Aedes* to host infection, host to *Culex* infection and *Culex* to host infection) the basic reproductive number obtained via next-generation method does not give the number of host infected by a single host if there an intermediate vector, but rather the geometric mean of the number of infections per generation [41]. Therefore, in our case the local stability of the disease-free equilibrium, X^0, (10) of the model is established through the Routh-Hurtwitz criteria [42,43], and the following result holds.

Theorem 5. *The model system (1,2,3) always has the disease-free equilibrium* X^0. *If* $\frac{b_1 q_1}{\mu_1} < 1 \wedge R_0^1 < 1 \wedge R_0^3 < 1 \wedge R_0 < 1$, *the disease-free equilibrium is locally asymptotically stable in* Ω^1.

Proof 4. *To prove the stability of the equilibrium point* X^0 *we use the Jacobian matrix (23) of the linearised system, which yield the following characteristic polynomial:*

$$x^4 + n_1 x^3 + n_2 x^2 + n_3 x + n_4 = 0 \quad (37)$$

where $n_1 = \mu_3 + \tilde{\varepsilon}_2 + \mu_2 + \varepsilon_2 + m_2 + \mu_2 + \mu_1 - b_1 q_1$, $n_2 = \mu_3(\tilde{\varepsilon}_2 + \mu_2)(1-c_1) + \mu_3(\varepsilon_2 + m_2 + \mu_2)(1-c_2) + (\mu_1 - b_1 q_1)(\tilde{\varepsilon}_2 + \mu_2)(1-c_3) + (\mu_1 - b_1 q_1)(\varepsilon_2 + m_2 + \mu_2)(1-c_4) + \mu_3(\mu_1 - b_1 q_1) + (\tilde{\varepsilon}_2 + \mu_2)(\varepsilon_2 + m_2 + \mu_2)$, $n_3 = (\mu_1 - b_1 q_1)(\tilde{\varepsilon}_2 + \mu_2)(\varepsilon_2 + m_2 + \mu_2)(1 - R_0^1) + \mu_3(\tilde{\varepsilon}_2 + \mu_2)(\varepsilon_2 + m_2 + \mu_2)(1 - R_0^3) + \mu_3(\mu_1 - b_1 q_1)(\tilde{\varepsilon}_2 + \mu_2)[1-(c_1+c_3)] + \mu_3(\mu_1 - b_1 q_1)(\varepsilon_2 + m_2 + \mu_2)[1-(c_2+c_4)]$, $n_4 = \mu_3(\mu_1 - b_1 q_1)(\tilde{\varepsilon}_2 + \mu_2)(\varepsilon_2 + m_2 + \mu_2)[1 - (c_1+c_2+c_3+c_4)]$
$= \mu_3(\mu_1 - b_1 q_1)(\tilde{\varepsilon}_2 + \mu_2)(\varepsilon_2 + m_2 + \mu_2)(1 - R_0)$,

with $\quad c_1 = \frac{(1-\theta_2)\gamma_3 g_4 g_6 S_2^0 S_3^0}{\mu_3(\gamma_3 + \mu_3)(\tilde{\varepsilon}_2 + \mu_2)}$, $c_2 = \frac{\theta_2\gamma_3 g_4 g_5 S_2^0 S_3^0}{\mu_3(\gamma_3 + \mu_3)(\varepsilon_2 + m_2 + \mu_2)}$,
$c_3 = \frac{(1-\theta_2)\gamma_1 g_1 g_3 S_1^0 S_2^0}{(\mu_1 - b_1 q_1)(\tilde{\varepsilon}_2 + \mu_2)}$, $c_4 = \frac{\theta_2\gamma_1 g_1 g_3 S_1^0 S_2^0}{(\mu_1 - b_1 q_1)(\varepsilon_2 + m_2 + \mu_2)}$, $R_0^3 =$
$c_1 + c_2 = \frac{\gamma_3 g_4 S_2}{\mu_3(\gamma_3 + \mu_3)}\left[\frac{(1-\theta_2)g_6 S_3^0}{\tilde{\varepsilon}_2 + \mu_2} + \frac{\theta_2 g_5 S_3^0}{\varepsilon_2 + m_2 + \mu_2}\right]$

Thus, $n_1 > 0$ *for* $\frac{b_1 q_1}{\mu_1} < 1$, $n_2 > 0$ *for* $\frac{b_1 q_1}{\mu_1} < 1 \wedge c_1 < 1$, $c_2 < 1, c_3 < 1, c_4 < 1$, $n_3 > 0$ *for* $\frac{b_1 q_1}{\mu_1} < 1 \wedge c_1 + c_3 < 1 c_2 + c_4 < 1$ *and* $n_4 > 0$ *for* $R_0^1 < 1 \wedge R_0^3 < 1 \wedge R_0 < 1$. *Thus the equation (37) has no root which is positive or zero (Descartes' rule of sign). Therefore equation (37) will only have negative roots or complex roots with negative real part if* $n_3(n_2 n_1 - n_3) - n_1^2 n_4 > 0$ *(according to Routh-Hurwitz criteria), that is,* $\frac{b_1 q_1}{\mu_1} < 1 \wedge R_0^1 < 1 \wedge R_0^3 < 1 \wedge R_0 < 1$. *Thus, the system (1,2,3) is locally asymptotically stable about the interior equilibrium* X^0.

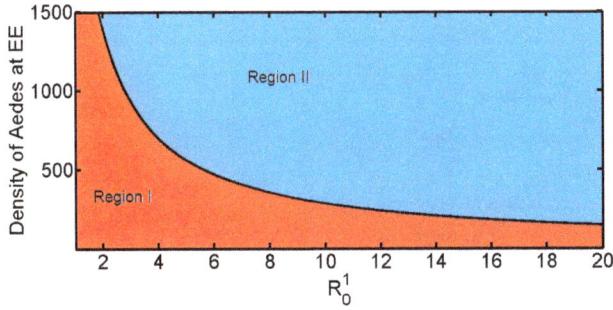

Figure 2. Based on equation (38), we represent the condition for existence of infected *Culex* mosquitoes at the endemic equilibrium (EE) state. The existence of infected *Culex* is impossible in region I. In region II both *Aedes* and *Culex* coexist. The border black line represents the threshold of coexistence, which is exactly $I_3^* = 100$.

0.6.1 Existence and uniqueness of endemic equilibrium,

X^*. The existence of the endemic equilibrium in Ω^1, is determined by equation (18). Taking $A = g_3 l_7, B = g_4 l_7$, $C = b_1 N_1 g_3 l_6, D = \mu_1 \mu_2 l_5$ and $E = b_1 N_1 g_4 l_6$, equation (18) can be written as

$$A(I_1^*)^2 + (BI_3^* + D - C)I_1^* + EI_3^* = 0. \qquad (38)$$

Solving equation (38) for $\{I_1^*, I_3^*\}$ we get $\{I_1^* > 0, I_3^* = -\frac{I_1^*(AI_1^* + D - C)}{I_1^* B - E}\}$ which gives $\{I_1^* > 0, I_3^* = \frac{g_3 \gamma_1 b_2 I_1^*(aR_0^1 - 1 - g_3 l_7 I_1^*)}{g_4[g_3 \gamma_1 b_2 l_7 I_1^* - \mu_1(\gamma_1 + \mu_1)R_0^1]}\}$, with $a = \frac{b_1 b_2}{\mu_2(\mu_1 - b_1 q_1)}$. The existence of positive I_3^* is given by the following inequalities:
$$\frac{E}{B} < I_1^* < \frac{C - D}{A} \vee \frac{C - D}{A} < I_1^* < \frac{E}{B}.$$
Since $\frac{E}{B} = \frac{b_1 N_1 g_4 l_6}{g_4 l_7} = \frac{b_1 N_1 l_6}{l_7}$ and $\frac{C - D}{A} = \frac{b_1 N_1 g_3 l_6 - \mu_1 \mu_2 l_5}{g_3 l_7}$
$= \frac{b_1 N_1 l_6}{l_7} - \frac{\mu_1 \mu_2 l_5}{g_3 l_7}$, we get that the meaningful inequality is
$\frac{C - D}{A} < I_1^* < \frac{E}{B}$, thus $\frac{aR_0^1 - 1}{g_3 l_7} < I_1^* < \frac{\mu_1(\gamma_1 + \mu_1)R_0^1}{g_3 \gamma_1 b_2 l_7}$.
Since $I_1^* > 0$, then $C - D$ should be positive. $C - D$ is the expression on the numerator of equation (25), which was verified to be positive whenever $R_0^1 > 1$ and $\frac{b_1 q_1}{\mu_1} < 1$. This gives the

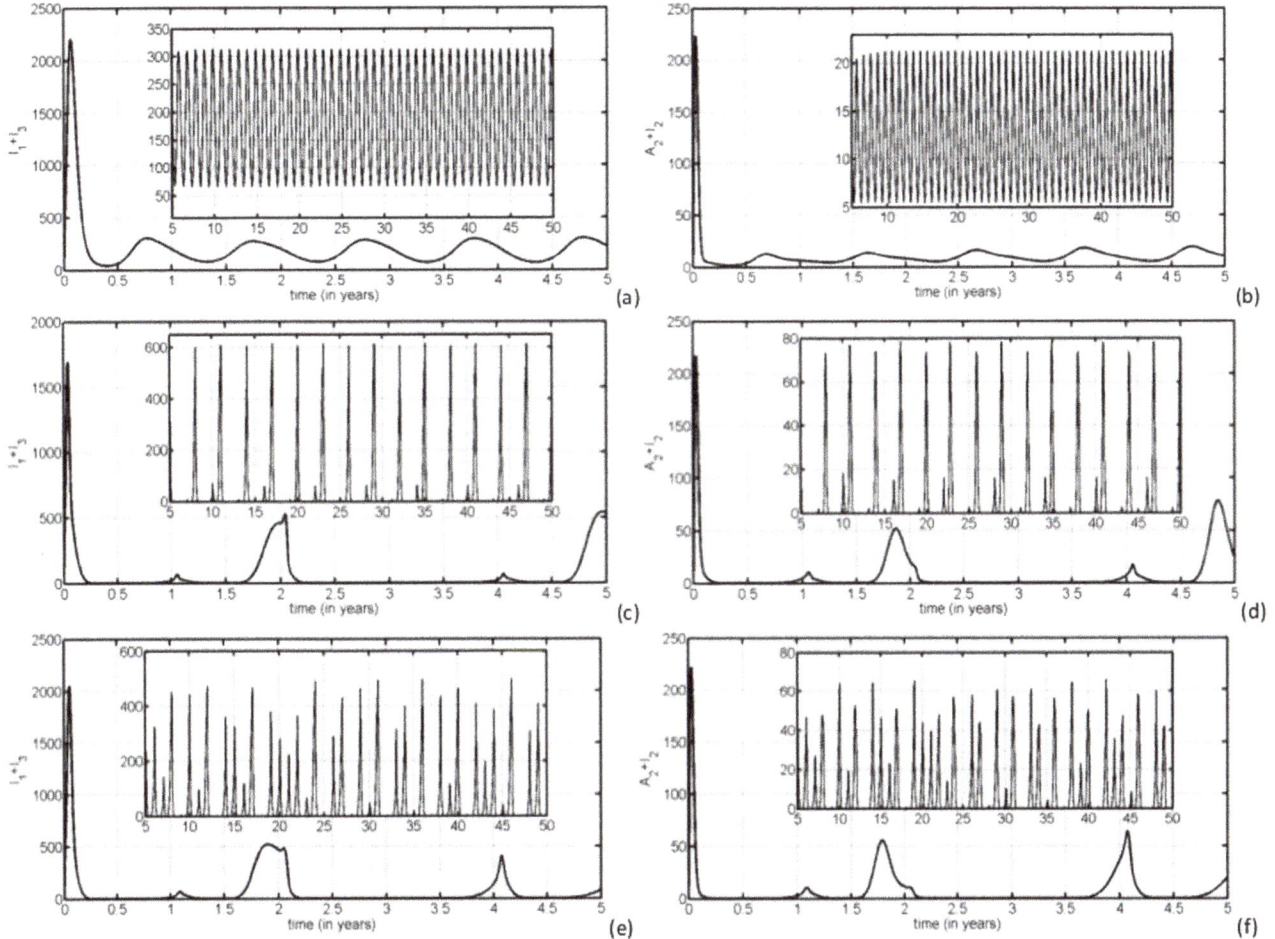

Figure 3. We display the time series of $(I_1 + I_3)$ left and $(A_2 + I_2)$ right. Parameters used for (a) and (b) are $\delta_1 = 0.6$, $\delta_3 = 0.6$, for (c) and (d) are $\delta_1 = 70$, $\delta_3 = 1.1$, finally for (e) and (f) are $\delta_1 = 24.7$, $\delta_3 = 1.1$. Figures (d) and (f) show a linear increase in livestock seroprevalence during post-epidemic which comes in cycles of 5 to 7 years approximately.

Table 2. Parameters description for the RVF model (1,2,3).

Parameter	Values	References	Parameters description and their dimensions
b_1	0.06	[9,13]	Per capita birth/death rate of *Aedes* mosquito species, Day^{-1}
b_2	0.0022	[12]	Per capita birth/death rate of livestock, Day^{-1}
b_3	0.06	[9,13]	Per capita birth/death rate of *Culex* mosquito species, Day^{-1}
q_1	0.1	[14]	Probability of vertical transmission from an infectious *Aedes* mosquito mother to its eggs, dimensionless
θ_a	0.20	Assumed	Development rate of mosquitoes, Day^{-1}, where $a=1$ and $a=3$
θ_2	0.6	[6,9]	Probability of an infected host moving to the symptomatic stage, dimensionless
$(1-\theta_2)$	0.4	[6,9]	Probability of an infected host moving to the asymptomatic stage, dimensionless
σ_1,σ_3	0.33	[5,9]	Number of times one *Aedes*, *Culex* mosquito would want to bite a host per Day, if it were freely available. This is a function of the mosquito's gonotrophic cycle (the amount of time a mosquito requires to produce eggs) and its preference for livestock blood, Day^{-1}
σ_2	19	[9]	The maximum number of mosquito bites a host can sustain per Day. This is a function of the host's exposed surface area, the efforts it takes to prevent mosquito bites (such as switching its tail), and any vector control interventions in place to kill mosquitoes encountering hosts or preventing bites, Day^{-1}
β_{2a}	0.21	[6,9]	Probability of transmission of infection from an infectious mosquito to a susceptible host given that a contact between the two occurs, dimensionless, where $a=1$ and $a=3$
β_{a2}	0.7,0.15	[6,9]	Probability of transmission of infection from an infectious host to a susceptible mosquito given that a contact between the two occurs, dimensionless, where $a=1$ and $a=3$
$\tilde{\beta}_{a2}$	0.30	[6,9]	Probability of transmission of infection from an asymptomatic host to a susceptible mosquito given that a contact between the two occurs, dimensionless
$1/\gamma_a$	6	[12,15]	is the average duration of the mosquitoes latent period, Days, where $a=1$ and $a=3$
$1/\varepsilon_2$	4	[5,9,16]	is the average duration of the infectious period I_2, Days
$1/\tilde{\varepsilon}_2$	4	[9,13,16]	is the average duration of the infectious asymptomatic period, Day^{-1}
m_2	0.1	[9,13,16]	Per capita disease-induced death rate for livestock, Day^{-1}
$1/\mu_1$	20	[9,13]	Lifespan of *Aedes* mosquitoes, Days
$1/\mu_2$	2190	[12]	Lifespan of livestock animals, Days
$1/\mu_3$	20	[9,13]	Lifespan of *Culex* mosquitoes, Days

threshold for the endemic persistence. Therefore the following result holds:

Theorem 6. *The RVF model (1,2,3) has a unique endemic equilibrium point* X^* *whenever* $R_0^1 > 1$ *and* $\dfrac{aR_0^1 - 1}{g_3 l_7} < I_1^*$

$< \dfrac{\mu_1(\gamma_1 + \mu_1)R_0^1}{g_3 \gamma_1 b_2 l_7}$.

The result in Theorem (6) indicates that depending on vertical transmission efficiency, if the *Aedes* basic reproduction number $R_0^1 > 1$ and I_1^* satisfy the inequality $\dfrac{aR_0^1 - 1}{g_3 l_7} < I_1^* < \dfrac{\mu_1(\gamma_1 + \mu_1)R_0^1}{g_3 \gamma_1 b_2 l_7}$, it is sufficient to cause an outbreak, since secondary vectors (*Culex* species) co-exist and serve as disease amplifiers. Figure 2 shows the region where I_3^* is strictly positive when varying both I_1^* and R_0^1. That is, in region II both infected *Aedes* and *Culex* co-exist while in region I only infected *Aedes* exist. This confirm the analytical results obtained above. The existence of infected *Culex* at endemic equilibrium depend on the existence infected *Aedes* and initial spread of the disease R_0^1. Thus, *Aedes* species have the potential to initiate the epidemic through transovarial transmission and the potential to sustain low levels of the disease during post epidemic periods.

0.7 Bifurcation and chaos investigation on the RVF model

To provide some numerical evidence for the qualitative dynamic behaviour of the model (1,2,3), time series with both transient and permanent regimes, phase portraits, Poincaré maps, bifurcation diagrams, Lyapunov exponents have been used to assess model sensitive dependence on initial conditions and return maps are used to illustrate the above analytical results and for determining new dynamics as the parameters vary. We start by introducing a simple case of seasonality on time dependent oviposition rates of mosquito populations (*Aedes* and *Culex*):

$$b_1(t) = b_1\left(1 + \delta_1 \sin\left(\frac{2\pi t}{T}\right)\right), b_3(t) = b_3\left(1 + \delta_3 \sin\left(\frac{2\pi t}{T}\right)\right) \quad (39)$$

where b_1 and b_3 are the baseline parameters of the oviposition rates of *Aedes* and *Culex* mosquitoes respectively, $T = 1$ year, δ_1 and δ_3 are the external forcing amplitudes for the two species of mosquitoes respectively, which represent the strength of seasonality that controls the magnitude of the fluctuations. When $\delta_1 = \delta_3 \equiv 0$, the model reduces to a non-seasonal model and the system possesses two types of equilibria: disease free and endemic equilibria. When the magnitude of the external forcing parameters δ_1, δ_3 is sufficiently small, $\delta_1, \delta_3 \in (0,1)$ the system responds with oscillations of the same annual period as external forces (see Figs.3 (a) and (b)). However with larger values (for instance $\delta_1 = 70, \delta_3 = 1.1$) the system shows other modes of oscillations (see Figs.3 (c) and (d)) with period 5 as confirmed by Poicaré maps Fig.4. In all this section, the system is integrated numerically with the fifth order Runge-Kutta algorithm [44]. The initials conditions

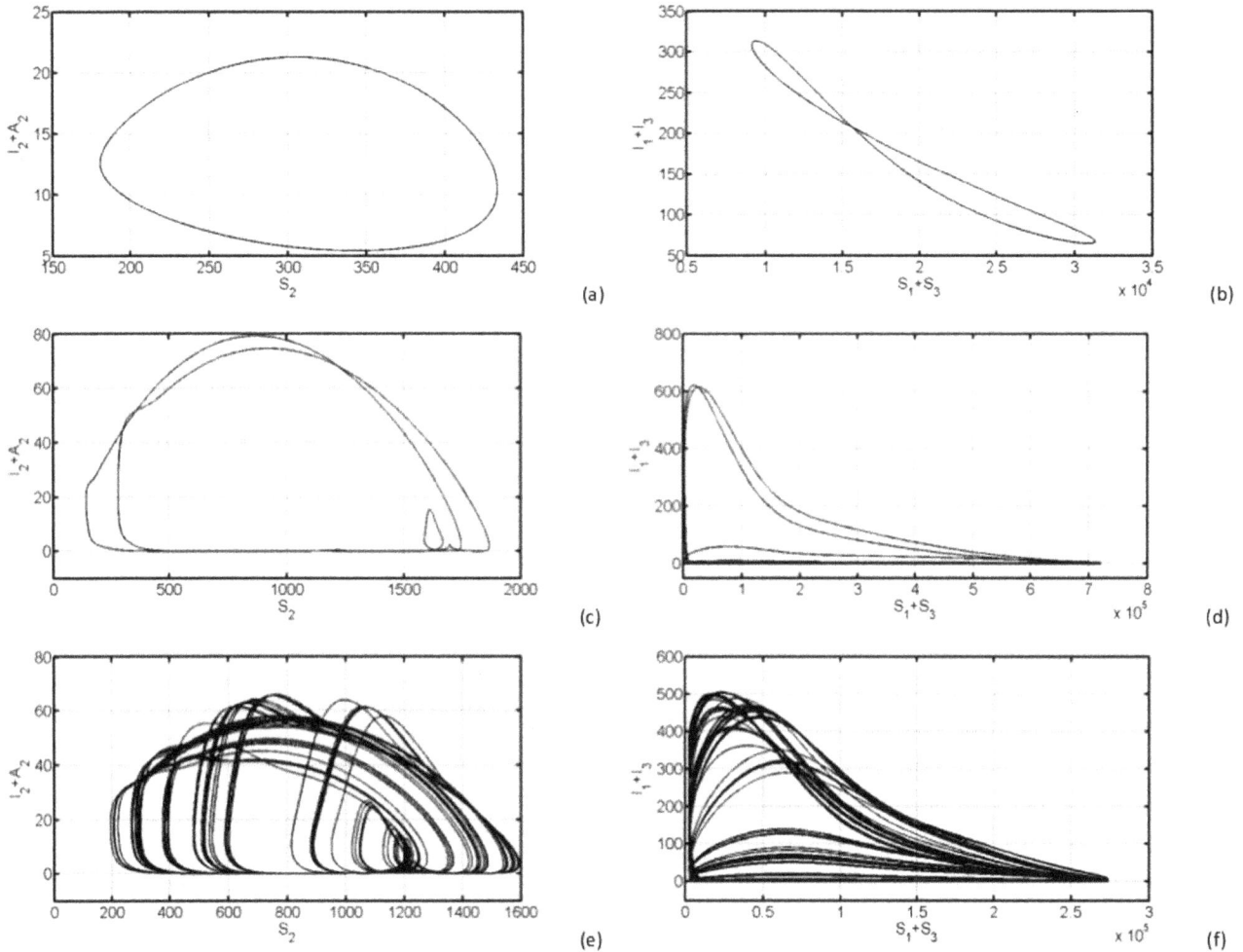

Figure 4. Phase portrait with couple $(I_2 + A_2, S_2)$ on the left and $(I_1 + I_3, S_1 + S_3)$ on the right. In (a) and (b), $\delta_1 = 0.6$, $\delta_3 = 0.6$, **the system is attracted by a limit cycle.** In (c) and (d), $\delta_1 = 70$, $\delta_3 = 1.1$, the system is multi-periodic. And in (e) and (f), $\delta_1 = 24.7$, $\delta_3 = 1.1$, the systems behave with higher multi periodicity.

and other values are $P_1(0) = 1000$, $U_1(0) = 999$, $E_1(0) = 0$, $I_1(0) = 1$, $S_2(0) = 1000$, $A_2(0) = 0$, $I_2(0) = 0$, $R_2(0) = 0$, $P_3(0) = 1000$, $S_3(0) = 5000$, $E_3(0) = 0$, $I_3(0) = 0$, $K_1 = 10000$, $K_2 = 2000$ and $K_3 = 10000$. The parameter values are shown in Table 2.

0.7.1 Time series simulations. Figure 3 depicts the time evolution of the sum of infectious *Aedes* and *Culex* mosquitoes, $I_1 + I_3$ and sum of infectious asymptomatic and symptomatic livestock for different values of $\delta_1 = 0.6, \delta_3 = 0.6$; $\delta_1 = 70, \delta_3 = 1.1$ and $\delta_1 = 24.7, \delta_3 = 1.1$. In (a) the number of infectious mosquitoes oscillates yearly reaching the same maximum. In (c) the quantity $I_1 + I_3$ also oscillates with first peak of above 500 around the second year. In (c) we notice a long lasting peak of about 500 infectious mosquitoes in the interval 18–25 months, which is likely to cause an inter-epidemic outbreak. Fig.3(b) shows a constant low oscillation, high peaks around second and fifth year in (d) and high peaks around second and fourth year in (f). Note that the internal figures describes the permanent regime which represent the dynamics where the system is expected to adapt to the external forcing. The time series for $\delta_1, \delta_3 \in (0,1)$, also show that the total of infected vectors $I_1 + I_3$ and infected livestock $A_2 + I_2$ stay quite away from zero, avoiding the chance of extinction in stochastic system with reasonable size (see Figs.3 (a) and (b)). This is due to

the fact that for $\delta_1, \delta_3 \in (0,1)$ vector oviposition continues throughout the year, albeit at lower rates during unfavourable seasons. This is not the case of East African region, where we have two rainy seasons (long and short) and a dry season, where under this former we expect stochastic extinction during some intervals of interepidemic periods.

In the region $\delta_1 > 1, \delta_2 > 1$, Figs.3 (c)–(f), we observe fluctuations in the total number of infected from reasonable small peaks (describing RVF post-epidemic activities) to very low values, which in this case drive almost surely the system to extinction.

0.7.2   Phase portrait diagrams and Poincaré maps. Instead of studying the entire complicated trajectories, important information is encoded in the phase plane. This approach allow us to analyse geometrically the total dynamics of the system. Varying δ_1, δ_3 the state space plots show a rich dynamical behaviour with bifurcations from limit cycles, multi-periodic oscillation to completely irregular behaviour which is usually the fingerprint of chaos (see Fig.4).

Poincaré map is a useful tool for analysing the dynamics of a nonlinear system. It allows good insight for global dynamics of the system by displaying the types of attractors of the system [45]. The successive iterations of the map are defined as:

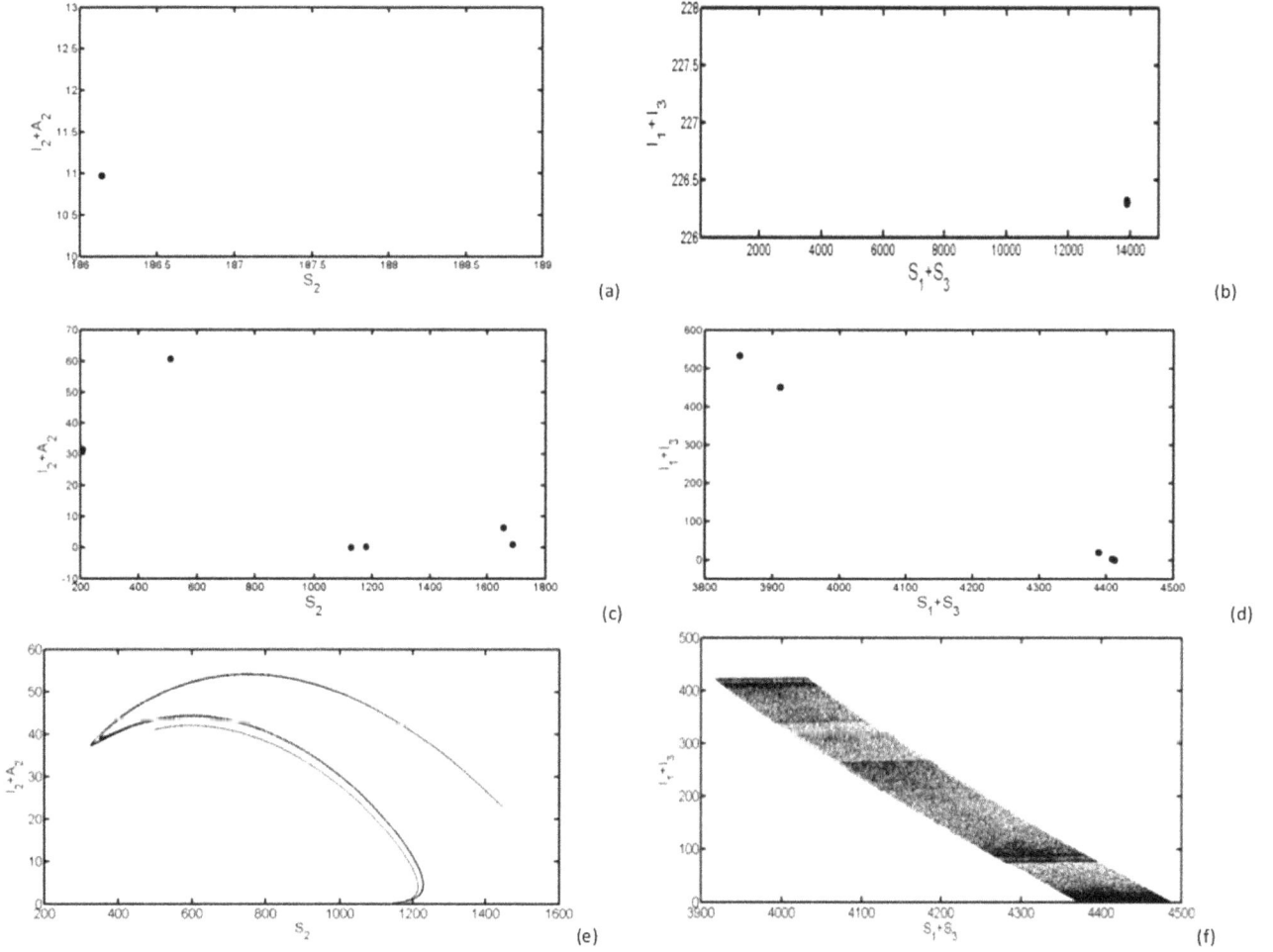

Figure 5. Poincaré maps with couple $(I_2 + A_2, S_2)$ on the left and $(I_1 + I_3, S_1 + S_3)$ on the right. In (a) and (b), $\delta_1 = 0.6$, $\delta_3 = 0.6$, in (c) and (d), $\delta_1 = 70$, $\delta_3 = 1.1$ and in (e) and (f), $\delta_1 = 24.7$, $\delta_3 = 1.1$.

$$P : \Sigma \to \Sigma$$

$$\Sigma = \left\{ \mathbf{X} | t = 0, \frac{2\pi}{\Omega}, \frac{4\pi}{\Omega}, \frac{8\pi}{\Omega}, \dots \right\} \in \mathbb{R}^{13} \qquad (40)$$

The attractor is generated by sampling the system stroboscopically at time corresponding to the multiple of the period $T = 2\pi/\Omega$. We have used 100,000 points and a period of one year. Figures 5 (a) and (b) with ($\delta_1 = 0.6$, $\delta_3 = 0.6$) show that the system is attracted by a limit cycle, because of the presence of a single dot. In this case the system is periodic. In (c) and (d) with ($\delta_1 = 70$, $\delta_3 = 1.1$) we notice a presence of a few dots, thus, the system is multi-periodic and in (e) and (f) with ($\delta_1 = 24.7$, $\delta_3 = 1.1$) we notice a strange attractor which is usually a sign of a chaotic system.

0.7.3 Maxima return maps of $I_1 + I_3, A_2 + I_2$ for state phase plots. We have used maxima return maps in order to get supplementary classification of different dynamics for parameters δ_1 and δ_3. For a time selected as t_{max}, at which $I_1 + I_3$ and $A_2 + I_2$ have a local maximum, we have plotted the number of infected mosquitoes and livestock respectively at time t_{max} and at the next local maximum $t_{returnmax}$. Figures 6 (a) and (b) show that all consecutive maxima coincide with themselves as shown by a single dot. In (c) and (d), we notice that consecutive maxima are few and different as a sign of irregularity, and in (e) and (f), we observe that a dot rarely comes back to the same point. Thus, the fingerprint of chaotic attractor is clearly visible now with the maxima return maps analysis.

0.7.4   Lyapunov   exponents   and   bifurcation diagrams.   The largest Lyapunov Exponent (LE) is quantitatively characterized by the average rate of separation of infinitesimally close trajectories in the phase space for a dynamic system. It can be used to determine how sensitive a dynamical system is to initial conditions [46]. In general for a N-dimensional dynamical system described by a set of equations $\frac{dX^i}{dt} = F^i(\mathbf{X}, t)$, the LEs are defined by [35]:

$$\lambda_i = \lim_{t \to \infty} \lim_{\delta X_0^i \to 0} \frac{1}{t} \ln \left(\frac{\|\delta X_t^i\|}{\|\delta X_0^i\|} \right), \qquad (41)$$

where λ_i is the ith LE and $\|\delta X_t^i\|$ is the distance between the trajectories of the ith component of the vector field F at time t.

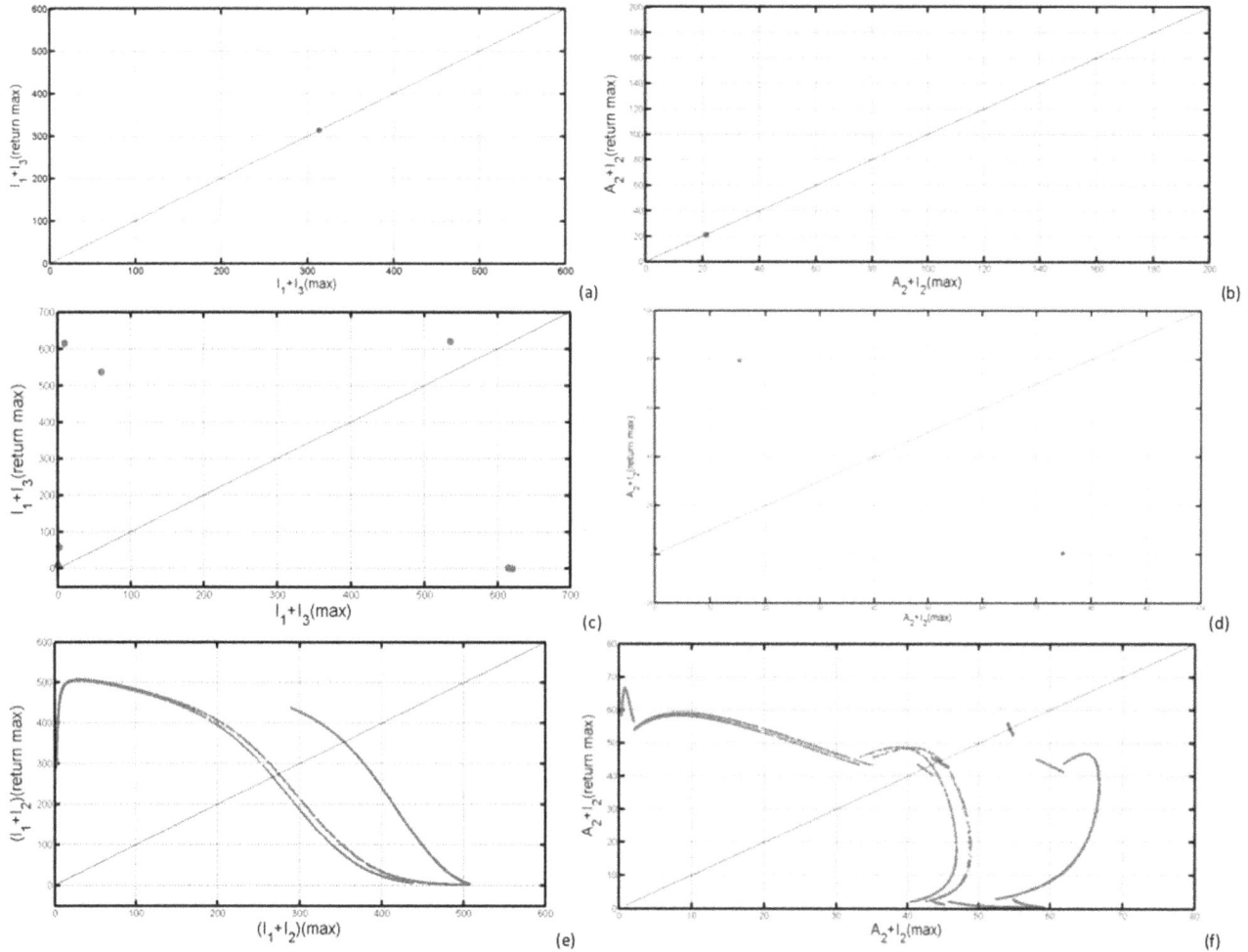

Figure 6. We display the maxima return map of $I_1 + I_3$ **and** $A_2 + I_2$ **with (a)–(b)** $\delta_1 = 0.1$, $\delta_3 = 0.1$, **(c)–(d)** $\delta_1 = 70$, $\delta_3 = 1.1$ **and (e)–(f)** $\delta_1 = 24.7$, $\delta_3 = 1.1$. The blanc line represents the first bisectrix of the plane.

Recall that exponential divergence in the phase space is given by the LEs. If the largest LE is less than or equal to zero, then the system may be regarded as periodic or quasi-periodic. Otherwise, if the largest LE is positive the system may have an irregular or chaotic behaviour. Another important fact to be mentioned is that negative LE does not, in general, indicate stability, and that positive largest LE does not, in general indicate chaos [47].

In Figs.7 (a)–(d) we have computed the bifurcation diagrams with respect to δ_1, the external forcing amplitude on the response of the RVF model. Figures (e) and (f) show the maximal LE after infinitesimal perturbation of 10^{-10} in the initial conditions. In Fig.7(e), the maximal LE is positive for $\delta_1 \gtrsim 60$ and around 50 and 25. In Fig.7(f), the maximal LE is positive for $15 \lesssim \delta_1 \lesssim 34$ and for $\delta_1 \gtrsim 85$.

Figure 7 shows the bifurcation diagrams of the local maxima of infectious mosquitoes and livestock undergoing forward forking bifurcation from period-1 to period-6 oscillatory type behaviour. In Fig.7(a), local maxima extrema I_1 of infectious *Aedes* species undergo irregular behaviour for $\delta_1 \gtrsim 65$, which is the fingerprint of chaos. Fig.7(b) shows irregular behaviour for $15 \lesssim \delta_1 \lesssim 34$ and $\delta_1 \gtrsim 85$, with large number of periods. In Figs.7 (c) and (d), we observe almost the same qualitative behaviour with the same parameters, but with notable difference in the value of the local maxima of the overall infectious mosquitoes fuelled by the

elevation of several secondary vectors which serve as disease amplifiers. When $\delta_3 = 1.1$ the local extrema $A_2 + I_2$ undergoes irregular behaviour for $15 \lesssim \delta_1 \lesssim 34$ and $\delta_1 \gtrsim 85$, with large number of periods Fig.7(h).

We observe from Fig.7(e) that for a fixed $\delta_3 = 0.1$ and varying δ_1 $(0 \leq \delta_1 \lesssim 62)$ the largest Lyapunov exponent is fairly negative indicating stable limit cycles and multi-periodicity with some shift to positive values as the system bifurcates through period doubling routes to chaos. Above $\delta_1 = 62$ a positive Lyapunov exponent clearly moves away from zero, indicating deterministically chaotic attractors. For a fixed $\delta_3 = 1.1$ and varying δ_1 Fig.7(f) the largest Lyaponov exponent fairly confirms the behaviour seen through bifurcation diagrams with positive values on the chaotic regions.

0.7.5 Interaction between *Culex* and *Aedes* oviposition rates. In the preceding section we have fixed the value of δ_3, while investigating the bifurcation behaviour when δ_1 is varying. In Figure 8 we have computed the maximal LE when those two parameters are varying. For $20 \lesssim \delta_1, \delta_3 \lesssim 100$, the maximal LE is negative, then the system is sensitive to initial conditions. For low values of δ_3 and $18 \lesssim \delta_1, \delta_3 \lesssim 45$, the maximal LE is positive. Another remarkable fact is observed when δ_1 is around 10 no matter the value of δ_3, the maximal LE will be positive. This shows i fact that, *Aedes* oviposition rate is predominant in leading

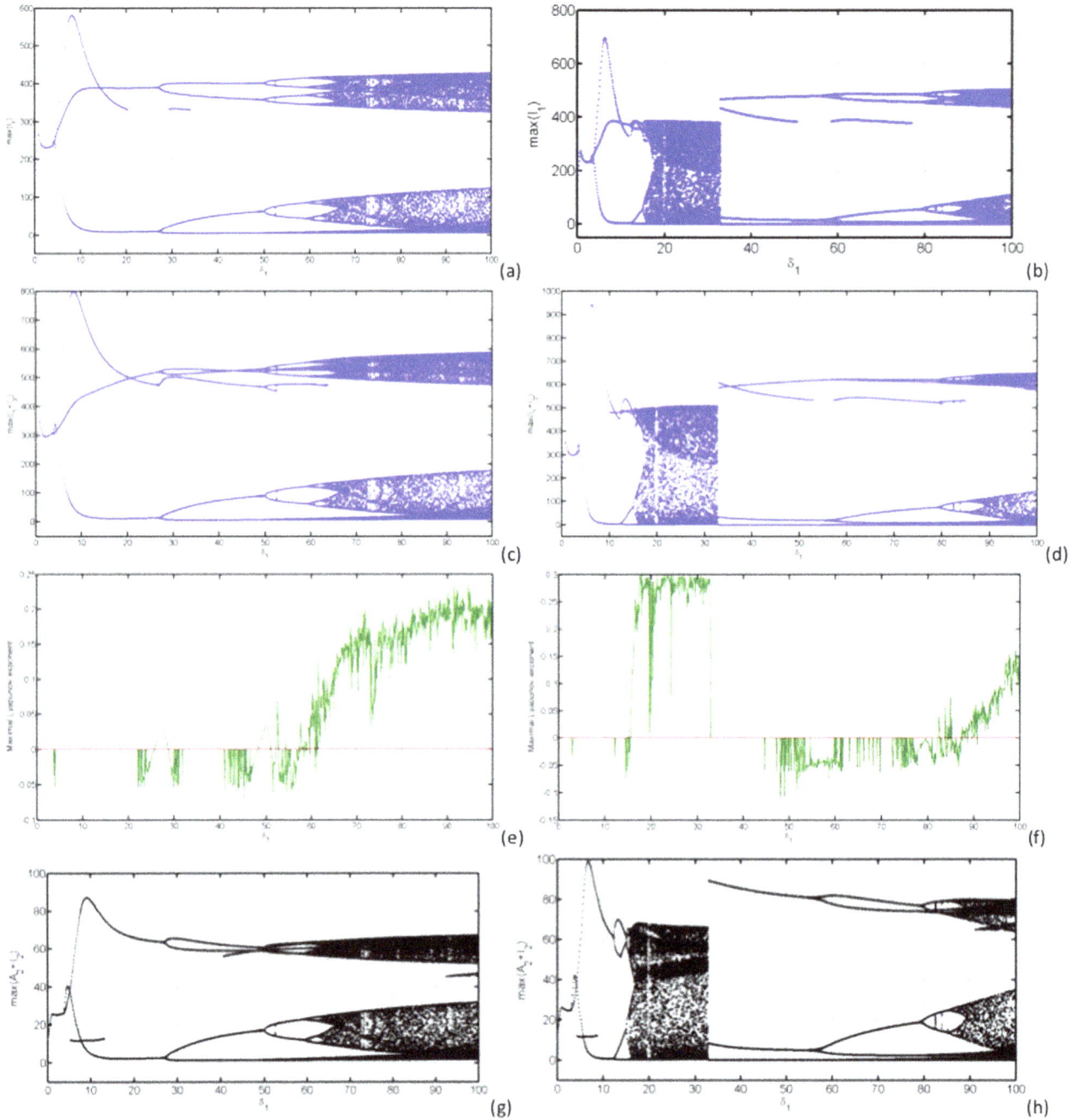

Figure 7. In (a) and (b), bifurcation diagrams for the local maximal quantities of I_1 **by varying the parameter** δ_1 **and fixing** $\delta_3 = 0.1$**(a) and** $\delta_3 = 1.1$**(b). In (c) and (d), bifurcation diagrams for the local maximal quantities of** $I_1 + I_3$ **by varying the parameter** δ_1 **and fixing** $\delta_3 = 0.1$**(c) and** $\delta_3 = 1.1$**(d). In (e) and (f), we have computed the largest LE for** $\delta_3 = 0.1$**(e) and** $\delta_3 = 1.1$**(f) and in (g) and (h), bifurcation diagrams for the local maximal quantities of** $A_2 + I_2$ **by varying the parameter** δ_1**, and fixing** $\delta_3 = 0.1$**(h) and** $\delta_3 = 1.1$**(f).**

irregular behaviour in our system, confirming that *Aedes* are indeed the RVF primary vectors.

Both maximal Lyapunov exponent functions of δ_1 and δ_3 and the Poincaré map of the set (δ_1, δ_3) fig.8 around $\delta_1 = 10$ agree with each other, confirming the analytical results obtained in Theorem 6.

Recall that in certain *Aedes* species of the subgenera *Neomelaniconion* and *Aedimorphus*, the female mosquitoes transmit RVF virus vertically to their eggs [3]. When these mosquitoes

lay their eggs in flooded areas, transovarially infected adults may emerge and transmit RVF virus to nearby domestic animals which may then lead to the infection of secondary arthropod vectors species including various *Culex* [48]. Thus, there is an initial quantity of primary infected vectors required to trigger an outbreak. Fig.8 shows that if the control magnitude of fluctuations in *Aedes* oviposition rate is around 10, and the number of newly transovarially infected mosquitoes is amplified by nearby domestic animals, then, the number of infected (in both host and vector) will

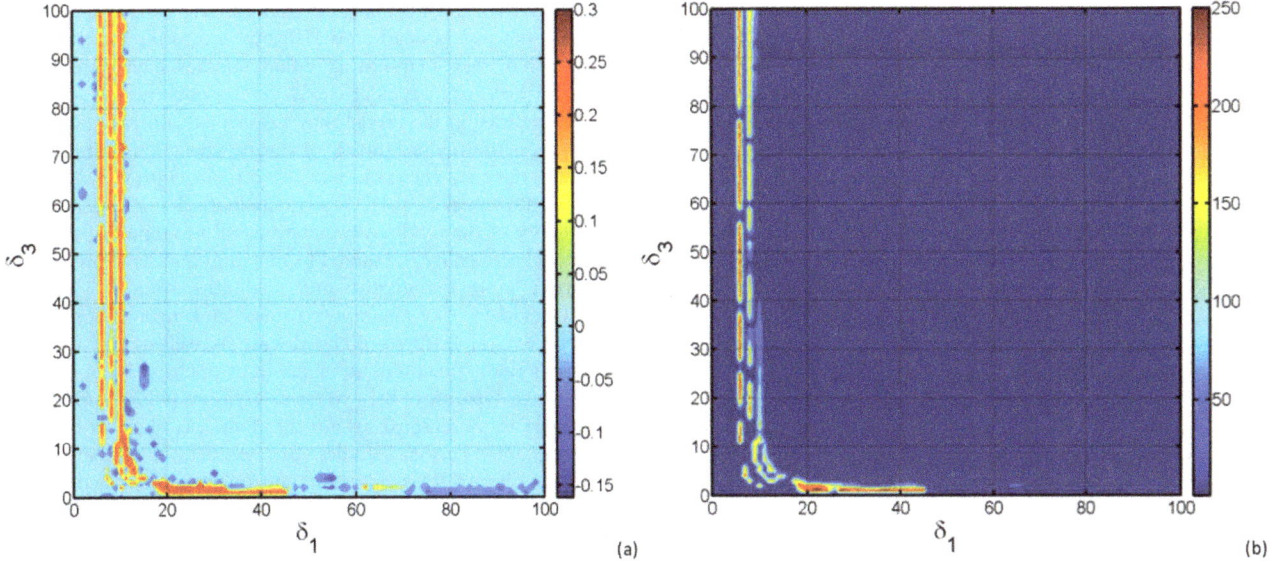

Figure 8. In (a) we display the maximal LE function of δ_1 **and** δ_3**.** The colorbar shows the value of the maximal LE. In (b) we display the number of points in the Poincaré map (the colorbar) according to the set of parameters (δ_1, δ_3).

be sufficiently enough to cause subsequent elevation of secondary vectors, including *Culex* species, and consequently trigger an outbreak.

Discussion and Conclusion

The proposed model accounts for the population dynamics of both livestock and mosquitoes (*Aedes* and *Culex*) and seasonal changes in weather that heavily affects the vector population size. Mosquito density varies over seasons, and the contact rates and vector oviposition rates vary dynamically based upon both host and vector densities since female mosquitoes need blood for oviposition. Qualitative analysis of the model showed that there exists a domain where the model is epidemiologically and mathematically well-posed. We then analysed the existence and stability of both disease free and endemic equilibria.

Dynamical analysis shows that when $R_0 < 1$, then the disease dies out and when $R_0 > 1$ the disease become endemic. A suitably constructed Lypunov function is used to determine the global stability of the endemic equilibrium of the model without *Culex* species and the existence of the endemic equilibrium of the overall model is seen to exist whenever $\frac{aR_0^1 - 1}{g_3 l_7} < I_1^* < \frac{\mu_1(\gamma_1 + \mu_1)R_0^1}{g_3 \gamma_1 b_2 l_7}$, meaning that the co-existence of the infectious host, *Aedes* and *Culex* mosquitoes is subjected to the number of infected *Aedes* mosquitoes.

We have used visualisation techniques to study the behaviour of RVF epidemic model under external forcing in the mosquito oviposition rates. The bifurcation diagrams show the emergence with increase in external forcing parameters δ_1, δ_3 of Hopf and pitchfork modes of bifurcation. That they have much larger amplification of infection levels that can take place if the system is encouraged to switch to multi-periodic mode. In transition, further amplification can occur if the multi-periodic mode becomes unstable and the system moves into chaotic state before finding an alternative stable periodic mode (e.g. Fig.7).

On the bifurcation diagrams the highest maximum number of infectious *Aedes* mosquitoes is only observed for values of δ_1

($\delta_1 < 10$) with different values of δ_3, meaning that for the disease to trigger an inter-epidemic a certain number of infectious *Aedes* mosquitoes is necessary. This confirm the analytical results obtain in section 0.6, as well as results obtained in [9] which showed that when mosquito populations follow seasonal patterns with large amplitudes, vertical transmission could play a significant role in long-term persistence of a pathogen. Another important conclusion is that even with a low maximum number of infectious individuals, the bifurcation diagrams show that if for fixed $\delta_3 = 1.1$ and varying δ_1 the system becomes chaotic in the interval $15 \lesssim \delta_1 \lesssim 35$, meaning that unpredictable and possibly uncontrolled low levels of inter-epidemic activities may occur, leading to higher morbidity in livestock. Hence observed fluctuations in RVF outbreak data and non deterministic nature of RVF inter-epidemic activities could now be better understood considering fluctuations on both rainy and dry season as significant factor.

A sero-survey study done in livestock approximately four years after the 2006/07 RVF outbreak in Tanzania, showed a linear increase in seroprevalence in the post-epidemic annual cohorts implying a constant exposure and presence of active foci transmission [10]. Figure 3 (d) and (f) demonstrate this behaviour which is shown to come in cycles of 5 to 7 years approximately, as well as fluctuations in the total number of infected from reasonable small peaks (describing RVF post-epidemic activities) to very low values. During these periods of low troughs for the total number of infected, the virus survive through vertical transmission in *Aedes* species and among wild animals as reservoirs [49]. Note that, this recurrent low level RVF virus activity during inter-epidemic periods, in East African region in particular, infects $1 - 3\%$ of livestock herds annually [50]. Generally, these infections pass undetected where there is no regular active surveillance in the livestock and human populations [10]. This suggests that RVF outbreaks partly result from build up RVF inter-epidemic activities for it has been observed that optimum climatic conditions (temperature and rainfall) only and presence of mosquitoes can not completely explain the RVF outbreaks [51].

Simulation of the interaction between the two populations densities of *Aedes* and *Culex* by varying the magnitudes of external forcing δ_1 and δ_3 of the oviposition rates b_1 and b_3 have opened a new window of research on the potential of *Aedes* species to initiate RVF outbreaks and sustain low endemic levels of the disease during inter-epidemic periods. This result concurs with the Chitnis et al. [9] suggestion that vertical transmission is required for inter-epidemic persistence.

One of the main objectives of this study was to investigate the possibility of prediction of RVF outbreaks with the aim of controlling RVF incidence. We have shown that seasonality may induce irregular behaviour on the disease dynamics. It has been shown that the interaction between oviposition rates of *Aedes* and *Culex* mosquitoes makes prediction more complex. In fact, higher irregularity are naturally expected in the higher seasonality forcing. However, our proposed model has shown that the complexity occurs even for a relatively low level of the magnitude of seasonal forces. We have also found that seasonal *Aedes* oviposition rate is most likely to generate uncontrollable behaviour than *Culex* seasonal oviposition rate. This study is of great epidemiological significance as it highlights a high uncertainty in RVF outbreak prediction by a simple theoretical mathematical model including seasonal influence in mosquito populations. In addition, the model including external seasonal forcing on mosquito oviposition rates shows ability to mimic the linear increase in livestock seroprevalence as reported in Sumaye et al. [10], with first post-epidemic peak around the second year, a following peak larger than the previous one around the fifth year (see Fig.3 (d) and (f)).

Currently, two types of RVF vaccine for animals exist: a live vaccine and inactivated vaccine. However, the current live vaccine can not be used for prevention and prevention using the inactivated vaccine is almost impossible to sustain in RVF affected countries for economic reasons [6,21,52]. Then, the possible alternative of controlling RVF transmission remains in keeping the vector population at the lowest levels. Therefore we argue that locations that may serve as RVF virus reservoirs should be eliminated or kept under control to prevent multi-periodic outbreaks and consequent chains of infections. We also recommend a systematic surveillance in the livestock or human population in order to monitor inter-epidemic RVF activities.

This study is not exhaustive and can be extend to include humans not just as dead ends [18] but also as disease amplifiers since it has been demonstrated that humans have potential to transmit the virus, particularly to *Aedes* mosquito species [8]. Also, including ticks on the model may help to explain and gain more insights on the understanding of disease dynamics and enhance control strategies, since ticks have been reported to play a role on disease transmission [51]. For mathematical convenience and tractability of the model, we made several assumptions, thus our results are driven by the model formulation and structure. A step toward a more quantitative and qualitative study is viable by relaxing some of the assumptions made and incorporating more epidemiological features of the disease as well as the use of a double periodic function and inclusion of stochasticity in order to capture the dynamic of the two rainfall seasons in East Africa (long and short rainy seasons), where the disease is likely to be more predominant. Further studies are needed to enhance the understanding of RVF epidemic and inter-epidemic activities in order to provide further insights in assessing the current and future control strategies.

Supporting Information

Appendix S1 A1. Computation of the basic reproduction number. A2. Computation of the basic reproduction number in periodic environments.

Acknowledgments

S.A. Pedro acknowledges with thanks the following institutions for support: German Academy Exchange Service (DAAD), International Center of Insect Physiology and Ecology (ICIPE), University of the Witwatersrand, Johannesburg, South Africa and Universidade Eduardo Mondlane, Mozambique. The conclusions are those of the authors and are not influenced by any institution.

Author Contributions

Conceived and designed the experiments: SAP HEZT RS SA. Performed the experiments: SAP FTN. Analyzed the data: SAP FTN. Contributed reagents/materials/analysis tools: SAP FTN. Wrote the paper: SAP FTN.

References

1. Megan JM, Bailey CL (1989) Rift Valley fever. Monath TP, ed. The Arboviruses: Epidemiology and Ecology. Volume IV. Boca Raton, FL: CRC Press Inc., pp.51–76.
2. Linthicum KJ, Anyamba A, Tucker CJ, Kelley PW (1999) Climate and satellite indicators to forecast Rift Valley fever epidemics in Kenya. Science: 285, pp.397–400.
3. Linthicum KJ, Davies FG, Kairo A, Bailey CL (1985) Rift Valley fever virus (family Bunyaviridae, genus Phlebovirus) isolations from Diptera collected during an interepizootic period in Kenya. J Hyg (Camb): 95, pp.197–209.
4. Logan TM, Linthicum KJ, Ksiazek TG, (1992) Isolation of Rift Valley fever virus from mosquitoes collected during an outbreak in domestic animals in Kenya. J Med Entomol 28: pp.293–295.
5. Ba Y, Diallo D, Kebe CMF, Dia I, and Diallo M (2005) Aspects of bioecology of two Rift Valley fever virus vectors in Senegal (West Africa): *Aedes vexans and Culex poicilipes* (Diptera: Culicidae). J. Med. Entomol. 42(5): pp.739–750.
6. Pépin M, Bouloy M, Bird BH, Kemp A, and Paweska J (2010) Rift Valley fever virus (Bunyaviridae: Phlebovirus): An update on pathogenesis, molecular epidemiology, vectors, diagnostics and prevention. Vet. Res. 41: p. 61.
7. Sang R, Kioko E, Lutomiah J, Warigia M, Ochieng C, (2010) Rift Valley Fever Virus Epidemic in Kenya, 2006/2007: The Entomologic Investigations. Am. J. Trop. Med. Hyg., 83(Suppl 2): pp.28–37.
8. Spickler AR (2006) Rift Valley Fever: infectious enzootic hepatitis of sheep and cattle. http://www.cfsph.iastate.edu/Factsheets/pdfs/riftvalleyfever.pdf.
9. Chitnis N, Hyman JM, Manore CA (2013) Modelling vertical transmission in vector-borne diseases with applications to Rift Valley fever. J. of Biological Dynamics, 7: 11–40, pp.1–4.
10. Sumaye RD, Geubbels E, Mbeyela E, Berkvens D (2013) Inter-epidemic Transmission of Rift Valley Fever in Livestock in the Kilombero River Valley,

Tanzania: A Cross-Sectional Survey. PLoS Negl Trop Dis 7(8): e2356, doi:10.1371/journal.pntd.0002356.
11. Bjornstad ON, Grenfell BT (2001) Noisy clockwork Time series analysis of population fluctuations in animals. Science 293: pp 638–643.
12. Gaff HD, Hartley DM, Leahy NP (2007) An epidemiological model of Rift Valley fever. Electron. J. Differ. Equ. (115): pp.1–12.
13. Kasari TR, Carr DA, Lynn TV, Weaver JT (2008) Evaluation of pathways for release of Rift Valley fever virus into domestic ruminant livestock, ruminant wildlife, and human populations in the continental United States. J. Am. Vet. Med. Assoc. 232(4): pp.514–529.
14. Romoser WS, Oviedo MN, Lerdthusnee K, Patrican LA, Turell MJ, et al (2011) Rift Valley fever virus-infected mosquito ova and associated pathology: Possible implications for endemic maintenance. Res. Rep. Trop. Med. 2: pp.121–127.
15. Turell MJ, Linthicum KJ, Patrican LA, Davies FG, Kairo A, et al (2008) Vector competence of selected African mosquito (diptera: Culicidae) species for Rift Valley fever virus. J. Med. Entomol. 45(1): pp.102–108.
16. Bird BH, Ksiazek TG, Nichol ST, MacLachlan NJ (2009) Rift Valley fever virus. J. Am. Vet. Med. Assoc. 234(7): pp.883–893.
17. Gaff H, Burgess C, Jackson J, Niu T, Papelis Y, et al (2011) Mathematical model to assess the relativebility of transmission of infection from an infectious mosquito to a susceptible & host given that a effectiveness of Rift Valley fever countermeasures. Int. J. Artif. Life Res. 2(2): pp.1–18.
18. Mpeshe SC, Haario H, Tchuenche JM (2011) A mathematical model of Rift Valley fever with human host. Acta Biotheor. 59(3–4): pp.231–250.
19. Parker MB (1986) Hatchability of eggs of Aedes taeniorhynchus(Diptera: Culicidae): effects of different temperatures and photoperiods during embryogenesis. Ann Entomol Soc Am 79: 925–930.

20. Rueda LM, Patel KJ, Axtell RC, Stinner RE (1990) Temperature-dependent development and survival rates of Culex quinquefasciatus and Aedes aegypti(Diptera: Culicidae). J Med Entomol 27: 892–898.
21. Mpeshe SC, Luboobi LS, Nkansah-Gyekye Y (2014) Modeling the Impact of Climate Change on the Dynamics of Rift Valley Fever. Computational and Mathematical Methods in Medicine, vol.2014, Article ID 627586, 12 pages.
22. Aguiar M, Paul R, Sakuntabai A, Stollenwork N (2014) Are we modelling the correct data? Minimizing false prediction for dengue fever in Thailand. Epidemiol. Infect. Cambridge University Press, pp 1–13.
23. Freud JA, Mieruch S, Scholze B, Wiltshire R, Freudel U (2006) Bloom dynamics in seasonally forced Phytoplankton-Zooplankton model: Trigger mechanism and timing effects. Ecol. Compl. 3: pp 129–139.
24. Greenman J, Kamo M, Boots M (2004) External forcing of Ecological and epidemiological systems: a resonance approach. Physica D 190: 136–151.
25. Ireland JM, Norman RA, Greenmann JV (2004) The effect of seasonal host birth rates on population dynamics The importance of resonance. J. Theor. Biol. 231: 229–238.
26. Davies FG, Martin V (2003) Recognizing Rift Valley Fever. FAO, Rome.
27. Geering WA, Davies FG, Martin V (2002) Preparation of Rift Valley Fever Contingency Plans. Food & Agriculture Organization of the UN (FAO), Rome.
28. Chevalier V, Rocque S, Baldet T, Vial L, Roger F (2004) Epidemiological processes involved in the emergence of vector-borne diseases: West Nile fever, Rift Valley fever, Japanese encephalitis and CrimeanCongo haemorrhagic fever. Rev. Sci. Tech. Office International des Epizooties 23(2): pp.535–556.
29. Turell MJ, Rossi CA, Bailey CL (1985) Effect of extrinsic incubation temperature on the ability of Aedes taeniorhynchus and Culex pipiens to transmit Rift Valley fever virus. Am. J. Trop. Med. Hyg. 34(6): pp.1211–1218.
30. Heffernan JM, Smith RJ, Wahl LM (2005) Perspectives on the basic reproductive ratio. J. R. Soc. Interface 2: 281–293.
31. Diekmann O, Heesterbeek JAP, Metz JAJ (1990) On the definition and the computation of the basic reproduction ratio R_0 in models for infectious diseases in heterogeneous populations. J. Math. Biol. 28(4): pp.365–382.
32. van den Driessche P, Watmough J (2002) Reproduction numbers and sub-threshold endemic equilibria for compartmental models of disease transmission. Math. Biosci. 180(1): pp.29–48.
33. Lipsitch M, Nowak MA, Ebert D, May RM (1995) The population dynamics of vertically and horizontally transmitted parasites. Proc. R. Soc. B 260: 321–327.
34. Grassly NC, Fraser C (2006) Seasonal infectious disease epidemiology. Proc. R. Soc. 273: 2541–2550.
35. Alligood KT, Sauer TD, York JA (1996) Chaos: An Introduction to Dynamical Systems. Springer-Verlag, New-York, Inc.
36. Bacaer N (2007) Approximation of the basic reproduction number R0 for vector-Borne diseases with a periodic vector population. Bull. Math. Biol. 69: 1067–1091.
37. Greenhalgh D, Griffiths M (2009) Backward bifurcation, equilibrium and stability phenomena in a three-stage extended BRSV epidemic model. J. Math. Biol. 59(1): 1–36.
38. Castillo-Chavez C, Feng Z, Huang W (2002) On the computation of R_0 and its Role on global stability. J. Math. Biol. 36: 227–248.
39. Korobeinikov A (2007) Global properties of infectious disease models with nonlinear incidence. Bull Math Biol 69: 1871–1886.
40. LaSalle JP (1976) The stability of dynamical systems. CBMS-NSF regional conference series in applied mathematics 25. SIAM, Philadelphia.
41. Li J, Blakeley D, Smith RJ (2011) The failure of R_0. Computational and Mathematical Methods in Medicine pp.1–17.
42. Fuchs BA, Levin BI (1961) Functions of a Complex Variable and Some of their Applications. vol. 2. Pergamon Press.
43. Pedro SA, Tchuenche JM (2010) HIV/AIDS dynamics: Impact of economic classes with transmission from poor clinical settings. Journal of Theoretical Biology 267: 471–485.
44. Press WH, Flannery BP, Teukolsky S, Vettering WT (1986) Numerical Recipes: The Art of Scientific Computing. Cambrige University Press.
45. Parker TS, Chua LO (1983) Practicals Numericals Algorithms for Chaotic Systems. Springer-Verlag, New-York Inc.
46. Gould H, Tobochnik J (1996) An Introduction to Computer Simulation Methods: Applications to Physical Systems. Second edition, Addison-Wesley, New-York.
47. Perron O (1930) Die Stabiltatsfrage bei differentialgleichumgen. Mathematische Zeitschrift bd. 32: pp 702–728.
48. Davies FG, Linthicum KJ, James AD (1985) Rainfall and epizootic Rift Valley fever. Bull World Health Organ 63: 941–943.
49. Munyua P, Murithi RM, Wainwright S, Githinji J, Hightower A, et al (2010) Rift Valley Fever Outbreak in Livestock in Kenya, 2006–2007. Am. J. Trop. Med. Hyg., 83(Suppl 2) pp.58–64.
50. Davies FG, Kilelu D, Linthicum KJ, Pegram RG (1992) Patterns of Rift Valley fever activity in Zambia. Epidemiol Infect 108: 185–191.
51. Nchu F. Rand A (2013) Rift Valley fever outbreaks: Possible implication of Hyalomma truncatum (Acari: Ixodidae). Afr. J. Microbiol. Res. Vol. 7(30): pp.3891–3894. DOI: 10.5897/AJMR12.2144.
52. FAO (2012) Rift Valley Fever: Vigilance Needed in the Coming Months. EMPRES WATCH, vol.27.

6

A Retrospective Study on the Epidemiology of Anthrax, Foot and Mouth Disease, Haemorrhagic Septicaemia, Peste des Petits Ruminants and Rabies in Bangladesh, 2010-2012

Shankar P. Mondal*¤, Mat Yamage

Food and Agriculture Organization of the United Nations, Dhaka, Bangladesh

Abstract

Anthrax, foot and mouth disease (FMD), haemorrhagic septicaemia (HS), peste des petits ruminants (PPR) and rabies are considered to be endemic in Bangladesh. This retrospective study was conducted to understand the geographic and seasonal distribution of these major infectious diseases in livestock based on data collected through passive surveillance from 1 January 2010 to 31 December 2012. Data analysis for this period revealed 5,937 cases of anthrax, 300,333 of FMD, 13,436 of HS, 247,783 of PPR and 14,085 cases of dog bite/rabies. While diseases were reported in almost every district of the country, the highest frequency of occurrence corresponded to the susceptible livestock population in the respective districts. There was no significant difference in the disease occurrences between districts bordering India/Myanmar and non-border districts (p>0.05). Significantly higher (p<0.01) numbers of anthrax (84.5%), FMD (88.3%), HS (84.9%) and dog bite/rabies (64.3%) cases were reported in cattle than any other species. PPR cases were reported mostly (94.8%) in goats with only isolated cases (5.2%) in sheep. The diseases occur throughout the year with peak numbers reported during June through September and lowest during December through April, with significant differences (p<0.01) between the months. The annual usages of vaccines for anthrax, FMD, HS and PPR were only 7.31%, 0.61%, 0.84% and 11.59% of the susceptible livestock population, respectively. Prophylactic vaccination against rabies was 21.16% of cases. There were significant differences (p<0.01) in the administration of anthrax, FMD and HS vaccines between border and non-border districts, but not PPR or rabies vaccines. We recommend that surveillance and reporting of these diseases need to be improved throughout the country. Furthermore, all suspected clinical cases should be confirmed by laboratory examination. The findings of this study can be used in the formulation of more effective disease management and control strategies, including appropriate vaccination policies in Bangladesh.

Editor: Jagat K. Roy, Banaras Hindu University, India

Funding: The study was supported by the United States Agency for International Development. The views expressed in this manuscript do not necessarily represent the position of the US Government. The funders had no role in study design, data collection and analysis, decision to publish, or preparation of the manuscript.

Competing Interests: The authors have declared that no competing interests exist.

* Email: shankarpm@yahoo.com

¤ Current address: Maxwell H. Gluck Equine Research Center, Department of Veterinary Science, University of Kentucky, Lexington, Kentucky, United States of America

Introduction

Bangladesh, located in South Asia, is one of the most densely populated countries in the world with an estimated 1,033 people/km^2 [1]. It also has the highest density of livestock (cattle, goats, sheep and buffaloes) in the world with an estimated 145 large ruminants/km^2 compared with 90 for India and 20 for Brazil [2]. Despite declining acreage of pasture land, the livestock population is growing steadily. Livestock are an integral component of agriculture in Bangladesh that includes the provision of draft power and manure. About 20% of the human population is directly and 50% is partly dependent on the livestock sector [3]. Bangladesh has an estimated 52.8 million livestock, mostly food producing cattle and goats [4]. Despite the significant livestock population, the current production of meat and milk is inadequate to meet current requirements of the human population and respective deficits have been estimated at 85.9% and 73.1% [5]. Infectious diseases are of critical importance in livestock production. Economic losses are attributable to decreased animal growth and productivity as well as frequent death of affected animals. Important diseases are foot and mouth disease (FMD), haemorrhagic septicaemia (HS), anthrax in large ruminants (cattle) and peste des petits ruminants (PPR) in small ruminants. Rabies has only begun to be addressed as a major public health threat.

FMD is one of the most important animal diseases currently causing severe economic losses in the South Asian region [6]. FMD, caused by a member of the *Aphthovirus* genus, family *Picornaviridae* [7], is an extremely contagious, acute viral disease primarily of all cloven-hoofed animals [8]. Annual losses due to FMD in Bangladesh are estimated at about US$62 million [9]. Recently, the country has confirmed outbreaks of FMD virus types O and A which are closely related to virus types active in India and

Nepal [10,11]. PPR is usually a disease of small ruminants [12], caused by a member of the *Morbillivirus* genus, family *Paramyxoviridae* [13]. PPR was first isolated in Bangladesh during a major occurrence in 1993 [14]. Since then, the disease has been recognized as endemic in goat. Outbreaks can be associated with up to 75% morbidity and 55% mortality in Black Bengal goats [15]. HS (caused by *Pasteurella multocida*) is another economically important bacterial disease of cattle and buffaloes [16] causing high rates of morbidity and mortality. HS, together with anthrax and black quarter (BQ; not included in this study), are responsible for an estimated economic loss of US$148.6 million each year [17]. Anthrax (caused by *Bacillus anthracis*) is endemic in South Asian countries including Bangladesh [18,19,20]. An anthrax outbreak occurred in 2009–2010 resulting in a serious problem in animals and humans; this led to the government declaring a "red alert" in 2010 [21]. Rabies, caused by a member of the *Lyssavirus* genus, family *Rhabdoviridae*, is transmitted mostly (>90%) by the bite of infected dogs to humans [22] and domestic animals [23] in Bangladesh, as in other Asian countries [24]. Bangladesh ranks third in the world after India and China in the number of rabies cases of livestock and/or humans [25]. Bangladesh continues to experience outbreaks of these diseases in livestock despite vaccination (except rabies) as part of a government effort to control them. Major factors to account for the continuing problem include inadequate monitoring, surveillance and disease reporting, lack of public awareness, lack of any controls over animal movements, inadequate management and vaccination strategies.

To effectively combat the threats posed by the selected and other diseases, there is a need for clear understanding of the epidemiology of the respective diseases [26]. The goal of an epidemiological study is to identify risk factors that need to be taken into consideration in the development of effective control measures. Information on the incidence of major infectious diseases (e.g., FMD) in livestock is available from a number of countries in which the diseases have been reported [27,28]. While there have been some studies of the incidence and distribution of FMD [29,30], PPR [31], HS [32,33], anthrax [19,20] and dog bite/rabies cases [23,33] in livestock in Bangladesh, the geographic areas and duration involved in such studies are too limited to reflect more accurately the national status. The Food and Agriculture Organization of the United Nations (FAO) provided technical assistance to the Government of Bangladesh (GoB) to undertake an analysis using passive surveillance data of the overall disease situation in livestock in the country. Accordingly, this study was conducted to investigate the geographic and seasonal distributions of anthrax, FMD, HS, PPR and dog bite/rabies in livestock throughout the country, based on available passive surveillance data for the period January 2010 to December 2012.

Methods

Geography of the study area

Bangladesh has a unique geographical location with an area of 147,570 km². The country is exceedingly flat, low-lying and subject to annual flooding, except for the narrow hilly regions in the northeast and southeast. It has one of the largest deltas of the world formed by two main rivers, Padma (Ganges in India) and Jamuna (Brahmaputra in India), which become confluent as a single river (Padma). The country has land boundaries totaling 4,246 km, of which the vast majority are with India and only 193 km at the southeastern border are with Myanmar (Figure 1). The existence of formal and informal cross-border movement of animals, animal products and feed is a traditional practice among the countries in the region. Bangladesh is divided into 7 divisions, 64 districts and 487 sub-districts or upazilas (an upazila is a lower administrative unit in the country). The livestock population is approximately 52.8 million, consisting of 23.2 million cattle, 1.4 million buffaloes, 25.1 million goats and 3.1 million sheep [4]. The majority of livestock are reared by smallholders in integrated agricultural farming systems.

Data source

For this study, passive surveillance animal disease data at the upazila level were determined from January 2010 to December 2012 (both months inclusive). Data were obtained from the Epidemiology Unit of the Department of Livestock Services (DLS), Dhaka, Bangladesh. The latter unit was established with technical support from the FAO after highly pathogenic avian influenza (HPAI) H5N1 virus was detected in the country in 2007. Bangladesh has a government-financed veterinary network that extends to the upazila level where it is headed by the Upazila Livestock Officer (ULO). Clinical records are kept at the upazila veterinary hospitals for all cases treated by staff veterinarians. Usually, animals seen by clinicians are sick animals presented by farmers. ULOs send monthly passive surveillance reports to the district level office (DLO), which in turn are sent to the Epidemiology Unit of DLS. This unit is responsible for carrying out outbreak investigations and specimen collection, compilation and analysis of disease reports. The current study was based on analysis of monthly reports for 2010 from 418 upazilas of 62 of the 64 districts (74% upazila coverage), for 2011 from 478 upazilas of all 64 districts (87% upazila coverage) and for 2012 from 471 upazilas of 63 districts (91% upazila coverage). No disease reports were available from Rangamati and Feni districts in 2010 and from Bandarban district in 2012.

For the purpose of this study, a case is defined as an animal with a history, clinical signs or lesions characteristic of anthrax, FMD, HS, PPR or dog bite/rabies; in some instances, there was supportive laboratory data from examination of pathological samples [34,35]. The term "dog bite" is used for a suspected rabies case as every animal bite (mostly dog bite) is potentially suspected as coming from a rabid animal. The signs/lesions are sufficient for registered veterinarians to make a provisional diagnosis of the endemic diseases in Bangladesh. Demographic data, such as date (month) animal was seen by clinicians, owner's address (upazila, district and division), animal species involved, disease diagnosed and utilization of vaccine were included in the reports. To avoid duplication with number of animals treated (especially in case of follow up visits), the status of the diseases is described using only newly reported cases.

Data analysis

Descriptive and temporal analysis. The data, obtained from DLS in Microsoft Access database, were transferred to a spreadsheet program (Excel 2007, Microsoft) (spreadsheet is available on request). Descriptive statistical analysis was conducted to examine the frequencies and annual patterns of anthrax, FMD, HS, PPR and dog bite/rabies occurrences. Three years' (2010 to 2012) data were aggregated into monthly estimated number of diagnosed cases, death cases and vaccination coverage against each disease; time series plots were created for each disease to visualize possible trends and seasonality. Each year was divided into the four main weather seasons in Bangladesh [36]: (1) pre-monsoon (March to May), (2) monsoon (June to August), (3) post-monsoon (September to November) and (4) winter (December to February). The seasonal distribution was assessed by summing the frequency of cases into these four seasons. The estimated number

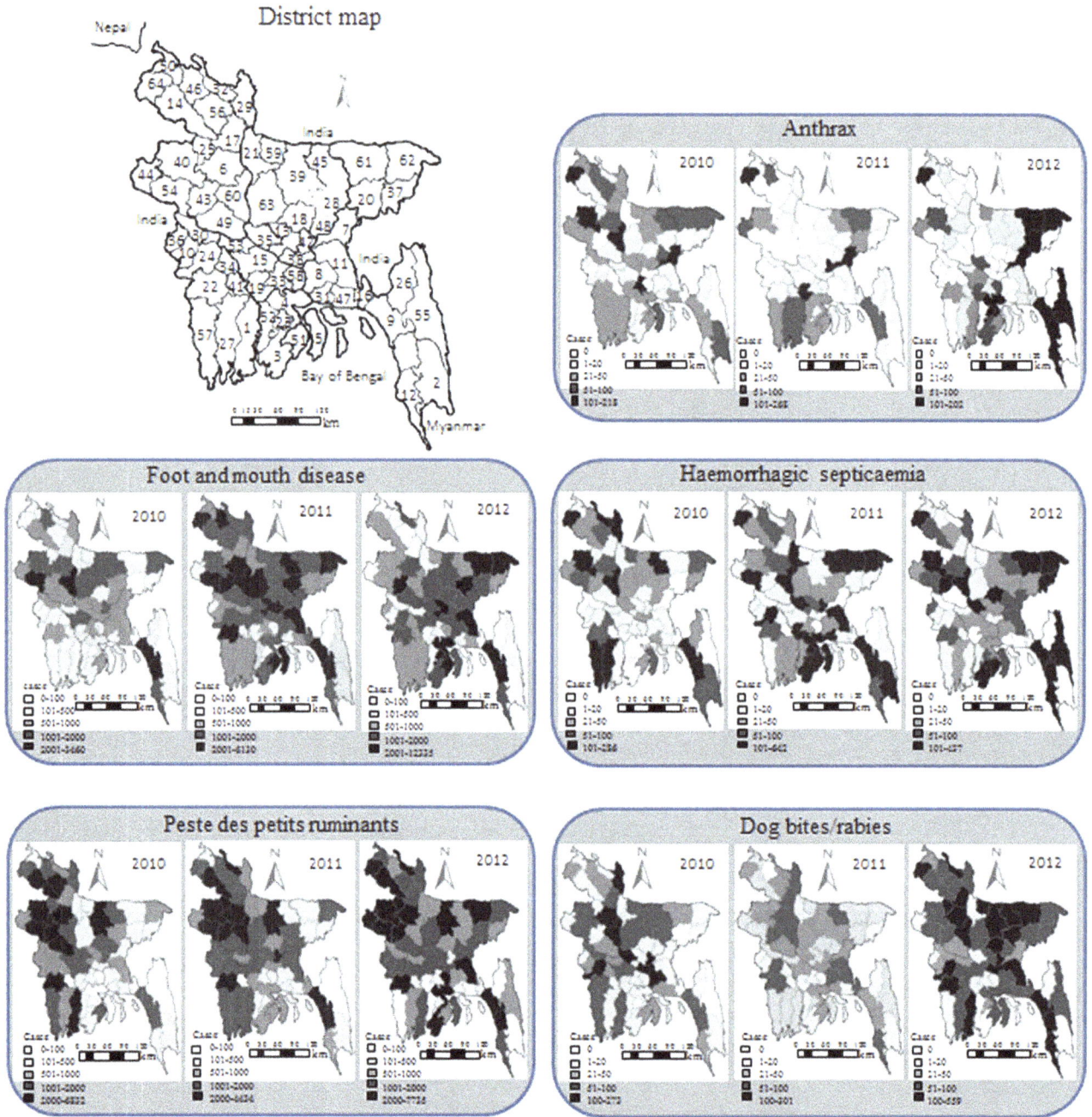

Figure 1. Map of Bangladesh showing 64 districts (top left): 1) Bagerhat, 2) Bandarban, 3) Barguna, 4) Barisal, 5) Bhola, 6) Bogra, 7) Brahmanbaria, 8) Chandpur, 9) Chittagong, 10) Chuadanga, 11) Comilla, 12) Cox's Bazar, 13) Dhaka (the capital), 14) Dinajpur, 15) Faridpur, 16) Feni, 17) Gaibandha, 18) Gazipur, 19) Gopalganj, 20) Habiganj, 21) Jamalpur, 22) Jessore, 23) Jhalokathi, 24) Jhenaidaha, 25) Joypurhat, 26) Khagrachhari, 27) Khulna, 28) Kishoreganj, 29) Kurigram, 30) Kushtia, 31) Laksmipur, 32) Lalmonirhat, 33) Madaripur, 34) Magura, 35) Manikganj, 36) Meherpur, 37) Moulvibazar, 38) Munshiganj, 39) Mymensingh, 40) Naogaon, 41) Narail, 42) Narayanganj, 43) Natore, 44) Nawabganj, 45) Netrokona, 46) Nilphamari, 47) Noakhali, 48) Norsingdi, 49) Pabna, 50) Panchgarh, 51) Patuakhali, 52) Pirojpur, 53) Rajbari, 54) Rajshahi, 55) Rangamati, 56) Rangour, 57) Satkhira, 58) Shariatpur, 59) Sherpur, 60) Sirajganj, 61) Sunamganj, 62) Sylhet, 63) Tangail, 64) Thakurgaon. The maps illustrate district distribution of the estimated number of diagnosed cases of anthrax, foot and mouth disease, haemorrhagic septicaemia, peste des petits ruminants and dog bite/rabies cases reported in livestock (cattle, goats, sheep and buffaloes) in the country, 2010–12.

of diagnosed cases was calculated under a null hypothesis that each disease report was independent of particular time of the year. Observed and expected numbers were computed by Chi-square test using GraphPad Software (www.graphpad.com/quickcalcs/index.cfm) to evaluate the association between the disease report

and time of the year. Analysis of level of significance was conducted for diagnosed/death cases per 1,000 animals examined and for vaccination rates per 10,000 susceptible animals.

Spatial analysis. Adobe Fireworks CS5.1 software program (Adobe Systems Inc., 345 Park Avenue San Jose, CA) was used to create maps for district distribution of the diseases in livestock in Bangladesh. Available case reports in any species of livestock (all ruminants for anthrax, FMD, HS and dog bite/rabies, and small ruminants for PPR) were aggregated at the district level and demonstrated in the map for yearly distribution of each disease (Figure 1). Since these diseases were reported from most of the districts of Bangladesh, the frequencies of cases in each district were presented separately for three years (2010 to 2012) to describe the annual distribution of reported cases in these districts.

Results

Descriptive analysis

From January 2010 through December 2012, records of 4,728,522 clinical cases in livestock (including 2,900,621 cattle, 1,545,831 goats, 141,707 sheep and 139,737 buffaloes) were collected from DLS veterinary clinics through a nation-wide passive surveillance program. Of the clinical diseases under study, the breakdown of numbers of reported cases are anthrax (5,937), FMD (300,333), HS (13,436), PPR (247,783) and dog bite/rabies (14,085) (Table 1). Except for anthrax, the number of reports of other diseases was higher in 2011 or 2012 than 2010. Anthrax cases were reported more in 2010 (n = 2,174) than 2011 (n = 1,668) or 2012 (n = 2,095). The mean reported prevalence rate (based on number of livestock examined) was highest for PPR (14.68%: 95% CI 14.63–14.74%), which was calculated based on the number of goats and sheep examined only, followed by FMD (6.35%: 6.33–6.37%), dog bite/rabies (0.30%: 0.29–0.30%), HS (0.28%: 0.28–0.29%) and anthrax (0.13%: 0.12–0.13%). The case fatality rate (CFR) was highest for cases of dog bite/rabies (24.32%: 95% CI 23.61–25.03%), followed by anthrax (13.49%: 12.62–14.37%), PPR (4.86%: 4.77–4.94%), HS (2.87%: 2.59–3.16%) and FMD (1.31%: 1.27–1.35%). The CFR of anthrax was reported higher in 2010 (19.92%) than in 2011 (10.37%) or 2012 (9.31%). Based on a livestock census conducted in 2005 in Bangladesh [5], reports of vaccination coverage against any of the five diseases were very low. The maximum coverage was against PPR (11.59%: 95% CI 11.58–11.60%) in susceptible small ruminants, followed by anthrax (7.31%: 7.31–7.32%), HS (0.84%: 0.83–0.84%) and FMD (0.61%: 0.60–0.61%) in all susceptible ruminants. Rabies vaccine used as post-exposure prophylaxis and calculated based on the number of total reported dog bite cases was 21.16% (95% CI 20.48–21.84%).

Geographic distribution

The spatial distribution of reported anthrax, FMD, HS, PPR and dog bite/rabies cases from January 2010 to December 2012 in livestock from different districts of Bangladesh is presented in Figure 1 and Tables S1–S3. Based on the overall data from 2010–2012, of the 487 upazilas in the country, anthrax and HS were reported in 169 (34%) and 186 (38%) upazilas from 61 of the 64 districts, respectively, and FMD, PPR and dog bite/rabies cases were reported in 445 (91%), 401 (82%) and 253 (52%) upazilas from all 64 districts of the country, respectively. The number of anthrax reports was highest in Thakurgaon (10%), Naogaon (8.4%), Bagerhat (7%), Sirajganj (5.1%) and Brahmanbaria (4.9%) districts in 2010; in Thakurgaon (16.1%), Narayanganj (12.3%), Brahmanbaria (8.5%) and Gopalganj (7.5%) districts in 2011; and in Rangamati (9.6%), Sunamganj (8.6%), Sylhet (8.5%), Brahmanbaria (7.4%) and Thakurgaon (6.9%) in 2012 (Figure 1 and Table S1); this accounted for 35.5%, 44.3% and 41.0% of all anthrax cases reported in the respective year. Sirajganj (a milk shed area) reported one of the highest number of anthrax cases in 2010, but this district did not have any reported cases of anthrax in

2011 or 2012. In all three years (2010 to 2012), stable and the highest number of FMD cases were reported in Chittagong, Sylhet, Rajshahi, Tangail, Bogra and Sirajganj districts; this accounted for 29.1%, 17.8% and 13.8% of all FMD cases reported, respectively. The Comilla district reported only a few FMD cases (1.8%) in 2010, but this district reported the highest number of FMD cases in 2011 (5.7%) and 2012 (7.6%). Thakurgaon, Chittagong and Sirajganj districts consistently reported the highest HS cases in all three years; this accounted for 18.8%, 16.7% and 13.9% of all HS cases reported in the respective year. The Barguna district reported none and Patuakhali reported only a few HS cases in 2010, but these two districts reported higher numbers of HS cases in 2011 (16.6%) and 2012 (17.2%). Consistently high PPR cases were reported in Jessore, Rajshahi, Bogra, Mymensingh, Naogaon and Chittagong districts during this three-year period; this accounted for 32.0%, 25.6% and 26.4% of all PPR cases reported, respectively. The number of dog bite/rabies reports was consistently high in Sirajganj, Munshiganj, Jhenaidaha, Bogra, Gaibandha, Narayanganj, Jessore and Chandpur districts in three years; this accounted for 42.5%, 32.9% and 34.9% of all dog bite/rabies cases reported, respectively. The two hilly districts Rangamati and Khagrachhari had the lowest number of disease cases. The annual patterns of the diseases in six upazilas with maximum reported cases are shown in Table S2. In 2010, Ranishankail upazila (Thakurgaon district) reported the highest number of both anthrax (n = 105, 4.83%) and HS (n = 232, 8.34%) cases, and Charghat (Rajshahi), Badarganj (Rangpur) and Lahajang (Munshiganj) reported the highest number of FMD (n = 1,664, 3.76%), PPR (n = 1,391, 2.0%) and dog bite/rabies (n = 240, 8.19%) cases, respectively. In 2011, Sonargaon upazila (Narayanganj district) reported the highest number of both anthrax (n = 183, 10.97%) and PPR (n = 1,459, 1.86%) cases, and Kaliganj (Lalmonirhat) and Patuakhali Sadar (Patuakhali) reported the highest number of FMD (n = 1,493, 1.59%) and HS (n = 373, 6.34%) cases, respectively. In 2012, Belaichhari (Rangamati district), Nalchhiti (Jhalokati), Baraigram (Natore) and Lalmonirhat Sadar (Lalmonirhat) reported the highest number of anthrax (n = 165, 7.88%), FMD (n = 4,830, 2.98%), HS (n = 434, 9.10%) and PPR (n = 2,790, 2.80%) cases, respectively. Shahjadpur upazila (Sirajganj district) reported the highest number of dog bites/rabies cases in both 2011 (n = 213, 5.46%) and 2012 (n = 329, 4.54%). Occurrence of the diseases corresponded to the number of susceptible livestock in the respective districts (Table S1). Further analysis showed that 50% of the districts (32/64) bordering India (31) and Myanmar (1) reported nearly equal numbers of cases compared to reports in non-border districts; there was no significant difference (p>0.05) between them (Table S3).

Species susceptibility

Table 2 shows the distribution of reported anthrax, FMD, HS, PPR and dog bite/rabies cases in different livestock species (cattle, goats, sheep and buffaloes) in Bangladesh. Data analysis showed that significantly higher (p<0.01) numbers of anthrax (84.5%), FMD (88.3%), HS (84.9%) and dog bite/rabies (64.3%) cases were reported in cattle than any other species. PPR cases were mostly reported in goats (94.8%) with the remainder in sheep (5.2%). The CFR of anthrax and dog bite/rabies were significantly higher (p<0.01) in cattle (15.5% and 31.4%, respectively) than other species (≤3.2% and ≤15.5%, respectively), but the CFR of HS was significantly higher (p<0.01) in buffaloes (7.9%) than cattle (2.0%) or goats/sheep (0%). The difference in the CFR of FMD or PPR between the species was not statistically significant (p>0.05).

Table 1. Estimated number of diagnosed cases, death cases and vaccination coverage of anthrax, foot and mouth disease, haemorrhagic septicaemia, peste des petits ruminants and dog bite/rabies in livestock (cattle, goats, sheep and buffaloes) in Bangladesh, 2010–2012.

Disease	2010	2011	2012	Total
Anthrax				
Diagnosed cases	2,174	1,668	2,095	5,937
Prevalence rate, % (95% CI*)	0.14 (0.13–0.15)[δ]	0.09 (0.08–0.09)	0.17 (0.16–0.18)	0.13 (0.12–0.13)
Death cases	433	173	195	801
Case fatality rate, % (95% CI)	19.92 (18.23–21.61)	10.37 (8.90–11.84)	9.31 (8.06–10.56)	13.49 (12.62–14.37)
Vaccination	2,602,967	3,417,136	3,325,525	9,345,628
Vaccination rate, % (95% CI)	6.11 (6.10–6.12)[†]	8.02 (8.01–8.03)	7.81 (7.80–7.82)	7.31 (7.31–7.32)
Foot and mouth disease				
Diagnosed cases	44,314	93,968	162,051	300,333
Prevalence rate, % (95% CI*)	2.81 (2.79–2.84)	4.95 (4.92–4.99)	12.91 (12.85–12.97)	6.35 (6.33–6.37)
Death cases	651	1,566	1,721	3,938
Case fatality rate, % (95% CI)	1.47 (1.36–1.58)	1.67 (1.58–1.75)	1.06 (1.01–1.11)	1.31 (1.27–1.35)
Vaccination	253,084	213,654	311,718	778,456
Vaccination rate, % (95% CI)	0.59 (0.59–0.60)	0.50 (0.49–0.50)	0.73 (0.73–0.74)	0.61 (0.60–0.61)
Haemorrhagic septicaemia				
Diagnosed cases	2,782	5,885	4,769	13,436
Prevalence rate, % (95% CI*)	0.18 (0.17–0.18)	0.31 (0.30–0.32)	0.38 (0.37–0.39)	0.28 (0.28–0.29)
Death cases	64	221	101	386
Case fatality rate, % (95% CI)	2.30 (1.74–2.86)	3.76 (3.27–4.24)	2.12 (1.71–2.53)	2.87 (2.59–3.16)
Vaccination	272,395	367,862	433,101	1,073,358
Vaccination rate, % (95% CI)	0.64 (0.63–0.64)	0.86 (0.86–0.87)	1.02 (1.01–1.02)	0.84 (0.83–0.84)
Peste des petits ruminants				
Diagnosed cases	69,684	78,441	99,658	247,783
Prevalence rate, % (95% CI*)	12.08 (11.99–12.16)	11.27 (11.20–11.35)	24.01 (23.88–24.14)	14.68 (14.63–14.74)
Death cases	4,417	4,094	3,523	12,034
Case fatality rate, % (95% CI)	6.34 (6.16–6.52)	5.22 (5.06–5.38)	3.54 (3.42–3.65)	4.86 (4.77–4.94)
Vaccination	1,514,476	2,127,698	2,427,648	6,069,822
Vaccination rate, % (95% CI)	8.67 (8.66–8.69)[‡]	12.19 (12.17–12.20)	13.91 (13.89–13.92)	11.59 (11.58–11.60)
Dog bite/rabies[θ]				
Diagnosed cases	2,930	3,904	7,251	14,085
Prevalence rate, % (95% CI*)	0.19 (0.17–0.19)	0.21 (0.20–0.21)	0.58 (0.56–0.59)	0.30 (0.29–0.30)
Death cases	781	1,159	1,485	3,425
Case fatality rate, % (95% CI)	26.66 (25.05–28.27)	29.69 (28.25–31.13)	20.48 (19.55–21.41)	24.32 (23.61–25.03)
Vaccination	579	767	1,634	2,980
Vaccination rate, % (95% CI)	19.76 (18.31–21.21)[‡]	19.64 (18.39–20.90)	23.54 (21.57–23.50)	21.16 (20.48–21.84)

*CI = Confidence intervals.
[δ]Calculated based on the number of livestock (cattle, buffaloes, sheep and goats) examined, which is 1,576,562 in 2010; 1,896,815 in 2011; and 1,255,145 in 2012 (only sheep and goats 576,936 in 2010; 695,845 in 2011; and 415,007 in 2012).
[†]Calculated based on susceptible livestock population (buffaloes, cattle, goats and sheep) in Bangladesh, which is 42,594,399 [5].
[‡]Calculated based on goat and sheep population only, which is 17,459,061 [5].
[θ]The term "dog bite" is used for a suspected rabies case as every animal bite (mostly dog bite) is potentially suspected as rabid animal bite, as the rabies control program in animals is nonexistent in Bangladesh [22].
Calculated based on reported dog bite cases assuming that all death cases are from rabies.

Temporal distribution

Monthly and seasonal distribution of anthrax, FMD, HS, PPR and dog bite/rabies reports from January 2010 through December 2012 are presented in Figure 2 and Table S4. All five diseases were reported throughout the year in livestock (Figure 2). The highest number of anthrax cases was reported in the month of August (n = 704, 11.9%) followed by July (11.3%); FMD in November (n = 37,204, 12.4%) followed by June (10.2%); HS in September (n = 1,893, 14.1%) followed by August (9.3%); PPR in June (n = 23,962, 9.7%) followed by August (9.3%); and dog bite/rabies in September (n = 1,612, 11.5%) followed by August (11.2%). The lowest number of anthrax, FMD, HS, PPR and dog bite/rabies reports

Table 2. Species distribution of estimated number of diagnosed cases and death cases of anthrax, foot and mouth disease, haemorrhagic septicaemia, peste des petits ruminants and dog bite/rabies in livestock in Bangladesh, 2010–2012.

Disease[δ]	Species	2010		2011		2012		Total	
		Diagnosed cases (%)	Death cases (CFR[θ], %)	Diagnosed cases (%)	Death cases (CFR, %)	Diagnosed cases (%)	Death cases (CFR, %)	Diagnosed cases (%)	Death cases (CFR, %)
Anthrax	Buffaloes	67 (3.1)	0	83 (5.0)	3 (3.6)	125 (5.97)	3 (2.4)	275 (4.63)	6 (2.18)
	Cattle	1879 (86.4)*	423 (22.5)*	1278 (76.6)*	165 (12.9)*	1858 (88.69)*	188 (10.12)*	5015 (84.47)*	776 (15.47)*
	Goats	220 (10.1)	10 (4.6)	270 (16.2)	5 (1.9)	112 (5.35)	4 (3.57)	602 (10.14)	19 (3.16)
	Sheep	8 (0.4)	0	37 (2.2)	0	0	0	45 (0.76)	0
FMD	Buffaloes	1015 (2.3)	2 (0.2)	3187 (3.4)	62 (2.0)	4596 (2.84)	4 (0.09)	8798 (2.93)	68 (0.77)
	Cattle	39694 (89.6)*	593 (1.5)	81515 (86.8)*	1277 (1.6)	143953 (88.83)*	1579 (1.10)	265162 (88.29)*	3449 (1.30)
	Goats	3444 (7.8)	56 (1.6)	8662 (9.2)	209 (2.4)	12287 (7.58)	134 (1.09)	24393 (8.12)	399 (1.64)
	Sheep	161 (0.3)	0	604 (0.6)	18 (3.0)	1215 (0.75)	4 (0.33)	1980 (0.66)	22 (1.11)
HS	Buffaloes	215 (7.7)	4 (1.9)	834 (14.2)	110 (13.2)*	907 (19.02)	41 (4.52)	1956 (14.56)	155 (7.92)*
	Cattle	2496 (89.7)*	60 (2.4)	5051 (85.8)*	111 (2.2)	3859 (80.92)*	60 (1.56)	11406 (84.89)*	231 (2.03)
	Goats	66 (2.4)	0	0	0	3 (0.06)	0	69 (0.51)	0
	Sheep	5 (0.2)	0	0	0	0	0	5 (0.04)	0
PPR	Goats	66717 (95.7)*	4229 (6.3)	73066 (93.1)*	3862 (5.3)	95096 (95.42)*	3414 (3.59)	234879 (94.79)*	11505 (4.90)
	Sheep	2967 (4.3)	188 (6.3)	5375 (6.9)	232 (4.3)	4562 (4.58)	109 (2.39)	12904 (5.21)	529 (4.10)
Dog bite	Buffaloes	33 (1.1)	0	32 (0.8)	9 (28.1)	64 (0.88)	11 (17.19)	129 (0.92)	20 (15.50)
/rabies	Cattle	2235 (76.3)*	705 (31.5)	2604 (66.7)*	939 (36.0)	4217 (58.16)*	1201 (28.48)*	9056 (64.30)*	2845 (31.42)*
	Goats	606 (20.7)	69 (11.4)	1133 (29.0)	209 (18.5)	2763 (38.11)	269 (9.74)	4502 (31.96)	547 (12.15)
	Sheep	56 (1.9)	7 (12.5)	135 (3.5)	2 (1.5)	207 (2.86)	4 (1.93)	398 (2.83)	13 (3.27)

[δ]Abbreviated: FMD = Foot and mouth disease, HS = Haemorrhagic septicaemia, PPR = Peste des petits ruminants.
[θ]CFR = Case fatality rate.
*Statistically significant at the $p < 0.01$ level.

was in December (5.4%), February (5.9%), April (5.4%), March (6.9%) and May (5.2%), respectively. There were significant differences between the months in the reported cases of each disease (p<0.01). When the overall data were grouped into the four main weather seasons in Bangladesh [36] (Table S4), the highest number of anthrax reports was observed in monsoon (34%), FMD in pre-monsoon (26.7%) followed by monsoon (26.3%), HS in post-monsoon (34%), PPR in monsoon (27.8%) and dog bite/rabies in post-monsoon (28.4%) followed by monsoon (26.7%). The lowest number of anthrax, FMD, HS, PPR and dog bite/rabies cases was reported in post-monsoon (20.5%), winter (20.9%), pre-monsoon (21.4%), winter (21.8%) and pre-monsoon (19.6%) season, respectively. There were significant differences (p<0.05) between the seasons on the occurrences of anthrax, HS, PPR and dog bite/rabies, but not FMD (p = 0.13). The highest number of death cases for each disease corresponded to the highest number of cases reported in the respective season. There was no significant differences (p> 0.05) in the CFR of anthrax, FMD, PPR or dog bite/rabies between the seasons, but the CFR for HS was significantly different between the seasons (p<0.01).

Vaccination

Geographic (border *vs.* non-border districts) and monthly distribution of vaccination coverage against anthrax, FMD, HS, PPR and rabies from January 2010 through December 2012 are presented in Figure 2 and Table S3. Based on the 2005 livestock census in Bangladesh [5], there were significant differences (p< 0.01) between border and non-border districts on the coverage of anthrax (6.14% and 8.91%, respectively), FMD (0.46% and 0.81%, respectively) and HS (0.69% 1.04%, respectively) vaccines, but not (p>0.05) PPR (12.24% and 10.60%, respectively) or rabies (19.68% and 23.51%, respectively) vaccines (Table S3). Sirajganj district reported the highest (>30%) coverage of anthrax vaccine in livestock in 2010. Significantly higher (p<0.0001) coverage of PPR vaccine was reported in southern Khulna and northern Rajshahi divisions (where the goat population is very high [5]) compared to the national average, which accounted for 16.8% of all vaccinations reported during this three-year period. The highest coverage of anthrax, FMD, HS, PPR and rabies vaccines was in June (13%), June (13.2%), October (12.4%) followed by June (11.2%), June (14.6%) and May (14.3%), respectively, and lowest in January (5.3%), July (4.8%), July (5.3%), July (5.8%) and October (5.1%), respectively (Figure 2).

Discussion

This is the first retrospective analysis of the geographic and seasonal distribution of anthrax, FMD, HS, PPR and dog bite/ rabies cases in livestock in Bangladesh. The data show that i) the diseases occur across the country irrespective of border and non-border districts, but the highest frequency of occurrence corresponded to the number of susceptible livestock in respective districts; ii) most of the reported anthrax, FMD, HS and dog bite/ rabies cases are in cattle and PPR in goats, the two predominant livestock species in the country [4]; iii) the diseases occur throughout the year but the highest frequency of occurrence are in the months of June through September (mostly during the monsoon season) and lowest in December through April (mostly during the winter season); and iv) the vaccination coverage against each of the diseases studied is inadequate, especially for anthrax, FMD and HS in the border districts. Therefore, it would be appropriate to target geographic areas and time of the year for future disease surveillance and control programs in the country.

When the reported data were analyzed based on geographic locations, consistently high numbers of cases for all five diseases were reported in Sirajganj, Narayanganj, Bogra, Chittagong, Thakurgaon and Naogaon districts (Figure 1 and Table S1), the latter three all border with India. The noted differences in disease occurrence could be due to high density of animal populations and widespread movement of animals between countries and within the country with mixing where animals are pastured or in animal markets. Sirajganj (a milk shed area) has a history of reporting high clinical cases of FMD (n = 3,708) in 1999 [37]; this district confirmed anthrax almost exclusively during 2009–2010 [19,20]. Whereas, Narayanganj is a small, densely human populated industrial area close to Dhaka (the capital); this has seen high numbers of cases of rabies during 2004–2008 [22] and in 2010 [38]. Data showed that the ratio of border/non-border cases with anthrax, FMD, HS, PPR or rabies infection was nearly equal (Table S3), with no significant difference between them (p>0.05). However, there is molecular evidence that the FMD virus (types O and A) recently isolated in Bangladesh were closely related to FMD viruses in circulation in India and Nepal [10,11]. Also, the recent PPR virus strains detected in Bangladesh and the neighboring countries including India, Nepal and Pakistan belong to the same lineage IV [39]. India and Nepal consume less meat especially beef, due to religious reasons. Therefore, the price differences encourage constant informal cross-border animal movement from India and Nepal to Bangladesh, with most animals being destined for the large cities. There are no border controls or animal quarantine [40] between the three countries. Moreover, cross-border movement of free-roaming dogs from India and Myanmar, two highly rabies-endemic countries in the world [41], could explain the persistent, high incidence of rabies in Bangladesh [22]. A considerable number of cattle come from Myanmar also. Several studies have confirmed cross-border animal movements as one of the main reasons for the spread and persistence of FMD [6,42], HS [16] and PPR [39,43]. During movement, these animals frequently infect local susceptible animal populations along the transportation routes [44]. The infected animals help to maintain virus circulation throughout the year. Live animal markets are held once or twice a week in most upazilas of Bangladesh. All disease-susceptible farm animals are sold at these markets. Previous studies have demonstrated a correlation between the market chain of livestock and the geographical spread of FMD [26] and PPR [45]. Animals receive minimum preventive veterinary care in Bangladesh, which further increases the risk of acquiring infections.

Cattle were the predominant species affected with anthrax (Table 2), which is consistent with anthrax reports from north-western Bangladesh during 2009–2010 [19]. Cattle are also known to be highly susceptible to inhalation of aerosolized FMD virus [46] and can become persistently infected [47]. This species was found to account for the highest number of cases of FMD in this study. This is consistent with the FMD epidemiology in Bhutan [28], India [48] and Nepal. Factors responsible may include the fact that cattle are the most populous species of livestock found in Bangladesh; cattle graze in plains (usually in large groups) whereas goats graze in the high lands (in small groups or individually); and, due to the higher economic value of cattle over goats and sheep, sick cattle are more often referred for veterinary attention. Buffaloes are more susceptible to HS than cattle [49], which explains the high CFR of HS in this species (Table 2). The overall low CFR of anthrax in all livestock species could be due to production of immunity by massive vaccination, early diagnosis and treatment of sick animals presented by farmers or the likely biases in the reporting system (see below). Rabies is not a notifiable

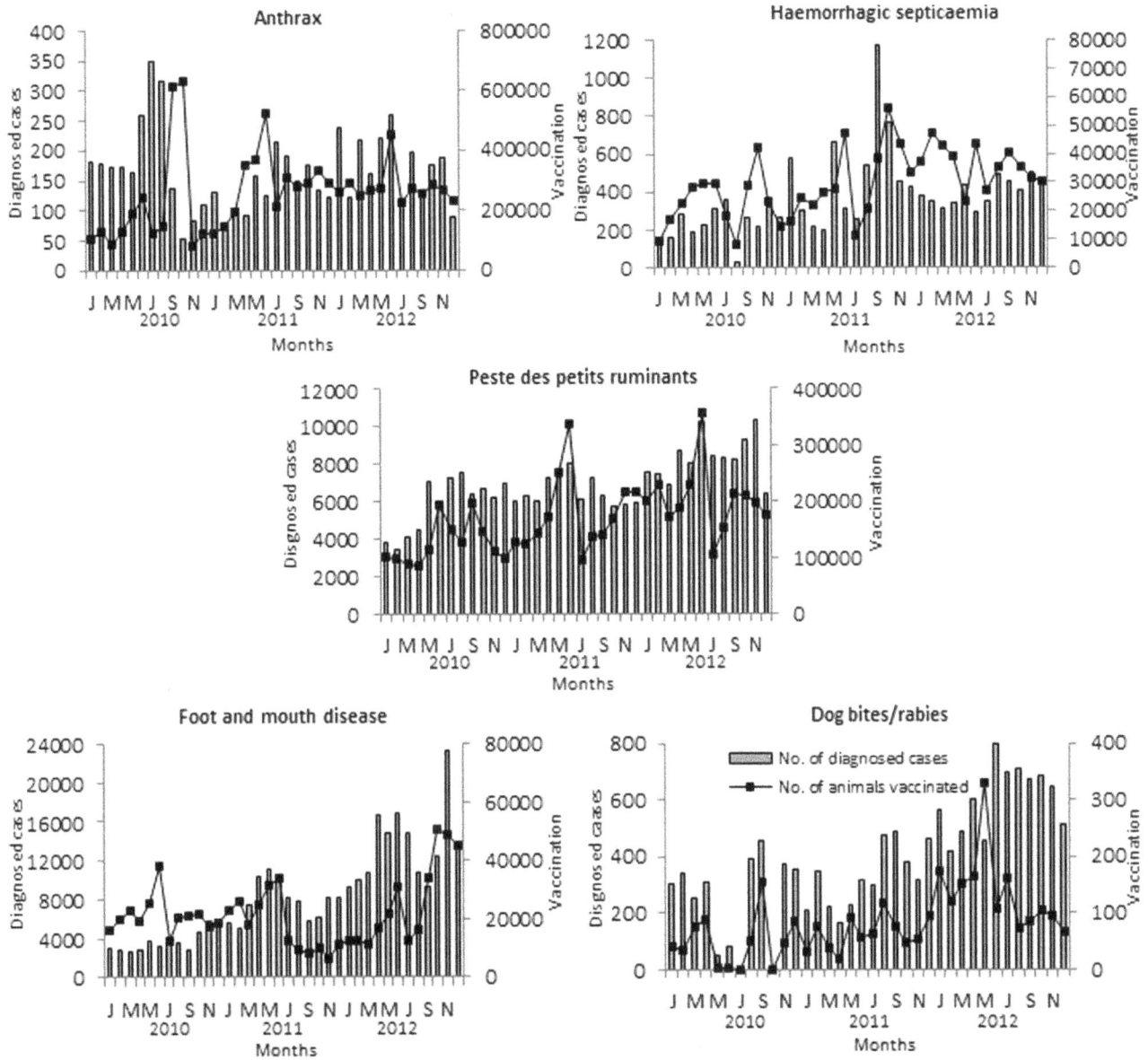

Figure 2. Monthly distribution of animal diseases and vaccination status in Bangladesh, 2010–2012. It represents the estimated number of diagnosed cases and vaccination of anthrax, foot and mouth disease, haemorrhagic septicaemia, peste des petits ruminants and dog bite/rabies reported in livestock (cattle, goats, sheep and buffaloes) in the country.

disease in Bangladesh, so the surveillance data in animals and humans are scarce. A comprehensive study by Hossain et al. [22] determined 732 human rabies cases (0.5%) out of 150,068 animal bite cases treated from 2005 through 2008, most of which were the result of dog bites (90.7%). In our study, 3,425 animal fatalities (24.32%) were reported out of 14,085 dog bites in livestock during 2010–2012. More dog bite/rabies cases were reported in goats than anthrax, FMD and HS cases probably due to more availability and easy access of this species by street dogs in village areas, or possibly more goat owners brought sick animals to the clinics. In Bangladesh, the proportion of goats to sheep is about 8:1 [4]. In this study, a higher number of PPR cases was observed in goats than sheep (16:1); this is consistent with the PPR epidemiology in India [44,45] suggesting that differences in the

virulence between species could be due to greater innate resistance in sheep.

In this study, reports of infectious disease occurrences throughout the year (mostly during the monsoon season) are consistent with the previous reports for anthrax [19], FMD [10,36], HS [33] and animal bite/rabies [22] cases in Bangladesh. Sudden anthrax outbreaks occurred in animals during July–August (monsoon) in 2010 (Figure 2). Environmental factors, including high ambient temperature and relative humidity that provide a milieu for germination of anthrax spores from infected carcasses thrown into flood waters or in open fields [20], may favor the presence of anthrax in Bangladesh [50]. During the rainy season, grass harvested along with roots might also harbor anthrax spores and when fed, livestock can become infected [19]. Moist conditions also prolong the survival of the HS organism (*P. multocida*), and thus the disease tends to spread more rapidly during the monsoon season when rice cultivation also brings about movements of animals [16]. Increased numbers of dog bite/rabies reports during post-monsoon and monsoon may be associated with the breeding season of dogs [51]. A significantly higher number of FMD cases during April–June (pre-monsoon) and November in 2012 (Figure 2) could be due to the increased movement of animals from outside and within the country for trade purposes during this particular year. The movement of livestock for management and husbandry purposes is important for local spread of disease [28]. Stress can also suppress the development of immunity and hence predispose an animal to infection [52]. In this study, more PPR cases in goats and sheep were also reported during the monsoon season (Table S4). This could be due to limited availability of feed during the summer and wet seasons and close confinement of goats in the households during this period of the year [44]. Introduction of new animals into the flocks could be another possibility. The feeding habits of goats are quite different from cattle (see above). Climate factors favorable for the survival and spread of the virus may also contribute to the seasonal distribution of PPR [53]. As opposed to our finding, a local study in Bangladesh reported highest PPR cases in the months of December–January and lowest in June–July [31]. This may not reflect the disease situation in the entire country. Therefore, it is difficult to draw any conclusions as the differences in sampling procedures may also affect conclusions [54]. Further studies may be necessary to better understand the seasonality of animal diseases in Bangladesh.

There is a routine anthrax, FMD, HS and PPR vaccination program for livestock in Bangladesh; however, the vaccination coverage was found to be very low (Table 1). The country has a capacity of annual production of only 3.4 million doses of anthrax vaccine, 0.4 million doses of bivalent (O, A) inactivated FMD vaccine, 0.8 million doses of formalin-killed HS vaccine and nearly 10 million doses of live attenuated PPR vaccine [55]. At present, Bangladesh is not producing any rabies vaccine. Tissue culture vaccine (TCV) is currently being imported from abroad mainly for humans [22]. For routine vaccination of livestock, DLS distributes locally produced animal vaccines (usually 100 ml/vial) at a subsidized rate of US$0.75 (50 taka). The abrupt decline in the numbers of anthrax cases in September–October in 2010 (Figure 2) could be due to production of immunity in many animals by massive vaccination by the government in particular areas (e.g., Sirajganj) of the country. Apparently, animals vaccinated against anthrax >6 months ago may not retain sufficient immunity resulting from the use of the attenuated Sterne strain vaccine in Bangladesh [56]. The efficacy of PPR vaccine is also a question due to its poor thermal stability and inadequate cold chain system in the country [57]. WHO recommends that 70% of a country's dog population should be vaccinated to eliminate or prevent outbreaks of rabies [58]; however, rabies vaccinations in dogs or stray dog elimination programs are very limited especially in rural parts of Bangladesh [25]. Development of a protective level of immunity against any disease requires effective vaccines. As part of vaccination campaigns, DLS should assess vaccine efficacy, develop a strategy to improve coverage and conduct serosurveillance to determine coverage and duration of immunity. There is a need for more accurate means to evaluate the dog population and good rabies vaccination coverage. The current government program on modernization of livestock vaccine production is expected to dramatically increase the production of quality vaccines, and the vaccination program will

be implemented in disease prevalent areas which will alter disease epidemiology.

Retrospective studies, based on data collected through passive surveillance, have contributed greatly in understanding animal disease epidemiology in Bhutan [28], India [48,59] and Laos [60]. For a resource limited country like Bangladesh, passive surveillance can also play an important role in the overall surveillance system. However, the findings in this study need to be interpreted with caution because of the likely biases in the reporting system. First, although there has been no dramatic change in the surveillance for the diseases during the 2010 through 2012 study period, some minor differences in the reporting system may have occurred. Apparently, more monthly reports were missing (e.g., Rangamati and Feni districts) from 2010 than from 2011 or 2012. Some over-reporting of disease data (e.g., anthrax cases) may have occurred from some upazilas depending on the level of enthusiasm of the responsible livestock authority, which is not unexpected in a disease endemic country [61]. Second, some underreporting (e.g., anthrax deaths) may have occurred due to a lack of awareness of farmers. We assumed these possible variables remained relatively constant during the study period. Third, the number of laboratory confirmed cases was not available; this may not be critical since anthrax, FMD, HS, PPR and rabies cases are not difficult to diagnose in endemic countries based on clinical signs. However, some reporting biases may have been associated with cattle because buffaloes generally show no/mild signs of FMD and can serve as silent spreaders of the disease. The biases occurring from clinical diagnosis of the FMD in cattle are expected to be low because cattle are the predominant species in Bangladesh and clinical signs are more discernible in this species compared to other FMD-susceptible species [62]. Fourth, sometimes bite status may not be associated with rabies cases in livestock, as smallholding farmers who raise their livestock in public fields or rice fields may not know whether their cattle had been bitten by a rabid animal [63]. Owner's interviews tend to be biased if the owners or their caretakers did not recognize abnormal changes in their animals. However, typical signs of rabies are very distinct and a misdiagnosis is unusual. The distinct late-stage clinical signs of rabies together with history of a dog bite mean that although misdiagnosis of other viral encephalitides remains a possibility, it is unlikely [64]. Fifth, the limited manpower restricts the ability of the veterinary authorities to respond to all reported cases. Introduction of web-based software, namely Livestock Disease Information System (LDIS), recently developed with the support from FAO ECTAD for reporting livestock diseases in Bangladesh, will enable tracking field cases of all diseases on a daily basis. Since use of the cell phone-Web based SMS-(Short Message Service) Gateway system has been successful with the surveillance of HPAI H5N1 in Bangladesh [65] and is popular nationally and internationally, this can also be of value for the surveillance of other important animal diseases.

In conclusion, this study provides information about the widespread distribution of anthrax, FMD, HS, PPR and dog bite/rabies in Bangladesh. The underlying factors could result from differences in the animal husbandry practices in different geographic locations, culture habits of animal uses, agro-climatic factors, lack of regulation of animal movements, lack of adequate vaccination and lack of knowledge about the epidemiology of the diseases. We recommend that the disease surveillance should be improved throughout the country, including a need for laboratory (serologic and molecular) confirmation of clinical cases. Probably, the most significant would be the identification and monitoring the circulation of the pathogens in the free-range and household animal populations. The findings from the present study constitute baseline data and provide the prompt for further investigation to better understand the epidemiology of important livestock diseases in Bangladesh.

Supporting Information

Table S1 District distribution of estimated number of diagnosed cases of anthrax, foot and mouth disease, haemorrhagic septicaemia, peste des petits ruminants and dog bite/rabies in livestock in Bangladesh, 2010–2012 (10 of the 64 districts with highest reported cases of each disease are highlighted as light grey for each year and as dark grey for three-year total).

Table S2 Upazila distribution of estimated number of diagnosed cases of anthrax, foot and mouth disease, haemorrhagic septicaemia, peste des petits ruminants and dog bite/rabies in livestock in Bangladesh, 2010–2012 (6 of the 487 upazilas in the country with maximum reported cases of each disease are presented).

Table S3 Geographic distribution (border *vs.* non-border districts) of estimated number of diagnosed cases and vaccination coverage of anthrax, foot and mouth disease, haemorrhagic septicaemia, peste des

petits ruminants and dog bite/rabies in livestock in Bangladesh, 2010–2012.

Table S4 Seasonal distribution of estimated number of diagnosed cases of anthrax, foot and mouth disease, haemorrhagic septicaemia, peste des petits ruminants and dog bite/rabies in livestock in Bangladesh, 2010–2012.

Acknowledgments

The authors are thankful to the Department of Livestock Services (DLS), Bangladesh for allowing use of this data for the current study and express gratitude to the staff members of the Epidemiology Unit and all field officers of DLS for their help in the disease reporting process. The authors would like to thank Alim-Al-Razi, Bimal Karmakar, Saiful Islam and Salma Khatun for their assistance with processing data, and Diane Furry for her support with creating the maps. Thanks are extended to Udeni Balasuriya, Peter Timoney, Roberta Dwyer and Kathleen Shuck for examining the manuscript.

Author Contributions

Conceived and designed the experiments: MY SPM. Performed the experiments: SPM. Analyzed the data: SPM. Contributed reagents/materials/analysis tools: SPM MY. Wrote the paper: SPM.

References

1. United Nations (2011) Department of Economic and Social Affairs, Population Division: World Population Prospects: The 2010 Revision. New York.
2. BARC Bangladesh (2010) Agricultural Research Priority: Vision-2030 and Beyond (Sub-sector: Livestock). Bangladesh Agriculture Research Council, Farmgate, Dhaka.
3. Bangladesh Economic Review (2009) Ministry of Finance, Government of Bangladesh.
4. Department of Livestock Services (2012) Ministry of Fisheries and Livestock Services, Government of Bangladesh.
5. Bangladesh Bureau of Statistics (2010) Agriculture Census 2005. Available: http://www.bbs.gov.bd/. Assessed May 2011.
6. Sumption K, Rweyemamu M, Wint W (2008) Incidence and distribution of foot-and-mouth disease in Asia, Africa and South America; combining expert opinion, official disease information and livestock populations to assist risk assessment. Transbound Emerg Dis 55: 5–13.
7. Mumford JA (2007) Vaccines and viral antigenic diversity. Rev Sci Tech 26: 69–90.
8. Grubman MJ, Baxt B (2004) Foot-and-mouth disease. Clin Microbiol Rev 17: 465–493.
9. FAO/OIE (2012) FMD virus pools and the regional programmes Virus Pool 2-South Asia. FAO/OIE Global Conference on foot and mouth disease control. Bangkok, Thailand, 27–29 June 2012.
10. Loth L, Osmani MG, Kalam MA, Chakraborty RK, Wadsworth J, et al. (2011) Molecular characterization of foot-and-mouth disease virus: implications for disease control in Bangladesh. Transbound Emerg Dis 58: 240–246.
11. Nandi SP, Rahman MZ, Momtaz S, Sultana M, Hossain MA (2013) Emergence and Distribution of Foot-and-Mouth Disease Virus Serotype A and O in Bangladesh. Transbound Emerg Dis. doi:10.1111/tbed.12113.
12. Lefèvre PC, Diallo A (1990) Peste des petits ruminants virus. Scientific and Technical Review. Office International des Epizooties 9: 951–965.
13. Gibbs EP, Taylor WP, Lawman MJ, Bryant J (1979) Classification of peste des petits ruminants virus as the fourth member of the genus Morbillivirus. Intervirology 11: 268–274.
14. Sil BK, Rahman MM, Taimur MJFA, Sarker AJ (1995) Observation of outbreaks of PPR in organized goat farms and its control strategy. In Proceedings of Annual Conference of the Bangladesh Society for Veterinary Education and Research. December 3, 2005, BARC, Dhaka.
15. Islam MR, Shamsuddin M, Rahman MA, Das PM, Dewan ML (2001) An outbreak of peste des petits ruminants in Black Bengal goats in Mymensingh, Bangladesh. The Bangladesh Veterinarian 18: 14–19.
16. De Alwis MCL, Wijewardana TG, Gomis AIU, Vipulasiri AA (1990) Persistence of the carrier state in haemorrhagic septicaemia (*Pasteurella multocida* serotype 6: B infection) in buffaloes. Trop Anim Health Pro 22: 185–194.
17. Ahmed S (1996) Status of some bacterial diseases of animals in Bangladesh. Asian Livest 21: 112–114.
18. Ray TK, Hutin YJ, Murhekar MV (2009) Cutaneous anthrax, West Bengal, India, 2007. Emerg Infect Dis 15: 497–499.
19. Biswas PK, Islam MZ, Shil SK, Chakraborty RK, Ahmed SS, et al. (2012) Risk factors associated with anthrax in cattle on smallholdings. Epidemiol Infect 140: 1888–1895.
20. Chakraborty A, Khan SU, Hasnat MA, Parveen S, Islam MS, et al. (2012) Anthrax outbreaks in Bangladesh, 2009–2010. Am J Trop Med Hyg 86: 703–710.
21. Siddiqui MA, Khan MA, Ahmed SS, Anwar KS, Akhtaruzzaman SM, et al. (2012) Recent outbreak of cutaneous anthrax in Bangladesh: clinico-demographic profile and treatment outcome of cases attended at Rajshahi Medical College Hospital. BMC Res Notes 5: 464.
22. Hossain M, Bulbul T, Ahmed K, Ahmed Z, Salimuzzaman M, et al. (2011) Five-year (January 2004–December 2008) surveillance on animal bite and rabies vaccine utilization in the Infectious Disease Hospital, Dhaka, Bangladesh. Vaccine 29: 1036–1040.
23. Rahman MS, Afroz1 MA, Roy U, Bari FY (2010) Analysis of Clinical Case Records from Some Villages Around Bangladesh Agricultural University (BAU) Veterinary Clinic. Int J BioRes 2: 17–20.
24. WHO 2011. http://www.searo.who.int/LinkFiles/CDS rabies.pdf.
25. Hossain M, Ahmed K, Marma AS, Hossain S, Ali MA, et al. (2013) A survey of the dog population in rural Bangladesh. Prev Vet Med 111: 134–138.
26. Perry BD, Gleeson LJ, Khounsey S, Bounma P, Blacksell SD (2002) The dynamics and impact of foot and mouth disease in smallholder farming systems in South-East Asia: a case study in Laos./Rev Sci Tech 21: 663–673.
27. Chhetri BK, Perez AM, Thurmond MC (2010) Factors associated with spatial clustering of foot-and-mouth disease in Nepal. Trop Anim Health Pro 42: 1441–1449.
28. Dukpa K, Robertson ID, Edwards JR, Ellis TM (2011) A retrospective study on the epidemiology of foot-and-mouth disease in Bhutan. Trop Anim Health Pro 43: 495–502.
29. Mannan MA, Siddique MP, Uddin MZ, Parvaz MM (2009) Prevalence of foot and mouth disease (FMD) in cattle at Meghna upazila in Comilla in Bangladesh. J Bangladesh Agril Univ 7: 317–319.
30. Sarker S, Talukder S, Islam MH, Gupta SD (2011) Epidemiological study of foot-and-mouth disease in cattle: Prevalence and risk factors assessment in Rajshahi, Bangladesh. Wayamba J Ani Sci. March 10, 2011.
31. Sarker S, Islam MH (2011) Prevalence and Risk Factor Assessment of Peste des petits ruminants in Goats in Rajshahi, Bangladesh. Vet World 4: 546–549.
32. Pharo HJ (1987) Analysis of Clinical Case Records from Dairy Co-operatives in Bangladesh. Trop Anim Health Pro 19: 136–142.
33. Debnath NC, Sil BK, Selim SA, Prodhan MAM, Howlader MMR (1990) A retrospective study of calf mortality and morbidity on smallholder traditional farms in Bangladesh. Prev Vet Med 9: 1–7.
34. Rosenberger G (1979) Clinical Examination of Cattle. 2nd ed., Verlag Paul Parey, Germany.
35. Samad MA (2000) Veterinary Practitioner's Guide. 1st pub., LEP pub. No. 07.BAU Campus, Mymensingh.

36. Chowdhury SMZH, Rahman MF, Rahman MB, Rahman MM (1993) Foot and mouth disease and its effects on mortality, morbidity, milk yield and draft power in Bangladesh. AJAS 6: 423–426.

37. Howlader MMR, Mahbub-E-Elahi ATM, Habib S, Bhuyian MJU, Siddique MAB, et al. (2004) Foot and Mouth Disease in Baghabari Milk Shed Area and It's Economic Loss in Bangladesh. J Biol Sci 4: 581–583.

38. Jamil KM, Ahmed K, Hossain M, Matsumoto T, Ali MA, et al. (2012) Arctic-like rabies virus, Bangladesh. Emerg Infect Dis 18: 2021–2024.

39. Banyard AC, Parida S, Batten C, Oura C, Kwiatek O, et al. (2010) Global distribution of peste des petits ruminants virus and prospects for improved diagnosis and Control. J Gen Virol 91: 2885–2897.

40. Gleeson LJ (2002) A review of the status of foot and mouth disease in South-East Asia and approaches to control and eradication. Rev Sci Tech 21: 465–745.

41. Gongal G, Wright AE (2011) Human Rabies in the WHO Southeast Asia Region: Forward Steps for Elimination. Adv Prev Med 2011: 383870.

42. Khounsy S, Conlan JV, Gleeson LJ, Westbury HA, Colling A, et al. (2009) Molecular epidemiology of foot-and-mouth disease viruses from South East Asia 1998–2006: the Lao perspective. Vet Microbiol 137: 178–183.

43. Dhar P, Sreenivasa BP, Barrett T, Corteyn M, Singh RP, et al. (2002) Recent epidemiology of peste des petits ruminants virus (PPRV). Vet Microbiol 88: 153–159.

44. Balamurugan V, Saravanan P, Sen A, Rajak KK, Venkatesan G, et al. (2012) Prevalence of peste des petits ruminants among sheep and goats in India. J Vet Sci 13: 279–285.

45. Singh RP, Saravanan P, Sreenivasa BP, Singh RK, Bandyopadhyay SK (2004) Prevalence and distribution of peste des petits ruminants virus infection in small ruminants in India. Rev Sci Tech 23: 807–819.

46. Kitching R (2002) Clinical variation in foot and mouth disease: cattle. Rev Sci Tech 21: 499–504.

47. Zhang ZD, Kitching RP (2001) The Localization of Persistent Foot and Mouth Disease Virus in the Epithelial Cells of the Soft Palate and Pharynx. J Comp Path 124: 89–94.

48. Bhattacharya S, Banerjee R, Ghosh R, Chattopadhayay AP, Chatterjee A (2005) Studies of the outbreaks of foot and mouth disease in West Bengal, India, between 1985 and 2002. Rev Sci Tech 24: 945–952.

49. Benkirane A, De Alwis MCL (2002) Haemorrhagic septicaemia, its significance, prevention and control in Asia. Vet Med – Czech 47: 234–240.

50. World Organisation for Animal Health (2010) World Animal Health Information Database. Available: http://www.oie.int/wahis/public.php?WAHIDPHPSESSID = adce2e623aeedddaa4b 858ff84f59f. Accessed August 12, 2010.

51. Malaga H, Nieto EL, Gambirazio C (1979) Canine rabies seasonality. Int J Epidemiol 8: 243–245.

52. Dohms JE, Metz A (1991) Stress-mechanisms of immunosuppression. Vet Immunol Immunopathol 30: 89–109.

53. Abubakar M, Jamal SM, Arshed MJ, Hussain M, Ali Q (2009) Peste des petits ruminants virus (PPRV) infection; its association with species, seasonal variations and geography. Trop Anim Health Pro 41: 1197–1202.

54. Ozkul A, Akca Y, Alkan F, Barrett T, Karaoglu T, et al. (2002) Prevalence, distribution, and host range of peste des petits ruminants virus, Turkey. Emerg infect Dis 8: 708–712.

55. Livestock Research Institute (2010) Annual Report on Production, Distribution and Balance of Vaccines in the Financial Year 2009–10, Bangladesh. Dhaka: Livestock Research Institute.

56. Food and Agriculture Organization (FAO) of the United Nations (2001) Anthrax in animals (http://www.fao.org/ag/magazine/0112sp.htm).Rome, Italy. Accessed 5 December 2010.

57. Rahman MA, Shadmin I, Noor M, Parvin R, Chowdhury EH, et al. (2011) Peste des petits ruminants virus infection of goats in Bangladesh: Pathological investigation, molecular detection and isolation of the virus. The Bangladesh Vet 28: 1–7.

58. Coleman PG, Dye C (1996) Immunization coverage required to prevent outbreaks of dog rabies. Vaccine 14: 185–186.

59. Verma AK, Pal BC, Singh CP, Udit J, Yadav SK, et al. (2008) Studies of the outbreaks of foot and mouth disease in Uttar Pradesh, India, between 2000 and 2006. Asian J Epidemiol 1: 40–46.

60. Khounsy S, Conlan JV, Gleeson LJ, Westbury HA, Colling A, et al. (2008) Foot and mouth disease in the Lao People's Democratic Republic: I. A review of recent outbreaks and lessons from control programmes. Scientific and Technical Review. Office International des Epizooties 27: 839–849.

61. Madin B (2002) An evaluation of Foot-and-Mouth Disease outbreak reporting in mainland South-East Asia from 2000 to 2010. Prev Vet Med 102: 230–241.

62. Davies G (2002) Foot and mouth disease. Res Vet Sci 73: 195–199.

63. Thiptara A, Atwill ER, Kongkaew W, Chomel BB (2011) Epidemiologic trends of rabies in domestic animals in southern Thailand, 1994–2008. Am J Trop Med Hyg 85: 138–145.

64. Plotkin SA (2000) Rabies. Clin Infect Dis 30: 4–12.

65. FAO (2011) Challenges of animal health information systems and surveillance for animal diseases and zoonoses. Proceedings of the international workshop organized by FAO, 23–26 November 2010, Rome, Italy.

7

Using Simulation to Interpret a Discrete Time Survival Model in a Complex Biological System: Fertility and Lameness in Dairy Cows

Christopher D. Hudson*, Jonathan N. Huxley, Martin J. Green

School of Veterinary Medicine and Science, University of Nottingham, Sutton Bonington Campus, Sutton Bonington, Leicestershire, United Kingdom

Abstract

The ever-growing volume of data routinely collected and stored in everyday life presents researchers with a number of opportunities to gain insight and make predictions. This study aimed to demonstrate the usefulness in a specific clinical context of a simulation-based technique called probabilistic sensitivity analysis (PSA) in interpreting the results of a discrete time survival model based on a large dataset of routinely collected dairy herd management data. Data from 12,515 dairy cows (from 39 herds) were used to construct a multilevel discrete time survival model in which the outcome was the probability of a cow becoming pregnant during a given two day period of risk, and presence or absence of a recorded lameness event during various time frames relative to the risk period amongst the potential explanatory variables. A separate simulation model was then constructed to evaluate the wider clinical implications of the model results (i.e. the potential for a herd's incidence rate of lameness to influence its overall reproductive performance) using PSA. Although the discrete time survival analysis revealed some relatively large associations between lameness events and risk of pregnancy (for example, occurrence of a lameness case within 14 days of a risk period was associated with a 25% reduction in the risk of the cow becoming pregnant during that risk period), PSA revealed that, when viewed in the context of a realistic clinical situation, a herd's lameness incidence rate is highly unlikely to influence its overall reproductive performance to a meaningful extent in the vast majority of situations. Construction of a simulation model within a PSA framework proved to be a very useful additional step to aid contextualisation of the results from a discrete time survival model, especially where the research is designed to guide on-farm management decisions at population (i.e. herd) rather than individual level.

Editor: Dawit Tesfaye, University of Bonn, Germany

Funding: This work was part of an internally (University of Nottingham) funded Ph.D. studentship. The funders had no role in study design, data collection and analysis, decision to publish, or preparation of the manuscript.

Competing Interests: The authors have declared that no competing interests exist.

* Email: chris.hudson@nottingham.ac.uk

Introduction

The ever-growing volume of data routinely collected and stored in everyday life presents researchers with a number of opportunities to gain insight and make predictions. Routine collection of data with potential research application is now very widespread, and is facilitating research using much larger sample sizes than in the past. One example of this is in agriculture, where widespread adoption of computerised recording systems has largely been driven by the need to manage larger enterprises and maximise efficiency, but is also creating an invaluable resource for researchers. A wide variety of traditional and new techniques have been applied to analysis of the large, retrospective datasets generated in this way, but in some cases more sophisticated and robust analytical techniques can yield results which are harder for the end user of the research to interpret and understand.

This study focuses on the relationship between a time-to-event outcome (in this case, the time between parturition and subsequent conception in a dairy cow) and a disease event (in this case lameness). Techniques for analysis of such data have evolved over the years, and this specific field has seen publications evaluating this relationship in a univariate way [1] using Kaplan-Meier survival analysis, and in a multivariate framework, using various

modifications of the Cox proportional hazards model [2–4]. However, accounting appropriately for time-dependent variables (for example, accounting for the possibility that a case of lameness may affect probability of conception within a specific frame of time around the case) using such approaches can be challenging, and model assumptions can be difficult to satisfy and are not always tested [5].

Another approach is discrete time survival analysis [6,7], where the dataset is amplified into smaller units of time for each individual animal and logistic regression is used to predict the probability of the outcome of interest at each time-point. This method is substantially more flexible, and more easily incorporates statistical advances such as multilevel regression using random effects to account for hierarchical clustering within data [7,8] (for example, of cows within herds), and Markov chain Monte Carlo sampling for parameter estimation within a Bayesian framework [9]. However, results from this type of analysis can be difficult to interpret, especially at the population level. For example, such analysis may yield an estimated odds ratio for the association between a lameness event and the probability of conception occurring during a given period of time, but there is no intuitive way to interpret the likely importance of this at the population level. In this context, on-farm interpretation is very important, because decision makers (e.g. a dairy herd's manager or veterinary clinician) need to be able to estimate the potential improvement in a herd's reproductive performance that could result from a reduction in lameness in order to conduct a cost benefit analysis for intervention. Simulation based approaches can be used to help address this issue, allowing the researcher to evaluate relationships between inputs and outputs of a given system across plausible scenarios. One such technique is known as probabilistic sensitivity analysis (PSA), and is commonly employed in health economic evaluations [10,11] to explore which inputs to a complex model have the most capacity to perturb the output. Such simulation models can also be used as the basis for decision support tools, an application common in the financial sector [12].

Good reproductive performance is essential for efficiency in dairy production [13], which in turn is increasingly important in the context of a global increase in demand and downward pressure on resource use [14]. A wide range of factors are known to affect dairy cow fertility, including incidence of clinical disease. Lameness is one of the most common endemic diseases in the modern dairy herd, with reported prevalence in the UK at over 35% [15], and has previously been associated with depressed reproductive performance in affected cows compared to unaffected controls [2,4,16,17]. However, a very high proportion of previous studies have been carried out using either a single herd or a small number of herds, and those deriving data from wider populations have often failed to detect an association [18,19], as did the most recent study in UK dairy cows [1]. Alongside this, a very wide variety of other factors are known to affect cow fertility. Therefore the clinician wishing to improve a herd's reproductive performance needs to interpret this research evidence in the context of the other influences on fertility when deciding how much weight should be given to control of lameness to improve reproduction.

In this study, the association between clinical lameness events and reproductive performance was evaluated using routinely collected management data from a group of dairy herds. The aim of the study was to explore the usefulness of simulation-based techniques as an aid to interpret the clinical significance of a discrete time survival model evaluating association between disease events and reproductive performance at herd level.

Materials and Methods

Data Collection and Restructuring

Routinely recorded farm management data were collected from 39 dairy herds across England and Wales. These were the subset of herds described in an earlier study [20] which demonstrated consistent recording of clinical lameness events (i.e. treatment of lame cows). Data collection, quality auditing and study inclusion criteria are described in detail by Hudson et al. [20]. Herds were not excluded on the basis of breed: 38 were mainly Holstein or Holstein–Friesian and one predominantly Guernsey. Detail regarding each event (for example, which limb was affected and the diagnosis made) was not evaluated in this study: all clinical lameness events were treated as equal. Where two lameness events were recorded for the same cow within 7 days, the second was removed (since both treatment records would have been likely to reflect the same disease event). Table 1 shows descriptive information for these herds.

Data were restructured into a format where each unit (line) of data was a two-day period during each lactation between 20 and 220 days after parturition (days in milk, DIM) where the cow was "at risk" of becoming pregnant (lactations were censored after

culling, death, sale or conception occurred). For each of these two-day risk periods, a binary variable was used to represent whether the cow became pregnant during the risk period. Clinical lameness records were used to determine whether a case of lameness was recorded at a variety of different time-frames relative to each risk period (see Table 2). Additional variables at both lactation level (e.g. parity of cow, lactation 305-day adjusted milk yield) and risk period level (e.g. DIM at beginning of risk period, month and year of risk period) were calculated for each risk period (Table 2). Where necessary, categorical variables were recoded to avoid categories containing small numbers of risk periods/lactations (e.g. animals of parity 5 or above were grouped as a single category). This generated a dataset consisting of 1,247,677 risk periods from 21,913 lactations in 12,515 cows from 39 herds. Initial data collation and restructuring was carried out using Microsoft Access 2010 (Microsoft Corp.), with further restructuring and variable calculation carried out using R v2.14 [21].

Discrete-time survival analysis

A multilevel discrete-time survival model [22] was constructed to evaluate the association between the probability of a cow becoming pregnant during a two-day risk period (the outcome) and the potential explanatory variables described in Table 2. A three-level hierarchical structure (with risk periods nested within cows nested within herds) was used to account for correlations between risk periods from the same cow and cows from the same herd.

The model took the standard form:

$$\text{Preg}_{tij} \sim \text{Bernoulli}\left(\text{mean} = \mu_{tij}\right)$$

$$\ln\left(\frac{\mu_{tij}}{1-\mu_{tij}}\right) = \alpha + \beta_1 \ln\text{DIM}_{tij} + \beta_2 \left(\ln\text{DIM}_{tij}\right)^2 \\ + \boldsymbol{\beta}_3 \mathbf{X}_{tij} + \boldsymbol{\beta}_4 \mathbf{X}_{ij} + \mathbf{u}_{ij} + \mathbf{v}_j \tag{1}$$

$$\mathbf{v}_i \sim N(0,\sigma_v^2) \tag{2}$$

$$\mathbf{u}_{ij} \sim N(0,\sigma_u^2) \tag{3}$$

where t represents a two-day risk period and i and j the ith cow in the jth herd; μ_{tij} the fitted probability of Preg_{tij} (the outcome of the ith cow in the jth herd becoming pregnant during risk period t); $\ln\text{DIM}_{tij}$ the natural logarithm of DIM at the beginning of risk period t; α the regression intercept; β_1 and β_2 the coefficients for the terms representing days in milk; $\mathbf{X}_{tij}$ the vector of risk period level covariates and $\boldsymbol{\beta}_3$ the corresponding vector of coefficients; $\mathbf{X}_{ij}$ the vector of cow-level covariates and $\boldsymbol{\beta}_4$ the corresponding vector of coefficients; u_{ij} the random effect to reflect variation between individual cows (e.g. due to genetic variation) and v_j the random effect representing variation between herds (e.g. due to nutritional management or environmental conditions of the herd), with σ_u^2

Table 1. Summary statistics of basic herd information for 39 dairy herds with good fertility and lameness records.

| | | | Percentiles | | | |
	Mean	Minimum	25%	50%	75%	Maximum
Herd size	243	88	153	202	292	669
Cull rate (%/year)	22	13	20	22	25	31
305 day adjusted milk yield (litres)	8329	4776	7366	8266	9566	11008
Incidence rate of clinical lameness (cases/cow-year)	0.40	0.10	0.22	0.30	0.41	1.88

and σ_v^2 the variances of the normal distributions of the respective random effects terms.

Model building and final parameter estimation was carried out using MLwiN v2.20 [23]. Model building and selection used the approach described in Hudson et al. [20], with Markov chain Monte Carlo (MCMC) sampling used for final parameter estimation [9] and retention in the model of variables where the 95% area of highest posterior density (HPD) for the variable's coefficient did not cover zero. Biologically plausible first order interaction terms were tested, and retained in the model only if their inclusion made a substantial difference to parameter estimates for coefficients of the main effects. Inclusion of herd-level random effects (slope variation) for the lameness-related model terms was also tested, to account for the possibility that the association between lameness and reproductive performance could vary between herds. These were again retained in the model only if they altered parameter estimates for main effects by more than 1%, or if between-herd variation was large relative to mean effect size (such that the variance of the herd-level random effect for the variable was more than 20% of the mean/overall effect).

Model sensitivity analysis revealed that the parameters of interest were not sensitive to choices made during data restructuring and model building (e.g. choice of risk period duration, choice of function to represent DIM or selection of timeframes for lameness events). Simulation-based posterior predictions were used to evaluate model fit as described in Hudson et al. [20], by subsetting the data in a variety of ways, using the model to predict probability of pregnancy for each risk period in the subset and

checking that the observed proportion of risk periods where pregnancy occurred lay within the 95% coverage interval of the predicted risk. Model results were illustrated as relative risks using a similar prediction-based approach [20]. Posterior predictions were carried out in R v2.14, using MCMC chains exported from MLwiN.

Probabilistic sensitivity analysis

In order to explore the relationship between herd reproductive performance and the incidence rate of lameness at herd level, a simulation model was developed. The aim of this part of the study was to evaluate the results of the discrete time survival analysis in a wider context to assess its potential usefulness to inform clinical on-farm management decisions.

Simulation model structure and process. The outline structure of the simulation model is shown in Figure 1. The model was constructed in Microsoft Excel 2010 (Microsoft Corp.), using Visual Basic for Applications (Microsoft Corp.) for process control. The explanatory variables in the final discrete-time survival model became input parameters for the herd-level simulation model, which was used to simulate 50,000 herds of 200 lactations each. Simulating a herd first involved drawing the herd-level input parameters (e.g. the herd's mean 305-day adjusted milk yield and incidence rate of clinical lameness) from the distributions shown in Table 3.

Simulation of the first cow-lactation in the herd was then commenced by drawing the lactation-level inputs (e.g. the parity of the cow) from the relevant distributions and simulating a clinical

Table 2. Potential explanatory variables calculated for each risk period in a study investigating the association between lameness and fertility in 39 dairy herds.

Variable	Level	Variable type
Parity (lactation number)	Lactation	Categorical (>4 recoded as single group)
305-day lactation milk yield	Lactation	Continuous
Year in which lactation began	Lactation	Categorical (<2003 recoded as single group)
DIM at start of risk period	Risk period	Continuous
Season of risk period	Risk period	Categorical (Jan-Mar, Apr-Jun, Jul-Sep, Oct-Dec)
Lame 71–100 d before risk period	Risk period	Binary (lameness case recorded or not)
Lame 43–70 d before risk period	Risk period	Binary (lameness case recorded or not)
Lame 15–42 d before risk period	Risk period	Binary (lameness case recorded or not)
Lame within 14 d of risk period	Risk period	Binary (lameness case recorded or not)
Lame 15–42 d after risk period	Risk period	Binary (lameness case recorded or not)
Lame 43–70 d after risk period	Risk period	Binary (lameness case recorded or not)
Lame 71–100 d after risk period	Risk period	Binary (lameness case recorded or not)

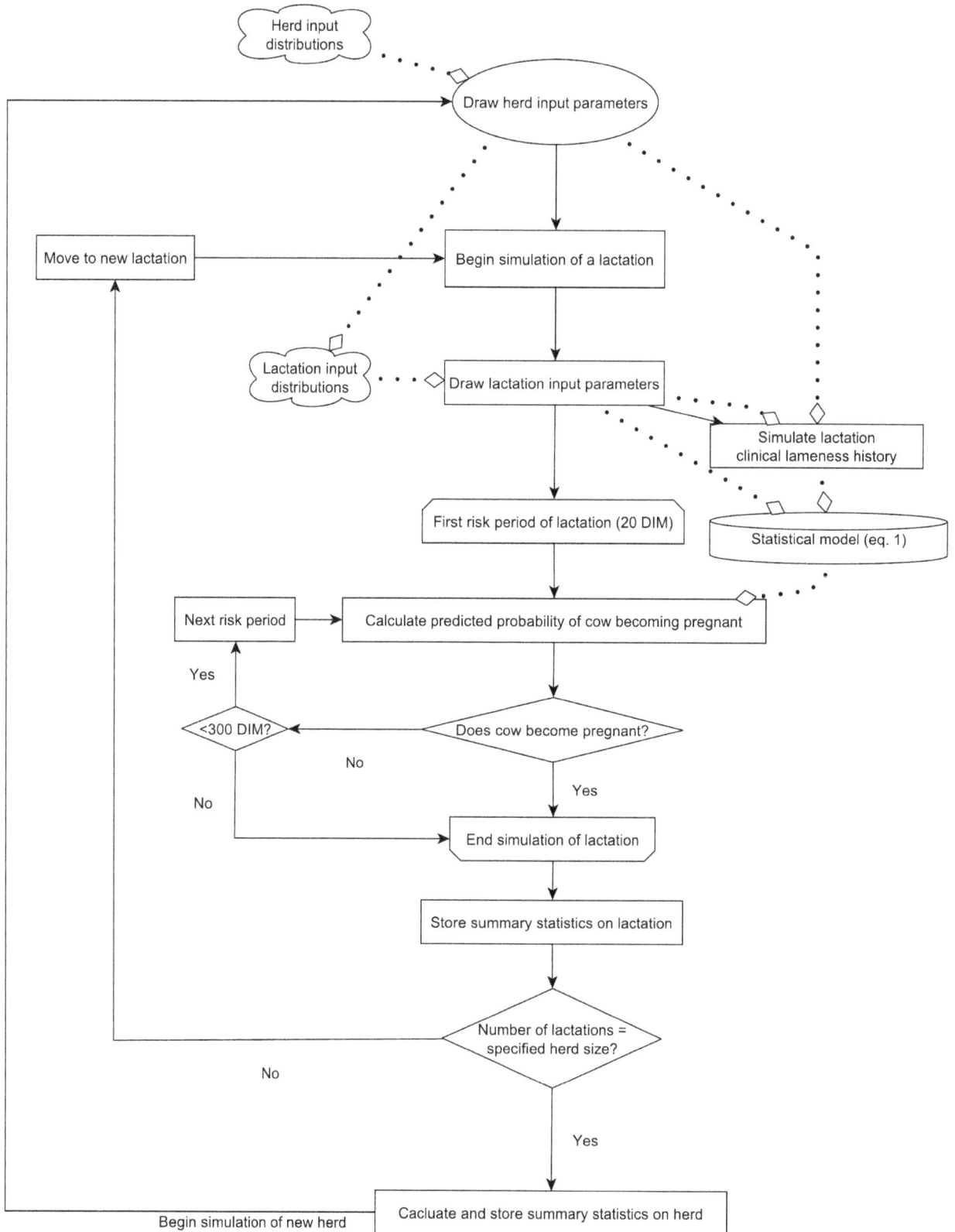

Figure 1. Structure of the simulation model used for probabilistic sensitivity analysis. Solid black lines indicate process flow, dotted lines indicate that information from the source of the line is used in the step of the process to which the line leads (denoted by a diamond).

Table 3. Input parameters used for each level of simulation in a study investigating the association between lameness and fertility.

Input variable	Level	Input distribution
Submission rate	Herd	Uniform, range 10–80%
Pregnancy rate	Herd	Uniform, range 10–60%
Herd average 305 d milk yield	Herd	Uniform, range 3000–12,500 litres
Proportion of herd in first lactation	Herd	Uniform, range 10–40%
Incidence rate of lameness	Herd	Uniform, range 0.1–1.5 cases/cow-year
Cost per extra empty day	Herd	Uniform, range £1.20–£4.20
Cost per failure to conceive cull	Herd	Uniform, range £550–£1750
Parity/lactation number	Lactation	Discrete, based on proportion of herd in first lactation
305 d lactation milk yield	Lactation	Beta, centred on herd average with standard deviation of 1,500 litres; adjusted for parity
Days in milk	Risk period	As described in text
Lame 43–70 d before risk period	Risk period	Binary, as described in text
Lame within 14 d of risk period	Risk period	Binary, as described in text
Lame 43–70 d after risk period	Risk period	Binary, as described in text
Lame 71–100 d after risk period	Risk period	Binary, as described in text

lameness history for the lactation. The latter was accomplished by using the distribution of DIM of all clinical lameness events from the original dataset (Figure 2) to assign a probability that a lameness event would occur at each two-day risk period through the lactation in a herd with a given overall lameness incidence rate. The discrete-time survival model described in the previous section was used to calculate the predicted probability of pregnancy occurring during each two-day risk period given the input parameters for that herd, lactation and risk period. This probability was adjusted to account for the herd's overall ("background") level of submission rate and pregnancy rate (i.e. the variation in these parameters not explained by lameness, milk yield or other model inputs). These are measures of specific aspects of a dairy herd's reproductive performance, submission rate being the proportion of eligible cows inseminated every 21 days (the normal length of the oestrous cycle) and pregnancy rate being the proportion of inseminations leading to a pregnancy. Both of these "background" herd fertility characteristics were represented as herd-level input parameters with a separate value for each simulated herd drawn from the relevant distribution.

A binary outcome to represent whether or not the cow became pregnant during the risk period was drawn from a binomial distribution based on this calculated probability. Repeated risk periods were simulated for each cow, until she either became pregnant or reached 300 DIM (a point at which farmers would commonly elect to remove cows from the herd if not pregnant), at which time simulation of the next lactation was begun. When 200 lactations had been simulated, the herd was considered complete. The mean number of DIM at pregnancy and the proportion of lactations ending without a pregnancy in each herd were stored along with the herd-level input parameters before beginning simulation of the next herd.

Simulation model inputs. Uniform input distributions were specified for all herd-level inputs, so that every potential combination of herd-level inputs was equally likely to be selected at each iteration of the simulation. The ranges for these distributions were selected based on the authors' clinical experience, such that they would be expected to cover the vast majority of realistic possibilities in UK dairy herds (Table 3). This was not considered to represent the true joint distributions of these

parameters across herds: the objective was not to speculate on which situations might occur most commonly, but to evaluate the potential impact of all different lameness incidence rates across as wide a variety of herd scenarios as possible. Some of the lactation-level inputs were drawn from non-uniform distributions so that the architecture of each simulated herd was realistic (so, for example, the milk yield for a lactation was drawn from a beta distribution parameterised such that a cow was likely to draw a lactation yield close to the herd average, and there was a smaller chance of drawing a yield much further from the average), as described in Table 3.

Simulation model outputs and analysis. A single herd-level outcome was devised to represent reproductive performance for each simulated herd (to allow evaluation of associations between this and the various input parameters). The mean number of DIM at pregnancy and the proportion of cows reaching 300 DIM without conceiving were combined using a modification of the method of Esslemont et al. [24] to produce a "modified FERTEX" (mFX) score. This involved comparing each value to a pre-set target (set at 60 days for the herd's mean DIM at pregnancy and zero for proportion of cows in the herd reaching 300 DIM without conceiving), and applying a unit cost to the difference from target for each. The sum of these two costs on a per-cow basis for each simulated herd gave that herd's mFX score. Since the cost of a culled cow and an additional empty day are widely acknowledged to vary from herd to herd, these were considered as herd-level inputs, and each drawn randomly for each herd from the distributions described in Table 3. The mFX score for each simulated herd was therefore a cost-based single measure of overall fertility performance (so that higher performing herds had lower mFX scores and vice versa).

Results from the simulations were analysed initially by illustrating associations between herd-level input parameters and mFX scores graphically using high-density scatterplots. Spearman rank correlation coefficients were calculated for the association between each herd-level input and mFX score (a non-parametric measure of correlation was selected as the mFX scores were positively skewed). Multiple regression (with the natural logarithm of mFX score as the outcome) was used to partition variance in mFX score between the various herd-level inputs. The resulting

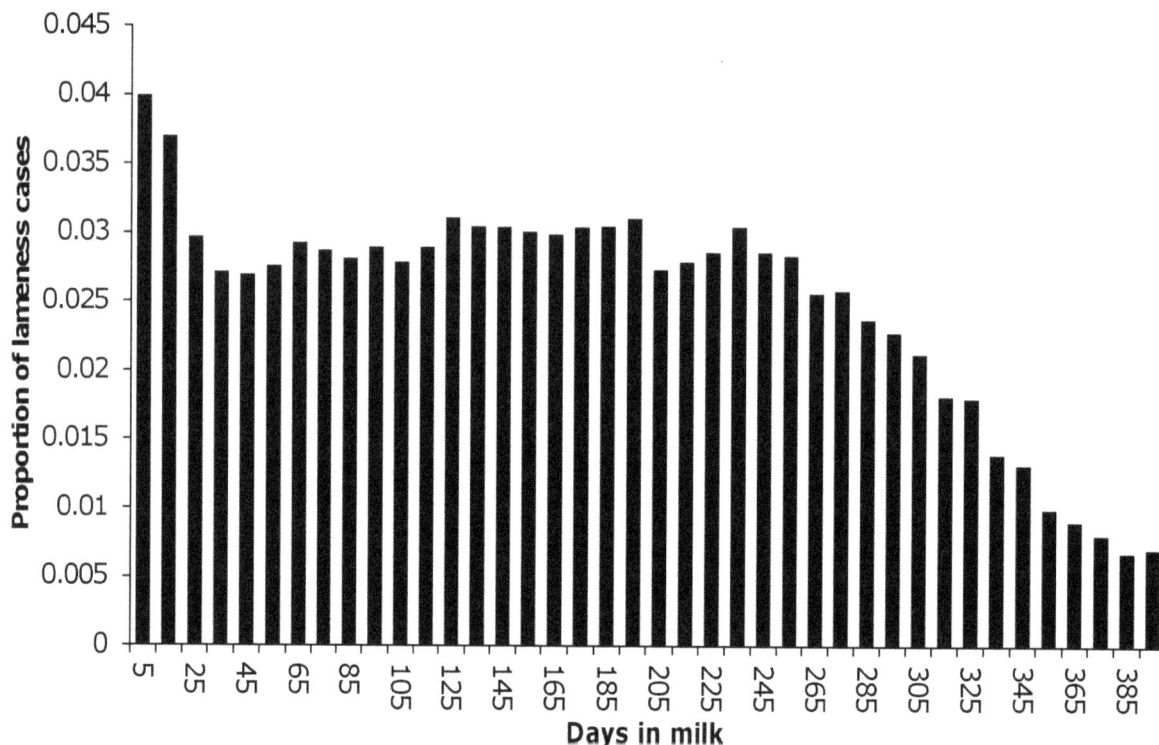

Figure 2. Distribution of lameness cases observed by days in milk.

regression model was also used to predict the effect on mFX score of increasing each individual input in turn from the middle of its input distribution to the upper quartile so that results could be displayed graphically as a tornado plot (a standard approach for presentation of PSA results).

Results

There were a total of 16,706 pregnancies from the 1,247,677 risk periods in the dataset, so that 1.34% of risk periods resulted in a pregnancy (corresponding to around 14% of cows becoming pregnant during each 21 day oestrous cycle). Of the 22,319 lactations in the dataset, 4,360 involved at least one case of lameness (corresponding to a lactational first case incidence rate of 19.5%).

Discrete-time survival analysis

Table 4 shows the parameter estimates for the regression model derived to predict the probability of pregnancy resulting during a two-day risk period. The predictor variables not directly associated with lameness showed very similar associations to those seen by Hudson et al. [20], with probability of pregnancy peaking at around 110 DIM, decreasing with increasing 305-day adjusted milk yield and lower predicted probabilities of pregnancy for cows in higher parities and during the months April to September. Clinical lameness events during four different time frames relative to the two-day risk period showed associations with the probability of pregnancy during the risk period. The largest association was seen when a lameness event was recorded within 14 days of the risk period, when the odds of pregnancy were reduced by almost 25% (odds ratio [OR] 0.76, area of 95% highest posterior density [HPD] 0.69–0.84). Lameness events recorded 43 to 70 days before, 43 to 70 days after and 71 to 100 days after a risk period

were all associated with a reduction in the odds of pregnancy during the risk period of around 15% (ORs 0.85, 0.88 and 0.86 respectively; areas of 95% HPD 0.76–0.95, 0.80–0.98 and 0.79–0.95 respectively). These associations are represented as posterior predicted relative risks in Figure 3. Predicted risks were also used to demonstrate that model fit was good. For each subset of data tested, the observed proportion of risk periods where pregnancy occurred fell within the 95% area of HPD of predicted risk for that subset (Figure 4).

Probabilistic sensitivity analysis

Univariate analysis. Univariate analysis of PSA results is presented using high-density scatterplots in Figure 5. These show that a herd's "background" level of submission and pregnancy rate were the individual inputs with the strongest influence on overall herd fertility performance, with both being moderately strongly correlated with herd mFX score (Spearman rank correlation coefficient −0.65 for submission rate and −0.59 for pregnancy rate). The herd incidence rate of clinical lameness had no clear relationship with mFX score, with a Spearman rank correlation coefficient of 0.028 and the scatterplot showing a square appearance with no clear trend in the area of highest point density.

Multivariate analysis. Analysis of the simulation results in a multivariate framework allows visualisation of results from the discrete time survival model in a clinical context. Table 5 shows that the herd's "background" level of submission and pregnancy rate explained the vast majority of the variation in herd mFX score, with 75% of overall variance explained by these two input parameters. It is important to remember that these inputs represent the marginal effect of between-herd variation in these aspects of fertility performance after the other model inputs have been accounted for (so, for example, a herd's "background" pregnancy rate would reflect its insemination success rate after

Table 4. Parameter estimates for discrete time survival model with pregnancy during a two-day risk period as the outcome, in a study investigating the association between lameness and fertility in 39 dairy herds.

Model term	n	coefficient	odds ratio	HPD[1] 2.5%	HPD[1] 97.5%
Intercept	1247677	−40.1		−40.3	−39.9
ln DIM	1247677	15.4		15.3	15.4
(ln DIM)^2	1247677	−1.62		−1.62	−1.61
Parity 1	325621		Reference		
Parity 2	288951		1.056	1.006	1.109
Parity 3	223118		0.978	0.923	1.034
Parity 4	153753		0.948	0.888	1.010
Parity >4	256234		0.761	0.720	0.805
Year: 2002 or earlier	148578		Reference		
Year: 2003	86158		1.000	0.924	1.088
Year: 2004	147847		0.901	0.831	0.970
Year: 2005	216142		0.928	0.864	1.000
Year: 2006	313278		0.858	0.796	0.923
Year: 2007–8	335674		0.897	0.833	0.967
Season 1: Jan–Mar	332357		Reference		
Season 2: Apr–Jun	278139		0.897	0.857	0.938
Season 3: Jul–Sept	266050		0.736	0.701	0.775
Season 4: Oct–Dec	371131		0.997	0.957	1.040
Centred 305 d yield (×1000 kg)	1247677		0.917	0.906	0.928
No lameness 70-43 d before	1219868		Reference		
Lameness case 70-43 d before	27809		0.850	0.760	0.948
No lameness within 14 d	1207760		Reference		
Lameness case within 14 d	39917		0.760	0.686	0.839
No lameness 43–70 d after	1207155		Reference		
Lameness case 43–70 d after	40522		0.880	0.803	0.968
No lameness 71–100 d after	1203737		Reference		
Lameness case 71–100 d after	43940		0.861	0.787	0.947

[1]HPD: interval of highest posterior density (so the range between HPD 2.5% and HPD 97.5% represents the 95% of the parameter space with highest posterior density).

accounting for any effects of milk yield, age structure and level of lameness).

Figure 6 shows the predicted change in herd mFX score which would result from a herd increasing each input parameter in turn from the middle of the range of the input distribution by 25% of the total range while the other inputs remain at the population median. For example, the top line on the plot shows that an increase in submission rate from the median value of the range of distribution for this input (45%) to the value representing the lower boundary of the upper quartile of the range (62.5%) would be expected to result in a decrease in mFX score (i.e. an improvement in overall reproductive performance) of around £100/cow/year. Increasing the herd's incidence rate of lameness cases from 80 to 115 cases/100 cow-years would be expected to increase herd mFX score by just over £5/cow/year. Therefore, a reduction in lameness incidence of 35 cases/100 cow-years (which would represent a large improvement, and may require substantial financial and time investment from the farmer) would be expected to lead to the same degree of improvement in fertility as an increase in submission rate of less than 1% (a small change, which would be expected to require substantially less investment).

Discussion

This study showed that relatively large associations between clinical lameness events and reproductive performance could be demonstrated at the level of a risk period within lactation (e.g. occurrence of a lameness case within 14 days of a risk period was associated with a 25% reduction in the risk of the cow becoming pregnant during the risk period, Figure 3). However, PSA revealed that a herd's incidence rate of lameness was highly unlikely to make a significant contribution to its overall level of reproductive performance when other factors affecting fertility were also taken into account. As the simulation model was constructed to represent a herd with even all-year-round calving, it is possible that the results will be less applicable to block calving herds, where cows may have a limited timeframe in which to conceive. It is plausible that clinical lameness events may have an increased importance in the latter situation, as even a modest reduction in risk of pregnancy during the breeding period could increase the risk of a cow being culled.

There is substantial variation in the conclusions of existing work evaluating the association between lameness and reproductive performance. A variety of previous studies have found associations between decreased fertility and either clinical lameness events

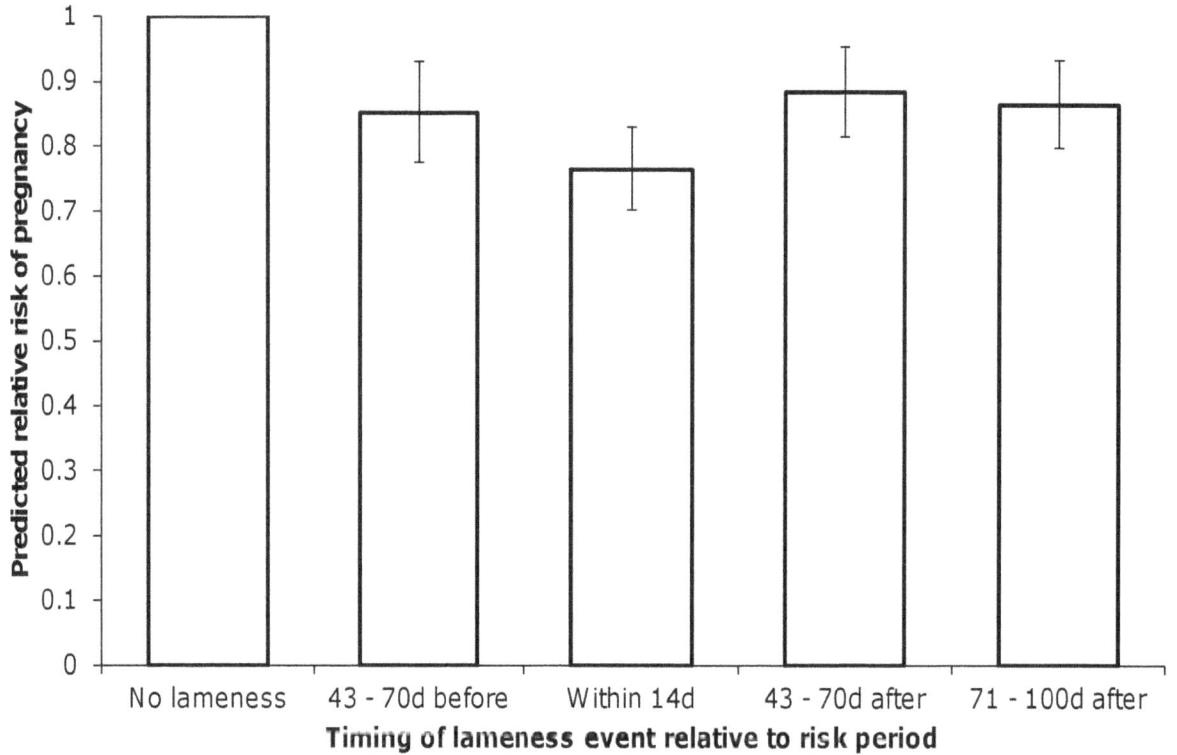

Figure 3. Association between predicted relative risk of pregnancy at a given risk period and clinical lameness. Error bars represent the 95% credible interval for each predicted relative risk.

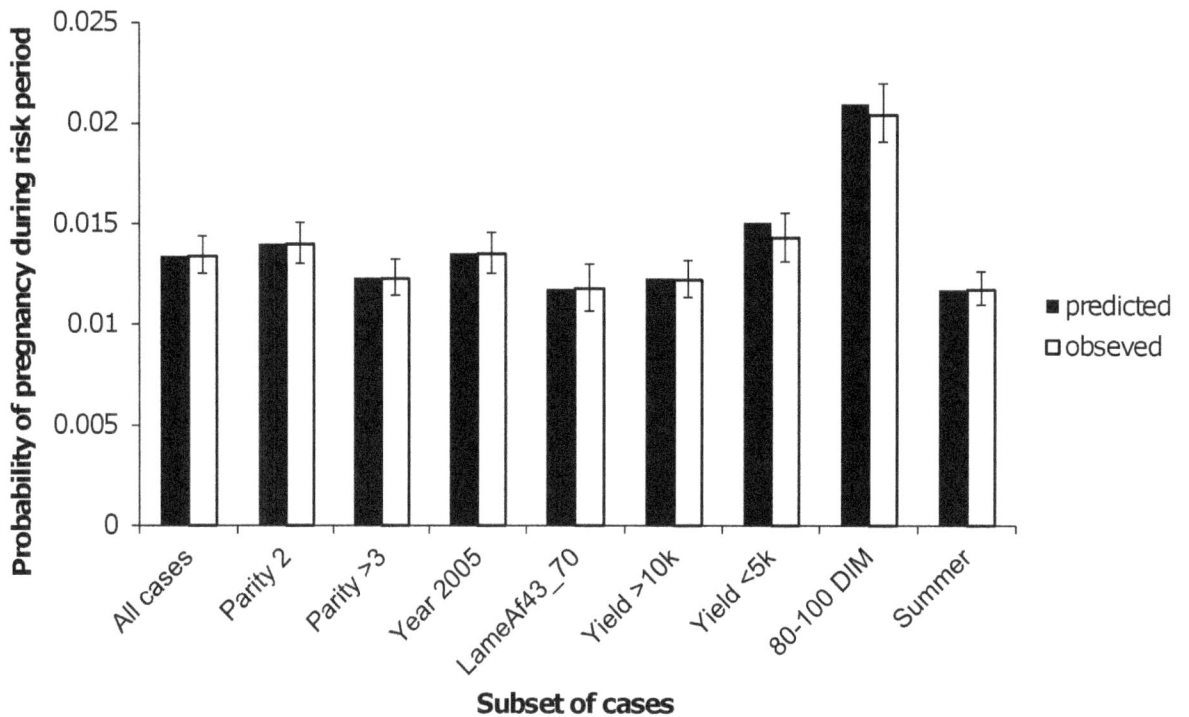

Figure 4. Predicted and observed risk of pregnancy across various categories. Predicted absolute risk of pregnancy (black bars) at risk periods in various categories (x-axis) compared to the observed proportion of risk periods in that category where a pregnancy occurred (white bars). Error bars represent the 95% credible interval for each predicted relative risk.

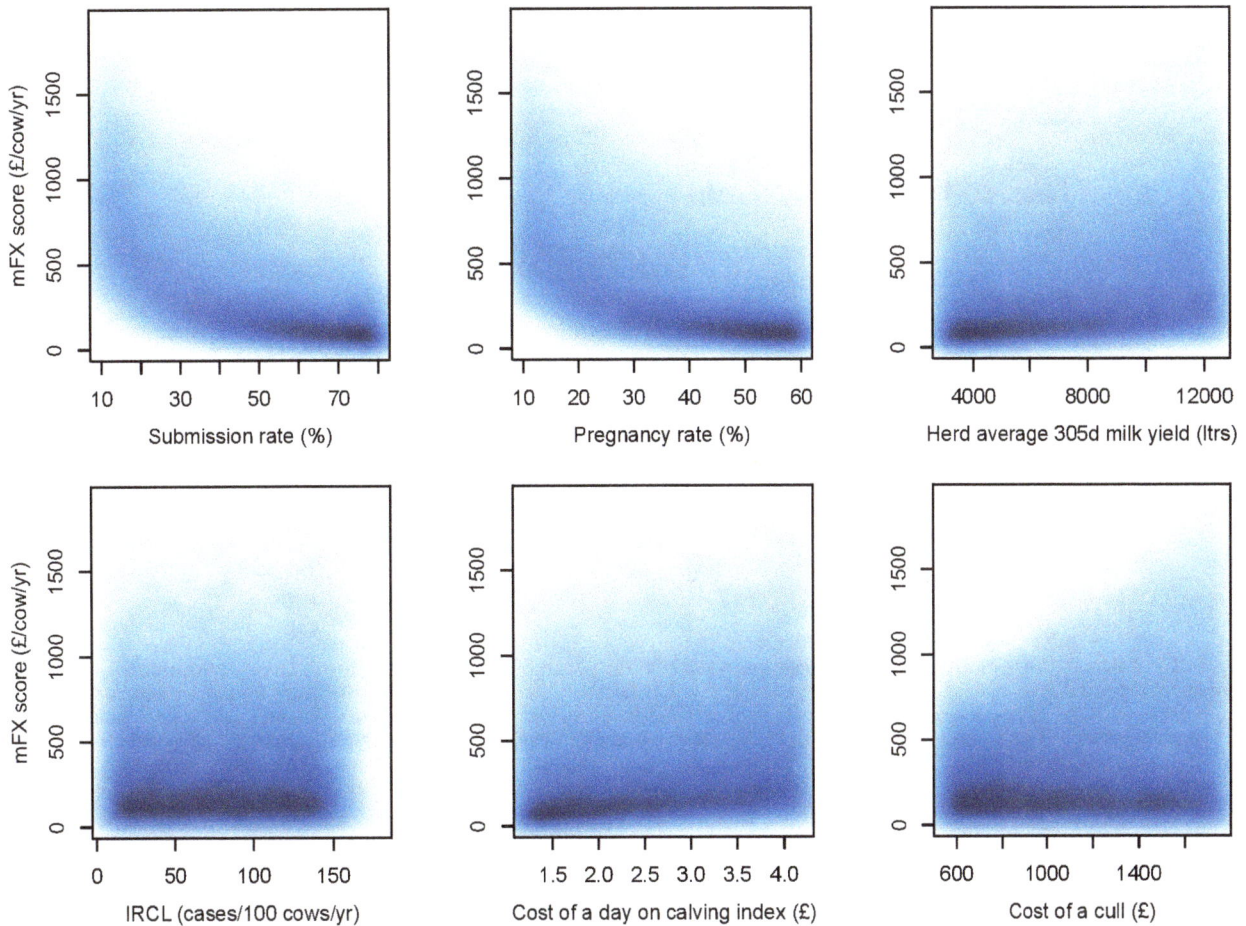

Figure 5. Associations between simulation inputs and overall herd-level reproductive performance. High density scatterplots showing the association between each simulated herd's reproductive performance (represented by modified FERTEX score, mFX, y-axis) and selected simulation input variables. Darker colours indicate areas of higher point density, IRCL: Incidence rate of clinical lameness.

[2,3,25] and/or identification of lameness through visual gait assessment [26,27]. In contrast, other studies have failed to reveal such an association [1,18,19]: notably there seems to be a tendency for studies involving larger numbers of herds to fail to identify significant associations. Many of the pre-existing papers in this area describe studies involving less than five herds (and most use a single herd); the notable exceptions to this are Loeffler et al. [18] (43 herds) and Sogstad et al. [19] (112 herds), neither of

which found significant associations between lameness events and reproductive outcomes. It is biologically plausible that any effect of lameness on reproductive performance will vary between herds (for example, due to the variation in the predominant causes of lameness in each herd and variation in the effectiveness of management of lame cows). The current study used data from 39 herds, but from a much larger number of cows compared to previous work. The possibility of between-herd variability in the

Table 5. Multiple regression derived partition of variance in modified FERTEX score across simulation input variables in a study evaluating associations between lameness and fertility in dairy herds.

Input parameter	Proportion of variance explained
Submission rate	41.4%
Pregnancy rate	34.2%
305-day adjusted lactation milk yield	8.9%
Cost per additional day on calving interval	5.7%
Cost per failure-to-conceive cull	2.0%
Incidence rate of clinical lameness	0.1%
Proportion of herd in lactation 1	0.0%

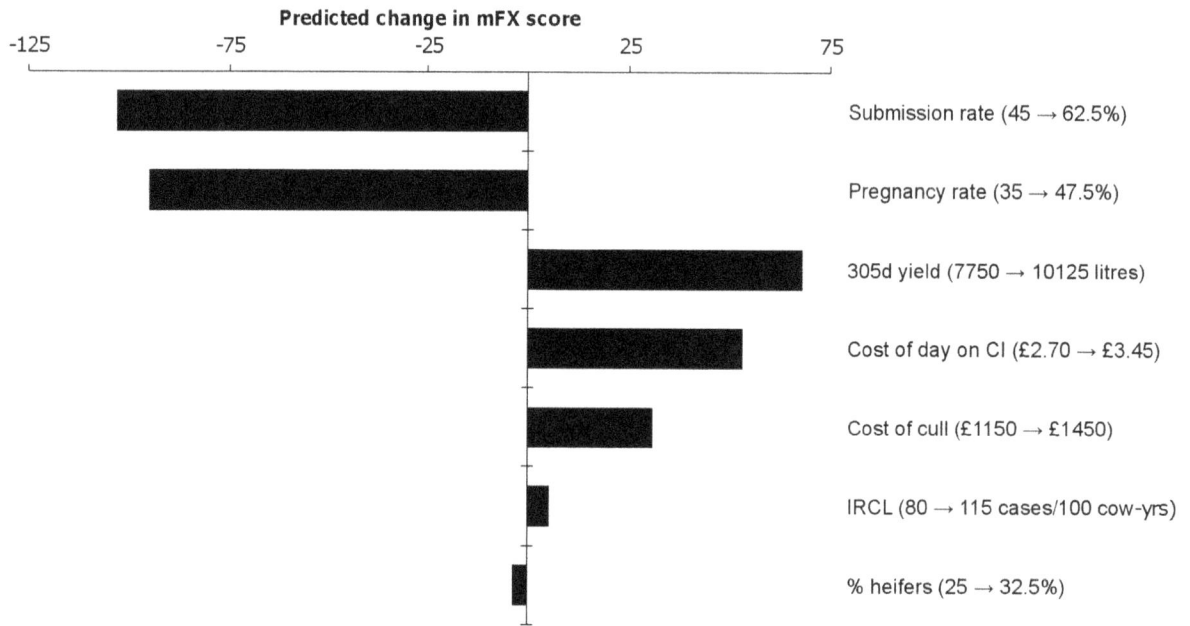

Figure 6. Predicted effect of an equivalent increase in each input parameter on overall reproductive performance. Tornado plot showing the predicted effect of increasing each input parameter in turn by a value representing 25% of the range of its input distribution from the median value, while the other input parameters are held at their population medians. The input parameters are listed on the right hand side of the graph, and the change in each input (from median to upper quartile) is given in parentheses. For example, the top bar shows that the predicted effect of moving from a submission rate of 45% (the median of the input distribution for this parameter) to 62.5% (the upper quartile of the input distribution) would be a decrease of just over £100/cow/year in the herd's modified FERTEX (mFX) score.

association between lameness events and fertility was explored here using herd-level random effects terms for the explanatory variables related to lameness. This revealed relatively little between-herd variability in effect within this group of herds. It is possible that somewhat different results would have been derived from building the statistical model using data from a different group of herds, but since the simulation model showed such a small potential for lameness to influence herd fertility, the difference in the statistical model results would have had to be extremely large in order to change the interpretation of the simulation results to any meaningful degree.

Some of the variation in previous published results may also be related to the way in which reproductive outcomes were measured: this study revealed significant associations between lameness events and the probability of pregnancy over a specific window of time relative to the lameness case, but when results were used to evaluate this within a PSA framework it transpired that lameness incidence rate was unlikely to influence overall herd reproductive performance. This means that previous studies focussing on particular categories or timings of lameness event and/or reproductive outcome may have been more likely to generate significant findings than those using broader categories or timeframes.

This study illustrates the usefulness of simulation-based techniques (such as PSA) to aid interpretation and contextualisation of model results. The approach we describe provides a potential route for researchers to facilitate better understanding of the results of their work and how they should be interpreted in a clinical context. This in turn can enhance research impact, and accelerate change in clinical practice. Although this example describes application of PSA to help interpret the results of a discrete time survival analysis, the technique would be equally applicable to other types of complex model, and to other analyses

based on logistic regression. In logistic regression, the model coefficients themselves can be difficult to interpret. Classically the coefficients are exponentiated to produce odds ratios (as shown in Table 4), but odds ratios themselves can be misleading because humans intuitively tend to think in terms of risk or probability rather than odds (and these can be quite different, especially where the risk is close to 0.5). This topic has been extensively explored in the medical literature [28–30], where results of such analyses must be interpreted by clinicians, some of whom may have a limited understanding of statistical methods. It is possible to convert an odds ratio to a relative risk for more intuitive interpretation (as shown in Figure 3), but where decisions are to be made at population level these can also be difficult to interpret. For example, in this case the relative risks would have been hard to interpret without a method to incorporate the likely range of herd-level lameness incidence rates and the distribution of lameness events through lactation. Here, the results from the discrete time survival model alone (along with some of the pre-existing literature) may have encouraged clinicians to place too much emphasis on control of lameness to improve herd-level reproductive performance.

This study highlights the usefulness of simulation-based techniques such as PSA as an extension of statistical modelling to help illustrate model results in an intuitive way within a clinical veterinary context. In this example, while there are associations between lameness events and reproductive performance at specific time-points, it is unlikely that a herd's incidence rate of lameness will have a substantial impact on herd fertility. This does not mean that lameness control is not important: lameness has significant impacts on both animal welfare and productivity [31]. Rather, our analysis suggests that herd lameness control is unlikely to lead to a significant improvement in overall reproductive performance in the majority of situations.

Acknowledgments

The authors acknowledge the assistance of the farmers and their veterinary surgeons who provided the data on which this work was based.

Author Contributions

Conceived and designed the experiments: CDH MJG JNH. Performed the experiments: CDH. Analyzed the data: CDH. Wrote the paper: CDH JNH MJG.

References

1. Peake KA, Biggs AM, Argo CM, Smith RF, Christley RM, et al. (2011) Effects of lameness, subclinical mastitis and loss of body condition on the reproductive performance of dairy cows. Vet Rec 168: 301.
2. Alawneh JI, Laven RA, Stevenson MA (2011) The effect of lameness on the fertility of dairy cattle in a seasonally breeding pasture-based system. J Dairy Sci 94: 5487–5493.
3. Hernandez J, Shearer JK, Webb DW (2001) Effect of lameness on the calving-to-conception interval in dairy cows. J Am Vet Med Assoc 218: 1611–1614.
4. Machado VS, Caixeta LS, McArt JAA, Bicalho RC (2010) The effect of claw horn disruption lesions and body condition score at dry-off on survivability, reproductive performance, and milk production in the subsequent lactation. J Dairy Sci 93: 4071–4078.
5. Bellera CA, MacGrogan G, Debled M, de Lara CT, Brouste V, et al. (2010) Variables with time-varying effects and the Cox model: some statistical concepts illustrated with a prognostic factor study in breast cancer. BMC Med Res Methodol 10: 20.
6. Singer JD, Willett JB (1993) It's about time: Using discrete-time survival analysis to study duration and the timing of events. J Educ Behav Stat 18: 155.
7. Steele F (2003) A discrete-time multilevel mixture model for event history data with long-term survivors, with an application to an analysis of contraceptive sterilization in Bangladesh. Lifetime Data Anal 9: 155–174.
8. Rasbash J, Steele F, Browne WJ, Goldstein H (2009) A User's Guide to MLwiN, v2.10. Centre for Multilevel Modelling, University of Bristol.
9. Browne WJ (2009) MCMC Estimation in MLwiN v2.20. Centre for Multilevel Modelling, University of Bristol.
10. Andronis L, Barton P, Bryan S (2009) Sensitivity analysis in economic evaluation: an audit of NICE current practice and a review of its use and value in decision-making. Health Technol Assess 13: 1–45.
11. Anderson K, Jacobson JS, Heitjan DF, Zivin JG, Hershman D, et al. (2006) Cost-effectiveness of preventive strategies for women with a BRCA1 or a BRCA2 mutation. Ann Intern Med 144: 397–406.
12. Evans GE, Jones B (2009) The application of Monte Carlo simulation in finance, economics and operations management. 2009 WRI World Congress on Computer Science and Information Engineering, CSIE 2009. Vol. 4. 379–383.
13. LeBlanc S (2007) Economics of improving reproductive performance in dairy herds. Adv Dairy Technol 19: 201–214.
14. Steinfeld H, Gerber P, Wassenaar T, Castel V, Rosales M, et al. (2006) Livestock's long shadow. Available: http://www.fao.org/docrep/010/a0701e/a0701e00.HTM. Accessed 25 April 2013.
15. Barker ZE, Leach KA, Whay HR, Bell NJ, Main DCJ (2010) Assessment of lameness prevalence and associated risk factors in dairy herds in England and Wales. J Dairy Sci 93: 932–941.
16. Garbarino EJ, Hernandez JA, Shearer JK, Risco CA, Thatcher WW (2004) Effect of lameness on ovarian activity in postpartum Holstein cows. J Dairy Sci 87: 4123–4131.
17. Melendez P, Bartolome J, Archbald LF, Donovan A (2003) The association between lameness, ovarian cysts and fertility in lactating dairy cows. Theriogenology 59: 927–937.
18. Loeffler SH, de Vries MJ, Schukken YH (1999) The effects of time of disease occurrence, milk yield, and body condition on fertility in dairy cows. J Dairy Sci 82: 2589–2604.
19. Sogstad AM, Østeraas O, Fjeldaas T (2006) Bovine claw and limb disorders related to reproductive performance and production diseases. J Dairy Sci 89: 2519–2528.
20. Hudson CD, Bradley AJ, Breen JE, Green MJ (2012) Associations between udder health and reproductive performance in United Kingdom dairy cows. J Dairy Sci 95: 3683–3697.
21. R Core Development Team (2010) R: A language and environment for statistical computing. Vienna, Austria: R Foundation for Statistical Computing. Available: http://www.R-project.org.
22. Yang M, Goldstein H (2003) Modelling survival data in MLwiN 1.20. Centre for Multilevel Modelling, University of Bristol.
23. Rasbash J, Charlton C, Browne WJ, Healy M, Cameron B (2010) MLwiN Version 2.2. UK: Centre for Multilevel Modelling, University of Bristol.
24. Esslemont RJ, Kossaibati M (2002) DAISY Research Report No. 5: The costs of poor fertility and disease in UK dairy herds - Trends in DAISY herds over 10 seasons. UK: University of Reading.
25. Bahonar AR, Azizzadeh M, Stevenson MA, Vojgani M, Mahmoudi M (2009) Factors affecting days open in Holstein dairy cattle in Khorasan Razavi province, Iran; A cox proportional hazard model. JAVA 8: 747–754.
26. Hernandez JA, Garbarino EJ, Shearer JK, Risco CA, Thatcher WW (2005) Comparison of the calving-to-conception interval in dairy cows with different degrees of lameness during the prebreeding postpartum period. J Am Vet Med Assoc 227: 1284–1291.
27. Bicalho RC, Vokey F, Erb HN, Guard CL (2007) Visual locomotion scoring in the first seventy days in milk: Impact on pregnancy and survival. J Dairy Sci 90: 4586–4591.
28. Zhang J, Yu KF (1998) What's the relative risk? A method of correcting the odds ratio in cohort studies of common outcomes. JAMA 280: 1690–1691.
29. Bland JM, Altman DG (2000) The odds ratio. BMJ 320: 1468.
30. Davies HTO, Crombie IK, Tavakoli M (1998) When can odds ratios mislead? BMJ 316: 989–991.
31. Huxley JN (2013) Impact of lameness and claw lesions in cows on health and production. Livest Sci 156: 64–70.

8

Genomic Prediction for Tuberculosis Resistance in Dairy Cattle

Smaragda Tsairidou[1]*, John A. Woolliams[1], Adrian R. Allen[2], Robin A. Skuce[2], Stewart H. McBride[2], David M. Wright[3], Mairead L. Bermingham[1], Ricardo Pong-Wong[1], Oswald Matika[1], Stanley W. J. McDowell[2], Elizabeth J. Glass[1], Stephen C. Bishop[1]

1 The Roslin Institute and RDVS, University of Edinburgh, Midlothian, United Kingdom, 2 Agri-Food and Biosciences Institute, Belfast, United Kingdom, 3 School of Biological Sciences, Queen's University of Belfast, Belfast, United Kingdom

Abstract

Background: The increasing prevalence of bovine tuberculosis (bTB) in the UK and the limitations of the currently available diagnostic and control methods require the development of complementary approaches to assist in the sustainable control of the disease. One potential approach is the identification of animals that are genetically more resistant to bTB, to enable breeding of animals with enhanced resistance. This paper focuses on prediction of resistance to bTB. We explore estimation of direct genomic estimated breeding values (DGVs) for bTB resistance in UK dairy cattle, using dense SNP chip data, and test these genomic predictions for situations when disease phenotypes are not available on selection candidates.

Methodology/Principal Findings: We estimated DGVs using genomic best linear unbiased prediction methodology, and assessed their predictive accuracies with a cross validation procedure and receiver operator characteristic (ROC) curves. Furthermore, these results were compared with theoretical expectations for prediction accuracy and area-under-the-ROC-curve (AUC). The dataset comprised 1151 Holstein-Friesian cows (bTB cases or controls). All individuals (592 cases and 559 controls) were genotyped for 727,252 loci (Illumina Bead Chip). The estimated observed heritability of bTB resistance was 0.23 ± 0.06 (0.34 on the liability scale) and five-fold cross validation, replicated six times, provided a prediction accuracy of 0.33 (95% C.I.: 0.26, 0.40). ROC curves, and the resulting AUC, gave a probability of 0.58, averaged across six replicates, of correctly classifying cows as diseased or as healthy based on SNP chip genotype alone using these data.

Conclusions/Significance: These results provide a first step in the investigation of the potential feasibility of genomic selection for bTB resistance using SNP data. Specifically, they demonstrate that genomic selection is possible, even in populations with no pedigree data and on animals lacking bTB phenotypes. However, a larger training population will be required to improve prediction accuracies.

Editor: Qin Zhang, China Agricultrual University, China

Funding: Smaragda Tsairidou gratefully acknowledges financial support from the Roslin Institute and the University of Edinburgh through the Principal's Career Development PhD, as well as the Greek State Scholarship Foundation. The authors also acknowledge the financial support of the Biotechnology and Biological Sciences Research Council, through CEDFAS initiative grants BB/E018335/1 & 2, and the Roslin Institute Strategic Programme Grant. The funders had no role in study design, data collection and analysis, decision to publish, or preparation of the manuscript.

Competing Interests: The authors have declared that no competing interests exist.

* E-mail: Smaragda.Tsairidou@roslin.ed.ac.uk

Introduction

Bovine tuberculosis (bTB) is caused by *Mycobacterium bovis*, an aerobic Gram$^+$ bacillus and member of the *M. tuberculosis complex*. Cattle (*Bos taurus*) predominantly become infected through the respiratory route and the main lesions observed are tubercles formed in the lungs and draining lymph nodes. BTB is a zoonotic disease and has the potential to impact on animal performance and welfare, causing significant financial losses to the dairy cattle industry worldwide due to production losses and the cost of eradication programmes [1].

Bovine tuberculosis eradication in the UK is impaired by limitations of the available diagnostic and control methods. Diagnosis is based on tuberculin skin testing (Single Intradermal Comparative Cervical test (SICCT) for the UK [2]), post-mortem examination in the abattoir and bacteriological confirmation of infection, all of which suffer imperfect sensitivity. Laboratory confirmation of tuberculin test reactors or suspect abattoir lesions is based on a combination of histology and mycobacterial culture; however, this is complicated by the highly specific requirements of the bacterium *in vitro*. Although the γ-interferon blood test (an alternative diagnostic test) has reportedly higher sensitivity than the standard interpretation SICCT, it has substantially lower specificity. Vaccination using Bacillus Calmette Guerin (BCG) is precluded because vaccinated animals would currently be indistinguishable from infected animals using standard tuberculin tests [3]. Eradication strategies may also be compromised by the presence of a wildlife reservoir, for example the Eurasian badger (*Meles meles*) in the UK and Ireland. Studies on the effectiveness of culling badgers in the UK to reduce bTB prevalence in cattle have shown both positive and negative effects [4].

Following exposure to *M. bovis* only a proportion of animals develop disease, implying variability among individuals in terms of response to infection [5]. Traditional selective breeding requires both phenotypes (i.e. bTB state) and pedigree information. Estimated breeding values (EBVs) can then be calculated using statistical techniques such as best linear unbiased prediction (BLUP). However, such selection would work only on the subset of animals in herds affected by bTB, or their close relatives, and it would require that the population be undergoing an epidemic. Even then, selection intensity would be low if only a small proportion of herds were affected [6]. Therefore, in the case of bTB resistance, it is appealing to be able to identify relatively resistant animals in the absence of phenotypic data from an epidemic.

In contrast to phenotypic selection, genomic selection is a new technology that addresses the problem of identifying relatively resistant individuals by obtaining EBVs for animals without observing phenotypes. Therefore, exposure to infection is not required, at least for several rounds of selection. Genomic selection utilises genomic EBVs estimated directly from SNP data rather than pedigree data (DGVs), calculated as the sum of the effects of genetic markers (Single Nucleotide Polymorphisms, SNPs) across the genome. One method for calculating DGVs is using genomic BLUP (GBLUP) [7,8]. Through genomic prediction methodology, DGVs may be estimated by combining knowledge on genotypes of the selection candidates and marker effects, and these can then be used as predictors of disease susceptibility for every animal. Genomic prediction in dairy cattle breeding presents certain advantages over phenotypic selection. In particular it improves the rate of genetic gain by shortening the generation intervals, since the DGVs can be calculated as soon as DNA samples are available. Hence, it also allows differentiation between full-sibs, (i.e. prediction of the Mendelian segregation term), without the delay of phenotypic recording [9,10].

Previous studies have confirmed the presence of potentially exploitable genetic variation in bTB susceptibility among dairy cattle [11,12]. The hypothesis in the present study is that genetic selection for disease resistance may offer a complementary bTB control strategy, by reducing infection risks and hence contributing to a reduction in herd-level incidence. The aim of this study was to estimate DGVs for bTB resistance by using dense SNP chip data on UK dairy cattle and to test these genomic predictions in the absence of disease phenotype. This is the first step in the investigation of the feasibility of genomic selection for bTB resistance on the basis of predicted DGVs.

Materials and Methods

Animals

Phenotypic data for 1,151 cows from 165 dairy cattle herds in Northern Ireland were collected in a case-control study design, with a sample prevalence of 0.51 in the compiled dataset [13]. Information available included bTB skin test data, as described below, the age of the cow on the day of the test, the year when the herd was tested, the season of the test, the reason for which the herd was tested and assigned breed. Animals were tested between August 2008 and September 2009, at a mean age of 4.8 years (ranging from 1 to 11 years); either as part of the annual herd test, herd check tests or reactor herd tests [14]. Most animals were assigned as Holstein

adult females, with a small number designated as Friesians (n = 164). A breakdown of data by these variables is given in Table 1.

The animal study was licensed by the Department of Health, Social Security and Public Safety for Northern Ireland (DHSSPSNI) under the UK Animals (Scientific Procedures) Act 1986 [ASPA], following a full Ethical Review Process by the Agri-Food & Biosciences Institute (AFBI) Veterinary Sciences Division (VSD) Ethical Review Committee. The study is covered by DHSSPSNI ASPA Project Licence (PPL-2638 'Host Genetic Factors in the Increasing Incidence of Bovine Tuberculosis'), and scientists and support staff working with live animals during the studies all hold DHSSPSNI ASPA Personal Licences.

Phenotype Definitions

Cattle that showed a positive reaction to the Single Intradermal Comparative Cervical test (SICCT), that had TB lesions confirmed by post-mortem examination of carcasses at slaughter and were confirmed as *M. bovis* positive by culture and molecular tests, were defined as cases (592 animals). In this study a positive SICCT was defined as a skin test reaction to *M. bovis* antigens (skin-fold thickness) that, after 72 h exceeds the reaction to *M. avium* antigens by at least 4 mm [2]. Controls were repeatedly SICCT negative and resident >6 months into the episode (559 animals), in herds where cases were observed [13]. Controls were age-matched and preferentially selected from herds with higher disease prevalence in order to increase their probability of exposure to the pathogen [15].

Genotyping

All individuals were genotyped using BovineHD Illumina Bead Chip. After quality control, 617,885 SNPs were retained for subsequent analysis. Quality control parameters applied included a minimum Gentrain Call (GC) score of 0.60, a minimum minor allele frequency of 0.05 and a minimum call rate of 0.90 for all loci. Animals with a call rate <90% were excluded. The map of the SNP positions was also available (bovine genome assembly *Bos taurus* UMD 3.0).

Structure Exploration

Principal component analysis (PCA) was used to explore data structure with principal components in *R* (*R version 2.14*). PCA allows discrimination of sample classes and identification of outlier groups representing subpopulations that are genetically distinct. PCA on the 1151×1151 identity-by-state (IBS) matrix of pairwise relatedness, followed by plotting the first principal component values against the second principal component revealed the presence of two clusters, the main one, and a secondary smaller cluster comprising 40 individuals (Figure S1 in [13]) none of which were described as Friesians. By using the BovineHD BeadChip genotypes no sub-structure due to designated animal breed was identified by PCA. Identification of the outliers showed that 39 of them originated from the same herd. Further enquiries revealed that cross-breeding with beef cattle breeds may have taken place in this herd. Thus, to address the possibility of breed differences these animals, along with one additional animal from a different herd that was also clustering with this group, were deleted in some of the following analyses as described in the definition of datasets, below.

Table 1. The number of animals in the dataset classified by year of test, season of test and reason for test.

	Year		Season			Test reason		
	2008	2009	Winter	Spring	Autumn	Annual	Herd check	Reactor herd
Cases	359	233	309	115	168	155	231	206
Controls	384	175	253	96	210	124	251	184
Totals	743	408	562	211	378	279	482	390

Definition of Datasets

Three slightly different datasets were used in this analysis. Firstly, the full dataset comprising all 1151 individuals was used. Secondly, a reduced dataset was derived from the full dataset, removing the 40 individuals that were identified as outliers by the PCA and for which there was information that they could be crossbreds. This was done in order to address the hypothesis that the presence of beef cross-bred animals may introduce genetic structure to the population and hence alter prediction accuracy. Finally, the analysis was repeated using only animals designated as being Holsteins, after having removed the animals reported by the farmers as Friesians (n = 164). For each analysis and dataset a new **G** matrix was calculated and the corresponding adjusted phenotypes and estimated heritability were obtained (for the analyses excluding the Friesians see details in Supplementary material).

Calculating Direct Genomic Estimated Breeding Values (DGV)

The aim of the analysis was to estimate the DGVs and then assess their predictive accuracy. To conduct a cross validation analysis, as described below, and to ensure that the sampling of phenotypes would not be biased by the fixed (non-genetic) effects, a two-step approach was used to calculate DGVs. Firstly, the data were pre-corrected for fixed effects, and then random genetic effects, or DGVs, were estimated using the pre-adjusted data [16].

1. Fixed effects model. An initial fixed effects model was used to obtain adjusted phenotypes, corrected for identifiable non-genetic factors. The fixed effects model included animal age, test year, season, test reason and breed as fixed effects, and was fitted using the ASReml package [17]:

$$Y_{ijkmpq} = \mu + a_i + D_j + S_k + R_m + B_p + e_{ijkmpq} \qquad (1)$$

where Y_{ijkmpq} represents the binary bTB status (0: control, 1: case) of the qth individual, μ is the overall mean, a_i is the age of the individual, D_j is the effect of the year of testing, S_k is the season of testing, R_m is the reason for which testing was initiated in the herd, B_p is the individual's breed and e_{ijkmpq} is the residual error. Since all the animals were female and since the controls were selected to originate from herds of higher prevalence, sex and herd of origin were not included in the fixed effects. The residual effects, which are independent of the fixed effects, were obtained and used as phenotypes for the subsequent analyses.

2. Random effects model. The genomic estimated breeding values were calculated for all individuals using the adjusted phenotypes from model (1). As pedigree relationships were unknown in this population, genetic similarities between animals were described using the marker-based IBS genomic

kinship (**G**) matrix which has the following elements:

$$f_{ij} = \frac{2}{n} \sum_{k=1}^{n} \frac{(x_{ik} - p_k)(x_{jk} - p_k)}{p_k(1 - p_k)}, (i \neq j)$$

$$f_{ij} = 1 + \frac{1}{n} \sum_{k=1}^{n} \frac{Obs(\# \, \mathrm{hom})_{ik} - E(\# \, \mathrm{hom})_k}{1 - E(\# \, \mathrm{hom})_k}, (i = j)$$

where x_{ik} (x_{jk}) is the genotype of the ith (j^{th}) animal at the kth SNP, n the total genomic SNPs, and p_k is the frequency of the B allele at the kth SNP. $Obs(\#hom)_{ik}$ and $E(\#hom)_k$ are the observed and expected number of homozygous genotypes for the ith animal at the kth SNP [18].

To construct **G**, SNPs found only in the homozygote state in the sample and those found on the X chromosome were removed (601,280 SNPs were finally retained in the analysis). From that, the inverse **G** matrix was obtained and used in the random effects model, fitted using the ASReml package, with the following model:

$$y_i = m + u_i + e_i \qquad (2)$$

where m is the overall mean, y_i is the residual effect for the ith individual as calculated from model (1), u_i is it is genomic estimated breeding value with $u \sim$ MVN $(0, \mathbf{G}\sigma_a^2)$ and e_i is its residual value with $e \sim$ MVN $(0, \mathbf{I}\sigma_e^2)$.

3. Full mixed model. For the purpose of estimating the heritability of bTB resistance from the full dataset, the fixed and random effects were fitted simultaneously in ASReml as follows:

$$y_i = \boldsymbol{\beta}_i + u_i + e_i \qquad (3)$$

where all the fixed effects ($\boldsymbol{\beta}$) from model (1) were fitted as before and the relationship information from the **G** matrix was incorporated as random effects.

Cross Validation

Genomic prediction accuracy can be assessed through cross validation, a non-parametric method that allows assessment of the predictive ability of a classifier [19]. By partitioning the data into a training set and a validation set, DGVs can be predicted for the validation set without reference to phenotypic information. Prediction accuracy can then be calculated by correlating the predicted breeding values and the observed phenotypes, corrected for trait heritability [20]. A five-fold cross validation was conducted as follows.

Firstly, to create the training set in each of the three datasets the individuals were partitioned into five random groups of near-equal size, with the randomization performed separately within the case and control sub-populations. Phenotypes were then masked for each subset in turn, creating five datasets (or folds) in which four-fifths of the animals had a phenotype (training-set, y_1), and one-fifth had no phenotype (validation-set, y_2).

Secondly using the GBLUP model (2), predicted DGVs were calculated for each validation-set in turn based on the **G** matrix alone, i.e. information recorded from the training-set animals, $(\hat{y}_2|y_1)$ [20–22].

For each of the five test-sets the correlation between the cross-validated predicted DGVs $(\hat{y})$ and the adjusted phenotypes (y), i.e. $r(y,\hat{y})$, was calculated. The expected accuracy $(r(g,\hat{g}))$ between the breeding value of an individual (g) and its estimate $(\hat{g})$, was derived from the correlation as $E[r(g,\hat{g})] \approx r(y, \hat{y})/h$, where h is the square root of the heritability [20,23]. The accuracy for each test set was calculated using the heritability obtained for each corresponding cross validation fold and then the average accuracy across all the individuals was obtained.

In order to reduce random sampling effects and assess the sampling properties of the accuracy, the cross validation analysis as described above was replicated six times, where for each replicate a new randomisation was performed so that the individuals comprising each of the groups were different. Finally the average accuracy across all six replications with its empirical 95% confidence interval was obtained, where the confidence interval was calculated from a one sample t-test for the six accuracy values obtained from the six replications.

Assessing Predictive Ability using ROC Curves

Genomic predictions can be further assessed through the properties of the Receiver Operator Characteristic (ROC) curves and the corresponding area-under-the-ROC-curve (AUC). A ROC curve is the plot of the probability of a positive test result given that the individual is diseased (sensitivity) versus the probability of a positive test result given that the individual is healthy (1-specificity) [24], for all successive thresholds. AUC represents the probability of correct assignment of individuals in the class of diseased or in the class of healthy on the basis of their genotype alone [24]. Using the R package, the predicted DGVs for each of the omitted (validation) groups from the cross validation procedure and the binary phenotype for all the 1,151 individuals were used to calculate the ROC curves, along with their corresponding AUC values, for each of the six randomisations for the full dataset.

Theoretical Expectations

AUC$_{max}$. Insight into the information obtained by calculating the ROC curves and their corresponding AUC can be gained by considering these values relative to the theoretical maximum AUC value that could be obtained given the characteristics of the trait and the population under study. Wray et al. (2010) [24] introduced the idea of a maximum AUC value (AUC$_{max}$) that would be achieved if the test classifier was a perfect predictor of genetic risk. This maximum is unique for each disease trait, since it depends on the disease prevalence (q) and the heritability of the trait on the underlying liability scale (h_L^2). h_L^2 can be estimated from the approximation $h_o^2 \sim h_L^2 q^2 i_q^2 [q(1-q)]^{-1}$ as introduced by Robertson and Lerner (1949), where h_o^2 is the heritability on the observed scale, q is the disease prevalence in the sample and i_q is the mean in standard deviation units of the proportion q of the population, assuming a normal distribution. The online

Table 2. Correlations between adjusted phenotypes and predicted DGVs, heritabilities and prediction accuracies.

	Full Dataset			Excluding minor cluster			Excluding Friesians		
	$r(\hat{y}_2, y_2)$	h^2	$r(g, \hat{g})$ SD	$r(\hat{y}_2, y_2)$	h^2	$r(g, \hat{g})$ SD	$r(\hat{y}_2, y_2)$	h^2	$r(g, \hat{g})$ SD
Run 1	0.10	0.21	0.22 0.12	0.13	0.21	0.29 0.05	0.13	0.18	0.34 0.22
Run 2	0.15	0.19	0.36 0.08	0.15	0.20	0.35 0.10	0.15	0.17	0.38 0.10
Run 3	0.15	0.20	0.34 0.14	0.12	0.21	0.29 0.17	0.14	0.18	0.35 0.18
Run 4	0.14	0.20	0.33 0.17	0.14	0.20	0.34 0.25	0.15	0.17	0.37 0.16
Run 5	0.13	0.20	0.31 0.11	0.16	0.19	0.40 0.21	0.15	0.17	0.37 0.18
Run 6	0.17	0.19	0.42 0.18	0.12	0.21	0.28 0.19	0.13	0.18	0.32 0.07
Average	**0.14**	**0.20**	**0.33 0.07**	**0.14**	**0.21**	**0.33 0.05**	**0.14**	**0.18**	**0.36 0.02**

$r(\hat{y}_2, y_2)$ is the average correlation between adjusted and predicted phenotypes, h^2 is the heritability estimate, and $r(g,\hat{g})$ is the prediction accuracy with corresponding standard deviation SD. In this table shown are the parameter values for each of the cross validation runs and the averages across all replications for the full data set, the reduced dataset after having removed the animals clustering separately in the PCA, and for the dataset without the animals designated as Friesians.

Table 3. Regression of phenotypes on predicted DGVs.

	Regression coefficient	SD	Regression coefficient	SD
Run 1	0.74	0.41	1.17	0.87
Run 2	1.14	0.27	1.31	0.45
Run 3	1.08	0.43	1.22	0.75
Run 4	1.16	0.78	1.26	0.55
Run 5	1.16	0.78	1.31	0.71
Run 6	1.42	0.75	1.06	0.24
Average	1.11	0.22	1.22	0.10

Average regression coefficients with the corresponding standard deviations among test sets for each of the cross validation runs and the average across all replications. Left part of the table: full data set, right part: dataset from which the Friesians were excluded.

calculator provided [24] was used to obtain expected values for AUC_{max} and AUC_{half}, which is defined as the AUC expected from a genomic profile that accounts for only a half of the known genetic variance. These values can be used as a basis of comparison for the actual AUC values obtained in the present study.

Prediction accuracy. Daetwyler at al. (2010) presented a formula for estimating the expected GBLUP accuracy [8]:

$$r_{g\hat{g}} = \sqrt{[N_P h^2/(N_P h^2 + \Sigma M_e)]} \qquad (4)$$

where N_P is the number of individuals in the training population, h^2 is the heritability on the observed scale, and M_e is defined as the number of independent chromosome segments which satisfies

$$\Sigma M_e = 2N_e L/ln(4N_e L) \qquad (5)$$

M_e depends on the genome length in Morgans L and on the effective population size N_e. Formulae (4) and (5) were applied to different putative effective population sizes for this sample of animals in order to obtain estimates for the number of independent chromosome segments and the expected corresponding prediction accuracy, for the full dataset and the dataset without the Friesians.

Results

GBLUP and Cross Validation

The GBLUP analysis gave an estimate for the heritability of bTB susceptibility of 0.23±0.06 on the observed scale ($h_L^2 = 0.34$) for the full data set, 0.23±0.07 ($h_L^2 = 0.34$) for the dataset after removing the 40 individuals identified as a distinct sub-population from the PCA and 0.21±0.07 ($h_L^2 = 0.34$) for the reduced data set with the Friesian individuals excluded. Table 2 shows the correlations between the adjusted phenotypes and the predicted DGVs, the corresponding heritability estimates and accuracy values with their standard deviations obtained as averages across the five cross validation groups for each of the six replications (detailed tables can be found in the supplementary material, Tables S1, S2, S3 in file S1). Accuracies of 0.33 (95% C.I.: 0.26, 0.40), 0.33 (95% C.I.: 0.28, 0.37), and 0.36 (95% C.I.: 0.33, 0.38) were obtained for the three datasets, respectively. As discussed below, these values are in line with theoretical

expectations given the size of the dataset. Further, for each of the cross validation folds and across the six replications, both for the full and the dataset without the Friesians, the observed phenotypes were regressed on the predicted DGVs (Table 3, detailed tables can be found in the Supplementary Material, Tables S4, S5 in file S1). These values are close to the expected value of 1.0.

ROC Curves and AUC Values

ROC curves, showing the utility of DGVs as predictors of the binary phenotype, are shown in Figure 1. In these ROC curve plots, the comparison of interest is with the outcome that would be expected by chance (diagonal line of no discrimination). The curves for all randomisations lie above this diagonal line. Therefore, for the population under study the use of genotypes provides information in the prediction of disease state, i.e. the markers help to predict resistance. The AUC values were 0.56, 0.59, 0.58, 0.57, 0.57 and 0.59 for the six different randomizations applied (Figure 1). Hence, there was a probability close to 0.58 of correctly classifying cows based on SNP chip genotype alone using these data. Examples of individual ROC curves for each of the five cross validation test sets within one cross validation run are shown in Figure S1 in file S1.

Theoretical Expectations

AUC values. For the data-set in the present study the disease prevalence was 0.51 (592 cases out of 1,151 animals in total) and h_L^2 was estimated to be 0.34 for a heritability on the observed scale of 0.23. For a prevalence $p = 0.5$, the selection intensity (i_q) would be 0.798 [25]. An $AUC_{max} = 0.77$ and $AUC_{half} = 0.69$, can then be obtained using the online calculator provided by Wray et al. (2010). Therefore, the maximum achievable accuracy in this dataset would be 0.77. Our AUC value of 0.58 is somewhat less than AUC_{half}, i.e. this is consistent with the accuracy value which also was less than 0.5.

Prediction accuracy. Expected accuracies of the genomic predictions are shown in Table 4. With N_P being the average number of individuals in the training population (920.8), h^2 the heritability on the observed scale (0.23), the number of independent chromosome segments M_e was calculated for different values of effective population size (Table 4). If ΔF_g is the rate of inbreeding per generation, then for a rate of inbreeding per year $\Delta F_y = 0.0017$ [26] and a five years generation interval for dairy cattle, $\Delta F_g \approx 0.01$, and thus, a

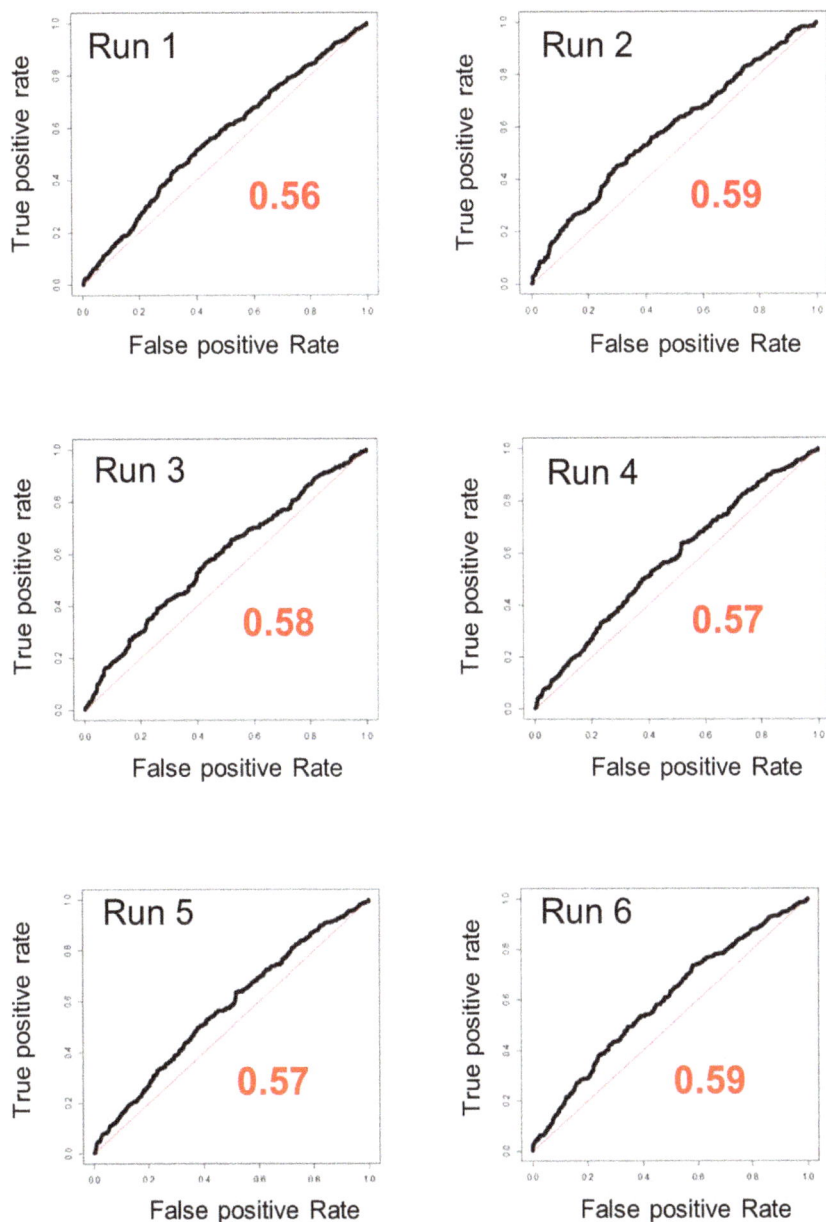

Figure 1. ROC curves for the six randomisations. ROC curves (a plot of true positive rate (Sensitivity) against false positive rate (1-Specificity)) and the corresponding AUC (the probability of correctly assigning an individual as diseased or as healthy on the basis of its genotype alone) for the six randomisation runs for the full dataset.

Table 4. Expected prediction accuracy for different values of effective population size.

Assumed N_e	Full dataset		Excluding Friesians	
	($N_P = 920.8$ and $h^2 = 0.23$)		($N_P = 789.6$ and $h^2 = 0.21$)	
	$\sum M_e$	$r_{g\hat{g}}$	$\sum M_e$	$r_{g\hat{g}}$
50	639.79	0.50	639.79	0.45
100	1136.53	0.40	1136.53	0.36
150	1600.18	0.34	1600.18	0.31

Training population size (N_p), heritability, number of independent chromosome segments ($\sum M_e$) and corresponding expected accuracy ($r_{g\hat{g}}$) for different assumed effective population sizes. Left part of the table: full data set, right part: dataset from which the Friesians were excluded.

suggestive value for the effective population size would be $N_e \approx 50$. Using formulas 4 and 5 with $N_e \approx 50$ ($M_e = 639.79$), the expected accuracy would be $r_{g\hat{g}} = 0.50$. Reversing the calculations, an expected accuracy of $r_{g\hat{g}} = 0.34$, gives an effective population size of $Ne \approx 150$. This value may not be an unreasonable value for the Holstein-Friesian cows in this sample, given that the population under study is a sample derived as a random selection of non-pedigree dairy cattle and hence possibly not as highly selected as cattle recorded in pedigree databases, and there are likely to be Friesian cows in the dataset along with the possibility of a small number of crossbred animals.

For the dataset with the animals designated as Friesians excluded, the expected accuracies were slightly lower, and the observed accuracy was consistent with an effective population size of ca. 100 individuals.

Discussion

This study provides evidence that genomic selection for bTB resistance is potentially feasible in populations where phenotypic information in unavailable for selection candidates, and even when no pedigree is available. Genomic selection can be considered as a two-step procedure. Initially, on a reference population with both phenotypic and genotypic information, DGVs can be calculated as the genome-wide sum of marker effects [21]. Then, for selection candidates the DGVs can be predicted without the need for phenotypes, since the marker effects have already been calculated in the relevant population [28]. With this design, the results of the present study are important in the context of bTB control. Predicting DGVs in the absence of phenotypes is highly beneficial in the case of bTB, since collection of appropriate phenotypic information requires that a population undergoes an epidemic and that all animals (including controls) are exposed to the pathogen [6]. These conditions can only be met for a subset of animals in the national population and will become increasingly difficult to satisfy as disease prevalence decreases.

The predictive accuracy of the DGVs is at levels that justify further studies on larger populations in order to obtain predictions that could be used in evaluation of selection candidates for their bTB resistance. In order to obtain an accuracy of 0.7, the theoretically required number of animals needed in the training population can be calculated by rearranging formula (4). Given a heritability of 0.23 and with $N_e = 50$, ~2,670 individuals would be needed in the training population. But if the N_e were to increase to 100, the size of the required training population would increase to ~4747 individuals, as might be expected. However, if the N_e was 100 but we targeted a prediction accuracy of 0.5, then the size of the training population needed would reduce to ~1647. Although in our study, the size of the training population (920.8) was somewhat smaller, the outcomes of the analyses suggest that genomic selection is potentially feasible. However, implementation of genomic selection should wait until we have a greater number of individuals in the training population, to enable us to achieve higher accuracy.

Estimated Heritability

The data set of UK dairy cattle analysed in this study through the GBLUP approach, provided a heritability estimate of 0.23 (0.34 on the liability scale) for the trait of tuberculosis resistance. This value indicates stronger evidence for genetic variation than previous estimates [11,12]. However,

direct comparison between studies with and without pedigree information should be undertaken with caution. Our estimate is lower than the value reported for deliberately challenged red deer [29]. Health traits often have low heritability due to problems of data collection and interpretation [6]. However, the intermediate heritability of tuberculosis resistance makes genomic selection for tuberculosis resistance an appealing approach to assist in bTB control.

ROC Curves Properties

A ROC curve is a representation of the different combinations of sensitivity and specificity for successive thresholds between a positive and a negative test result. For a pair of infected and healthy individuals, the probability of correctly identifying the case is represented by the AUC [30]. Although the ROC curves and their AUCs based on genotypic information in this study show only a modest increase in the probability of correctly classifying cases or controls compared to random expectations, these values should also be considered relative to the AUC_{max} [24]. This represents an upper limit of predictive ability given the properties of the dataset and the trait under study, assuming that the classifier (i.e. the DGVs) were a perfect predictor of genetic risk. Since AUC_{max} depends on disease prevalence and trait heritability, the authors argue that prediction accuracy measure should be preferred for genomic prediction evaluation [31], as it is independent of the epidemic properties.

Cross Validation Prediction Accuracy

Random error due to sampling effects was minimized by averaging the accuracies across several replications with different randomizations so that the individuals comprising each of the five groups were different each time. The differences observed between the randomizations indicate that even with ca. 1000 individuals, random sampling effects still contribute significantly to the cross validation outcomes. Conducting more randomisations was preferred to increasing the number of groups i.e. cross validation folds, because the test set would be reduced, increasing variability across the cross validation folds.

When the full dataset was used, the accuracy obtained was consistent with the theoretical accuracy obtained using the formula by Daetwyler et al. (2008) for an effective population size of $N_e = 150$, given the properties of the dataset (i.e. sample size and trait heritability). This N_e value is somewhat higher than that often suggested for the Holstein cattle population (c.f. N_e ca. 50 [27]), but may have been inflated due to the structure present in the dataset revealed by PCA, and also from the designation of several individuals as Friesian. Both factors would increase the apparent N_e. Further, the population under study is not a pedigree or a highly selected population, with the animals included in the study sampled from random commercial farms.

It should be noted that results from the different variations of the datasets used were coherent across the analyses. When the cows designated as Friesians were removed, in addition to giving slightly increased accuracy, the dataset behaved more consistently across replicates, and the corresponding implied N_e was reduced (N_e ca. 100). This was despite the fact that the dataset was smaller; presumably reflecting a more uniform population with linkage disequilibrium extending across longer chromosomal regions. Removing the PCA outliers had little impact on the prediction accuracy, however the number removed (14 cases and 26 controls) may have been too few to affect the results.

Phenotypic selection based on EBVs remains a possibility for bTB, but collection of enough phenotypic data to accurately estimate EBVs across an entire population is challenging since it requires the presence of an epidemic. Even if pedigree-recorded herds were affected, providing complete and good quality data, as is the case in the UK, analysing these data would only provide results with an application to specific sub-populations, i.e. animals that are more closely related to the herd. For animals that are more distantly related by pedigree to the ones in the epidemic, accuracy of the pedigree-based EBVs would be poor. Genomic selection for bTB resistance overcomes this problem and thus is potentially very useful, even if prediction accuracy is only modest.

Finally it has been estimated that the basic reproductive number (R_0), i.e. the average number of cases generated by one infectious individual, for bTB in the UK is only slightly greater than 1 (1.07) and so even a modest intervention would be sufficient to substantially reduce the risks or severities of bTB breakdowns [32]. Similarly, even when R_0 is substantially greater than one as in the case of the UK foot-and-mouth disease epidemic, a combination of intervention strategies can substantially contribute towards bringing the epidemic under control [33]. Selection to make animals more resistant would help to reduce R_0 for bTB.

Conclusion

Our results demonstrate that genomic selection is potentially feasible for bTB resistance even in populations with no pedigree data available, and it can be applied to animals lacking bTB phenotypes. Potentially this technique could also be applied to other diseases such as Paratuberculosis (Johne's disease). Access to a greater number of animal phenotypes, thereby creating larger training sets, would help to improve potential prediction accuracies and open up opportunities for implementation.

Supporting Information

File S1 File S1 includes the following: Figure S1. ROC curves for each of the five cross validation test groups. For the full data set, the ROC curves for each of the five cross validation test groups are presented for the first randomisation. **Table S1. Detailed accuracy tables for the six randomisations for the data set including all the individuals.** For the data set including all the individuals, the correlation, heritability with its standard error and corresponding prediction accuracy for each of the five test-groups from the Cross Validation procedure are presented for the six different randomization replications. **Table S2.**

Detailed accuracy tables for the six randomisations for the data set in which animals clustering separately in the PCA were removed. For the data set in which animals clustering separately in the PCA were removed, the correlation, heritability with its standard error and corresponding prediction accuracy for each of the five test-groups from the Cross Validation procedure are presented for the six different randomisation replications. **Table S3. Detailed accuracy tables for the six randomisations for the data set when the 164 animals designated as Friesians were removed.** The correlation, heritability with its standard errors and corresponding prediction accuracy for each of the five test groups in the Cross Validation procedure resulting from the six randomisation replications when the 164 animals designated as Friesians were removed. The data for the remaining 987 animals were re-randomised to training and test sets, which were ~790 and ~198 respectively. In the initial fixed effects model breed was removed from the fixed effects and a new **G** matrix calculated only for the Holsteins was used. **Table S4. Detailed results for the regression analysis on the full dataset.** For the full datset, intercept (a) and regression coefficients (b) for the regresison of adjusted phenotypes (observed) on cross-validated EBVs (predicted), for each cross validation fold across the six replication runs, with corresponding standard deviations. **Table S5. Detailed results for the regression analysis on the datset without the Friesians.** For the datset without the Friesians, intercept (a) and regression coefficients (b) for the regression of adjusted phenotypes (observed) on cross validated EBVs (predicted), for each cross validation fold across the six replication runs, with corresponding standard deviations.

Acknowledgments

We would like to thank Richard Talbot, David Morrice and their colleagues from ARK-Genomics, Roslin Institute, for the timely and efficient DNA extraction and genotyping, and excellent technical support throughout the project; Department of Agriculture and Rural Development for access to Animal and Public Health Information System data; the support provided by Will Barker and DARD Veterinary Service, staff at WD Meats and Veterinary Sciences Division Farm Staff who delivered all the abattoir case sampling and farm control sampling; herd-keepers who gave permission to sample their control cattle; VSD-AFBI specialist histology/pathology and bacteriology staff involved in TB case confirmation.

Author Contributions

Conceived and designed the experiments: SB ST EG JW RS SHM AA. Performed the experiments: AA RS SHM DW MB SWM EG SB JW. Analyzed the data: ST. Contributed reagents/materials/analysis tools: RP OM. Wrote the paper: ST SB JW RS AA DW.

References

1. Allen AR, Minozzi G, Glass EJ, Skuce RA, McDowell SWJ, et al. (2010) Bovine tuberculosis: the genetic basis of host susceptibility. Proceedings of the Royal Society B: Biological Sciences 277(1695): 2737.
2. de la Rua-Domenech R, Goodchild AT, Vordermeier HM, Hewinson RG, Christiansen KH, et al. (2006) Ante mortem diagnosis of tuberculosis in cattle: a review of the tuberculin tests, gamma-interferon assay and other ancillary diagnostic techniques. Res Vet Sci 81: 190–210.
3. Buddle BM, Pollock JM, Skinner MA, Wedlock DN (2003) Development of vaccines to control bovine tuberculosis in cattle and relationship to vaccine development for other intracellular pathogens. International Journal for Parasitology 33: 555–566.
4. Donnelly CA, Wei G, Johnston WT, Cox DR, Woodroffe R, et al. (2007) Impacts of widespread badger culling on cattle tuberculosis: concluding analyses from a large-scale field trial. Int J Infect Dis 11: 300–308.
5. Pollock JM, Neill SD (2002) Mycobacterium bovis infection and tuberculosis in cattle. Vet J 163: 115–127.
6. Bishop SC, Woolliams JA (2010) On the genetic interpretation of disease data. PLoS One 5: 0008940.
7. Meuwissen TH, Hayes BJ, Goddard ME (2001) Prediction of total genetic value using genome-wide dense marker maps. Genetics 157: 1819–1829.
8. Daetwyler HD, Pong-Wong R, Villanueva B, Woolliams JA (2010) The Impact of Genetic Architecture on Genome-Wide Evaluation Methods. Genetics 185: 1021–1031.

9. Hayes BJ, Visscher PM, Goddard ME (2009) Increased accuracy of artificial selection by using the realized relationship matrix. Genet Res 91: 47–60.

10. Daetwyler HD, Villanueva B, Woolliams JA, Daetwyler HD, Villanueva B, et al. (2008) Accuracy of Predicting the Genetic Risk of Disease Using a Genome-Wide Approach. PLoS One 3: e3395.

11. Bermingham ML, More SJ, Good M, Cromie AR, Higgins IM, et al. (2009) Genetics of tuberculosis in Irish Holstein-Friesian dairy herds. J Dairy Sci 92: 3447–3456.

12. Brotherstone S, White IM, Coffey M, Downs SH, Mitchell AP, et al. (2010) Evidence of genetic resistance of cattle to infection with Mycobacterium bovis. J Dairy Sci 93: 1234–1242.

13. Bermingham ML, Bishop SC, Woolliams JA, Pong-Wong R, Allen AR, et al. (2014) Genome-wide association study identifies novel loci associated with resistance to bovine tuberculosis. Heredity E-pub 5 February.

14. Abernethy DA, Denny GO, Menzies FD, McGuckian P, Honhold N, et al. (2006) The Northern Ireland programme for the control and eradication of Mycobacterium bovis. Veterinary Microbiology 112: 231–237.

15. Bishop SC, Doeschl-Wilson AB, Woolliams JA (2012) Uses and implications of field disease data for livestock genomic and genetics studies. Front Genet 3: 00114.

16. de los Campos G, Hickey JM, Pong-Wong R, Daetwyler HD, Calus MPL (2012) Whole Genome Regression and Prediction Methods Applied to Plant and Animal Breeding. Genetics.

17. Gilmour A, Gogel B, Cullis B, Thompson (2009) ASReml User Guide Release 3.0. VSN International Ltd. Hemel Hempstead, HP1 1ES, UK.

18. Uemoto Y, Pong-Wong R, Navarro P, Vitart V, Hayward C, et al. (2013) The power of regional heritability analysis for rare and common variant detection: simulations and application to eye biometrical traits. Front Genet 4: 00232.

19. Hastie T, Tibshirani R, Friedman J (2003) The Elements of Statistical Learning: Data Mining, Inference, and Prediction: Springer.

20. Legarra A, Robert-Granié C, Manfredi E, Elsen J-M (2008) Performance of Genomic Selection in Mice. Genetics 180: 611–618.

21. Luan T, Woolliams JA, Lien S, Kent M, Svendsen M, et al. (2009) The accuracy of Genomic Selection in Norwegian red cattle assessed by cross-validation. Genetics 183: 1119–1126.

22. Daetwyler HD, Calus MPL, Pong-Wong R, de los Campos G, Hickey JM (2013) Genomic Prediction in Animals and Plants: Simulation of Data, Validation, Reporting and Benchmarking. Genetics 193(2): 347–65.

23. Quilez J, Martinez V, Woolliams JA, Sanchez A, Pong-Wong R, et al. (2012) Genetic Control of Canine Leishmaniasis: Genome-Wide Association Study and Genomic Selection Analysis. PLoS One 7: e35349.

24. Wray NR, Yang J, Goddard ME, Visscher PM (2010) The Genetic Interpretation of Area under the ROC Curve in Genomic Profiling. PLoS Genet 6: e1000864.

25. Falconer DS, Mackay TFC (1997) Introduction to Quantitative Genetics. Ed 4. Longmans Green, Harlow, Essex, UK.

26. Kearney JF, Wall E, Villanueva B, Coffey MP (2004) Inbreeding trends and application of optimized selection in the UK Holstein population. J Dairy Sci 87: 3503–3509.

27. McParland S, Kearney JF, Rath M, Berry DP (2007) Inbreeding trends and pedigree analysis of Irish dairy and beef cattle populations. J Anim Sci 85: 322–331.

28. Habier D, Fernando RL, Dekkers JC (2007) The impact of genetic relationship information on genome-assisted breeding values. Genetics 177: 2389–2397.

29. Mackintosh CG, Qureshi T, Waldrup K, Labes RE, Dodds KG, et al. (2000) Genetic Resistance to Experimental Infection with Mycobacterium bovis in Red Deer (Cervus elaphus). Infection and Immunity 68: 1620–1625.

30. Janssens AC, Aulchenko YS, Elefante S, Borsboom GJ, Steyerberg EW, et al. (2006) Predictive testing for complex diseases using multiple genes: fact or fiction? Genet Med 8: 395–400.

31. Wray NR, Goddard ME, Visscher PM (2007) Prediction of individual genetic risk to disease from genome-wide association studies. Genome Res 17: 1520–1528.

32. Cox DR, Donnelly CA, Bourne FJ, Gettinby G, McInerney JP, et al. (2005) Simple model for tuberculosis in cattle and badgers. Proceedings of the National Academy of Sciences of the United States of America 102: 17588–17593.

33. Ferguson NM, Donnelly CA, Anderson RM (2001) Transmission intensity and impact of control policies on the foot and mouth epidemic in Great Britain. Nature 413: 542–548.

9

Simulation Modelling of Population Dynamics of Mosquito Vectors for Rift Valley Fever Virus in a Disease Epidemic Setting

Clement N. Mweya[1,4]*, Niels Holst[2], Leonard E. G. Mboera[3], Sharadhuli I. Kimera[4]

1 National Institute for Medical Research, Tukuyu, Tanzania, **2** Department of Agroecology, Aarhus University, Slagelse, Denmark, **3** National Institute for Medical Research, Dar es salaam, Tanzania, **4** Department of Veterinary Medicine and Public Health, Sokoine University of Agriculture, Morogoro, Tanzania

Abstract

Background: Rift Valley Fever (RVF) is weather dependent arboviral infection of livestock and humans. Population dynamics of mosquito vectors is associated with disease epidemics. In our study, we use daily temperature and rainfall as model inputs to simulate dynamics of mosquito vectors population in relation to disease epidemics.

Methods/Findings: Time-varying distributed delays (TVDD) and multi-way functional response equations were implemented to simulate mosquito vectors and hosts developmental stages and to establish interactions between stages and phases of mosquito vectors in relation to vertebrate hosts for infection introduction in compartmental phases. An open-source modelling platforms, Universal Simulator and Qt integrated development environment were used to develop models in C++ programming language. Developed models include source codes for mosquito fecundity, host fecundity, water level, mosquito infection, host infection, interactions, and egg time. Extensible Markup Language (XML) files were used as recipes to integrate source codes in Qt creator with Universal Simulator plug-in. We observed that Floodwater Aedines and Culicine population continued to fluctuate with temperature and water level over simulation period while controlled by availability of host for blood feeding. Infection in the system was introduced by floodwater Aedines. Culicines pick infection from infected host once to amplify disease epidemic. Simulated mosquito population show sudden unusual increase between December 1997 and January 1998 a similar period when RVF outbreak occurred in Ngorongoro district.

Conclusion/Significance: Findings presented here provide new opportunities for weather-driven RVF epidemic simulation modelling. This is an ideal approach for understanding disease transmission dynamics towards epidemics prediction, prevention and control. This approach can be used as an alternative source for generation of calibrated RVF epidemics data in different settings.

Editor: Jens H. Kuhn, Division of Clinical Research, United States of America

Funding: This project was supported by Health Research Users Trust Fund of the National Institute for Medical Research (NIMR) under human capacity development strategy for training of CNM. The funders had no role in study design, decision to publish, or preparation of the manuscript.

Competing Interests: The authors have declared that no competing interests exist.

* Email: cmweya@nimr.or.tz

Introduction

Rift Valley fever (RVF) is an infection caused by arbovirus belonging to genus *Phlebovirus* of the family *Bunyaviridae*. The viruses use arthropod vectors such as mosquitoes and sand flies for infection transfer to livestock and humans [1]. Since its first description in 1930 in Kenya [2,3], the virus has occurred as epidemic disease in Sub-Saharan Africa primarily in eastern and southern Africa, North Africa, Arabian Peninsula and Madagascar [4,5] and poses a potential threat to Europe [6]. In all recorded epidemics, the disease had socio-economic impact due to high animal and human morbidity and mortality. The major outbreaks in Kenya, Tanzania and Somalia were in 1997–1998 and 2006–2007 [7,8], with human deaths totalling 478 and 318 in years 1998

and 2007 respectively [9]. During the 2006–2007 outbreaks in Kenya and Tanzania, a reported number of 16,973 cattle, 20,193 goats, and 12,124 sheep died of the disease, with spontaneous abortions observed for 15,726 cattle, 19,199 goats, and 11,085 sheep [9–11]. Similar to other arboviral infection, RVF virus is passed from generation to generation of Aedine mosquitoes trans-ovarially [12–14]. This vertical disease transmission permits the virus to survive over prolonged periods because eggs can survive for several years in dry conditions [12,15–17].

Emergence of infected mosquito populations and amplification of the virus are determined by changes in weather conditions [15,18,19]. In East Africa, RVFV epidemics are known to be associated with patterns of unusually heavy rainfall [20]. This led the World Health Organization (WHO) and Food and Agriculture

Organization (FAO) to developed RVF forecasting models centred on cyclical patterns of the El Niño/Southern Oscillation (ENSO) [18,21]. These models incorporate measurements of global and regional elevated sea surface temperatures, rainfall and satellite derived-normalized difference vegetation index data [22–24] which derive from Remote Sensing Satellite Imagery (RSSD), including use of Landsat, SPOT and Synthetic Aperture Radar and Cold Cloud Density (CCD) which allow use of more sophisticated tools to predict RVF virus epizootic activity over much wider areas [24–26]. Predictions were corroborated through entomological field investigations of mosquitoes and virus activity in the suspected area [27] as a key element in controlling RVF [28]. However, recent climate-driven prediction results in 2012 for some areas in Kenya and Tanzania [29] indicating foreseeable challenges due to the complexity of the disease (virus, vectors, and hosts) involved and their interactions with the environment hence a need to incorporate more tools.

Mathematical models have been developed for RVFV epidemics to complement available weather only dependent prediction models [30–33]. Many of them are based on previously developed epidemiological model of RVF that focus mainly on animals and vectors population dynamics with hypothetical consideration of infection dynamics [32]. Further development of this model incorporated the role of vaccination and vector control to describe epidemiology of RVFV in areas of intense transmission [34,35]. Other developments for this model associate exclusion of a vertical

transmission in vectors and inclusion of animal movements for spatial spread of disease [36–38]. Some models associate epidemics with cryptic cycles of the virus within animal hosts [39] and a more improved vertical transmission in vectors that include seasonality [31]. The role of daily weather data such as temperature and rainfall as model input to determine vector populations have not previously been directly considered. This limits their further applicability in predictive epidemiology due to insufficient incorporation of weather data and on-the-ground biological processes related to RVF disease.

Development of prediction models for RVFV epidemics faces many challenges like lack of reliable data. Absence of field-based rapid diagnostic tools results in the disease first being detected when it is actually beginning to decline from within the infected populations. RVF epidemics preparedness teams are therefore less effective for counter-measure against the impact of the disease. It is well documented that in order for disease to be controlled by vaccination, animals need to be vaccinated 4–6 weeks before stress and risk periods [40] to ensure that the vaccinated population have developed enough immunity against the virus [29,41]. We therefore present a simulation modelling approach that incorporate weather data to simulate on-the-ground entomological data on mosquito abundances in relation to their hosts as previously recommended [11].

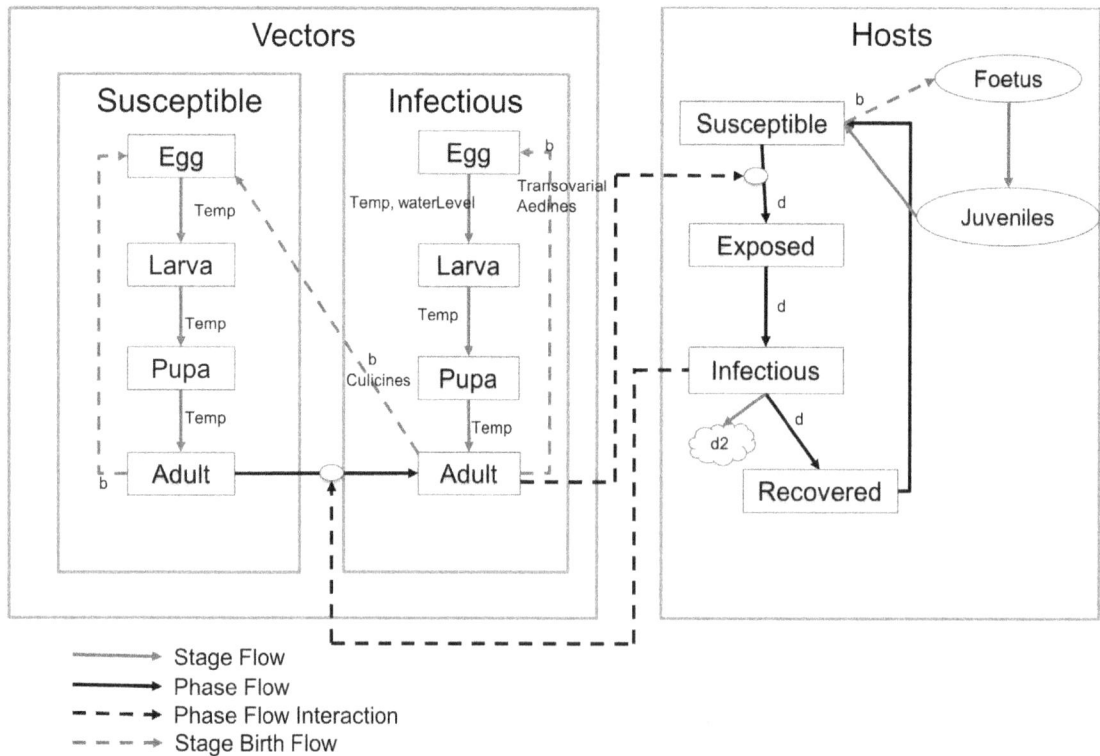

Figure 1. Diagrammatic presentation of RVF vector population dynamics simulation model. Adult mosquitoes lay eggs directly in breeding sites or in soil above water level (the latter remain inactive for many years). Hatching of inactive floodwater Aedes eggs depend on water level in breeding sites which in-turn depends on amount of daily rainfall. Our model considers mosquito growth and mortality in each developmental stage depend on temperature, water level and host availability. Mosquitoes move from susceptible to infectious phase after contact with infectious host. Hosts remain in the susceptible phase until after effective contact with infectious mosquitoes, and then hosts flow from susceptible to exposed, infectious and recovered phases. **Abbreviations**: b = births, d = natural mortality, d_2 = mortality due to disease, temp = depends on temperature, waterLevel = depends on water in breeding sites, transovarial = transovarial transmission.

Table 1. Parameters description.

Parameter	Description	Value range	Details	Reference
aedesLongevity	Longevity of females Aedes	30.0–45.8 days		[58]
aedesFecundity	Eggs laid per female Aedes per day	25–35 egg per day		[59]
aedesEggMortality	Number eggs dead per day in a stage	11.3–12.9%	failure to hatch	[55,59,60]
aedesHatchRate	Hatch rate for Aedes	85–95%		[59]
aedesLarvalSurvival	Larvae survival rates	90–100%		[59]
aedesLarvaeMortality		13.97–16.7%	Endogenous causes	[59]
aedesPupaMortality		17–30%	Endogenous causes	[59]
sexRatio	Proportion of female mosquitoes for both Aedes and Culex spp	1:1		[58,59]
transovarial	Virus transovarial transmission rate	Range from 0 to 1	RVF virus vertical transmission in Aedes mosquitoes is still not known	[31]
gonotrophicCycles	Gonotrophic cycles or number of blood meals per female	5–9 times	Cycle after every 3–5 days	[58]
culexLongevity	Survival or longevity (females Culex)	25.2–36.9 days		[61], [62]
culexFecundity	Culex fecundity	21–69 eggs per day	63–200 eggs after every 3 to 5 days	[63]
culexHatchRate	Egg hatching (Culex)	75.2–89.0%		[62]
culexEggMortality	Egg mortality (Culex)	10.9–24.9%		[62]
culexPupaGrowth	Larva pupation (Culex)	47.8–68.5%		[62]
culexLarvaeMortality	Larvae mortality (Culex)	15.9–31.8%		[62]
culexPupaMortality	Pupae mortality (Culex)	5.62–6.13%		[62]
activationRate	Infectious eggs hatch from soil per day	10–100%		[64]
waterLevelThreshold	Minimum amount of water in mosquito breeding sites required to activate infectious eggs		Adjusted based on parameter sensitivity analysis	
dailyLoss	Amount of water lost per day	Fixed/Manually adjusted	Adjusted based on parameter sensitivity analysis	
daysDegreesLarvae	Cumulative temperature for larvae growth	206 Celsius degrees		[55,59,60,65–67]
daysDegreesPupae	Cumulative temperature for pupa growth	74 Celsius degrees		[55,59,60,65–67]
sheepLifeSpan	Longevity of females sheep	6 to 11 years		[68]
lambAge	Age period for lamb	365 days		[68]
gestationPeriod	Period for foetus development	152 days		[68]
carryingCapacity	Environment's maximum load	200 sheep per square kilometre	Calculated from sheep population in specific areas	
sheepAbortions	Foetus die per day due to RVF	90–100%		[69,70]
lambMortality	Lamb die per day due to RVF	Less than 50%		[69,70]
adultMortality	Adult sheep die per day due to RVF	20–30%		[69,70]

Materials and Methods

Study scenario and data source

The Ngorongoro district in Tanzania was purposely selected as the main study scenario. The district is part of the Serengeti-Masai Mara Ecosystem, which is defined by the limits of the annual wildlife migration linking with a neighbour country, Kenya experiencing similar disease epidemics. The district represents unique interaction between livestock, wildlife and human interface with animal migrations. The area has experienced several records of RVFV outbreaks. According to 2006–2007 outbreaks, high animal mortality was recorded in this area [5]. Freely accessible daily rainfall and temperature data from 1994–1999 for Ngor-

ongoro with Narok ecosystem, Mwanza and Musoma regions downloaded from http://www.ncdc.noaa.gov/cdo-web.

Assumptions for simulation model

The assumptions for model development include; Floodwater Aedine mosquitoes are responsible for maintenance of the virus with vertical transmission and Culicine mosquitoes play a major role in virus amplification during epidemics. Water level in potential breeding sites determines hatching of Floodwater Aedine eggs. Increased water level in breeding sites is required to allow infected eggs laid further in the soil to hatch. Mosquito developmental stages use cumulative temperature as important

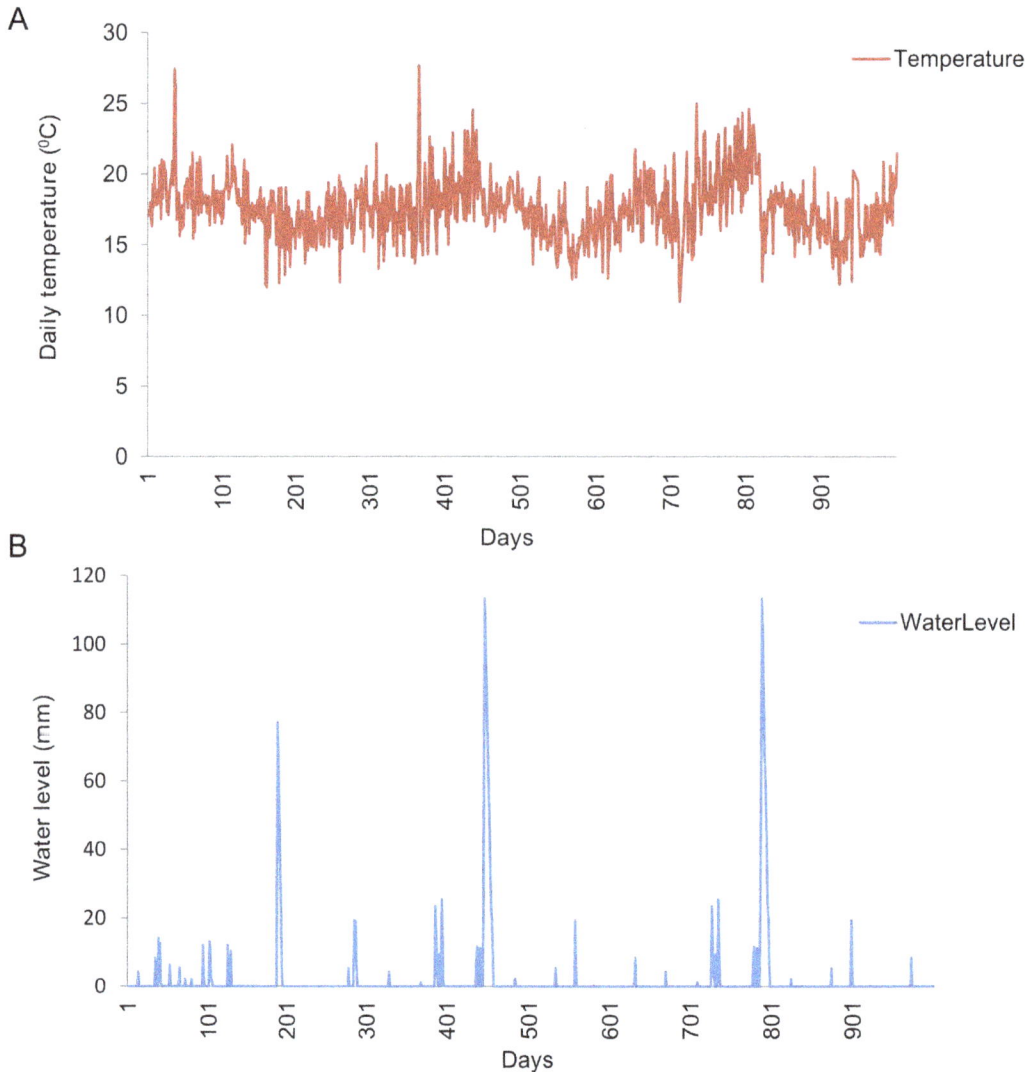

Figure 2. Daily weather data for Ngorongoro district from 1994–1999 only for the first 1000 days. (A) Daily temperature in °C. (B) Water level in breeding sites (millimetres) calculated from daily rainfall data.

model input factor to determine maturation time and adults survival. Mosquito search for a blood meal is a function of availability of hosts and that the probability of a successful blood meal is a function of the availability of host. During feeding, a mosquito has the probability of transferring viral infection to a host, or becoming infected by taking a blood meal from a viremic host. Flow of infection in mosquitoes and host is governed in compartmental phases. RVFV infection is initiated in a single phase small population of Floodwater Aedine mosquitoes before reaching the amplifying Culicine mosquitoes (Figure 1).

Formulation for simulation model

1-D and 2-D time-varying distributed delay (TVDD) equations were used to formulate the models [42–45]. These time-variant distribution delay equations were initially developed in 1970s based on a kth order time-invariant distributed delay and later on applied as stage structured population dynamics models. TVDD models emphasize that delay in the distribution from one stage or phase to another is the quality of the output given some input parameters. All entities that enter the delay process at the input

either leave at the output or remain stored inside the process. The 2-D TVDD are implemented similar to 1-D TVDD in a way that stages and phases are capable of interacting simultaneously [46]. Details on how these mathematical models were implemented in C++ programming language are indicated in Text S1. Four developmental stages such as eggs, larvae, pupae and adults with host age groups were modelled using 1-D TVDD. 2-D TVDD were used to model distribution compartmental phases of mosquitoes and hosts. Mosquitoes were categorised in two phases; Susceptible (S) and Infectious (I). Hosts were categorised in four phases; Susceptible (S), Exposed (E), Infectious (I) and Recovered (R) (Figure 1). We have included the exposed stage because we need model predictions to be accurate to the nearest day by accounting for the time lag between infection and the onset of infectiousness.

During each mosquito developmental stage temperature dependence delays were used [44,45]. The mean delay time for mosquitoes to pass through a stage of growth is calculated as a total required number of degree days given as cumulative temperature. A simplified water balance model was used to

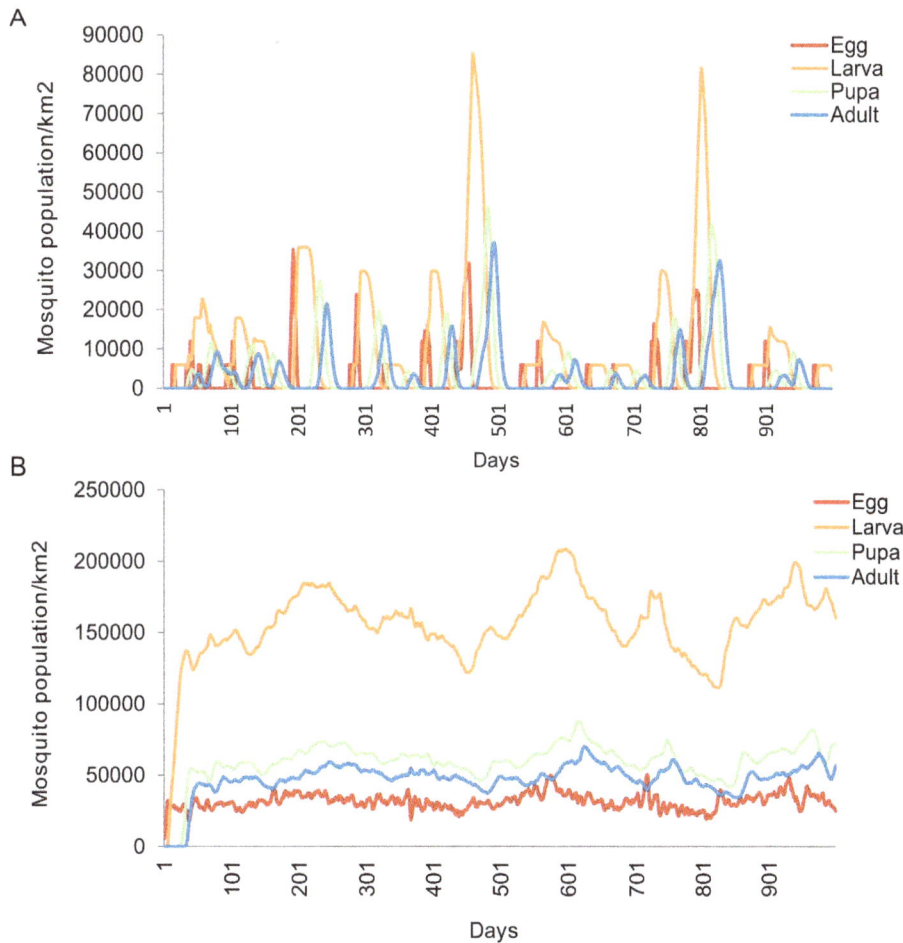

Figure 3. Simulated RVF vector population dynamics showing developmental stages from eggs, larvae, pupae and adults. (A) Floodwater Aedines depending on water level in breeding sites and host availability. (B) Culicines.

simulate daily variations in amount of water in potential breeding sites for floodwater Aedine mosquitoes. Daily rainfall data was used as model input to determine cumulative amount of water in breeding sites after deduction of daily water loss due to other factors such as evaporation. We applied water balance equation that uses the principles of conservation of mass in a closed system as previously described [47,48] but with added simplicity to reflect mosquito breeding behaviour. Cumulative amount of water in breeding sites determined hatching of floodwater Aedine eggs laid on the soil above water level in breeding sites (Figure 1).

Multi-way functional response equations previously described for predator prey relations [49] were modified to reflect vector-host interactions in a disease setting as indicated in Text S1. Mult-way functional responses were used to determine how host search for blood meal influenced mosquito fecundity. Mosquito vector phases (susceptible or infectious) were allowed to take a blood meal from all phases and stages of a host. Interaction between infectious mosquito vectors with susceptible host caused a phase outflow to exposed hosts. Interaction between susceptible mosquito vectors with infectious host caused a phase outflow to infectious vectors. Infectious Floodwater Aedine mosquitoes were allowed to lay infectious eggs timed to hatch depending on cumulative water level in breeding sites above threshold. Infectious Culicines laid eggs hatching susceptible mosquitoes as they lack transovarial transmission. Infection transfer to hosts was calculated automat-

ically as indicated in Text S1. Phase outflow for the host from exposure phase to infectious and then recovered take consideration of host mortality due to disease and recovered host were allowed to flow into a susceptible phase (Figure 1). RVFV don't induce lifelong immunity like measles, recovered animals should be at risk of getting infection again but it is still not known how long it takes before they become susceptible again.

Development of simulation model

Model algorithms were developed using an open-source Universal Simulator and Qt Integrated Development Environment in C++ programming language [50]. We followed procedures for installation and use of Qt creator, Universal Simulator end user and developer's versions as provided in the Universal Simulator website (http://www.ecolmod.org). Source codes for mosquito fecundity, host fecundity, water level, mosquito infection, host infection and Aedines eggs time were prepared. Extensible Markup Language (XML) files were prepared as recipe to integrate source codes in Qt creator with Universal Simulator plug-in. Source codes incorporated control structures for hatching of infectious inactive egg laid in the soil due to water level increase in breeding sites and RVFV infection initiation from Floodwater Aedine mosquitoes to susceptible host and then to Culicine mosquitoes for virus amplification. Details of parameters used are as shown in Table 1 and source codes are shown in Text S1.

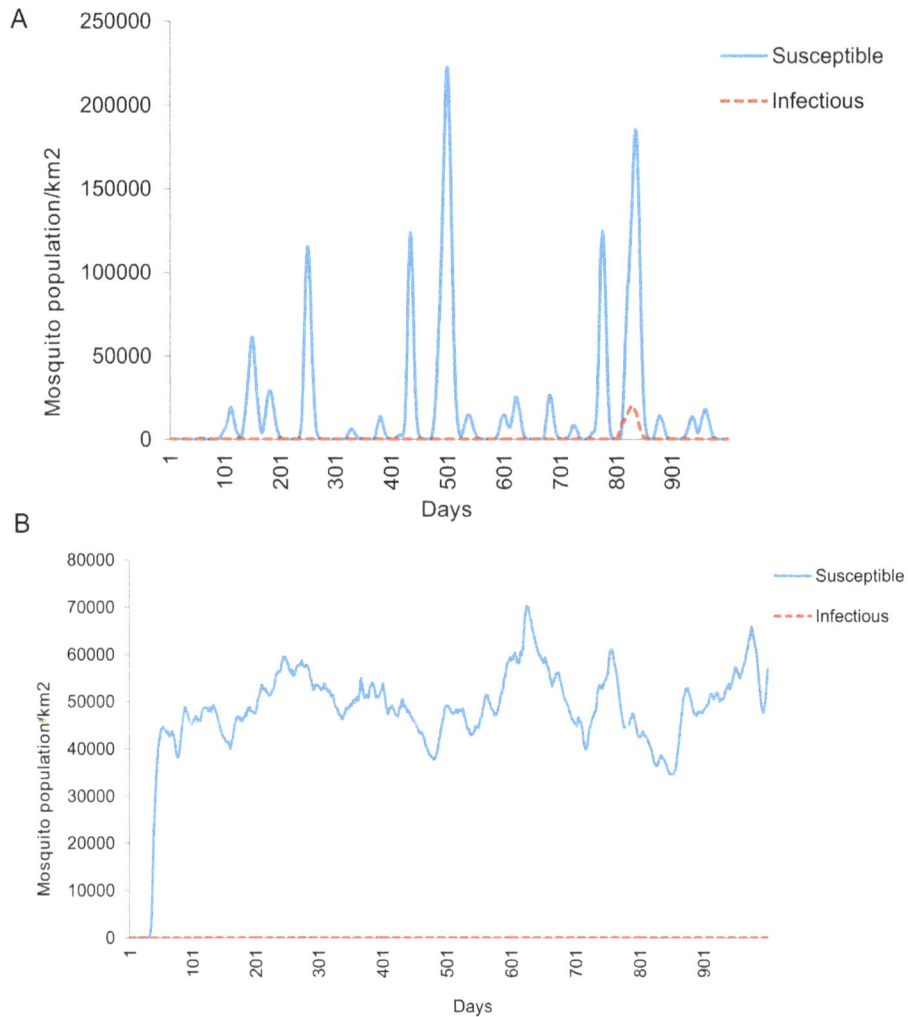

Figure 4. Simulated infection initiation before virus amplification. (A) Floodwater Aedines initiate infection. (B) Culicines without infection from infected sheep to prevent virus amplification.

Parameter sensitivity and calibration

In order to understand the influence of many time based processes in this model, sensitivity analysis of model outputs due to variation in input parameters was assessed during simulation period. Stochastic random normal distribution was applied to quantify the sensitivity of the outputs [51]. Sensitivities were assessed on daily time-step spanning 100 steps of simulation. The influence of temperature, water level thresholds, infection period, incubation period and vector-host interactions on time-dependent sensitivities were quantified. Generated sensitivity data was then used to calibrate the models output to reflect the actual number that would have been trapped in the same period based on independent mosquito population dataset [52].

Results

During simulations, the following initial conditions were prescribed to run once; 50 adult Floodwater Aedine and Culicine mosquitoes that were allowed to lay eggs and initiated growth to larvae, pupae and adult mosquitoes under appropriate conditions. Similarly, initial population for host sheep was 50 lamb and 100 adults with the environmental carrying capacity of 200 sheep per

square kilometer (Table 1). Mosquito population dynamics simulated for both floodwater Aedines and Culicine showed relationship with daily temperatures and rainfall fluctuate over a period from 1994 to January 1999 (Figure 2A) and rainfall data used to determine estimated amount of water in breeding sites for Aedine mosquitoes (Figure 2B).

Selected parameters were sensitive to substantial changes with vector-host population's simulation time. Low temperature thresholds had a significant impact on larvae by delaying transfer of larvae to pupae. High temperature caused high mortality in larvae and reduces adult survival days. Water level thresholds that depended on daily rainfall influenced the emergence of floodwater Aedine mosquitoes and hatching of infectious eggs laid in the soil above water level in the breeding site. At low water level thresholds, population of floodwater Aedine mosquitoes varied similar with Culicine which did not depend on water level for mosquito emergence. In this light, water level threshold for emergence of infectious floodwater is adjusted to reflect the biological role of floodwater Aedine in RVF epidemics.

Mosquito attack rates for blood meal and infection introduction during vector-host interactions were sensitive to determine stage and phase flows. Vector-host interactions were influenced by

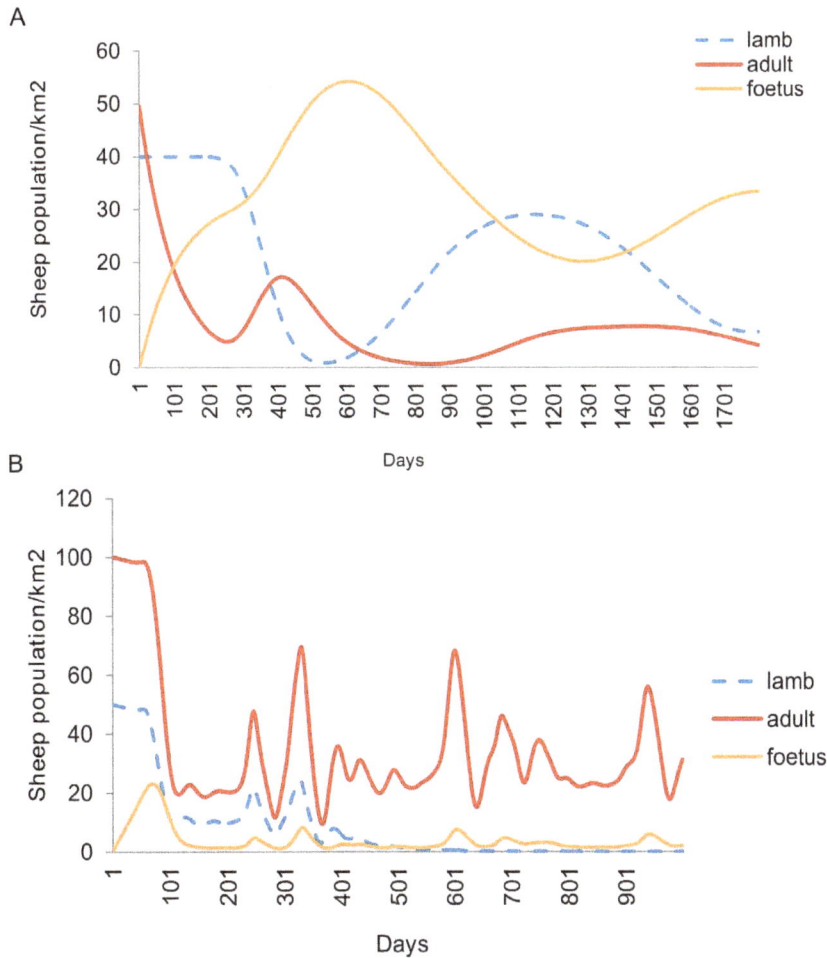

Figure 5. Sheep population dynamics controlled at the environmental carrying capacity of 200 sheep per square kilometre. (A) Growth stages without infection. (B Growth stages after introduction of controlled infection within Aedines mosquitoes only.

infection period and RVFV incubation period in hosts. Infectious period in mosquito vectors and hosts influenced the pattern and peak size of the simulated epidemic, longer infectious period extended the duration of the epidemic. For mosquitoes, this duration was set to the lifespan of the mosquito in order to reflect the actual duration of RVF epidemic whereas in hosts ranged from three to six days. Longer disease incubation period within hosts showed a delayed increase in the number of infectious hosts and therefore a later peak in the epidemic than when the incubation period is assumed to be short. Knowing the infection and incubation period appeared to be important in predicting dynamics of a simulated epidemic.

Simulation results yielded equilibrium over time with a stable and consistent number of mosquitoes, regardless of the initial starting point of the adult population following model calibration. Floodwater Aedines and Culicine vector population continued to fluctuate with temperature and water level over the entire period while controlled by availability of host for blood feeding (Figure 3A, B). In order to initiate infection, emergence of infectious floodwater Aedines was set at different water level threshold (Figure 4A, B). Culicines only pick infection from infected sheep once in order to amplify disease epidemic (Figure 4B).

Sheep population provided as lamb and adults were allowed to fluctuate over the whole simulation period. Sheep remained in the susceptible phase until had contact from infectious Floodwater mosquitoes (Figure 5A, B). Following infection introduction in the exposure phase, sheep were allowed to flow to infectious and recovered phases. Mortality due to disease was also calculated and simulated at a given time. Mortality provided varied with age group of sheep and sex to indicate high abortions in natural environment as indicator for RVF epidemic (Figure 6).

Controlled simulation of mosquito population dynamics without influence of host availability for a period from 1994 to 1999 showed sudden increase after about 1450 days of simulation, a period between December 1997 and January 1998, similar to the time in which Ngorongoro district experienced a RVF disease outbreak (Figure 7). However, this sudden increase in mosquito population was not observed in Mwanza region where RVF outbreak did not occurred in the same period (Figure 7). This unusual pattern in vector population increase could be associated with potential of RVFV outbreaks. The early stage of the simulated potential disease outbreak was characterized by an abnormal decline in vector population as a potential future epidemic indicator.

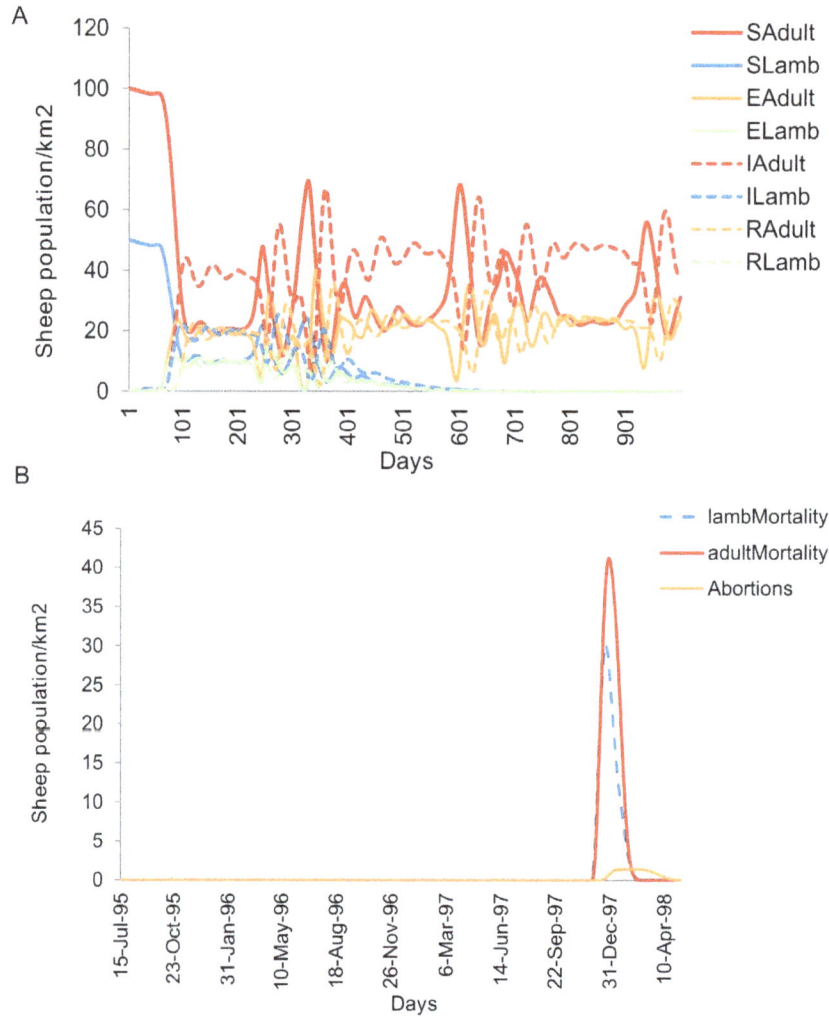

Figure 6. Simulated RVF epidemic. (A) Compartmental phases after allowing infection to flow from Aedines to Culicines for virus amplification, recovered hosts are not allowed to flow back into the susceptible hosts. (B) Calculated host mortality per developmental stages due to infection with RVF virus. **Abbreviations**: SAdult = Susceptible adults, SLamb = Susceptible lamb, EAdult = Exposed adult, ELamb = Exposed lamb, IAdult = Infectious adult, ILamb = Infectious lamb, RAdult = Recovered adult, RLamb = Recovered lamb.

Discussion

Our simulation modelling strategy was to produce useful tool for studying effects of daily rainfall and temperature on vector life stages in terms of stage-specific growth and death rates. Conditions that result in unusual abundance of vector mosquito species have been shown to have a positive association with RVFV epidemics [53]. The model that we developed provides understanding of the dynamics of RVFV vector population by implementing time dependent distribution delay and functional response modelling approaches for aggregated systems. These models have previously had broad applications in predicting life cycles of insects, animals, plants, trees, and capital goods in economics, but not in previously published RVF modelling papers [43,46,49]. Assessment of the value of the underlying biological processes allows us to examine potential variability in RVFV infections in animal and human populations given the vectors for both maintenance and amplification of the virus in the population.

Studying RVFV transmission dynamics poses a big challenge among scientists, as disease outbreaks are associated with abnormal changes in weather conditions which are essential

components for prediction of disease epidemics. Choosing the right modelling procedure for this complex disease can be quite challenging. Simulation modelling of RVFV vector populations dynamic remains a useful tool in understanding these transmission dynamics. In our simulation model, we attempt to replicate the actual biological processes related to dynamics of the relevant disease vectors in a local endemic setting. This model takes advantage of previously developed mathematical equations for modelling disease vectors and hosts stages at different phases of infection but with careful selection of useful parameter in relation with the biology of RVFV [54-56].

The current procedures for simulations development are highly flexible to allow inclusion of factors that might accelerate the emergence and decline of Aedine population by not only considering availability of water in respective breeding sites. However, we carefully avoided including other factors such as landscape features [57] and soil types in relation with vectors distribution. Although Aedine populations may play important role of RVFV infection initialization, we limited our simulation procedure to generalized presentation of vectors for maintenance of the virus by Aedines and amplification during epidemics by

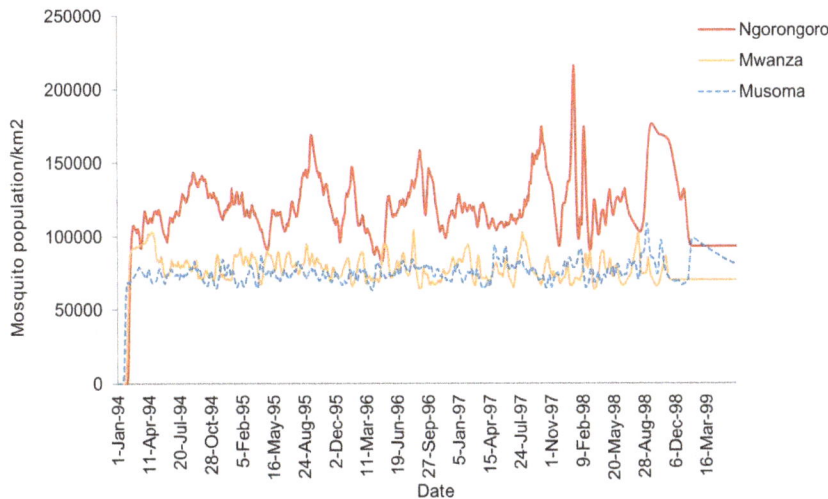

Figure 7. Vector population dynamics simulation results indicating unusual increase in mosquito population in late 1997 and early 1998. Similar period to when large-scale RVF outbreak occurred in Ngorongoro district. Disease outbreak did not occur in Mwanza and Musoma areas during the same period.

Culicines. Despite this simplicity, our model produced reasonable vector population values and generated trajectories that were consistent with expectations for years from 1994 to 1999 based on only freely accessed weather data. This model provides flexibility for inclusion of more hosts and vectors interactions as would appear in disease epidemics setting.

While developing models for RVF disease prediction is highly useful, significant work is needed for further improvement in this modelling approach. We agree on simplification of some parameter estimation such as trans-ovarial transmission within Aedes mosquitoes due to the lack of more information. RVF virus vertical transmission in Aedes mosquitoes is still not known [31]. This simulation required inclusion of more relevant numerical information and use of the advanced calendar module in order to be able to clearly mark simulation dates linking biological processes with simulation output. Further model improvements should include need for separate models handling animal and human population dynamics and addition of spatial distribution of vectors and host in relation to disease distribution.

Simulation outputs from this study provide new insights for weather-driven RVFV epidemic modelling. This study shows that daily temperature and rainfall are key ecological factors to include in models that predict episodes related to RVFV outbreak [20]. Simulations provide an ideal approach for understanding the important parameters in virus transmission dynamics with important insights to be gained in prevention and control of such epidemics. This approach can be used as an alternative source for generation of RVFV epidemics data in different scenario for use in advanced computational analyses and can be modified for use to other diseases. Final version of this simulation model is available for download as a Universal Simulator plug-in in both the end user version and source code from http://www.ecolmod.org/download.html.

Supporting Information

Text S1 File containing instructions to guide installation and use of therein attached RVF plug-in source codes.

Acknowledgments

We sincerely acknowledge participation of CNM to a three month online course on participatory ecological modelling for PhD students under the Graduate School of Science and Technology (GSST), Flakkebjerg Research Center, Aarhus University, Denmark.

Author Contributions

Conceived and designed the experiments: CNM NH SIK LEGM. Performed the experiments: CNM NH. Wrote the paper: CNM NH SIK LEGM. Verified simulation modelling biological concept: LEGM SIK.

References

1. Bishop DH, Beaty BJ (1988) Molecular and biochemical studies of the evolution, infection and transmission of insect bunyaviruses. Philos Trans R Soc Lond B Biol Sci 321: 463–483.
2. Daubney R, Hudson JR, Garnham PC (1931) Enzootic hepatitis or Rift Valley fever: an undescribed disease of sheep, cattle and man from east Africa. Journal of Pathology and Bacteriology 34: 545–579.
3. Davies FG (1975) Observations on the epidemiology of Rift Valley fever in Kenya. J Hyg (Lond) 75: 219–230.
4. Meegan JM, Moussa MI, el-Mour AF, Toppouzzada RH, Wyess RN (1978) Ecological and epidemiological studies of Rift Valley fever in Egypt. J Egypt Public Health Assoc 53: 173–175.
5. Mohamed M, Mosha F, Mghamba J, Zaki SR, Shieh WJ et al. (2010) Epidemiologic and clinical aspects of a Rift Valley fever outbreak in humans in Tanzania, 2007. Am J Trop Med Hyg 83: 22–27. 83/2_Suppl/22 [pii]; doi:10.4269/ajtmh.2010.09-0318.
6. Chevalier V (2013) Relevance of Rift Valley fever to public health in the European Union. Clin Microbiol Infect 19: 705–708.
7. Kebede S, Duales S, Yokouide A, Alemu W (2010) Trends of major disease outbreaks in the African region, 2003–2007. East Afr J Public Health 7: 20–29.
8. Clements AC, Pfeiffer DU, Martin V, Otte MJ (2007) A Rift Valley fever atlas for Africa. Prev Vet Med 82: 72–82. S0167-5877(07)00111-0 [pii]; doi:10.1016/j.prevetmed.2007.05.006.
9. Dar O, McIntyre S, Hogarth S, Heymann D (2013) Rift Valley fever and a new paradigm of research and development for zoonotic disease control. Emerg Infect Dis 19: 189–193. doi:10.3201/eid1902.120941.
10. Mweya CN, Kimera SI, Kija JB, Mboera LE (2013) Predicting distribution of Aedes aegypti and Culex pipiens complex, potential vectors of Rift Valley fever virus in relation to disease epidemics in East Africa. Infect Ecol Epidemiol 3. doi:10.3402/iee.v3i0.21748;21748 [pii].

11. Jost CC, Nzietchueng S, Kihu S, Bett B, Njogu G et al. (2010) Epidemiological assessment of the Rift Valley fever outbreak in Kenya and Tanzania in 2006 and 2007. Am J Trop Med Hyg 83: 65–72. 83/2_Suppl/65 [pii]; doi:10.4269/ajtmh.2010.09-0290.

12. Logan TM, Linthicum KJ, Thande PC, Wagateh JN, Nelson GO et al. (1991) Egg hatching of Aedes mosquitoes during successive floodings in a Rift Valley fever endemic area in Kenya. J Am Mosq Control Assoc 7: 109–112.

13. Diallo M, Lochouarn L, Ba K, Sall AA, Mondo M et al. (2000) First isolation of the Rift Valley fever virus from Culex poicilipes (Diptera: Culicidae) in nature. Am J Trop Med Hyg 62: 702–704.

14. Romoser WS, Oviedo MN, Lerdthusnee K, Patrican LA, Turell MJ et al. (2011) Rift Valley fever virus-infected mosquito ova and associated pathology: possible implications for endemic maintenance. Res Rep Trop Med 121–127.

15. Nguku PM, Sharif SK, Mutonga D, Amwayi S, Omolo J et al. (2010) An investigation of a major outbreak of Rift Valley fever in Kenya: 2006–2007. Am J Trop Med Hyg 83: 5–13. 83/2_Suppl/05 [pii]; doi:10.4269/ajtmh.2010.09-0288.

16. Linthicum KJ, Anyamba A, Tucker CJ, Kelley PW, Myers MF et al. (1999) Climate and satellite indicators to forecast Rift Valley fever epidemics in Kenya. Science 285: 397–400. 7614 [pii].

17. Gerdes GH (2002) Rift valley fever. Vet Clin North Am Food Anim Pract 18: 549–555.

18. Anyamba A, Linthicum KJ, Small JL, Collins KM, Tucker CJ et al. (2012) Climate teleconnections and recent patterns of human and animal disease outbreaks. PLoS Negl Trop Dis 6: e1465. doi:10.1371/journal.pntd.0001465;PNTD-D-11-00034 [pii].

19. Tabachnick WJ (2010) Challenges in predicting climate and environmental effects on vector-borne disease episystems in a changing world. J Exp Biol 213: 946–954. 213/6/946 [pii]; doi:10.1242/jeb.037564.

20. Soti V, Tran A, Degenne P, Chevalier V, Lo SD et al. (2012) Combining hydrology and mosquito population models to identify the drivers of Rift Valley fever emergence in semi-arid regions of West Africa. PLoS Negl Trop Dis 6: e1795. doi:10.1371/journal.pntd.0001795;PNTD-D-12-00330 [pii].

21. Anyamba A, Chretien JP, Small J, Tucker CJ, Linthicum KJ (2006) Developing global climate anomalies suggest potential disease risks for 2006–2007. Int J Health Geogr 5: 60. 1476-072X-5-60 [pii]; doi:10.1186/1476-072X-5-60.

22. Anyamba A, Linthicum KJ, Small J, Britch SC, Pak E et al. (2010) Prediction, assessment of the Rift Valley fever activity in East and Southern Africa 2006–2008 and possible vector control strategies. Am J Trop Med Hyg 83: 43–51. 83/2_Suppl/43 [pii]; doi:10.4269/ajtmh.2010.09-0289.

23. Linthicum KJ, Anyamba A, Britch SC, Chretien JP, Erickson RL et al. (2007) A Rift Valley fever risk surveillance system for Africa using remotely sensed data: potential for use on other continents. Vet Ital 43: 663–674.

24. Pin-Diop R, Toure I, Lancelot R, Ndiaye M, Chavernac D (2007) Remote sensing and geographic information systems to predict the density of ruminants, hosts of Rift Valley fever virus in the Sahel. Vet Ital 43: 675–686.

25. Tourre YM, Lacaux JP, Vignolles C, Lafaye M (2009) Climate impacts on environmental risks evaluated from space: a conceptual approach to the case of Rift Valley Fever in Senegal. Glob Health Action 2. doi:10.3402/gha.v2i0.2053.

26. Witt CJ, Richards AL, Masuoka PM, Foley DH, Buczak AL et al. (2011) The AFHSC-Division of GEIS Operations Predictive Surveillance Program: a multidisciplinary approach for the early detection and response to disease outbreaks. BMC Public Health 11 Suppl 2: S10. 1471-2458-11-S2-S10 [pii]; doi:10.1186/1471-2458-11-S2-S10.

27. Mohamed M, Mosha F, Mghamba J, Zaki SR, Shieh WJ et al. (2010) Epidemiologic and clinical aspects of a Rift Valley fever outbreak in humans in Tanzania, 2007. Am J Trop Med Hyg 83: 22–27. 83/2_Suppl/22 [pii]; doi:10.4269/ajtmh.2010.09-0318.

28. Hall RA, Blitvich BJ, Johansen CA, Blacksell SD (2012) Advances in arbovirus surveillance, detection and diagnosis. J Biomed Biotechnol 2012: 512969. doi:10.1155/2012/512969.

29. FAO (2012) Rift Valley Fever. Vigilance needed in the coming months. Food and Agriculture Organization of the United Nations (FAO). EMPRES WATCH 27.

30. Barker CM, Niu T, Reisen WK, Hartley DM (2013) Data-driven modeling to assess receptivity for Rift Valley Fever virus. PLoS Negl Trop Dis 7: e2515. doi:10.1371/journal.pntd.0002515;PNTD-D-13-00095 [pii].

31. Chitnis N, Hyman JM, Manore CA (2013) Modelling vertical transmission in vector-borne diseases with applications to Rift Valley fever. J Biol Dyn 7: 11–40. doi:10.1080/17513758.2012.733427.

32. Gaff HD, Hartley DM, Leahy NP (2007) An epidemiological model of Rift Valley fever. Electron J Differ Equ (EJDE) [electronic only] 15: 12. doi:10.1089/vbz.2010.0084.

33. Gao D, Cosner C, Cantrell RS, Beier JC, Ruan S (2013) Modeling the spatial spread of Rift Valley fever in Egypt. Bull Math Biol 75: 523–542. doi:10.1007/s11538-013-9818-5.

34. Gaff H, Burgess C, Jackson J, Niu T, Papelis Y et al. (2011) Mathematical Model to Assess the Relative Effectiveness of Rift Valley Fever Countermeasures. Int J Artificial Life Res 2: 1–18.

35. Gaff H, Schaefer E (2009) Optimal control applied to vaccination and treatment strategies for various epidemiological models. Math Biosci Eng 6: 469–492.

36. Niu T, Gaff HD, Papelis YE, Hartley DM (2012) An epidemiological model of Rift Valley fever with spatial dynamics. Comput Math Methods Med 2012: 138757. doi:10.1155/2012/138757.

37. Mpeshe SC, Haario H, Tchuenche JM (2011) A mathematical model of Rift Valley Fever with human host. Acta Biotheor 59: 231–250. doi:10.1007/s10441-011-9132-2.

38. Xue L, Scott HM, Cohnstaedt LW, Scoglio C (2012) A network-based meta-population approach to model Rift Valley fever epidemics. J Theor Biol 306: 129–144. S0022-5193(12)00210-X [pii]; doi:10.1016/j.jtbi.2012.04.029.

39. Manore CA, Beechler BR (2013) Inter-Epidemic and Between-Season Persistence of Rift Valley Fever: Vertical Transmission or Cryptic Cycling? Transbound Emerg Dis. doi:10.1111/tbed.12082.

40. OBP (2013) Immunisation schedules. Onderstepoort Biological Products SOC (Ltd). Available:http://www.obpvaccines.co.za/Cms_Data/Contents/OBPDB/Media/downloads/Immune-program-feb2012.pdf. Accessed 05 August 2014.

41. Ikegami T, Makino S (2009) Rift valley fever vaccines. Vaccine 27 Suppl 4: D69–D72. S0264-410X(09)01054-8 [pii]; doi:10.1016/j.vaccine.2009.07.046.

42. Vansickle J (1977) Attrition in Distributed Delay Models. IEEE Transactions on Systems, Man and Cybernetics SMC-7: 635–638.

43. Manetsch TJ (1976) Time-Varying Distributed Delays and Their Use in Aggregative Models of Large Systems. IEEE Transactions on Systems, Man and Cybernetics SMC-6: 547–553.

44. Fouque F, Baumgartner J (1996) Simulating development and survival of Aedes vexans (Diptera: Culicidae) preimaginal stages under field conditions. J Med Entomol 33: 32–38.

45. Loncaric Z, Hackenberger K (2013) Stage and age structured Aedes vexans and Culex pipiens (Diptera: Culicidae) climate-dependent matrix population model. Theor Popul Biol 83: 82–94. S0040-5809(12)00081-0 [pii]; doi:10.1016/j.tpb.2012.08.002.

46. Larkin TS, Carruthers RI, Legaspi BC (2000) Two-dimensional distributed delays for simulating two competing biological processes. Transactions of the Society for Computer Simulation International 17: 25–33.

47. Arnell NW (1999) A simple water balance model for the simulation of streamflow over a large geographic domain. Journal of Hydrology 217: 314–335.

48. Schaake JC, Koren VI, Duan QY, Mitchell K, Chen F (1996) Simple water balance model for estimating runoff at different spatial and temporal scales. J Geophys Res 101: 7461–7475.

49. Gutierrez AP (1992) Physiological-Basis of Ratio-Dependent Predator Prey Theory - the Metabolic Pool Model As A Paradigm. Ecology 73: 1552–1563.

50. Holst N (2013) A universal simulator for ecological models. Ecological Informatics 13: 70–76.

51. Muller A (2001) Stochastic Ordering of Multivariate Normal Distributions. Ann Inst Stat Math 53: 567–575.

52. Mweya CN, Kimera SI, Karimuribo ED, Mboera LE (2013) Comparison of sampling techniques for Rift Valley Fever virus potential vectors, Aedes aegypti and Culex pipiens complex, in Ngorongoro District in northern Tanzania. Tanzan J Health Res 15. doi:10.4314/thrb.v15i3.89438;89438 [pii].

53. Elfadil AA, Hasab-Allah KA, Dafa-Allah OM (2006) Factors associated with rift valley fever in south-west Saudi Arabia. Rev Sci Tech 25: 1137–1145.

54. Yusoff N, Budin H, Ismail S (2012) Simulation of Population Dynamics of Aedes aegypti using Climate Dependent Model. International Journal of Medical and Biological Sciences 6: 97–102.

55. Kokkinn MJ, Duval DJ, Williams CR (2009) Modelling the ecology of the coastal mosquitoes Aedes vigilax and Aedes camptorhynchus at Port Pirie, South Australia. Med Vet Entomol 23: 85–91. MVE787 [pii]; doi:10.1111/j.1365-2915.2008.00787.x.

56. Soti V, Tran A, Degenne P, Chevalier V, Lo SD et al. (2012) Combining hydrology and mosquito population models to identify the drivers of Rift Valley fever emergence in semi-arid regions of West Africa. PLoS Negl Trop Dis 6: e1795. doi:10.1371/journal.pntd.0001795;PNTD-D-12-00330 [pii].

57. Soti V, Chevalier V, Maura J, Begue A, Lelong C et al. (2013) Identifying landscape features associated with Rift Valley fever virus transmission, Ferlo region, Senegal, using very high resolution satellite imagery. Int J Health Geogr 12: 10. 1476-072X-12-10 [pii]; doi:10.1186/1476-072X-12-10.

58. Tsuda Y, Takagi M, Suzuki A, Wada Y (1994) A comparative Study on Life Table Characteristics of Two Strains of Aedes albopictus from Japan and Thailand. Trop Med 36: 15–20.

59. Aida HN, Dieng H, Ahmad AH, Satho T, Nurita A et al. (2011) The biology and demographic parameters of Aedes albopictus in northern peninsular Malaysia. Asian Pac J Trop Biomed 1: 472–477. doi:10.1016/S2221-1691(11)60103-2;apjtb-01-06-472 [pii].

60. Aytekin S, Aytekin AM, Alten B (2009) Effect of different larval rearing temperatures on the productivity (R o) and morphology of the malaria vector Anopheles superpictus Grassi (Diptera: Culicidae) using geometric morphometrics. J Vector Ecol 34: 32–42. JVEC5 [pii]; doi:10.1111/j.1948-7134.2009.00005.x.

61. Suman DS, Tikar SN, Mendki MJ, Sukumaran D, Agrawal OP et al. (2011) Variations in life tables of geographically isolated strains of the mosquito Culex quinquefasciatus. Med Vet Entomol 25: 276–288. doi:10.1111/j.1365-2915.2010.00939.x.

62. Gomez C, Rabinovich JE, Machado-Allison CE (1977) Population analysis of Culex pipiens fatigans Wied. (Diptera: Culicidae) under laboratory conditions. J Med Entomol 13: 453–463.

63. Yao CQ, Ning CX, Xu XD (1988) Studies on life table characteristics of Culex pipiens quinquefasciatus Wuhan strain. J Tongji Med Univ 8: 249–252.

64. Freier JE, Rosen L (1987) Vertical transmission of dengue viruses by mosquitoes of the Aedes scutellaris group. Am J Trop Med Hyg 37: 640–647.

65. Tauthong P, Brust TA (1977) The effect of temperature on the development and survival of two populations of *Aedes campestris* Dyar and Knab (Diptera: Culicidae). Can J Zool 55: 135–137.

66. Turell MJ, Rossi CA, Bailey CL (1985) Effect of extrinsic incubation temperature on the ability of *Aedes taeniorhynchus* and *Culex pipiens* to transmit Rift Valley fever virus. Am J Trop Med Hyg 34: 1211–1218.

67. Mohammed A, Chadee DD (2011) Effects of different temperature regimens on the development of *Aedes aegypti* (L.) (Diptera: Culicidae) mosquitoes. Acta Trop 119: 38–43. S0001-706X(11)00074-X [pii]; doi:10.1016/j.actatropica.2011.04.004.

68. Yunmei L, Xiaoming W (2000) A study of blue sheep population life table and its group structure of different seasons in Helan Mountain. Acta Theriologica Sinica 20: 258–262.

69. Gerdes GH (2004) Rift Valley fever. Rev Sci Tech 23: 613–623.

70. Yedloutschnig RJ, Dardiri AH, Mebus CA, Walker JS (1981) Abortion in vaccinated sheep and cattle after challenge with Rift Valley fever virus. Vet Rec 109: 383–384.

10

Preliminary Validation of Direct Detection of Foot-And-Mouth Disease Virus within Clinical Samples Using Reverse Transcription Loop-Mediated Isothermal Amplification Coupled with a Simple Lateral Flow Device for Detection

Ryan A. Waters[1], Veronica L. Fowler[1]*, Bryony Armson[1], Noel Nelson[2], John Gloster[2], David J. Paton[1], Donald P. King[1]

1 Livestock Viral Disease Program, The Pirbright Institute, Pirbright, Guildford, Surrey, United Kingdom, **2** Atmospheric Dispersion and Air Quality, The Meteorological Office, Exeter, United Kingdom

Abstract

Rapid, field-based diagnostic assays are desirable tools for the control of foot-and-mouth disease (FMD). Current approaches involve either; 1) Detection of FMD virus (FMDV) with immuochromatographic antigen lateral flow devices (LFD), which have relatively low analytical sensitivity, or 2) portable RT-qPCR that has high analytical sensitivity but is expensive. Loop-mediated isothermal amplification (LAMP) may provide a platform upon which to develop field based assays without these drawbacks. The objective of this study was to modify an FMDV-specific reverse transcription–LAMP (RT-LAMP) assay to enable detection of dual labelled LAMP products with an LFD, and to evaluate simple sample processing protocols without nucleic acid extraction. The limit of detection of this assay was demonstrated to be equivalent to that of a laboratory based real-time RT-qPCR assay and to have a 10,000 fold higher analytical sensitivity than the FMDV-specific antigen LFD currently used in the field. Importantly, this study demonstrated that FMDV RNA could be detected from epithelial suspensions without the need for prior RNA extraction, utilising a rudimentary heat source for amplification. Once optimised, this RT-LAMP-LFD protocol was able to detect multiple serotypes from field epithelial samples, in addition to detecting FMDV in the air surrounding infected cattle, pigs and sheep, including pre-clinical detection. This study describes the development and evaluation of an assay format, which may be used as a future basis for rapid and low cost detection of FMDV. In addition it provides providing "proof of concept" for the future use of LAMP assays to tackle other challenging diagnostic scenarios encompassing veterinary and human health.

Editor: Luis Menéndez-Arias, Centro de Biología Molecular Severo Ochoa (CSIC-UAM), Spain

Funding: This study was supported by United Kingdom Department for the Environment Food and Rural Affairs (Defra project SE1127) and funding from the European Union FP7-KBBE-2011-5 under grant agreement no. 289364 (RAPIDIA-Field). In addition this material is based upon work supported by the United States Department of Homeland Security under Award Number HSHQDC-12-J-00415 through Texas A & M AgriLife Research and the Institute for Infectious Diseases (IIAD). The views and conclusions contained in this document are those of the authors and should not be interpreted as necessarily representing the official policies, either expressed or implied, of the United States Department of Homeland Security. The funders had no role in the study design, data collection and analysis, decision to publish, or preparation of the manuscript.

Competing Interests: The authors have declared that no competing interests exist.

* Email: veronica.fowler@pirbirght.ac.uk

Introduction

Incursions of foot-and-mouth disease (FMD) into countries or zones with FMD-free status has devastating impacts. Although the clinical manifestations of FMD can be severe, the primary impact of an outbreak is that there is an immediate restriction on international trade of animals and animal products. An outbreak therefore has a huge economic consequences on the country, a result of both direct and indirect monetary losses. For example the 2001 UK FMDV outbreak was estimated to have cost over £8 billion [1] with a resultant drop of national GDP in that year of

0.2%. As a result of the economic impact in the event of an incursion of FMD, the primary goal is to return to FMD free status as quickly as possible after the first case is identified to minimise these impacts upon national livestock industries.

Rapid and accurate detection of FMDV is one of the first steps in the control pathway and therefore central to minimising spread of the disease. Samples from suspected outbreaks can be tested for the presence of virus by (i) RT-qPCR [2], (ii) FMDV antigen ELISA [3], and (iii) virus isolation [4]. Although some of these tests are rapid, they all rely upon the transport of samples from suspect cases to centralised laboratories which can add a significant time delay from sample collection to arrival at the laboratory. This is especially relevant if the distances involved are large. In addition to rapidity, the ability to detect pre-clinical infection is also desirable to maximise the impact of subsequent control measures. Due to the required rapidity of responses to the UK 2001 outbreak demanded at the time, many premises were slaughtered without confirmatory laboratory diagnosis. Retrospective analysis of samples collected on these premises could not find any evidence of FMD circulation on 23% of the farms designated as infected [5]. Moreover, the widespread dissemination of FMD in the UK in 2001 has been largely attributed to the silent spread in sheep [6], which would render field based assays reliant upon clinical signs useless in this species as sheep are well documented to often show minimal to no clinical signs associated with FMDV infection [7].

Two of the main reports published after the UK 2001 outbreak recommended the development of rapid field based diagnostics [8,9]. The benefits of such assays are not only restricted to previously free countries either. Many endemic countries in the developing world have relatively poor infrastructure and under-funded laboratory facilities. Accurate, rapid, and cheap diagnostic tests which are able to be implemented on farm would enable the majority of clinical cases suspected to be FMD, to be confirmed and reported to a central facility with relative ease and confidence. Accumulation of this outbreak data has been recognised as an essential first step in both longer term progressive control of the disease and also of an early warning system for nascent outbreaks of FMD within an endemic country [10].

To date, two main technologies exploiting either antigen or nucleic acid detection methods have been targeted for incorporation into portable diagnostic platforms [11,12]. An immuno-chromatographic lateral flow device (LFD) to directly detect viral antigen, with equivalent diagnostic sensitivity to the laboratory based antigen ELISA, has been developed for use in the field as a pen side test [13]. This assay is extremely portable and easy to use, giving a result in as little as 10 minutes. However, only a limited number of sample types can be tested using the LFD which must contain large amounts of FMD viral antigen in order to generate a positive result. These factors restrict the usefulness of this test to the acute clinical phase of FMD where diseased epithelium is collectable (up to 3–4 days after the onset of lesions) and contains large amounts of intact FMDV antigen. Beyond this time, either no epithelium is available to process, or viral antigen has degraded to a level no longer detectable by the test (Unpublished field observations). As described previously, some animals may not show obvious clinical signs during the entirety of infection with FMDV, making the use of this LFD redundant in these situations and by extension during the incubation period.

Detection of viral nucleic acid using real time RT-qPCR is recognised as having a much higher analytical sensitivity than antibody-based assays for the detection of FMDV [14]. Because very small quantities of viral RNA are able to be detected with the real time RT-qPCR, the diagnostic window applicable to this test is much wider than for the LFD, including the ability to detect FMDV RNA during the pre-clinical phase of infection. This, therefore, results in it having a much higher diagnostic sensitivity than the LFD. Indeed pre-clinical detection of FMDV in animals was demonstrated in the field during the 2007 FMD outbreak in the UK using RT-qPCR [15].

FMDV-specific real-time RT-qPCR assay chemistry has been transferred into portable PCR platforms and evaluated for diagnostic use [16–19]. These assays maintain high analytical sensitivity equivalent to that of a laboratory based test [19], and also a higher diagnostic sensitivity than the LFD. The hardware required for these assays is, however, relatively expensive since it uses a complex protocol for nucleic acid extraction and also needs precision temperature control for the amplification step. Furthermore, decontamination of such complex instrumentation is difficult. In light of these drawbacks, it is likely that such an assay would not be used as an on-farm pen side test, but would rather be positioned in regional veterinary laboratories close to (or within) the outbreak foci [12]. Given these limitations, a more cost-effective format for molecular diagnostics of FMD on farm, whilst maintaining the highest analytical sensitivity, is required.

In 2000, a novel nucleic acid amplification chemistry was developed called Loop-mediated isothermal AMPlification (LAMP). LAMP amplifies a nucleic acid target at a single constant temperature, relying on the strand displacement activity of a *Bst* DNA polymerase enzyme, negating the need for thermal cycling [20]. LAMP methods have been shown to have similar analytical sensitivity to RT-qPCR or PCR and do not require an expensive thermal cycler for the amplification of target sequences. LAMP assays have now been developed for the detection of multiple infectious disease organisms including bacteria [21], protozoa [22] and viruses [23]. An FMDV-specific RT-LAMP assay has previously been developed, which was able to rapidly detect FMDV RNA extracted from lesion material with equivalent analytical sensitivity to the laboratory based RT-qPCR [24]. Detection of RT-LAMP products was achieved either by analysis using agarose gel electrophoresis or utilisation of an intercalating dye combined with real-time PCR machines, both of which were effective but not practical to use as a pen side method. Turbidity [25] and colour change detection formats have been reported as more portable and simple direct visual methods for the detection of LAMP products for other pathogens, but are sometimes difficult to interpret.

Detection of LAMP products has been done by using LFD end point detection techniques [26–29] but have drawbacks of relatively fastidious conditions. More recently, detection of dual labelled LAMP products has been demonstrated using bespoke low cost LFDs operating on a much simpler antigen-antibody interaction. This simple approach enabled simple LAMP assay detection of African Swine Fever Virus (ASFV) [30]. Unequivocal positive or negative results that can be interpreted by a non-specialist can thus be obtained at low cost.

Here, we describe the modification of a previously reported FMDV-specific RT-LAMP assay, to allow detection of dual labelled LAMP products with a commercially available LFD. Furthermore, this study also investigated the practicality of simple methods that could be applied for sample preparation in the field.

Results

Development and validation of RT-LAMP-LFD assay using RNA standards

The limit of detection for the one step RT-qPCR assay was established using FMDV RNA standards (O/UKG/34/2001). RNA standards of concentrations from 10^7 copies/μl to 10^1 copies/μl (inclusive) were consistently detected (Figure 1a). At higher dilutions, 50% of reactions containing 10^0 copies/μl RNA standards were detected, while all of the dilutions at 10^{-1} copies/μl were negative. In light of this data, four dilutions spanning consistently positive (10^2 and 10^1), intermediate (10^0) and negative (10^{-1}) by RT-qPCR were taken forward to subsequently evaluate the performance of the RT-LAMP assay.

Preliminary experiments examined the performance of the already existing RT-LAMP chemistry compared to RT-qPCR. In these experiments where the RT-LAMP was performed using a

10-fold dilutions of FMDV 3D RNA standards

Copies / µL	10^3	10^2	10^1	10^0	10^{-1}
a) Ct Value	29.4	32.1	35.2	+/−	-
b) Tp Value	23.1	27.2	30.7	+/−	-
c) AGE result	+	+	+	+/−	-
d) LAMP-LFD				+/−	

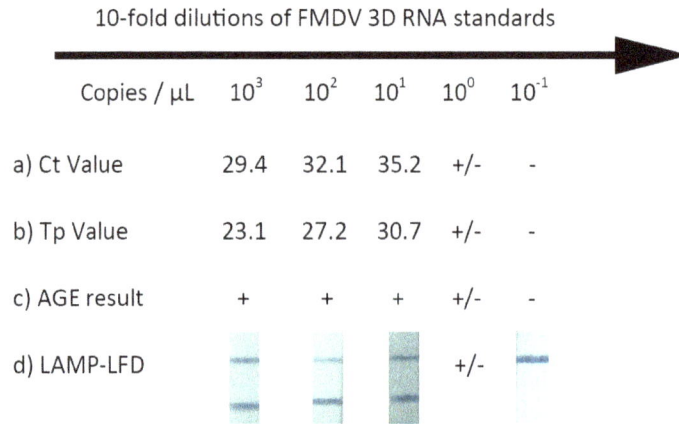

Figure 1. Limit of detection between the RT-qPCR (Ct value), RT-LAMP (Tp value) and RT-LAMP LFD assays. (a) RT-qPCR amplification Ct values corresponding to each of the 10-fold dilutions of RNA standards; (b) RT-LAMP amplification result with Tp values given for each RNA copy number; (c) AGE analysis of RT-LAMP-LFD reaction, spanning the same RNA standards as in (a) and (b); (d) The RT-LAMP-LFD reactions from (c) applied to the LFD device. +/− indicates that out of 4 identical replicates of a given RNA concentration applied to a specific assay (a–d), there were a mixture of positive and negative results.

real-time PCR machine, the limit of detection between the RT-LAMP and RT-qPCR assay were equivalent (Figure 1b). Furthermore, agarose gel electrophoresis (AGE) end-point examination of RT-LAMP products agreed with these results generated on a real-time PCR machine with PicoGreen as an indicator of amplified LAMP products (Figure 1c). However, in these experiments it was not possible to evaluate the RT-LAMP-LFD assay using the real-time PCR machine due to interference of the fluorescein (flc) labelled primers with PicoGreen detection. Therefore these results using the labelled primers were visualized using LFD's and AGE. Biotin and fluorescein labelling of the oligos used in the RT-LAMP assay (termed RT-LAMP-LFD) had no effect on the limit of detection of the assay when the reactions were analysed by both AGE and the LFD (Figure 1d). Of note was the fact that the intensity (and thus quantity) of the positive bands on AGE from the RT-LAMP-LFD were all similar, and did not reduce in intensity as the limit of detection was approached, reflecting a clear positive-negative distinction. Importantly, when these reaction products were applied to the LFD, negative and positive results completely matched those revealed by AGE, with equivalent intensity of positive bands being noted (Figure 1d). The positive bands, when present, were evident within one minute of application to the LFD.

Determination of the optimum temperature range for the RT-LAMP and RT-LAMP-LFD assays

The impact of varying the incubation temperature from 55–75°C upon assay sensitivity was assessed for the RT-LAMP and RT-LAMP-LFD assays. Each assay was performed at a range of temperatures and amplification products detected using AGE. The RT-LAMP reaction maintained a limit of detection comparable to that of the RT-qPCR assay when incubated at temperatures between 55.3 and 63.2°C (Table 1). Amplification appeared to be non-specific below 55.3°C, while at 71°C and higher, no amplification was observed with any of the RNA samples tested. The RT-LAMP-LFD maintained the same limit of detection as the RT-qPCR between 55.3 to 63.2°C, a slightly narrower window than the RT-LAMP assay (Table 1). At 65.9°C and 68.5°C, the limit of detection was reduced 10 fold to 10^1 copies RNA, with no amplification observed at 71.0°C and above. The reaction products from the RT-LAMP-LFD were also tested using

the LFD: all products that yielded positive results for AGE were also positive using the LFD, while all reactions negative using AGE were also negative when using a LFD. All positive LFD results could be seen within one minute after application of the amplification product to the device.

Detection of FMDV RNA by RT-LAMP-LFD in a simple format

Based on the results above, a water bath set to 60°C was able to act as the heat source for the RT-LAMP-LFD reactions (Figure 2). After an incubation period of 60 minutes, the dual-labelled reaction products were analysed by LFD and results were confirmed using AGE. Using these conditions, the RT-LAMP-LFD assay consistently detected the RNA standards at 10^1 copies/ µl (Figure 2). Samples run in parallel on an electronic heat block gave identical results (data not shown).

Due to the reported insensitivity of the LAMP chemistry to inhibiting factors that might be present in clinical samples [31], the ability to perform the RT-LAMP-LFD directly on epithelial samples containing FMDV was evaluated. FMDV spiked 10% epithelial suspension, and non-spiked (negative) 10% epithelial solutions were each used neat or pre-diluted 1 in 3 and 1 in 5 in nuclease free water. Five µl of each dilution of the spiked and non-spiked suspensions were analysed using the RT-LAMP-LFD assay using a water bath and an incubation step of 60°C for 60 minutes. Positive RT-LAMP-LFD results were obtained for all dilutions of the positive epithelium suspension (Figure 3). Intermittent DNA AGE patterns, not consistent with RT-LAMP products were detected in neat negative epithelial suspensions and those diluted 1 in 3 indicative of non-specific reactions. Furthermore, these reactions, when run on the LFD, always generated negative results. All negative epithelial suspensions analysed at a 1 in 5 dilution, gave no AGE bands and were also negative after LFD interrogation. As a result, all 10% epithelial suspensions were pre-diluted 1 in 5 with nuclease free water before all subsequent RT-LAMP-LFD analyses.

Limit of detection of the pen-side RT-LAMP-LFD assay

The performance of the optimised RT-LAMP-LFD assay was compared against the RT-qPCR, as well as the FMDV antigen LFD (SVANODIP FMDV-Ag, Svanova) currently marketed for

Table 1. The effect of isothermal temperature on the end point limit of detection of both the RT-LAMP (un-labelled internal primers) and RT-LAMP-LFD (labelled internal primers) reaction.

RNA copies/μl	Mean Ct Value	RT-LAMP - temperature/°C											
		55	55.3	56.5	58.3	60.6	63.2	65.9	68.5	71	73.1	74.6	75.4
10^2	32.3	+	+	+	+	+	+	+	+	–	–	–	–
10^1	35.5	+	+	+	+	+	+	+	–	–	–	–	–
10^0	+/–	+	+	+/–	+/–	+/–	+/–	–	+/–	–	–	–	–
10^{-1}	–	+	–	–	–	–	–	–	–	–	–	–	–
Neg control	–	+	–	–	–	–	–	–	–	–	–	–	–

RNA copies/μl	Mean Ct Value	RT-LAMP-LFD - temperature/°C											
		55	55.3	56.5	58.3	60.6	63.2	65.9	68.5	71	73.1	74.6	75.4
10^2	32.3	+	+	+	+	+	+	+	+	–	–	–	–
10^1	35.5	+	+	+	+	+	+	–	+	–	–	–	–
10^0	+/–	+/–	+/–	+/–	+/–	+	+	–	–	–	–	–	–
10^{-1}	–	–	–	–	–	–	–	–	–	–	–	–	–
Neg control	–	–	–	–	–	–	–	–	–	–	–	–	–

RNA standards were used to define the limit of detection, with the RT-qPCR Ct values being displayed for each RNA dilution. The RNA standards span the limit of detection of the RT-qPCR assay. + indicates reaction was positive by gel electrophoresis and PicoGreen fluorescence analysis (for un-labelled primers) or by LFD analysis (for labelled primers). +/– indicates variable positivity amongst quadruplicates analysed for a given RNA copy number.

a)

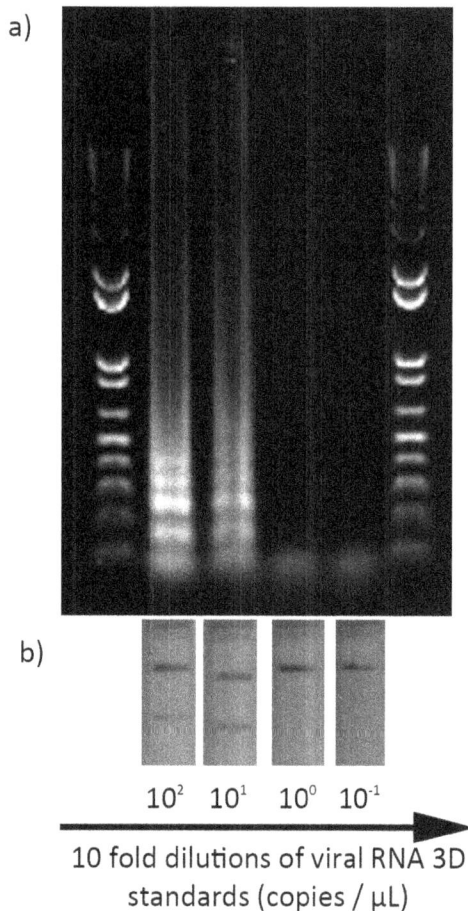

b)

10^2 10^1 10^0 10^{-1}

10 fold dilutions of viral RNA 3D
standards (copies / µL)

Figure 2. RT-LAMP-LFD reactions utilising a simple desk top water bath as the isothermal heat source. (a) RT-LAMP-LFD products analysed using AGE; (b) The RT-LAMP-LFD products from (a) applied to the LFD.

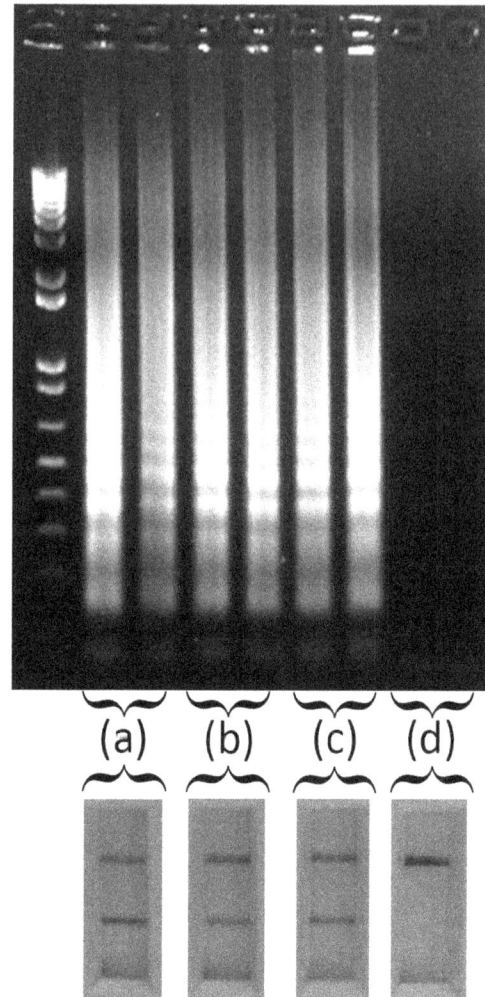

(a) (b) (c) (d)

Figure 3. Titration of epithelial suspensions and subsequent analysis with the RT-LAMP-LFD assay. A 10% epithelial homogenate (w/v) containing 10^6 TCID$_{50}$/mL FMDV was diluted in nuclease free water as described below. These dilutions were each assayed in duplicate with the RT-LAMP-LFD protocol, and analysed with AGE and on an LFD. (a) Application of 5 uL of the "neat" 10% epithelial homogenate added directly to the RT-LAMP-LFD reaction, (b) 1 in 3 dilution, and (c) 1 in 5 dilution, (d) 5 ul of nuclease free water added to the reaction mixture.

field diagnosis of FMD [13]. Using a decimal dilution series of FMDV spiked 10% epithelial suspensions as the starting sample, the ability of these different assays to detect FMDV was compared. The antigen LFD gave positive results when neat and 10^{-1} dilutions of epithelium were analysed; however, all other dilutions were negative (Figure 4a). RNA robotically extracted from the spiked epithelial suspension dilution series gave positive signals from the neat to the 10^{-5} dilutions of the epithelial suspensions (Figure 4b). The optimised RT-LAMP assay had an equivalent limit of detection as the RT-qPCR assay on detecting this extracted RNA, when analysed on the real-time PCR machine and Tp values examined (Figure 4c). Independent processing of this dilution series was undertaken using the optimised RT-LAMP-LFD assay including pre dilution of each epithelial suspension 1 in 5 with nuclease-free water, isothermal amplification using a water bath and detection the RT-LAMP products with the LFD (Figure 4d). RT-LAMP-LFD was found to generate concordant results to those obtained using automated real-time RT-qPCR, with clear detection of FMDV RNA within the dilution range of neat to 10^{-5}.

Direct detection of FMDV from field samples

Epithelial suspensions representing four serotypes (A, Asia 1, SAT1 and SAT2) were analysed using the direct RT-LAMP-LFD

protocol. Following the 60 minute water bath incubation at 60°C, the dual labelled reaction products were visualised by LFD and results confirmed by AGE (Table 2c). For comparison total nucleic acid was extracted from the original epithelial suspensions using a robot (MagNA pure LC, Roche). This RNA (5 µl) was then assayed in parallel by real-time PCR and RT-LAMP using a PCR machine (Stratagene) and visualised by fluorescence. In addition the epithelial suspensions were applied directly to the FMDV antigen LFD (Table 2d). FMDV was detected by all assays from all four serotypes assessed (Table 2), with the negative controls all negative.

Direct detection of FMDV RNA in air samples

Following successful evaluation of the finalized RT-LAMP-LFD assay on field epithelial samples, air samples collected with one of two portable air samplers during experimental FMDV transmission experiments were also analysed. Parallel testing of these

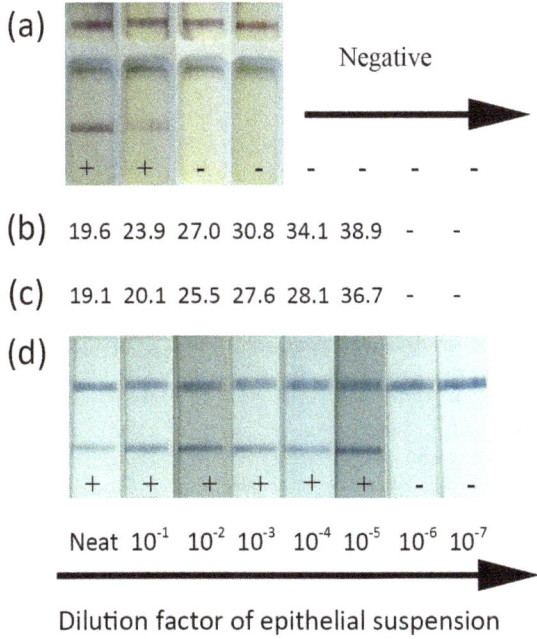

(a)   Negative →   +   +   −   −   −   −   −   −

(b)   19.6 23.9 27.0 30.8 34.1 38.9   −   −

(c)   19.1 20.1 25.5 27.6 28.1 36.7   −   −

(d)   +   +   +   +   +   +   −   −

Neat 10^{-1} 10^{-2} 10^{-3} 10^{-4} 10^{-5} 10^{-6} 10^{-7} →

Dilution factor of epithelial suspension

Figure 4. Comparative limit of detection between Svanova LFD, RT-qPCR, RT-LAMP-LFD and the RT-LAMP assays. 10 fold dilutions of FMDV containing epithelial suspensions were analysed using the Svanova LFD device (a) by applying the suspensions directly to the device. RNA was extracted from each suspension and subsequently analysed using either the RT-qPCR (giving a Ct value) (b) the RT-LAMP assay read using PicoGreen fluorescence(giving a Tp value) (c) or by mixing each 10 fold dilution 1:5 with nuclease free water, and directly adding this to the RT-LAMP-LFD assay for subsequent detection with the LFD (d).

samples was carried out using automated real-time RT-qPCR and the results are summarised in Table 3. The real-time RT-qPCR assay detected viral RNA, collected using a Biocapture 650 over a period of 30 minutes, from the air of a box containing five sheep at both one and two days post infection (dpi). FMDV RNA could also be detected using the real-time RT-qPCR assay in air samples collected in the same way in a box housing cattle at two dpi. Air samples from a box containing five pigs were positive for viral RNA when analysed using the real-time RT-qPCR assay on all days (one, two, three and four dpi). These same samples were analysed using the RT-LAMP-LFD assay, by adding 5 ul of the aqueous sample directly into the RT-LAMP-LFD reaction mix. Apart from an air sample collected from the sheep box (at two dpi), there was complete concordance between the results generated by the RT-LAMP-LFD and the real-time RT-qPCR (Table 3). The aforementioned discrepant result had the lowest recorded positive signal for any of the real-time RT-qPCR positive samples (Table 3). These results were irrespective of whether the air samples had been collected with either the Biobadge 100 (3 hour run time or 20 hour run time) or Biocapture 650. Furthermore, positive RT-LAMP-LFD results were generated for pigs (at one dpi) that were not showing overt clinical signs.

Discussion

A range of LAMP and RT-LAMP assays have been developed to detect nucleic acids from a wide variety of different pathogens that impact upon veterinary and human health. The development of portable hardware and companion protocols to enable LAMP

Table 2. Comparison between the RT-qPCR, RT-LAMP and RT-LAMP-LFD assays from field epithelial suspensions.

Epithelial suspension		Asia 1	A				SAT 1	SAT 2	
		TUR 2/2013	PAK 21/2012	IRN 24/2012	TUR 7/2013	TUR 4/2013	TAN 50/2012	TAN 14/2012	BOT 15/2012
(a) RT-qPCR (Ct)	No Ct	12.52	12.54	13.93	12.6	19.33	25.65	14.75	18.79
(b) RT-LAMP (Tp)	No Ct	26.41	20.34	23.21	17.74	30.63	47.82	21.44	27.88
(c) AGE	−	+	+	+	+	+	+	+	+
(d) Svanova LFD	−	+	+	+	+	+	+	+	+
(e) RT-LAMP-LFD	−	+	+	+	+	+	+	+	+

(a) RT-qPCR amplification Ct values corresponding to each of the 1:5 dilutions of FMDV epithelial suspensions from a range of serotypes; (b) RT-LAMP amplification result with Tp values given for each epithelial suspension; (c) AGE analysis of LAMP-LFD reaction, spanning the same epithelial suspensions as in (a) and (b); (d) epithelial suspension analysed by Svanova antigen LFD; (e) The RT-LAMP-LFD reactions from (c) applied to the LFD device.

Table 3. RT-LAMP-LFD Detection of FMDV in air samples collected with 2 different portable air samplers (Biobadge 100 and Biocapture 650).

Species infected	Air sampling instrument used	Assay utilised	Sample collection/days post infection				
			0	1	2	3	4
Pig	Biobadge (short Run ~3 hrs)	RT-qPCR (Ct Value)	No Ct	25.8	23.52	30.07	27.66
		LAMP-LFD	–	+	+	+	+
	Biobadge (long run ~20 hrs)	RT-qPCR (Ct Value)	No Ct	20.74	23.51	24.02	28.19
		LAMP-LFD	–	+	+	+	+
	Biocapture (~30 mins)	RT-qPCR (Ct Value)	No Ct	22.41	23.49	23.68	29.74
		LAMP-LFD	–	+	+	+	+
Cattle	Biocapture (~30 mins)	RT-qPCR (Ct Value)	No Ct	No Ct	33.84	No Ct	No Ct
		LAMP-LFD	–	–	+	–	–
Sheep	Biocapture (~30 mins)	RT-qPCR (Ct Value)	No Ct	35.78	37.31	No Ct	No Ct
		LAMP-LFD	–	+	+	–	–

RNA was extracted and analysed using the RT-qPCR assay, with Ct values being displayed. Raw air samples were applied to the RT-LAMP-LFD assay, and analysed using the LFD. Air samples were collected from day 0 (day of inoculation), every day, until day 4. Species sampled were pigs, cattle and sheep.

assays to be deployed into the field (or clinic), however, has taken lower priority to date. LAMP has a number of characteristics that are particularly suitable for incorporation into a simple assay format. These include: synthesis of large amounts of DNA which can be readily detected using agarose-gel electrophoresis, or using a fluorescence plate reader in combination with fluorescent intercalating dyes (such as a real-time PCR machine). These approaches are not currently suitable as the basis for a simple test that could be used in the field. Alternative methods that are being considered for simple detection of LAMP include the use of turbidity equipment to monitor the accumulation of insoluble magnesium pyrophosphate that is generated as a white precipitated bi-product of the LAMP amplification [25], or the use of dyes such as hydroxynaphthol blue that respond to changes in cation (Mg^{2+}) concentration associated with LAMP amplification [32]. However, these indirect measurements of LAMP products are prone to generating false negative results and are not currently robust enough for field use. Furthermore, without specific hardware, these forms of detection fail to generate a binary positive/negative result.

In this study, we have modified an existing FMDV RT-LAMP assay in such a way that the entire process can be performed without the use of expensive equipment. The labelling of the primers to allow direct detection of the RT-LAMP products had no effect on assay limit of detection. It should be pointed out, however, that the primer pair which were conjugated to Flc/Biotin to enable successful LFD detection of products in the study described here were the forward and backward internal primers (FIP/BIP). Preliminary experiments were undertaken using a different Flc/Biotin labelled primer pair, namely the forward and reverse loop primers (Floop/Bloop). This approach was initially tried due to success utilising this approach in development of an ASFV LAMP-LFD assay [30]. Whilst successful for the ASFV-LAMP assay, it failed when applied to the FMDV-LAMP assay, hence the ultimate switch to using the labelled FIP/BIP approach. This disparity most likely reflects differences in the ratios to which the different primer sets are incorporated into the complex array of RT-LAMP products, which itself will be related to the identity of the specific primer sequences. This is an important consideration whilst adapting LAMP assays to this LFD format. The limit of detection of the direct simplified assay was such that it was equivalent to that of a validated real-time RT-qPCR assay used for diagnosis in National and International FMD Reference laboratories. The similar intensities of positive bands on both AGE analysed RT-LAMP and RT-LAMP-LFD products illustrated that when amplification does occur, a similar amount of end product is generated, regardless of the input copy number. Importantly, because this polarized digital nature of product quantity was mirrored by the LFD analysis of RT-LAMP-LFD, it meant that interpretation of these devices was straight forward and less open to subjective interpretation, even when samples at the limit of detection were examined. These results are in contrast to assay results generated using an FMDV antigen LFD (SVANODIP FMDV-Ag, Svanova) where the intensity of the band was proportional to the amount of viral antigen in the sample and results can be difficult to interpret when tested samples comprise FMDV at, or near to, the limit of detection. The implication of this is that the RT-LAMP-LFD assay most likely has a wider diagnostic window than the antigen LFD, being able to detect viral RNA for much longer time points post infection than the antigen LFD. This hypothesis should be investigated by testing a multitude of sample types and multiple time points post infection using both the antigen LFD and the RT-LAMP-LFD.

We observed 100% concordance between the results generated using the LFD and AGE methods for both positive and negative samples, demonstrating that a LFD approach to the analysis of RT-LAMP reactions is both sensitive and robust.

In addition to a simple and inexpensive method to detect RT-LAMP reaction products, this study has also demonstrated that cDNA amplification by RT-LAMP is not reliant upon a stringent isothermal incubation step, since the analytical sensitivities of the RT-LAMP assays were maintained over a wide range of temperatures ($8.2°C$ for the unlabelled and labelled RT-LAMP assays). This allows RT-LAMP amplification to be performed in a water bath set to $60°C$ as the heat source. The successful amplification and detection of the RNA targets using these conditions, whilst having no impact upon the limit of detection of the assay, provides a practical demonstration that a tightly controlled temperature afforded by a thermal cycler is not necessary for the RT-LAMP-LFD assay. These findings are important since, when compared to the requirement for precise thermal incubation steps, functionality of the assay over a wide temperature range has the potential to reduce the cost of a portable heat source that might be used as the basis for an assay deployed into the field. Furthermore, the ability for amplification to be efficient at multiple temperatures may allow a wider number of heat sources, for example the use of exothermic reactions.

The production of template nucleic acid free of tissue-derived PCR inhibitory factors is an important consideration when developing molecular assays for the detection pathogens in the field. This aspect has previously been recognised as a limitation to field deployment of molecular methods for pathogen detection [18]. Unlike PCR, previous studies have indicated that LAMP is not inhibited to the same extent by contaminants that might be carried over from the sample [33] allowing amplification even with relatively crude extraction procedures [34]. Our study provides evidence that simply diluting the raw epithelial suspension with nuclease-free water is sufficient for the efficient amplification of FMDV using RT-LAMP-LFD. Similarly, air sample fluid from a portable air sampler can be added directly to the RT-LAMP-LFD reaction mix without compromising analytical sensitivity when compared to a diagnostic real-time RT-qPCR assay. Dispensing with complex RNA extraction methods is a major step forward in portable nucleic acid detection platforms, as all that is required is a heat source, an LFD and the RT-LAMP-LFD reaction master mix.

This study compares the performance of front line tests that can be used for FMD diagnosis including an antigen LFD (SVANO-DIP FMDV-Ag, Svanova) and real-time RT-qPCR with the RT-LAMP-LFD assay. Our results show that the simplified RT-LAMP-LFD assay utilising a raw sample is 10^4 times more sensitive at detecting the presence of FMDV compared with the FMDV-specific antigen LFD (SVANODIP FMDV-Ag, Svanova). Furthermore, when compared to current "portable" real time RT-qPCR assays/equipment, there is a much wider scope for higher throughput of the LAMP-LFD assay described here, due to robust chemistry conditions, no need for RNA extraction, and simple detection methodology. FMDV RNA could be detected using the finalised RT-LAMP-LFD protocol, from field samples containing four currently circulating serotypes of FMDV from around the world. This demonstrates a potential geographical and serotypic robustness of this assay and its use as a diagnostic tool in multiple endemic countries. Furthermore, these data suggest that the RT-LAMP-LFD assay may also have a longer diagnostic temporal window in which FMDV can be detected, compared to the antigen LFD. In part, this conclusion is supported by the ability of the RT-LAMP-LFD assay to detect low amounts of FMDV in air

samples collected with portable samplers, including air samples from groups of infected pigs in the pre-clinical stage of disease. In addition to the obvious value of this assay in the urgent detection of FMD cases in normally FMD free countries, field detection of FMD will also assist the diagnosis of the disease in developing countries that have limited laboratory capability and/or difficult transport links that do not facilitate rapid submission of clinical samples.

In conclusion, we present the development and evaluation of a robust FMDV diagnostic assay using RT-LAMP chemistry, the results of which can be observed using a simple LFD. The unequivocal nature of the positive and negative readings is important for field based formats where subjective interpretation of test results is undesirable. There is no requirement for prior RNA extraction, thus allowing the simple addition of raw epithelial homogenates and raw air samples containing FMDV to the assay directly, whilst maintaining a similar limit of detection as the "gold standard" real-time RT-qPCR assay after extraction of RNA. The assay also has a wide operating temperature, negating the need for strict temperature regulation. These are ideal characteristics for a pen-side assay for FMDV. Further work is now required to formulate this assay into a kit format suitable for routine use, in addition to continuing validation and assessment of further sample types. The findings presented here for the detection of FMDV may also impact upon diagnostic scenarios for other veterinary and human diseases where the rapid and simple detection of nucleic acid targets are warranted.

Methods

Ethics statement

All animal samples utilised in this paper were archival samples from previous studies approved by The Pirbright Institute ethical review committee under the auspices of the Animal Scientific Procedures Act (ASPA) 1986 (as amended).

Epithelial suspensions and air samples

Spiked epithelial suspensions. A 10% tongue epithelial homogenate in sample preparation buffer (SVANODIP, Svanova) was prepared from uninfected sheep epithelium. To prepare the spiked epithelium suspension, the 10% tongue suspension was spiked 1:100 with 10^8 TCID$_{50}$/ml of FMDV UKG 34/2001, to create a "neat" stock of 10% tongue homogenate containing a titre of 10^6 TCID$_{50}$/ml FMDV.

Field sample epithelial suspensions. Epithelial suspensions prepared from samples submitted to The World Reference Laboratory for FMD (Pirbright, UK), representing serotypes A (TUR 2/2013; PAK 21/2012), Asia 1 (IRN 24/2012; TUR 7/2013; TUR 4/2013), SAT 1 (TAN 50/2012) and SAT2 (TAN 14/2012; BOT 15/2012) were used to evaluate the direct RT-LAMP-LFD assay. These epithelial suspensions were diluted 1 in 5 in nuclease free water prior to running 5 μl of each epithelial suspension (in duplicate) on the RT-LAMP-LFD assay.

Air samples used in this study were archival samples collected with portable air sampling devices during a previous animal study, the virus being of serotype Asia-1 [35].

Preparation of RNA standards

Synthetic viral RNA was generated from plasmid pT73S containing full-length FMDV by *in vitro* transcription using a commercially available T7 RNA polymerase kit (Ambion, UK) as described by [36]. This plasmid contained the target sequences of both the one step real-time RT-PCR assay used in this study [15] as well as the region amplified by the RT-LAMP assay [24]. The resultant viral RNA was resuspended in DEPC treated water and quantified at A_{260} using a NanoDrop ND-1000 spectrophotometer. The RNA copy number concentration was calculated and adjusted to 10^9 copies/μl.

RNA extraction

Unless otherwise stated, total RNA was extracted by an automated procedure on a MagNA Pure LC using the total nucleic acid kit reagents following manufacturer's guidelines.

Reverse transcription quantitative PCR (RT-qPCR)

The RT-PCR assay used was a one-step assay that amplifies a 107 nucleotide fragment within the highly conserved 3D region of the FMDV genome, as previously described [15]. All samples assayed using this method were tested in triplicate.

Reverse transcription LAMP (RT-LAMP)

The RT-LAMP assay used was as previously described [24], with the following modifications. The primer sequences were identical to those reported by Dukes et al [24], and given in Table S1, targeting the highly conserved RNA polymerase region of the FMDV genome (3D). The total reaction mixture was 25 μl, consisting of the following components: 2.5 μl of 10x Thermopol buffer (New England Biolabs), 1 μl of a forward internal primer (FIP)/Backward internal primer (BIP) stock mix (50 μM of each FIP/and BIP), 1 μl of an F3/B3 stock mix (5 μM each), 1 μl of each of an F Loop/B Loop stock mix (25 uM each), 0.5 μl of dNTP stock mixture (10 mM of each), 0.5 μl of $MgSO_4$ (stock is 100 mM), 5 μl of Betaine (5 M stock solution), 2.2 μl of enzyme mix (Bst DNA Polymerase (New England Biolabs) 8 u/μl mixed with AMV Reverse Transcriptase (Promega) 10 u/μl in a volumetric ratio of 100:1), 5 μl of a PicroGreen dye mix (molecular probes) 1.3 μl of nuclease free H_2O and 5 μl of template RNA (or epithelial suspension). Samples were tested in triplicate. RT-LAMP reactions were run on a Stratagene Mx3005p PCR machine (Agilent Technologies) and visualised using fluorescence generated by PicoGreen intercalation and agarose gel electrophoresis imaging (AGE). Raw fluorescence was collected at one minute intervals for 60 minutes at a given incubation temperature. Exponential increase in fluorescence (δR) indicated a positive RT-LAMP reaction, irrespective of time of onset during the 60 minute incubation period [24]. The time elapsed at which point this fluorescence was detected was noted at the time to positivity (Tp).

Reverse transcription LAMP combined with lateral flow detection (RT-LAMP-LFD)

Additional modifications which were made to the RT-LAMP assay to enable detection of the product with an LFD consisted of labelling the FIP and BIP at the 5' terminus with fluorescein (Flc) and biotin (Btn), respectively. The subsequent reaction was referred to as RT-LAMP-LFD to distinguish it from the RT-LAMP reaction containing no labelled IP's. RT-LAMP-LFD reactions were run using either a heat block, gradient heat block (for determining optimum temperature range 55–75°C) or using a water bath set at 60°C for one hour.

RT-LAMP-LFD reactions were visualized using agarose gel electrophoresis in combination with an immunochromatographic LFD (Forsite Diagnostics, York, UK). This device had been used in a previous study to detect LAMP products from an ASFV LAMP assay, which also incorporated biotin and fluorescein labelled primers [30]. After the 60 minute incubation step, 2 μl of the resultant RT-LAMP-LFD reaction product was added to 200 μl of LFD-Buffer C (Forsite diagnostics, York, UK) mixed well, and 75 μl of this mix was applied to the loading window of the LFD device. The mix was wicked along the device to the test line and control line. A positive result was indicated by the presence of two lines (test line and control line, respectively), while a negative result only generated a single band (control line). If no lines appeared on the LFD then it meant the test was invalid and must be run again with a new device.

Acknowledgments

The authors thank Lee Murray and Professor Wataru Yamazaki for their helpful discussions in the laboratory and colleagues in the World Reference Laboratory for FMD, The Pirbright Institute, for the supply of field epithelial suspensions.

Author Contributions

Conceived and designed the experiments: RAW DPK VLF. Performed the experiments: RAW VLF BA. Analyzed the data: RAW DPK VLF. Contributed reagents/materials/analysis tools: RAW VLF BA NN JG. Contributed to the writing of the manuscript: RAW VLF BA. Critical review of the manuscript: VLF DPK DJP NN JG.

References

1. Office NA (2002) The 2001 outbreak of foot-and-mouth disease: report by the Comptroller and Auditor General.
2. Shaw AE, Reid SM, Ebert K, Hutchings GH, Ferris NP, et al. (2007) Implementation of a one-step real-time RT-PCR protocol for diagnosis of foot-and-mouth disease. J Virol Methods 143: 81–85.
3. Ferris NP, Dawson M (1988) Routine Application of Enzyme-Linked Immunosorbent-Assay in Comparison with Complement-Fixation for the Diagnosis of Foot-and-Mouth and Swine Vesicular Diseases. Veterinary Microbiology 16: 201–209.
4. Snowdon WA (1966) Growth of foot-and mouth disease virus in monolayer cultures of calf thyroid cells. Nature 210: 1079–1080.
5. Ferris NP, King DP, Reid SM, Shaw AE, Hutchings GH (2006) Comparisons of original laboratory results and retrospective analysis by real-time reverse transcriptase-PCR of virological samples collected from confirmed cases of foot-and-mouth disease in the UK in 2001. Vet Rec 159: 373–378.
6. Gibbens JC, Sharpe CE, Wilesmith JW, Mansley LM, Michalopoulou E, et al. (2001) Descriptive epidemiology of the 2001 foot-and-mouth disease epidemic in Great Britain: the first five months. Vet Rec 149: 729–743.
7. Geering WA (1967) Foot-and-mouth disease in sheep. Australian Veterinary Journal 43: 485–489.
8. Anderson I (2002) Foot and Mouth Disease 2001: Lessons to be Learned Inquiry Report. Report to the Prime Minister and the Secretary of State for Environment Food and Rural Affairs. London, The Stationery Office.
9. Society TR (2002) Infectious Diseases in Livestock. London, Royal Society.
10. Sumption K, Domenech J, Ferrari G (2012) Progressive control of FMD on a global scale. Vet Rec 170: 637–639.
11. Heesters BA, Chatterjee P, Kim YA, Gonzalez SF, Kuligowski MP, et al. (2013) Endocytosis and recycling of immune complexes by follicular dendritic cells enhances B cell antigen binding and activation. Immunity 38: 1164–1175.
12. Sammin D, Ryan E, Ferris NP, King DP, Zientara S, et al. (2010) Options for decentralized testing of suspected secondary outbreaks of foot-and-mouth disease. Transbound Emerg Dis 57: 237–243.
13. Ferris NP, Nordengrahn A, Hutchings GH, Reid SM, King DP, et al. (2009) Development and laboratory validation of a lateral flow device for the detection of foot-and-mouth disease virus in clinical samples. J Virol Methods 155: 10–17.
14. Shaw AE, Reid SM, King DP, Hutchings GH, Ferris NP (2004) Enhanced laboratory diagnosis of foot and mouth disease by real-time polymerase chain reaction. Rev Sci Tech 23: 1003–1009.

15. Ryan E, Gloster J, Reid SM, Li Y, Ferris NP, et al. (2008) Clinical and laboratory investigations of the outbreaks of foot-and-mouth disease in southern England in 2007. Vet Rec 163: 139–147.

16. Callahan JD, Brown F, Osorio FA, Sur JH, Kramer E, et al. (2002) Use of a portable real-time reverse transcriptase-polymerase chain reaction assay for rapid detection of foot-and-mouth disease virus. J Am Vet Med Assoc 220: 1636–1642.

17. Hearps A, Zhang Z, Alexandersen S (2002) Evaluation of the portable Cepheid SmartCycler real-time PCR machine for the rapid diagnosis of foot-and-mouth disease. Vet Rec 150: 625–628.

18. King DP, Dukes JP, Reid SM, Ebert K, Shaw AE, et al. (2008) Prospects for rapid diagnosis of foot-and-mouth disease in the field using reverse transcriptase-PCR. Vet Rec 162: 315–316.

19. Madi M, Hamilton A, Squirrell D, Mioulet V, Evans P, et al. (2012) Rapid detection of foot-and-mouth disease virus using a field-portable nucleic acid extraction and real-time PCR amplification platform. Vet J 193: 67–72.

20. Notomi T, Okayama H, Masubuchi H, Yonekawa T, Watanabe K, et al. (2000) Loop-mediated isothermal amplification of DNA. Nucleic Acids Res 28: E63.

21. Iwamoto T, Sonobe T, Hayashi K (2003) Loop-mediated isothermal amplification for direct detection of Mycobacterium tuberculosis complex, M. avium, and M. intracellulare in sputum samples. J Clin Microbiol 41: 2616–2622.

22. Njiru ZK, Mikosza AS, Armstrong T, Enyaru JC, Ndung'u JM, et al. (2008) Loop-mediated isothermal amplification (LAMP) method for rapid detection of Trypanosoma brucei rhodesiense. PLoS Negl Trop Dis 2: e147.

23. Fukuta S, Kato S, Yoshida K, Mizukami Y, Ishida A, et al. (2003) Detection of tomato yellow leaf curl virus by loop-mediated isothermal amplification reaction. J Virol Methods 112: 35–40.

24. Dukes JP, King DP, Alexandersen S (2006) Novel reverse transcription loop-mediated isothermal amplification for rapid detection of foot-and-mouth disease virus. Arch Virol 151: 1093–1106.

25. Mori Y, Nagamine K, Tomita N, Notomi T (2001) Detection of loop-mediated isothermal amplification reaction by turbidity derived from magnesium pyrophosphate formation. Biochem Biophys Res Commun 289: 150–154.

26. Kiatpathomchai W, Jaroenram W, Arunrut N, Jitrapakdee S, Flegel TW (2008) Shrimp Taura syndrome virus detection by reverse transcription loop-mediated isothermal amplification combined with a lateral flow dipstick. J Virol Methods 153: 214–217.

27. Nimitphak T, Kiatpathomchai W, Flegel TW (2008) Shrimp hepatopancreatic parvovirus detection by combining loop-mediated isothermal amplification with a lateral flow dipstick. J Virol Methods 154: 56–60.

28. Nimitphak T, Meemetta W, Arunrut N, Senapin S, Kiatpathomchai W (2010) Rapid and sensitive detection of Penaeus monodon nucleopolyhedrovirus (PemoNPV) by loop-mediated isothermal amplification combined with a lateral-flow dipstick. Mol Cell Probes 24: 1–5.

29. Jaroenram W, Kiatpathomchai W, Flegel TW (2009) Rapid and sensitive detection of white spot syndrome virus by loop-mediated isothermal amplification combined with a lateral flow dipstick. Mol Cell Probes 23: 65–70.

30. James HE, Ebert K, McGonigle R, Reid SM, Boonham N, et al. (2010) Detection of African swine fever virus by loop mediated isothermal amplification. J Virol Methods 164: 68–74.

31. Francois P, Tangomo M, Hibbs J, Bonetti EJ, Boehme CC, et al. (2011) Robustness of a loop-mediated isothermal amplification reaction for diagnostic applications. FEMS Immunol Med Microbiol 62: 41–48.

32. Bearinger JP, Dugan LC, Baker BR, Hall SB, Ebert K, et al. (2011) Development and initial results of a low cost, disposable, point-of-care testing device for pathogen detection. IEEE Trans Biomed Eng 58: 805–808.

33. Blomstrom AL, Hakhverdyan M, Reid SM, Dukes JP, King DP, et al. (2008) A one-step reverse transcriptase loop-mediated isothermal amplification assay for simple and rapid detection of swine vesicular disease virus. J Virol Methods 147: 188–193.

34. Fukuta S, Iida T, Mizukami Y, Ishida A, Ueda J, et al. (2003) Detection of Japanese yam mosaic virus by RT-LAMP. Arch Virol 148: 1713–1720.

35. Ryan E, Wright C, Gloster J (2009) Measurement of airborne foot-and-mouth disease virus: preliminary evaluation of two portable air sampling devices. Vet J 179: 458–461.

36. Zhang ZD, Hutching G, Kitching P, Alexandersen S (2002) The effects of gamma interferon on replication of foot-and-mouth disease virus in persistently infected bovine cells. Arch Virol 147: 2157–2167.

11

The Risk of Disease to Great Apes: Simulating Disease Spread in Orang-Utan (*Pongo pygmaeus wurmbii*) and Chimpanzee (*Pan troglodytes schweinfurthii*) Association Networks

Charlotte Carne[1]*, Stuart Semple[1], Helen Morrogh-Bernard[2,3], Klaus Zuberbühler[4,5], Julia Lehmann[1]

1 Centre for Research in Evolutionary and Environmental Anthropology, University of Roehampton, London, United Kingdom, 2 The Orang-utan Tropical Peatland Project, Centre for International Cooperation in Sustainable Management of Tropical Peatland, Universitas Palangka Raya, Palangka Raya, Central Kalimantan, Indonesia, 3 Centre for Research in Animal Behaviour, College of Life and Environmental Sciences, University of Exeter, Exeter, United Kingdom, 4 School of Psychology and Neuroscience, University of St Andrews, St Andrews, Fife, United Kingdom, 5 Cognitive Science Centre, University of Neuchâtel, Neuchâtel, Switzerland

Abstract

All great ape species are endangered, and infectious diseases are thought to pose a particular threat to their survival. As great ape species vary substantially in social organisation and gregariousness, there are likely to be differences in susceptibility to disease types and spread. Understanding the relation between social variables and disease is therefore crucial for implementing effective conservation measures. Here, we simulate the transmission of a range of diseases in a population of orang-utans in Sabangau Forest (Central Kalimantan) and a community of chimpanzees in Budongo Forest (Uganda), by systematically varying transmission likelihood and probability of subsequent recovery. Both species have fission-fusion social systems, but differ considerably in their level of gregariousness. We used long-term behavioural data to create networks of association patterns on which the spread of different diseases was simulated. We found that chimpanzees were generally far more susceptible to the spread of diseases than orang-utans. When simulating different diseases that varied widely in their probability of transmission and recovery, it was found that the chimpanzee community was widely and strongly affected, while in orang-utans even highly infectious diseases had limited spread. Furthermore, when comparing the observed association network with a mean-field network (equal contact probability between group members), we found no major difference in simulated disease spread, suggesting that patterns of social bonding in orang-utans are not an important determinant of susceptibility to disease. In chimpanzees, the predicted size of the epidemic was smaller on the actual association network than on the mean-field network, indicating that patterns of social bonding have important effects on susceptibility to disease. We conclude that social networks are a potentially powerful tool to model the risk of disease transmission in great apes, and that chimpanzees are particularly threatened by infectious disease outbreaks as a result of their social structure.

Editor: Cheryl S. Rosenfeld, University of Missouri, United States of America

Funding: Charlotte Carne was funded by a scholarship from the University of Roehampton (http://www.roehampton.ac.uk/home/). The Royal Zoological Society of Scotland (http://www.rzss.org.uk/) provided core funding for the Budongo Conservation Field Station. The orang-utan field research was funded by the Wildlife Conservation Society (WCS: http://www.wcs.org/), the US Fish and Wildlife Service Great Ape Conservation Fund (http://www.fws.gov/international/wildlife-without-borders/great-ape-conservationfund.html), Orang-utan Tropical Peatland Project (OuTrop: http://www.outrop.com/), Primate Conservation Inc. (http://www.primate.org/), and the L.S.B. Leakey Foundation (http://leakeyfoundation.org/). The funders had no role in study design, data collection and analysis, decision to publish, or preparation of the manuscript.

Competing Interests: The authors have declared that no competing interests exist.

* E-mail: charlotte.carne@roehampton.ac.uk

Introduction

Great apes are susceptible to a wide range of diseases, including Ebola [1], polio-like diseases and mange [2], measles and scabies [3], influenza [4], tuberculosis [5] and various respiratory diseases [2,6–9]. Because all apes have a long life history, populations need considerable time to recover from epidemics [9]. Although not all long-term chimpanzee (*Pan troglodytes spp.*) field sites have been affected by lethal epidemics, some have suffered great losses due to diseases. Respiratory epidemics have affected a number of study sites [2,6–9], with indications that some infections have been transmitted from humans [8,10]. In chimpanzees, morbidity varied from 20 to 98%, with death rates of between 3 and 17%

[7,9]; such disease outbreaks are therefore of great concern to researchers and conservationists. As a response, various study sites have put in place a range of rules to try to prevent disease transmission despite the difficulties of enforcing them [3,11]. In contrast to chimpanzees, there are no documented large scale epidemics in orang-utans (*Pongo spp.*), although there are reports of disease transmission from humans. For example at Ketambe, Sumatra, an influenza type disease and conjunctivitis have been passed from human caretakers to rehabilitant orang-utans, with the former then passed on to two wild orang-utans [4]. Orang-utan rehabilitation sites often host tourists who, if ill and infectious, pose a serious health risk to the animals [12]. While disease transmission from humans to great apes has become an inherent

problem associated with ecotourism and scientific research, natural diseases that affect great apes in the absence of humans will also continue to be a threat [1,13,14]. In conclusion, understanding how diseases spread within groups and populations of great apes is of vital importance to implement effective preventative measures and to minimise the risk of losing individuals, and ultimately the species, to diseases.

Patterns of disease spread are influenced by a number of parameters, most importantly by the social organisation of a species and disease-specific parameters, such as transmission mode, infectiousness and time to recovery. For example, data from humans suggest that highly infectious diseases, such as Ebola, measles or influenza, have infectious periods lasting for 10 days, 6–7 days and 2–3 days respectively, while tuberculosis is less infectious but has a longer infectious period [15–17]. In order to react and plan adequately it is therefore important to make informed predictions of how different diseases are likely to spread within different social groupings. This type of information could help to identify the most effective strategies for both responding to and preventing epidemics.

So far, virtually no epidemiological models exist for great apes, although social network-based approaches of disease transmission have been used for African buffalo (*Syncerus caffer*) [18], brushtail possums (*Trichosurus vulpecula*) [19] and killer whales (*Orcinus orca*) [20]. For African buffaloes, the model predicted that slowly spreading diseases would affect more individuals than rapidly spreading diseases, as a result of the movement of individuals between groups over time [18]. In possums, contact patterns predicted that bovine tuberculosis would spread within the entire population if more than 8% of contacts led to secondary infections [19], while killer whales were shown to be highly susceptible to disease spread as a result of both the topology of the network and the strength of relationships within it [20]. These models provide first predictions of the way that diseases with different properties would spread within wildlife populations and as such give indications as to which might cause the largest loss of individuals.

In this study, we use epidemiological modelling to explore disease spread in chimpanzees and orang-utans. Both species are characterised by fission-fusion social systems; relationships are fluid, with individuals assembling in temporary parties that regularly change in composition [21,22]. Within this general classification, orang-utans and chimpanzees lie at opposite ends of the spectrum in terms of gregariousness. Chimpanzees spend a far larger proportion of time in association, while orang-utans spend the majority of their time alone or with dependent offspring [4,23–26]. This difference is likely to affect the risk that disease poses to each species. Traditional disease models are typically based on homogenously mixed populations, in which all individuals are equally likely to interact with all other individuals, so called mean-field models [15], thereby ignoring the details of species-specific social dynamics. More recent models have incorporated the natural heterogeneity of contact patterns using social network analysis. A typical finding is that the topology of the network can have a considerable impact on the predicted disease spread [18,27–29]. For example, simulations of disease transmission in African buffalo indicated a much faster spread of disease on a mean-field network than on actual association networks [18]. Despite the advantages and presumably greater precision in predictions of the social network approach, it has not yet been employed widely in wildlife epidemiological models as it is data intensive and requires detailed behavioural observations.

Here, we used a social network approach to simulate predicted disease spread in wild orang-utans and chimpanzees, in order to assess the threat that disease poses to these species. We focused specifically on diseases that are transmitted through close proximity or direct contact between individuals, such as respiratory diseases. We employed a susceptible-infected-recovered network modelling approach to investigate the potential spread of disease in association networks from a population of 37 orang-utans from the Sabangau forest, Indonesia, and 55 members of a chimpanzee community from Budongo, Uganda. Our aims were (i) to determine the susceptibility of the orang-utan and chimpanzee networks to the spread of diseases with differing infectiousness and probability of recovery, (ii) to compare the association network approach with the more traditional mean-field approach, to determine if the topology of the network impacted predicted disease spread, and (iii) to compare the results between the species to highlight the impact of gregariousness on the threat of disease.

Methods

Ethics Statement

Permits and ethical approval for the field studies were obtained from the Indonesian Institute of Sciences and the Ministry of Research and Technology and the Uganda National Council for Science and Technology, the Ugandan Wildlife Authority and the National Forestry Authority.

Association Data and Network Construction

We constructed networks for both species using association data, i.e. presence in the same party, where a party was defined as all individuals within 50 m of each other. The orang-utan data were collected from 2003–2011 as part of the OuTrop multidisciplinary research project in collaboration with CIMTROP, in the Natural Laboratory for the Study of Peat Swamp Forests (2°19'S 114°00'E). The population comprised 46 individuals: four adolescent females, 10 adult females, two adolescent males, 16 unflanged males and 14 flanged males. Nine of these orang-utans were never observed in association with other individuals and so were excluded from the analyses, as this study focuses on diseases that are transmitted through close proximity between individuals or through direct individual-to-individual contact. Data were collected during focal follows that lasted for as long as 10 consecutive days. Association data were recorded using instantaneous sampling every five minutes. In total, 165,717 focal scans were recorded.

The chimpanzee data were collected between August 2007 and July 2010 on 55 members of the Sonso community of Budongo Forest: 12 adolescent females, 24 adult females, eight adolescent males and 11 adult males. Data were collected during focal follows and association data recorded using scan samples every 15 minutes. In total, 34,143 focal scans were recorded.

Weighted association networks were constructed from the association data, using Dyadic Association Indices (DAIs) as the weights of the edges:

$$DAI = \frac{AB}{A + B - AB}$$

where A is the total number of times that A was observed, either alone or with other independent individuals, B is the total number of times B was observed and AB is the total number of times that A and B were observed together. Association indices range from zero

A

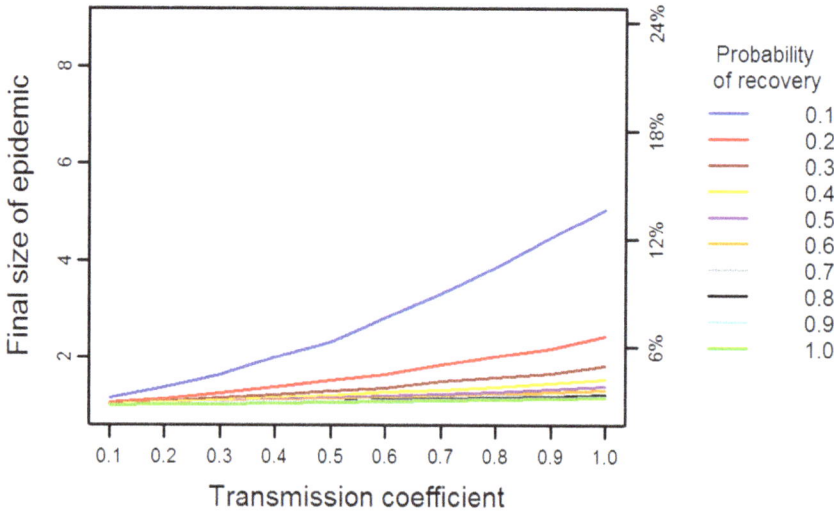

B

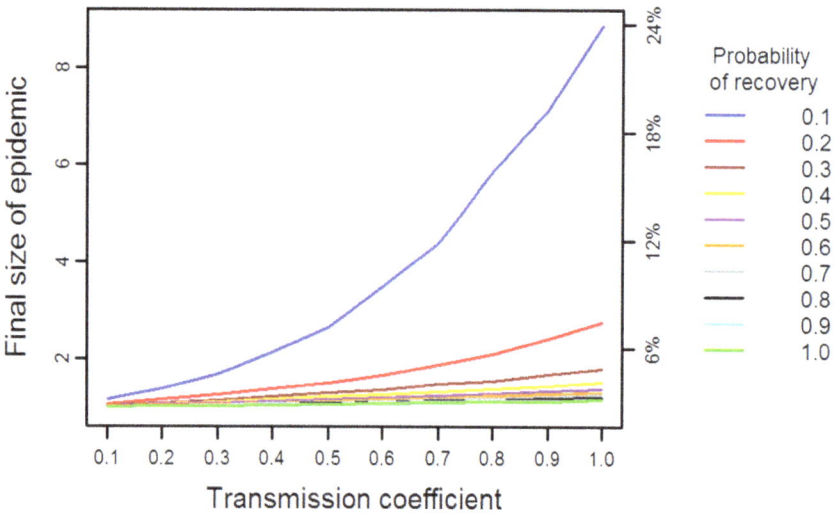

Figure 1. Predicted disease spread in the orangutan network. The final size of the epidemic in terms of absolute size and the percentage of the population, for diseases with different combinations of transmission and recovery probabilities in (a) the orang-utan association network and (b) the mean-field network.

to one, with zero indicating that two individuals were never observed together and one indicating that they were always observed together.

Disease Simulations: Susceptible-infected-recovered Models

We simulated the spread of disease using a susceptible-infected-recovered model. This involved allocating each individual in the network one of three states at all times: susceptible, infected or recovered. The simulation begins with the infection of one individual in the network, patient zero; this individual is selected at random. All other individuals start the simulation as susceptible.

The spread of disease from patient zero to its contacts is assumed to be a function of the transmission coefficient β, representing the infectiousness of the disease, and the dyadic association index, representing the probability that a dyad will associate. At each time step, disease spreads from infected to susceptible individuals with a probability that is the product of these two variables. Once infected, individuals recover with a probability γ, the recovery coefficient, and do not return to susceptible status. It is important to note that conceptually, recovered individuals are equivalent to dead individuals. In all cases the individual is removed from the network and can no longer transmit disease. In terms of modelling subsequent disease spread it is consequently not important to distinguish the number of individuals that recover from the number that die and so here both states will be referred to as recovered.

Simulating the Spread of Different Diseases

We ran all simulations using tnet [30] in R [31]. The simulations were run with a range of values for the transmission and recovery coefficients, to simulate the spread of diseases with differing levels of infectiousness and recovery. We varied the transmission coefficient and the probability of recovery from 0.1 to 1.0 at intervals of 0.1 and simulated the spread of diseases with all 100 combinations of values (i.e. 0.1 and 0.1, 0.1 and 0.2, 0.1 and 0.3 etc.). Each simulation stops when disease has stopped spreading and all infected individuals have recovered. At this stage, the total number of individuals that were infected is calculated to give the final size of the epidemic. For each combination of parameters we ran the simulation 10,000 times and calculated the mean final size of the epidemic.

The Effect of Network Topology on Predictions

We explored the effect of network topology on the spread of disease by comparing the size of the epidemics predicted on the association networks with the size of the epidemics predicted on mean-field networks, where individuals mix homogeneously. In the mean-field network, all individuals were connected to all others and each dyad associated with an association index that was equivalent to the mean of the association indices in the actual network. This ensured that the overall force of infection in the mean-field model was the same as that in the association network [18]. Again, we varied the transmission and recovery coefficients between 0.1 and 1.0 and tested all 100 combinations of parameters. We simulated the spread of disease on the mean-field networks 10,000 times for each combination of parameters and calculated the final size of the epidemic.

Results

The Spread of Disease in the Orang-utan Network

Simulating the spread of diseases with differing transmission coefficients and probabilities of recovery on the orang-utan association network indicated that disease does not spread extensively under any combination of these parameters (Figure 1a). Even with a very low probability of recovery of 0.1 per time step and a very high transmission coefficient of 1.0, on average only five of the orang-utans (ca. 14% of the population) became infected.

The spread of disease across the mean-field network (Figure 1b) was very similar to that across the association network. All combinations of the transmission coefficient and the probability of recovery produced almost identical results on the mean-field network as those on the association network. The only exception was diseases with very low recovery ($\gamma = 0.1$) and high infectiousness ($\beta > 0.6$), but even here, the greatest difference found between the predictions was less than four individuals (ca.10% of the population). Thus, for orang-utans association data appear to be irrelevant to predict the number of individuals infected, regardless of disease type.

The Spread of Disease in the Chimpanzee Network

Simulations on the chimpanzee network indicated a much higher degree of vulnerability to disease than predicted for the orang-utan (Figure 2a). Diseases with a high probability of transmission, i.e. highly infectious diseases, spread to almost all members of the network even when combined with a high recovery probability. Indeed, even if recovery was certain at each time step ($\gamma = 1.0$), a disease only needed a transmission probability of 0.5 in order to reach over 40 members (73%) of the chimpanzee community on average. Diseases with a low probability of transmission and a high probability of recovery did not spread as much in the network; entering a minimum transmission probability of 0.1 and a maximum recovery probability of 1.0 generated a final epidemic size of 9.76 individuals (17.7% of the community). Increasing the transmission coefficient led to large relative increases in the final size of the epidemic, while increasing the probability of recovery had a smaller effect on total number infected by the epidemic. The chimpanzee network therefore appears to be susceptible to diseases with a range of parameters, but particularly to those with intermediate to high transmission coefficients.

Comparing the spread of disease on the chimpanzee association network with that on the mean-field network produced very different results to those seen in the simulations for orang-utans. Regardless of parameter combinations, the final size of the epidemic on the mean-field network was higher than that on the association network (Figure 2b). Only diseases with very high recovery rates ($\gamma > 0.7$) and low transmission coefficients ($\beta = 0.1$) spread more on the association network than on the mean-field network. Excluding these extreme cases, on average an additional 7.53 chimpanzees, or 14% of the community (range 1–22%), were predicted to become infected on the mean-field network compared to the association network. Incorporating heterogeneity in contact patterns therefore has an important effect on the predicted disease spread.

Discussion

The spread of a range of diseases with differing infection and recovery parameters was simulated in a community of chimpanzees and a population of orang-utans, to assess the vulnerability of these species to epidemics. While disease was not predicted to spread rapidly or extensively through the orang-utan population, the chimpanzee community was predicted to be extremely vulnerable to disease. Furthermore, the topology of the association network was found to have an important effect on the predictions of disease spread for chimpanzees, but not for orang-utans. It is important to note that the simulations were based on association networks using data collected over nine years for the orang-utans and three years for the chimpanzees. Although this difference prevents any detailed quantitative comparisons being made between the two species, the markedly different overall patterns that emerged highlight differences in how disease is likely to spread in each species. Overall, our results are relevant for the planning of conservation initiatives and disease prevention measures. While disease risk should not be ignored for orang-utans, infectious diseases represent a particularly major threat for wild chimpanzees and effective measures to prevent disease from entering communities should therefore be implemented, especially in habituated populations.

As with all modelling approaches, there are a number of simplifications/generalisations that needed to be made, which are important to discuss. The definition of social contact employed here may have important influences on the inferences that can be drawn. Both orang-utans and chimpanzees were said to be associating if they were within 50 metres of one another (a commonly used definition by field workers). Although for much of the measured association time individuals will in fact be in much closer proximity than the 50 metre cut-off distance, in reality many diseases require very close contact for transmission to take place

A

B

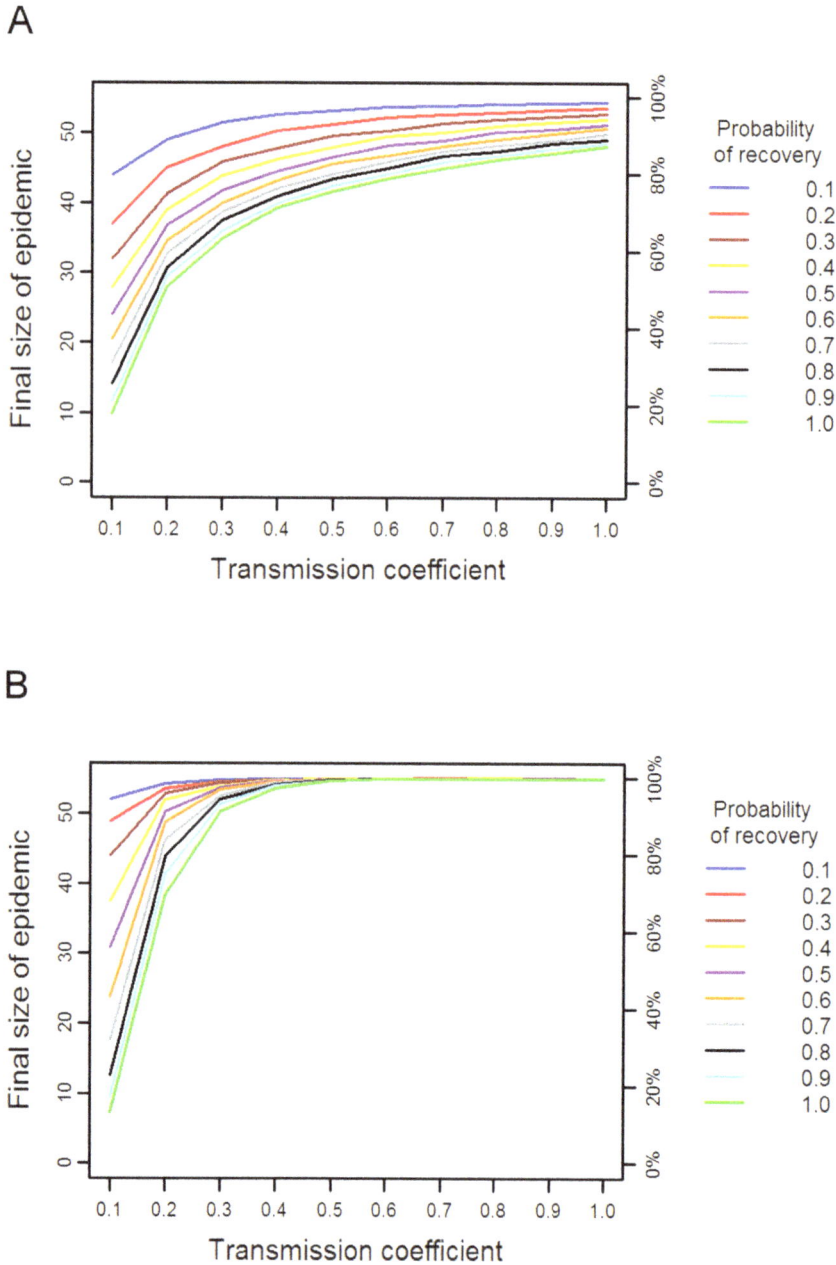

Figure 2. Predicted disease spread in the chimpanzee network. The final size of the epidemic in terms of absolute size and the percentage of the population, for diseases with different combinations of transmission and recovery probabilities in (a) the chimpanzee association network and (b) the mean-field network.

[32]. Examples include sexually transmitted diseases and those caused by parasites, which are also further complicated by stages of the life cycle spent outside the host and the number of parasites infecting each host [15,33]. In addition, many diseases are spread through the faecal-oral route where the link between association and transmission is less clear; for example, viruses causing diseases such as polio can survive for several months in the soil [32] and so may be transmitted between individuals that have never been in proximity. In some cases, using contact networks instead of association networks might be more appropriate, and similar models to those used here could be run on these other types of networks. Our results do, however, provide a general model of the spread of respiratory diseases, which are both relatively common

and extremely threatening to great apes [2,9]. Improving our understanding of the spread of respiratory disease is important for these species, especially in regards to the appropriate management of both research and ecotourism sites.

The simulations used here were based on static association networks, as opposed to dynamic networks which include temporal changes in contact patterns [34]. Static networks are assumed to provide an accurate representation of the relationships between individuals in the population or community, and hence of the overall social organisation [20]. Although our networks may be biased towards core individuals that are sampled more often, a model run on a static network is assumed to provide an indication of the way in which disease would be expected to spread on average, based on the overall structure of the society. This may be misleading as it fails to account for short-term relationships that change as a result of ecology or demography, which could have an important effect on the pattern of disease transmission [35]. Therefore, it may be useful to also analyse dynamic networks, in which relationships vary over shorter periods of time and disease spreads in accordance with the contact patterns present during that particular time period [18]. However, this would require a large amount of data collected over short periods of time to ensure that relationships are adequately sampled. As such extensive databases are rare, most network models to date have been static [36]. The orang-utan social system in particular, with individuals dispersed over large areas and spending considerable amounts of time alone, would be extremely difficult to sample sufficiently to create a reliable dynamic model. Using data collected over a long period of time ensures that rare relationships are included, producing a more accurate representation of the general social structure (and hence patterns of disease spread) [37].

The Impact of Gregariousness on Predicted Disease Spread

The disease simulations described in this paper, using a range of transmission and recovery parameters, provide clear evidence of the impact that differences in gregariousness between the orang-utans and chimpanzees have on predicted vulnerability to disease spread. Even diseases with very high infectiousness and slow recovery did not infect more than five of the 37 orang-utans (14%). A highly infectious disease associated with low recovery is, however, clearly a worst-case scenario, although it should be emphasised that the loss of five individuals could have an important impact on the population. The chimpanzee network, by contrast, was highly susceptible to diseases with a broad range of transmission and recovery parameters, particularly those with medium to high transmission coefficients. At a number of study sites, respiratory epidemics have indeed been shown to affect the majority of chimpanzees [8,38]. This demonstrates that chimpanzee communities are likely to be extremely susceptible to even moderately contagious diseases, while very contagious diseases such as measles and pertussis [39] may have catastrophic consequences. Even diseases with low infectivity and rapid recovery, a best case scenario in terms of disease parameters, spread to a high number of chimpanzees (18%). Chimpanzees are clearly susceptible to disease spread, and the extent of this vulnerability, encompassing diseases varying widely in transmission and recovery parameters, is a serious conservation concern. The spread of diseases from humans has already been implicated in a number of epidemics in chimpanzees [2,7] and mortality from disease is often high [9]. Ecotourism has many associated benefits, such as providing finances and local support for the conservation of great apes [32], and so it is not practical to recommend the complete cessation of great ape tourism. However, the speed with which diseases can spread between chimpanzees is a clear warning that strict hygiene measures must be enforced to prevent the introduction of disease into the chimpanzee communities.

The relative lack of disease spread predicted among orang-utans, particularly in comparison to the chimpanzee, suggests that orang-utans are unlikely to be regularly affected by infectious disease, as a result of their social system. Further studies should investigate the extent to which this finding applies to orang-utans in rehabilitation centres, which live at much higher densities than those in the wild [40]. In these conditions, it is possible that orang-utan social structure is in fact closer to that of the chimpanzee than wild orang-utans, leading to a much higher risk of disease spread.

The Impact of Network Topology on Predicted Disease Spread

Although models with the most realistic parameters should produce the most accurate predictions, it is often impossible or excessively time consuming (in terms of data collection) to obtain sufficiently detailed data. For these reasons, in network epidemiological models, mean-field networks are often used instead of actual association or interaction networks. Our results show that for orang-utans, the mean-field network produced similar results to those from the association network for almost all combinations of parameters tested. This indicates that the fine-grained structure of the orang-utan network has little impact on predicted transmission patterns, with the exception of diseases with long recovery times and high infectiousness. It seems likely that the low levels of association between orang-utans in the network limit the spread of disease, regardless of the exact topology of the network. Consequently, the predictions produced here are likely to be widely applicable to other populations of Bornean orang-utans, which are known to spend a comparable amount of time alone as the population studied here [24,25]. Orang-utans in Sumatra have been found to be more gregarious than those in Borneo [4,22] and so these populations may face a somewhat higher risk of disease transmission, but this is still likely to be lower than that found for the chimpanzee.

The results from the mean-field network for the chimpanzee provide support for the value of using an actual association network approach in disease simulations for this species, as the predicted final sizes of the epidemics on the mean-field network differed considerably from those on the association networks, in most cases being greater. It is likely that there is a threshold level of association above which it becomes useful to incorporate association data. Without data from a wider variety of social systems it is difficult to estimate where this threshold may lie; however, it is clear that for highly gregarious species such as chimpanzees, the inclusion of (ideally fine-grained) association data can have important effects on predictions.

Wider Implications of Modelling Results: Information Flow and Culture

The models presented here to assess disease spread dynamics can also be interpreted as models for the spread of social information and the evolution of culture [41]. The results can be directly interpreted in terms of the ease of information flow, and suggest that information is likely to flow faster and to a greater number of individuals among chimpanzees than orang-utans. This adds to the current debate about the spread and acquisition of traditions in chimpanzees and orang-utans. Both species have been shown to exhibit a range of behaviours, such as using tools to obtain social insects or using leaves to collect drinking water, that could be classed as traditions or culture [42,43]. Geographical variation in these behaviours has not been explained by genetic or ecological differences and has therefore been attributed to local innovations and social learning [44,45]. Observations show that chimpanzees have a larger cultural repertoire than orang-utans, and it has been suggested that this may result from greater opportunities for social learning as a consequence of higher overall gregariousness [42,43,45]. This hypothesis seems to be supported by our findings, although the spread of cultural behaviours might differ slightly from that of disease in that individuals are unlikely to forget a learned behaviour (i.e. recover). However, even at very low recovery rates (which would indicate a very high probability of retaining a behaviour) disease did not spread widely between orang-utans, despite the fact that nine years of data were used to compile the association network. This implies that there are indeed limited opportunities for the transmission of social information between orang-utans, which may help to explain why they are characterised by fewer traditions.

Conclusion

The results of this study indicate that while orang-utans seem to be at low risk of suffering disease epidemics, for chimpanzees disease represents a major threat. Once a single chimpanzee is exposed to a contagious pathogen, our model predicts rapid and extensive spread within the community. This emphasises the importance of this issue for the future conservation of the chimpanzee, and highlights the value of modelling approaches to the study of wildlife diseases.

References

1. Bermejo M, Rodriguez-Teijeiro JD, Illera G, Barroso A, Vila C, et al. (2006) Ebola outbreak killed 5000 gorillas. Science 314: 1564–1564.
2. Pusey AE, Wilson ML, Collins DA (2008) Human impacts, disease risk, and population dynamics in the chimpanzees of Gombe National Park, Tanzania. American Journal of Primatology 70: 738–744.
3. Wallis J, Lee DR (1999) Primate conservation: The prevention of disease transmission. International Journal of Primatology 20: 803–826.
4. Rijksen HD (1978) A field study on Sumatran orang utans (Pongo pygmaeus abelu Lesson 1827): ecology, behaviour and conservation. Wageningen: H. Veenman Zonen BV.
5. Russon A (2009) Orangutan rehabilitation and reintroduction. In: Wich SA, Utami SS, Mitra Setia T, van Schaik CP, editors. Orangutans: Geographic Variation in Behavioral Ecology and Conservation. Oxford: Oxford University Press. 327–350.
6. Cranfield MR (2008) Mountain Gorilla research: The risk of disease transmission relative to the benefit from the perspective of ecosystem health. American Journal of Primatology 70: 751–754.
7. Kaur T, Singh J (2008) Up close and personal with Mahale chimpanzees - A path forward. American Journal of Primatology 70: 729–733.
8. Koendgen S, Kuehl H, N'Goran PK, Walsh PD, Schenk S, et al. (2008) Pandemic human viruses cause decline of endangered great apes. Current Biology 18: 260–264.
9. Williams JM, Lonsdorf EV, Wilson ML, Schumacher-Stankey J, Goodall J, et al. (2008) Causes of death in the Kasekela chimpanzees of Gombe National Park, Tanzania. American Journal of Primatology 70: 766–777.
10. Kaur T, Singh J, Tong S, Humphrey C, Clevenger D, et al. (2008) Descriptive epidemiology of fatal respiratory outbreaks and detection of a human-related metapneumovirus in wild chimpanzees (Pan troglodytes) at Mahale Mountains National Park, western Tanzania. American Journal of Primatology 70: 755–765.
11. Lukasik-Braum M, Spelman L (2008) Chimpanzee respiratory disease and visitation rules at Mahale and Gombe National Parks in Tanzania. American Journal of Primatology 70: 734–737.
12. Muehlenbein MP, Martinez LA, Lemke AA, Ambu L, Nathan S, et al. (2010) Unhealthy travelers present challenges to sustainable primate ecotourism. Travel Medicine and Infectious Disease 8: 169–175.
13. Kilbourn AM, Karesh WB, Wolfe ND, Bosi EJ, Cook RA, et al. (2003) Health evaluation of free-ranging and semi-captive orangutans (Pongo pygmaeus pygmaeus) in Sabah, Malaysia. Journal of Wildlife Diseases 39: 73–83.
14. Leendertz FH, Yumlu S, Pauli G, Boesch C, Couacy-Hymann E, et al. (2006) A new Bacillus anthracis found in wild chimpanzees and a gorilla from West and Central Africa. PLoS Pathog 2: e8.
15. Anderson RM, May RM (1991) Infectious Diseases of Humans: Dynamics and Control. Oxford: Oxford University Press.
16. Baxter T (1993) Low infectivity of tuberculosis. The Lancet 342: 371.
17. Dowell SF, Mukunu R, Ksiazek TG, Khan AS, Rollin PE, et al. (1999) Transmission of Ebola Hemorrhagic Fever: A study of risk factors in family members, Kikwit, Democratic Republic of the Congo, 1995. Journal of Infectious Diseases 179: S87–S91.
18. Cross PC, Lloyd-Smith JO, Bowers JA, Hay CT, Hofmeyr M, et al. (2004) Integrating association data and disease dynamics in a social ungulate: Bovine tuberculosis in African buffalo in the Kruger National Park. Ann Zool Fennici 41: 879–892.
19. Porphyre T, Stevenson M, Jackson R, McKenzie J (2008) Influence of contact heterogeneity on TB reproduction ratio R-0 in a free-living brushtail possum Trichosurus vulpecula population. Veterinary Research 39: 31.
20. Guimaraes PR, de Menezes MA, Baird RW, Lusseau D, Guimaraes P, et al. (2007) Vulnerability of a killer whale social network to disease outbreaks. Physical Review E 76: 042901.
21. Mitani JC, Watts DP, Muller MN (2002) Recent developments in the study of wild chimpanzee behavior. Evolutionary Anthropology 11: 9–25.
22. van Schaik CP (1999) The socioecology of fission-fusion sociality in orangutans. Primates 40: 69–86.
23. Doran D (1997) Influence of seasonality on activity patterns, feeding behavior, ranging, and grouping patterns in Tai chimpanzees. International Journal of Primatology 18: 183–206.
24. Galdikas BMF (1985) Orangutan sociality at Tanjung-Puting. American Journal of Primatology 9: 101–119.
25. Mackinnon J (1974) Behavior and ecology of wild orangutans (Pongo-pygmaeus). Animal Behaviour 22: 3–74.
26. Wrangham RW (1980) Sex differences in the behavioural ecology of chimpanzees in Gombe National Park, Tanzania. J Reprod Fert 28: 13–31.
27. Duncan AJ, Gunn GJ, Lewis FI, Umstatter C, Humphry RW (2012) The influence of empirical contact networks on modelling diseases in cattle. Epidemics 4: 117–123.
28. Griffin RH, Nunn CL (2012) Community structure and the spread of infectious disease in primate social networks. Evolutionary Ecology 26: 779–800.
29. Moreno Y, Pastor-Satorras R, Vespignani A (2002) Epidemic outbreaks in complex heterogeneous networks. European Physical Journal B 26: 521–529.
30. Opsahl T (2009) Structure and Evolution of Weighted Networks: University of London (Queen Mary College).
31. Team RDC (2011) R: A language and environment for statistical computing R Foundation for Statistical Computing, Vienna, Austria. ISBN 3-900051-900007-900050.
32. Homsy J (1999) Ape tourism and human diseases: how close should we get? Critical review of the rules and regulations governing park management and tourism for the wild mountain gorilla, Gorilla gorilla beringei.
33. Nunn CL, Altizer SM (2006) Infectious Diseases in Primates: Behavior, Ecology and Evolution. Oxford: Oxford University Press.
34. Danon L, Ford AP, House T, Jewell CP, Keeling MJ, et al. (2011) Networks and the epidemiology of infectious disease. Interdisciplinary perspectives on infectious diseases 2011: 284909.
35. Craft ME, Caillaud D (2011) Network models: an underutilized tool in wildlife epidemiology? Interdisciplinary perspectives on infectious diseases 2011: 676949–676949.
36. Cross P, Drewe J, Patrek V, Pearce G, Samuel M, et al. (2009) Host population structure and implications for disease management. In: Delahay R, Smith G, Hutchings M, editors. Management of Disease in Wild Mammals. Tokyo: Springer-Verlag Tokyo, Inc. 9–30.
37. Croft DP, James R, Krause J (2008) Exploring Animal Social Networks. Princeton: Princeton University Press.
38. Reynolds V (2005) The chimpanzees of the Budongo Forest: ecology, behaviour, and conservation. Oxford: Oxford University Press.
39. Crowcroft NS, Pebody RG (2006) Recent developments in pertussis. Lancet 367: 1926–1936.
40. Wolfe ND, Karesh WB, Kilbourn AM, Cox-Singh J, Bosi EJ, et al. (2002) The impact of ecological conditions on the prevalence of malaria among orangutans. Vector Borne and Zoonotic Diseases 2: 97–103.
41. Voelkl B, Noe R (2008) The influence of social structure on the propagation of social information in artificial primate groups: A graph-based simulation approach. Journal of Theoretical Biology 252: 77–86.

Acknowledgments

We thank all staff at the Budongo Conservation Field Station for their support and UNCST, UWA, NFA for permission to carry out the study in Budongo Forest. We also thank the Indonesian Institute of Sciences, LIPI, and RISTEK (Ministry of Research and Technology) for granting permission to undertake the research in Sabangau. We thank Dr. Suwido Limin, Director of CIMTROP (Centre of International Co-operation in Management of Tropical Peatlands) and the Rektor of the University of Palangkaraya for supporting our research in the 'Natural Laboritory' (LHAG). Special thanks to all our field assistants in Sabangau who helped collecting data especially Santi, Twenty, Thomas, Zeri, Otto, Iwan, Adul, Azes, Mark Harrison, Carly Waterman, Nick Marchant, Ben Buckley and Osamu for all their hard work in the field.

Author Contributions

Conceived and designed the experiments: CC SS JL. Performed the experiments: CC HMB KZ. Analyzed the data: CC. Contributed reagents/materials/analysis tools: HMB KZ. Wrote the paper: CC SS HMB KZ JL.

42. van Schaik CP, Ancrenaz M, Djojoasmoro R, Knott CD, Morrogh-Bernard HC, et al. (2009) Orangutan cultures revisited. In: Wich SA, Utami Atmoko SS, Mitra Setia T, van Schaik CP, editors. Orangutans: Geographic Variation in Behavioral Ecology and Conservation. Oxford: Oxford University Press. 299–309.

43. Whiten A, Goodall J, McGrew WC, Nishida T, Reynolds V, et al. (1999) Cultures in chimpanzees. Nature 399: 682–685.

44. Krützen M, Willems EP, van Schaik CP (2011) Culture and Geographic Variation in Orangutan Behavior. Current Biology 21: 1808–1812.

45. Whiten A, van Schaik CP (2007) The evolution of animal 'cultures' and social intelligence. Philosophical Transactions of the Royal Society B-Biological Sciences 362: 603–620.

12

Prioritizing Zoonoses: A Proposed One Health Tool for Collaborative Decision-Making

Cassidy Logan Rist⁹, Carmen Sofia Arriola⁹, Carol Rubin*⁹

Centers for Disease Control and Prevention, Atlanta, Georgia, United States of America

Abstract

Emerging and re-emerging zoonotic diseases pose a threat to both humans and animals. This common threat is an opportunity for human and animal health agencies to coordinate across sectors in a more effective response to zoonotic diseases. An initial step in the collaborative process is identification of diseases or pathogens of greatest concern so that limited financial and personnel resources can be effectively focused. Unfortunately, in many countries where zoonotic diseases pose the greatest risk, surveillance information that clearly defines burden of disease is not available. We have created a semi-quantitative tool for prioritizing zoonoses in the absence of comprehensive prevalence data. Our tool requires that human and animal health agency representatives jointly identify criteria (e.g., pandemic potential, human morbidity or mortality, economic impact) that are locally appropriate for defining a disease as being of concern. The outcome of this process is a ranked disease list that both human and animal sectors can support for collaborative surveillance, laboratory capacity enhancement, or other identified activities. The tool is described in a five-step process and its utility is demonstrated for the reader.

Editor: Tara C. Smith, Kent State University, United States of America

Funding: The authors have no support or funding to report.

Competing Interests: The authors have declared that no competing interests exist.

* Email: chr1@cdc.gov

⁹ These authors contributed equally to this work.

Introduction

The majority of emerging or reemerging infectious diseases originate in animals [1,2], with over 250 zoonoses documented in the literature as newly discovered or rapidly increasing in incidence or geographical range in the past 70 years [3,4]. In addition to the emergence of zoonotic pathogens, an estimated 20% of all human illness and death in the least developed countries are attributable to endemic zoonoses [5]. Globally, the top 13 zoonoses deemed most impactful to poor livestock keepers in developing countries are responsible for an estimated 2.7 million deaths and 2.4 billion cases of human illness each year; the majority of these diseases also have negative effects on livestock production [4]. The global impact of emerging and endemic zoonoses on both human and animal populations make their control and prevention a natural starting point for collaboration between human and animal health sectors. As collaboration efforts move forward, identifying zoonotic disease priorities of jurisdictional importance to governments and institutions becomes critical.

Given the realities of finite fiscal and personnel resources for both public health and animal health institutions in all countries, joint prioritization of zoonoses has the potential to benefit both sectors as efforts are made to conduct efficient and effective surveillance, develop laboratory capacity, target outbreak response, implement disease control strategies, and identify research activities. However, accomplishing the task of prioritization in a manner that is transparent and useful for all stakeholders can be challenging even in the best of situations; the paucity of quantitative data for decision-making and lack of framework required for multi-sectoral collaboration can significantly impede the process. Taking a collaborative approach to the priority-setting process ensures equal input from stakeholders in both human and animal health sectors, and ideally results in a ranked list of zoonoses that can inform joint efforts in areas of overlapping interest.

Historically recognized methods for prioritization have been adapted by health officials to identify infectious diseases, of both public and animal health importance, for national surveillance and risk-assessment [6–12]; several publications have focused specifically on the prioritization of zoonoses [13–22]. In general, after determining the pathogens to be prioritized, the ranking processes have employed a hybrid of methods to 1) select the criteria used to define the importance of pathogens, 2) apply weights to individual criteria, and 3) to score the pathogens within each criterion. Criteria weights and associated criteria scores are then combined in some manner to produce the final ranked list of pathogens. The various methods used for criteria selection and weighting, and the scoring of pathogens are often described as qualitative, quantitative, or semi-quantitative in nature based on the scoring system used and the type of data required (Table 1).

Published descriptions of infectious disease prioritization processes vary by the number of pathogens ranked, the number of criteria chosen and the methods used for ranking criteria and

Table 1. Methods used for criteria selection, weighting and scoring of pathogens.

Method	Definition	Examples
Qualitative	Qualitative methods rely on subjective individual preference and, in group settings, are often based on a process that creates consensus among group members	Delphi method [28]; Subject matter expert opinion
Semi-quantitative	Semi-quantitative methods also rely on individual preference, but allow choices to be ranked relative to each other using a numerical scale	Analytic Hierarchy Process [25]; Las Vegas method [29]
Quantitative	Quantitative methods rely on numerical scales that are designed to reflect objective values (e.g. prevalence or incidence)	Decision Tree Analysis* [30]

*The nature of the questions used in the decision tree will determine if the process is quantitative or semi-quantitative.

scoring pathogens (Table 2). Most recent publications have moved toward using more quantitative methods for prioritization, however all still rely on subject matter expert (SME) opinion at some time during the process. Although a few of the recent publications are focused on prioritization in developing countries [20–22], efforts overall remain limited to a small subset of health institutions, particularly to those located in developed countries with greater access to scientific expertise and specific disease prevalence data [13–19].

One Health Zoonotic Disease Prioritization Tool

In contrast to existing prioritization processes, the One Health Zoonotic Disease Prioritization (OHZDP) Tool was developed specifically to meet the needs of those working in areas where quantitative data on zoonoses are scarce and ties between the human and animal health sectors may be underutilized. Using established qualitative, semi-quantitative and quantitative methods, the OHZDP Tool seeks to build collaboration between diverse stakeholders and provide a dynamic list of prioritized zoonoses that can be used to justify research and allocate funding. Four important requirements of the prioritization tool were identified during the development process. Specifically, the Tool is designed to:

1) Allow equal input from stakeholders in all invested sectors using transparent methods.

2) Accommodate diversity in location (i.e. globally), scale (i.e. local, national, regional), and intended purpose (i.e. project development, surveillance, research activities, etc.) of the prioritization process.

3) Acknowledge data limitations and utilize alternative disease data to create a prioritized list of zoonotic diseases when data specific to the region are not available.

4) Provide outcomes in a timely manner so that participants may give immediate feedback and capitalize on collaborations built during the prioritization process.

Methods

The OHZDP Tool addresses the above requirements in a series of five steps (Figure 1). Some of the steps involve group work, while others can be performed by a single individual or subset of the group. The setting in which the group work takes place is assumed to be in-person, as discussion is key to several steps in the process. A moderator familiar with the Tool is optimal to facilitate group discussion and to compile and present results.

In order to provide a clear understanding of the process, an example of the expected outcome is provided after each step in the process is described below. The example is not representative of any specific government or country institution, but is intended to give the reader an idea of how the process proceeds stepwise.

Step One–Prepare for Group Work

Once the need for joint prioritization is recognized and the intent for the product of the prioritization process is agreed upon (i.e. how the prioritized list will be used for collaboration by the stakeholders), a group of suitable representatives of all stakeholders is identified and asked to participate. Based on focus group research, the recommended number of participants should be between 6 and 12 people in order to balance variation in opinion with a manageable group size [23,24]; Stakeholder groups should be equally represented in the final group selection. Selected representatives should have a strong working knowledge of their sector's current zoonotic disease activities and ability to advocate for the use of the final prioritized list in future collaborative efforts.

With the purpose of the prioritization in mind, a list of zoonoses of jurisdictional importance to the stakeholders is generated. This list can be compiled by a single person or group (not necessarily the selected stakeholder representatives), and should make use of all available internal and external sources. The list should be thoughtfully generated and include zoonoses and vector-borne diseases with animal reservoirs suspected to be of local importance; rather than an exhaustive enumeration of all possible zoonotic diseases. The list is brought to the table at the beginning of the group meeting, and may consist of diseases (e.g. Salmonellosis), pathogens (e.g. *Salmonella enteritidis*), and/or groups of pathogens (e.g. food-borne gastrointestinal illness) depending on the level of detail desired. Optimally, the list will include about 15–30 diseases or pathogens.

Example:

• Purpose: To determine which zoonoses will receive funding for joint surveillance projects between a human health agency and an animal health agency in 'Country X'.

• Stakeholders include both the human and animal health agencies. Each agency chooses five representatives to participate in the prioritization process for a total of 10 participants.

• Prior to the scheduled group work, one representative from both the human and animal health agency work together to develop the list of zoonoses to be ranked. The list includes: all zoonotic pathogens currently under surveillance by either the human or animal health agency; and any zoonoses known to be present in the human or animal population in Country X or

Table 2. Summary of publications on the prioritization of infectious diseases at the national or regional level*.

Author	Purpose of Prioritization (Country/Region)	No. of Pathogens Ranked	No. of Criteria Used	Methods Used — To Select Criteria	To Rank/Weight Criteria	To Score Pathogens	To Determine Final Pathogen Rank
Doherty J, 2000 [7]	To establish priorities for national communicable disease surveillance (Canada)	43	10	Discussion by 10 SMEs	Equal weight	Consensus scoring using the Delphi method [28] by 10 SMEs using a semi-quantitative scale: 0–5	Sum of pathogen scores
McKenzie J et al., 2007 [8]	To prioritize pathogens for a wildlife disease surveillance strategy (New Zealand)	82	3	Not stated	Equal weight	Individual scoring by unstated number of team members using both quantitative and semi-quantitative scales. Each pathogen scored by only one person	Multiplication of all three criteria scores
Cardoen S et al., 2009 [19]	To prioritize food-and water-borne zoonoses most relevant as hazards in the food chain (Belgium)	51	5	Not stated	Weights assigned by 7 risk managers using the semi-quantitative Las Vegas method [29]. Mean score used as final weight	Individual scoring by 35 SMEs using a semi-quantitative scale: 0–4. Mean score used in final analysis	Sum [criterion weight × pathogen score]

Table 2. Cont.

Author	Purpose of Prioritization (Country/Region)	No. of Pathogens Ranked	No. of Criteria Used	Methods Used		To Rank/Weight Criteria	To Score Pathogens	To Determine Final Pathogen Rank
				To Select Criteria	To Rank/Weight Criteria			
Havelaar AT et al., 2010 [17]	To support the development of national surveillance systems for emerging zoonoses (Netherlands)	86	7	Not stated	Weights assigned by 7 risk managers, 11 SMEs, and 11 medical and veterinary students using the quantitative method of probabilistic inversion [13]	Scored using a quantitative natural scale with 4–5 levels for each criterion. Point score representing central value in range used for final analysis	Linear model used to combine criteria weights with transformed point scores for each pathogen
Balabanova Y et al., 2011 [10]	To rank common pathogens based on their importance for national surveillance and epidemiological research in order to guide future research (Germany)	127	10	Not stated	Weights assigned by 86 SMEs using semi-quantitative scoring scale 0–10. Average of median score used as final weight	Consensus scoring using the Delphi method [28] by 20 SMEs using three-tiered semi-quantitative scoring system: −1, 0, 1	Sum [criterion weight × pathogen score]
Humblet MF et al., 2012 [18]	To prioritize 100 animal diseases and zoonoses (Europe)	100	57 divided into 1 of 5 categories	Discussion by SMEs	Weights assigned by 40 SMEs using the semi-quantitative Las Vegas method [29] for categories and criteria. Mean scores used as final weights	Individual scoring by 40 SMEs using a semi-quantitative scale: 0–7. Mean score used in final analysis	Sum [5 category scores] where: Category score = Sum [criterion weight × pathogen score] × category weight

Table 2. Cont.

Author	Purpose of Prioritization (Country/Region)	No. of Pathogens Ranked	No. of Criteria Used	Methods Used — To Select Criteria	To Rank/Weight Criteria	To Score Pathogens	To Determine Final Pathogen Rank
Ng V and Sargeant JM, 2012 [15]	To describe a systematic and quantitative approach to the prioritization of zoonoses in North America involving public participants (United States and Canada)	62	21	Nominal group technique [31] used in focus groups with 54 participants from medical, veterinary and non-health backgrounds	Criteria scores determined by emailed surveys to 1,539 members of the public using the quantitative Conjoint Analysis method [33]	Scored using quantitative 3–4 level scale defined based on range of values exhibited in the literature	Hierarchical Bayes models fitted to derive CA-weighted scores
Ng V and Sargeant JM, 2013 [16]	To develop a point-scoring system to derive a recommended list of zoonoses for prioritization (United States and Canada)	62	21	Nominal group technique used in focus groups with 54 participants from medical, veterinary and non-health backgrounds	Criteria scores determined by emailed surveys to 1,471 health professionals using the quantitative Conjoint Analysis method [33]	Scored using quantitative 3–4 level scale defined based on range of values exhibited in the literature	Hierarchical Bayes models fitted to derive CA-weighted scores
Cediel N et al., 2013 [20]	To establish priorities for zoonoses surveillance, prevention and control (Colombia)	32	12	Based on criteria developed by Krause et al., 2009 [32]	Weights assigned by 12 SMEs using semi-quantitative scoring scale 0–12. Average of median scores used as final weight	Consensus scoring using the Delphi method [28] by 12 SMEs using three-tiered semi-quantitative scoring system: −1, 0, 1	Sum [criterion weight × pathogen score]
Batzukh Z et al., 2013 [22]	To strengthen surveillance and response activities and laboratory capacity between human, animal and environmental sectors (Mongolia)	29	Not stated	Not stated	Not stated	Not stated	Not stated

*Only publications that include a final ranked list of pathogens are referenced in the table.

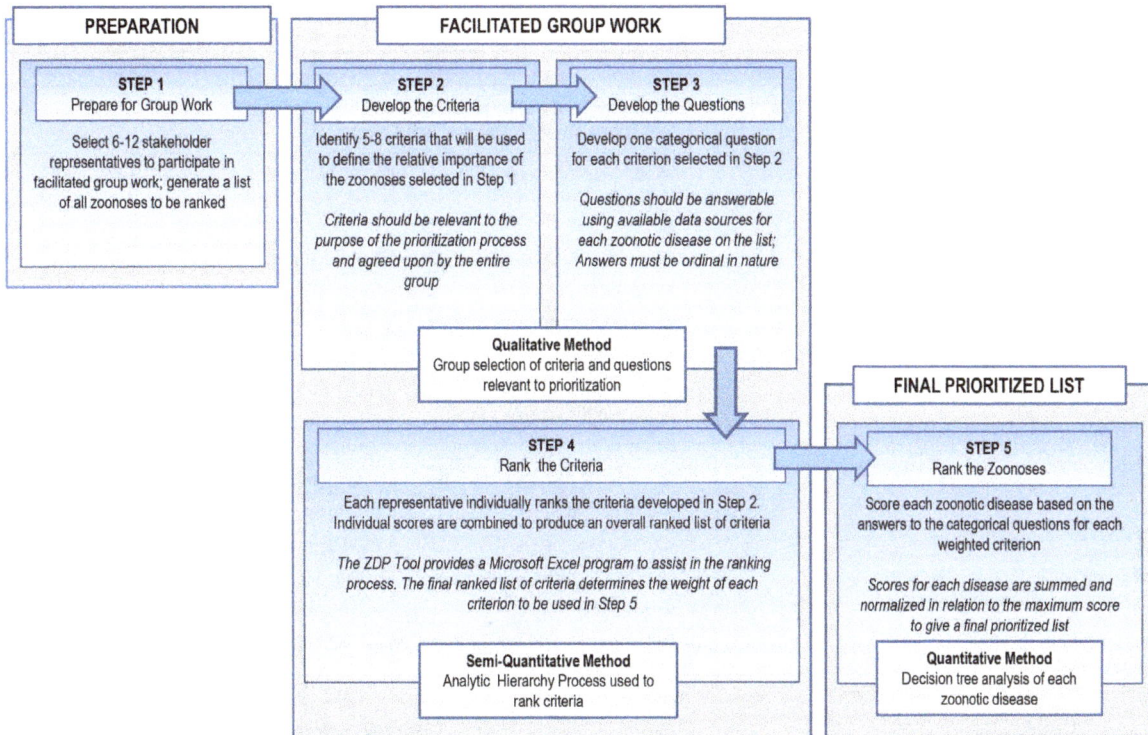

Figure 1. The five steps of the prioritization process using the One Health Zoonotic Disease Prioritization Tool.

in any bordering country as determined by a PubMed literature search, reports to ProMED-mail, the World Health Organization (WHO) and the World Organisation for Animal Health (known as OIE for its acronym in French). The list generated includes 20 zoonoses, all of which are categorized as individual pathogens except for several bacterial foodborne zoonoses (*Escherichia coli, Salmonella spp., and Campylobacter spp.,*), which are included as a single category of "Bacterial Food-Borne Zoonoses".

Step Two–Develop the Criteria

The selected group of 6–12 stakeholder representatives meets to brainstorm and develop a list of criteria that will be used to define what qualifies a zoonosis as being important. Five to nine criteria are agreed upon through moderated discussion, but not ranked at this time. The range in number of criteria [5–9] has been recognized as optimum for use in the ranking process used in Step 4 of the Tool [25]. The list of criteria is generated by subjective assessment, however the moderator provides examples of criteria used in other published methods for disease prioritization to the group in order to encourage careful consideration of all potentially useful criteria (Table 3).

Example:

- The ten representatives meet and select the following criteria (not listed in any specific order) as important to determining joint surveillance priorities: Bioterrorism potential, severity of illness in humans, economic burden of disease, amenability to collaborate, and epidemic potential.

Step Three–Develop a Question for Each Criterion

One categorical question is composed for each criterion using the same group of representatives. The questions can have binomial (e.g. yes/no) or multinomial answers that must be ordinal in nature (e.g. <10%, 10–50%, >50–75%, >75%). The ordinal nature of the answers is necessary for the scoring process used in the decision-tree analysis described in Step 5. Numerical cutoff values should be selected carefully, as different cut points will alter scores for some pathogens, and should provide good discrimination among diseases. In order to simplify the process, no more than 5 ordinal categories are recommended; this is consistent with the quantitative scales used by previously described methods [15–17].

The Tool provides a list of sample categorical questions for each of the criteria listed (Table 3), however these can and should be modified based on group preference and relevance to the particular purpose of the process. Questions must be structured in such a way that they can be answered by a single person or group using data sources available for all of the pathogens on the initial list. Sources of data to answer the questions are identified or defined at this point, according to the respective question (e.g. CDC website, PubMed literature search, country outbreak or surveillance data, OIE website, WHO website, etc.). Ensuring that questions are answerable provides the qualitative component of the prioritization method and may require unique or innovative thinking during question development, especially in settings where traditional disease data such as prevalence and incidence are lacking.

Example:

The ten representatives develop the following questions and answers to represent criteria selected in Step 2:

- Bioterrorism Potential:

Table 3. Example criteria and categorical questions used in Steps 2 and 3 of the OHZDP Tool to prioritize zoonotic diseases (ZD).

Examples of Criteria for Selection*	Examples of Candidate Categorical Questions Used to Define Each Criteria[†]
Transmission potential between humans and animals	**Q:** Has the ZD caused outbreaks in the country involving animals and humans within the last XX years?
	A: Yes or No
Epidemic/pandemic potential in humans	**Q:** Has the ZD caused epidemics in the past XX years?
	A: Yes or No
	Q: Has the ZD caused pandemics in the past XX years?
	A: Yes or No
	Q: Has the ZD pathogen been detected in a new location or population (human or animal) in the country in the past XX years?
	A: Yes or No
	Q: Is the ZD pathogen capable of sustained human-to-human transmission?
	A1: Yes or No
	A2: Three categories: Never reported, Rare/close contact only, Sustained
Bioterrorism potential	**Q:** Is the ZD listed as select agent (Lists A, B, and C)?
	A: Yes or No
Amenability to collaborate/collaboration already established	**Q:** Do both the Ministry of Health (MoH) and Ministry of Agriculture (MoA) have surveillance/control measures for the ZD?
	A1: Yes or No
	A2: Three categories: Neither, Either MoH or MoA, Both MoH and MoA
Economic burden of disease	**Q:** What is the ZD case fatality rate in animals without treatment?
	A: Four categories: 0–1%, >1–10%, >10–25%, >25%
	Q: Is the ZD listed on the OIE list of reportable animal diseases?
	A: Yes or No
	Q: Does the ZD cause significant (>XX%) decrease in animal productivity?
	A: Yes or No
Severity of illness in humans	**Q:** What is the ZD case fatality rate in humans without treatment?
	A: Three categories: 0–1%, >1–10%, >10%
	Q: Is the ZD case fatality rate >XX% in humans?
	A: Yes or No
	Q: Can the ZD result in long-term disability?
	A: Yes or No
	Q: Is case fatality rate greater than XX%, or does the pathogen cause long-term disability in greater than XX% of those infected?
	A: Yes or No
Ability to prevent/control the zoonotic disease in the country	**Q:** Is the ZD listed in country-specific surveillance programs for humans or animals?
	A1: Yes or No
	A2: Three categories: Neither, human or animal, both human and animal
	Q: Is there a known wildlife reservoir for the pathogen?
	A: Yes or No
	Q: Is there an effective vaccine for the ZD in the primary animal reservoir?
	A: Yes or No

*The handout is provided to participants to stimulate conversation and is not intended as an exhaustive list of possibilities.
[†]Only one categorical question is chosen to represent each criterion.

Q: Is the pathogen listed as a select agent (Lists A, B, or C)?
A: Yes or No
Source: As referenced by CDC website.

- Severity of Illness in Humans:

Q: Is the case fatality rate for the pathogen/disease in humans greater than 10%?
A: Yes or No
Source: As referenced by WHO website or published literature specific to the country.

- Economic Burden of Disease:

  Q: Does the pathogen cause more than 10% mortality in the animal population or more than a 10% decrease in animal productivity?
  A: Yes or No
  Source: As referenced by OIE website or published literature specific to the country.

- Epidemic Potential:

  Q: Has the pathogen been detected in a new location or population (human or animal) within Country X or any bordering country within the past 5 years?
  A: Yes or No
  Source: As referenced by Country X outbreak and/or surveillance data, confirmed reports on ProMED mail website, confirmed reports to WHO or OIE.

- Amenability to Collaborate:

  Q: Do human or animal health laboratories have diagnostic capacity available for the pathogen in Country X?
  A: Three categories: (Neither) or (At least one- human or animal) **or** (Both human **and** animal labs have capacity)
  Source: Confirmation from Country X laboratory personnel

Step Four–Rank the Criteria

The selected criteria are ranked using the semi-quantitative Analytic Hierarchy Process (AHP) [25]. First, each group member individually ranks the criteria using a series of pairwise comparisons of the criteria with a Microsoft Excel program developed as part of the OHZDP Tool to help guide participants through the ranking process. Next, the moderator uses the Excel program to merge responses of all participants, thus creating a ranked list of the criteria determined by the scores provided by each individual. Finally, a sequential (from largest to smallest) weight is assigned for the highest to lowest ranked criterion (e.g. for five selected criteria, the highest ranking criterion is assigned a weight of 5, the second highest a 4, down to the lowest ranking criterion which receives a weight of 1).

Example:

Each of the ten representatives individually ranks the criteria developed in Step 2 using the AHP process with the assistance of the Excel program. The individual scores are combined to produce a final ranked list of criteria, and are given weights based on their rank:

1) Severity of Illness in Humans (weight = 5)
2) Bioterrorism Potential (weight = 4)
3) Economic Burden of Disease (weight = 3)
4) Capacity to Collaborate (weight = 2)
5) Epidemic Potential (weight = 1)

Step Five–Rank the Zoonotic Diseases

A decision tree is built in Microsoft Excel using the highest ranked criterion as the first node, the second highest ranked criterion as the second node, and so on. The previously formulated

categorical questions and answers delineate the path that diseases will follow. The pathogens identified in Step 1 move through the decision tree based on responses to the categorical questions at each node. Responses or "decision branches" are weighted based on the weight given to each criterion in Step 4. When answers are binomial, a score of 1 is applied to one answer and a score of 0 is given to the other answer. The answer given a '1' will receive the full weight of the criterion. For questions with multinomial answers, scores are given in increasing levels determined by dividing the answer's ordinal position by the total number of answers to the question (e.g. A question with 4 ordinal answers: score for $<10\% = 1 \div 4 = 0.25$; score for $10-50\% = 2 \div 4 = 0.5$; score for $>50-75\% = 3 \div 4 = 0.75$; $>75\% = 4 \div 4 = 1$). The weight corresponding to the criterion is then multiplied by the answer's score to get the weighted score for the question (e.g. if the answer to the question was 10–50% and the weight of the criterion was 3, then the weighted score for the question $= (2 \div 4) x 3 = 1.5$). Weighted scores for all questions are summed for each pathogen and normalized in relation to the maximum score to generate the final prioritized list of pathogens. The final product is a list of the original pathogens, presented in a ranked order that is determined by the weighted criteria deemed important by the group.

Example (Figure 2):

- The question for the first criterion (severity of illness in humans) has a binomial answer (yes/no); it was decided that the 'yes' answer receives the score of 1. For the example of rabies, the answer to question 1– "Is the case fatality rate in humans greater than 10%?"– is 'yes,' therefore the score of 1 is multiplied by the weight of the criterion (weight = 5) and the weighted score = 5. This process is applied to all questions with binomial answers.

- The question for the fourth criterion (capacity to collaborate) has a multinomial answer (neither/at least one/both), with 'neither' receiving the lowest score ($1 \div 3 = 0.33$), 'at least one' receiving the second highest score ($2 \div 3 = 0.67$) and 'both' receiving the highest score ($3 \div 3 = 1$). For the example of rabies, the answer to question 4– "Do the human or animal laboratories have diagnostic capacity available for the pathogen in Country X?"–is 'both', therefore the score of $3 \div 3$ is multiplied by the weight of the criterion (weight = 2), and the weighted score = 2. If the answer was 'at least one' then the weighted score would be $= (2 \div 3) x 4 = 1.34$.

The final score for rabies is 8, or the sum of the weighted scores for each question $(5 + 0 + 0 + 2 + 1 = 8)$. Each of the original 20 zoonoses on the list is scored with this method and the final scores are normalized in relation to the highest score. After all pathogens are scored based on the results of decision tree analysis, the agencies in this fictitious example agree to use available funding to support the top 5 zoonoses on the ranked list to support joint surveillance activities.

Discussion

As governments and institutions move toward a multi-sectoral approach to zoonotic disease prevention, control, and research, effective channels for collaboration are required. Methods for joint prioritization can provide the means to open communication and build trust as well as provide transparency in the priority decision-making process. The proposed OHZDP Tool provides a process through which a prioritized list of zoonotic pathogens is generated by combining a qualitative method for determining criteria to be used, the semi-quantitative method of the AHP to rank criteria, and the quantitative technique of decision tree analysis to rank the

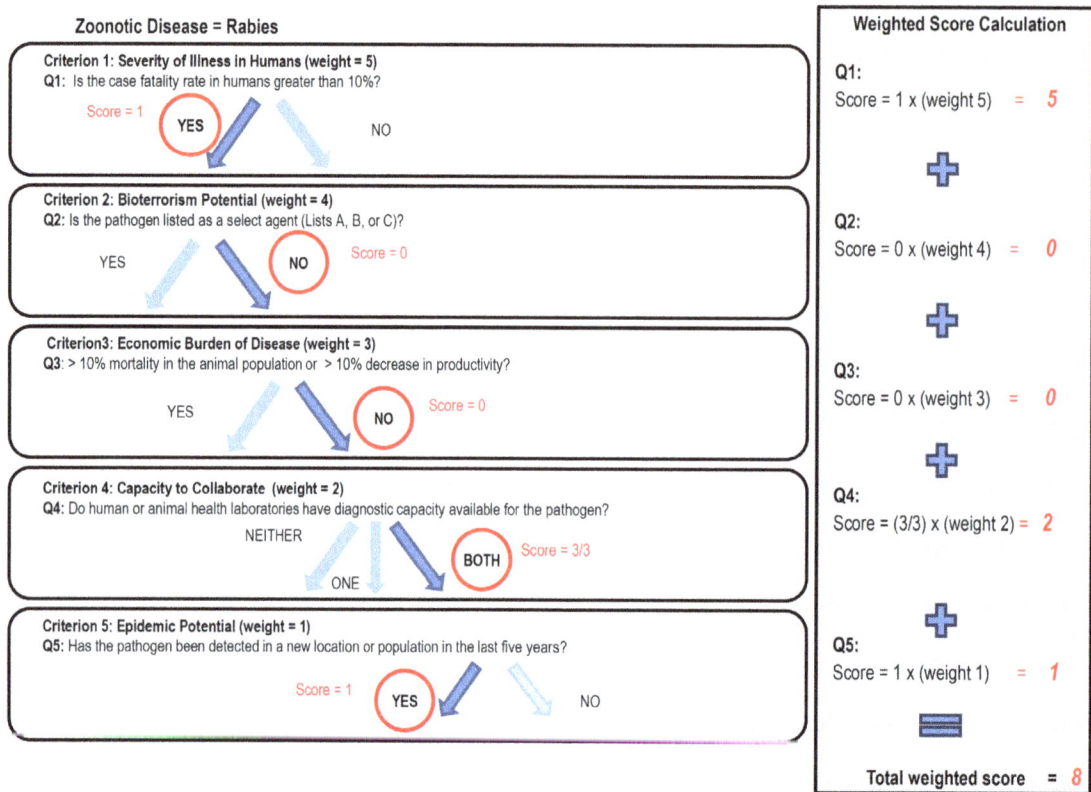

Figure 2. An example of decision tree analysis (Step 5 in the OHZDP Tool) for rabies. The criteria and questions shown are examples only, provided to show the process of how each zoonotic disease is scored. Criteria and questions are developed and given weights by the stakeholder representatives during the facilitated group work in Steps 2–5. Weighted scores for each question are summed to give the total weighted score for each pathogen; total weighted scores are normalized in relation to the maximum pathogen score to give a final ranked list.

pathogens. The process and methods employed meet the four requirements that were identified during the development phase.

Equal input from all participants is achieved in steps 2 through 4, combining group discussion and individual ranking to generate a weighted set of criteria and associated questions to be used in the decision tree analysis. Although qualitative methods, in this case group agreement on criteria and questions, have been criticized for lack of transparency and for the potential introduction of bias that can occur when employed in group settings [8], the semi-quantitative method of the AHP used to create the combined ranked list of criteria ultimately limits the influence any one person or perspective can have over the decision-making process. However, decisions made based on qualitative and semi-quantitative methods still rely on the selection of participants who may or may not be representative of all stakeholders [26,27]; thus, the appropriate selection and balance of stakeholders is explicitly emphasized as part of the prioritization process.

The OHZDP Tool provides flexibility to diverse stakeholders invested at local, national, or regional levels by allowing the group to first determine the purpose of the prioritization process and then define criteria and questions relevant for ranking the list of zoonoses. The example of 'Country X' used in this paper defines its purpose as 'funding allocation for disease surveillance at the national level' and creates a list of all zoonotic pathogens that are geographically relevant and of national interest. Alternatively, the Tool could be used by a university or research institution to determine which zoonotic diseases should be the focus of the upcoming funding cycle. In this case, the list may be smaller and limited to the current investigators' pathogens of interest or current research.

Strictly quantitative methods provide a more unbiased approach to decision-making because choices are based on data. For example, in health decision-making, people can examine health parameters for different diseases and prioritize them based on burden of disease estimates, provided good quality data are available. Quantitative methods have been applied to prioritize diseases, specifically in developed countries [15–17]. However, the methods have rarely been employed in developing countries, where, in general, public health surveillance data are lacking [20–22]. The OHZDP Tool uses decision tree analysis in a quantitative manner, relying on the categorical questions to be answerable based on objective data. Because questions are not fixed as they are for most other described methods [7,10,13,15–20], this allows participants to make use of disease data they know to be available for the scope and purpose of the prioritization process.

Integral components of collaborative work include respect for time and the ability to act on decisions made by the group. Although the OHZDP Tool was designed with the desired outcome of a prioritized list in mind, it also builds collaboration through the process. By coming together as a group, representatives are able to understand how other stakeholders view the importance of zoonoses to their relative sectors; developing criteria together helps to frame the zoonoses in relation to group priorities. The OHZDP Tool provides Microsoft Excel programs to assist in group ranking of criteria (Step 2) and in the final ranking of pathogens in the decision tree process (Step 5), which together with facilitated group work results in a rapid and transparent method for zoonoses prioritization.

In the pilot trials of the tool, Steps 2–4 could be completed in a one-day time period. The decision tree process, which can be completed primarily by the facilitator or other assigned individuals, can take up to another half or full day of time depending on the number of zoonoses selected for analysis. This means that participants know the results of the ranked criteria at the end of the first group session, and the results for the final ranked pathogen list can be ready within 24 hours. Rapid turnaround allows further discussion and a timely output that can be used immediately for its intended purpose.

To provide further clarification for the five steps in the OHZDP Tool, the complete output from one pilot study is provided in the supporting information. For this particular pilot study, the authors brought together six professionals currently active in zoonotic disease research. Three of the participants were asked to assume the role of representatives from a fictional country's Ministry of Health and three from the Ministry of Agriculture. They were provided a list of 17 zoonoses (Table S1) and assisted through Steps 2–4 of the OHZDP Tool (Tables S2, S3). Step 5 was completed by the authors (Table S4, S5), and the final prioritized list is presented in Table S6.

The authors are aware that further validation of the OHZDP Tool is an optimal next step; however, the OHZDP Tool is similar to other tools in its design, as each step of the prioritization process (selection of criteria, weighting of criteria, scoring of pathogens, and final determination of pathogen rank), employs a previously validated prioritization method (Table 2). Quantitative comparison with the tools that already exist may be difficult as the majority require at least basic surveillance data [7,10,15–19]. The OHZDP Tool is designed to be used in countries where surveillance data are lacking and even expert opinion may not be sufficient to accurately estimate zoonotic disease prevalence or incidence in human and/or animal populations.

Future pilots of the Tool will assess its internal validity by repeating the process using different representatives from the same stakeholder groups and comparing the final prioritized lists using non-parametric tests. In addition, results of sensitivity tests for the impact of each criterion and the importance of assigned criteria weights will be documented to assess their influence on the final ranking of the diseases. And finally, although the range of number of participants, criteria and categories for questions were provided using documented sources [23–25], the robustness of the Tool can be further evaluated by altering these values and comparing results. A Facilitator Manual for the OHZDP Tool, including

instructions for the Excel programs is available from the authors upon request for those interested in participating in ongoing evaluation and validation of the Tool.

In summary, the OHZDP Tool was developed for use by organizations or institutions interested in prioritizing zoonoses; the purpose of the prioritization can vary based on stakeholder needs, but can ultimately serve to identify areas of overlapping interest, focus the use of limited resources, and maximize the impact of zoonotic disease related activities. The Tool presented here differs from others in its ability to combine individual and group decision making processes together with limited disease data in a manner that is flexible enough to meet the needs of multi-sectoral groups with differing levels of jurisdictional reach. The authors feel the tool offers a transparent and timely process for those who wish to prioritize zoonoses using a collaborative approach and welcome any questions or comments on the Tool's potential utility.

Supporting Information

Table S1 Step 1: List of zoonotic diseases compiled for pilot testing of the OHZDP Tool.

Table S2 Steps 2 and 3: Criteria and associated questions selected by the pilot group.

Table S3 Step 4: Excel program for group ranking of criteria using the Analytic Hierarchy Process.

Table S4 Step 5: Answers to the questions for each of the 17 selected zoonoses.

Table S5 Step 5: Excel program used to rank the pathogens using decision tree analysis.

Table S6 Step 5: Prioritized list of the 17 zoonoses based on their final, normalized scores in the decision-tree analysis.

Author Contributions

Conceived and designed the experiments: CLR CSA CR. Analyzed the data: CLR CSA CR. Wrote the paper: CLR CSA CR.

References

1. Taylor LH, Latham SM, Woolhouse ME (2001) Risk factors for human disease emergence. Phil Trans R Soc Lond B 356: 983–9. doi:10.1098/rstb.2001.0888.
2. Woolhouse M, Gowtage-Sequeria S (2005) Host range and emerging and reemerging pathogens. Emerg Infect Dis 12: 1842–7. doi:10.3201/eid1112.050997.
3. Jones KE, Patel NG, Levy MA, Storeygard (2008) Global trends in emerging infectious disease. Nature 451: 990–993. doi:10.1038/nature06536.
4. Grace D, Mutua F, Ochungo P, Kruska R, Jones K, et al. (2012) Mapping of poverty and likely zoonoses hotspots. Zoonoses Project 4. Report to the UK Department for International Development. Nairobi, Kenya: ILRI.
5. Grace D, Jones B, McKeever D, Pfeiffer D, Mutua F, et al. (2011) Zoonoses: Wildlife/livestock interactions. Zoonoses Project 1. Report to the UK Department for International Development and ILRI. Nairobi, Kenya: ILRI, and London, UK: Royal Veterinary College.
6. Rushdy A, O'Mahony M (1998) PHLS overview of communicable diseases 1997: results of a priority setting exercise. Commun Dis Rep CDR Suppl 8(5): S1–12.
7. Doherty JA (2000) Establishing priorities for national communicable disease surveillance. Can J Infect Dis 11(1): 21–4.

8. McKenzie J, Simpson H, Langstaff I (2007) Development of methodology to prioritize wildlife pathogens for surveillance. Prev Vet Med 81(1–3): 194–210.
9. Krause G (2008) How can infectious diseases be prioritized in public health? EMBO Rep 9 (Suppl 1): S22–S27. doi:10.1038/embor.2008.76.
10. Balabanova Y, Gilsdorf A, Buda S, Burger R, Eckmanns T, et al. (2011) Communicable diseases prioritized for surveillance and epidemiological research: results of a standardized prioritization procedure in Germany, 2011. PloS One 6(10). Available: http://www.plosone.org/article/info%3Adoi%2F10.1371%2Fjournal.pone.0025691. Accessed 2013 Apr 23.
11. Maino M, Perez P, Oviedo P, Sotomayor G, Abalos P (2012) The analytic hierarchy process in decisionmaking for caprine health programmes. Rev Sci Tech 31(3): 889–97.
12. Mourits MC, van Asseldonk MA, Huirne RB (2010) Multi Criteria Decision Making to evaluate control strategies of contagious animal diseases. Prev Vet Med 96(3–4): 201–10. doi:10.1016/j.prevetmed.2010.06.010.
13. Kurowicka D, Bucura C, Cooke R, Havelaar A (2010) Probabilistic inversion in priority setting of emerging zoonoses. Risk Analysis 30(5): 715–723. doi:10.1111/j.1539-6924.2010.01378.x.
14. Ng V, Sargeant JM (2012) A stakeholder-informed approach to the identification of criteria for the prioritization of zoonoses in Canada. PloS One 7(11).

Available: http://www.plosone.org/article/info%3Adoi%2F10.1371%2Fjournal.pone.0029752. Accessed 2013 Apr 25.

15. Ng V, Sargeant JM (2012) A quantitative and novel approach to the prioritization of zoonotic diseases in North America: a public perspective. PloS 7(11). Available: http://www.plosone.org/article/info%3Adoi%2F10.1371%2Fjournal.pone.0048519. Accessed 2013 Apr 25.

16. Ng V, Sargeant JM (2013) A quantitative and novel approach to the prioritization of zoonotic diseases in North America: a health professionals' perspective. PloS One 8(8). Available: http://www.ncbi.nlm.nih.gov/pmc/articles/PMC3749166/. Accessed 2013 Dec 10.

17. Havelaar AH, van Rosse F, Bucura C, Toetenel MA, Haagsma JA, et al. (2010) Prioritizing emerging zoonoses in the Netherlands. PloS One 5(11). Available: http://www.plosone.org/article/info%3Adoi%2F10.1371%2Fjournal.pone.0013965. Accessed 2013 Apr 23.

18. Humblet MF, Vandeputte S, Albert A, Gosset C, Kirschvink N, et al. (2012) Multidisciplinary and evidence-based method for prioritizing diseases of food-producing animals and zoonoses. Emerg Infect Dis 18(4). Available: http://wwwnc.cdc.gov/eid/article/18/4/11-1151_article. Accessed 2013 Apr 25.

19. Cardoen S, Van Huffel X, Berkvens D, Quoilin S, Ducoffre G, et al. (2009) Evidence-based semiquantitative methodology for prioritization of foodborne zoonoses. Foodborne Pathog Dis 6(9): 1083–96. doi:10.1089/fpd.2009.0291.

20. Cediel N, Villamil LC, Romero J, Renteria L, De Meneghi D (2013) Setting priorities for surveillance, prevention, and control of zoonoses in Bogota, Colombia. Rev Panam Salud Publica 33(5): 316–24.

21. Sekar N, Shah NK, Abbas SS, Kakkar M (2011) Research options for controlling zoonotic disease in India, 2010–1015. PloS One 6(2). Available: http://www.plosone.org/article/info%3Adoi%2F10.1371%2Fjournal.pone.0017120. Accessed 2013 Apr 23.

22. Batsukh Z, Tsolmon B, Otgonbaatar D, Undraa B, Dolgorkhand A, et al. (2013) One Health in Mongolia. In: Mackenzie JS, Jeggo M, daszak, Richt JA, editors. One Health: The Human-Animal-Environment Interfaces in Emerging Infectious Diseases. Curr Top Microbiol Immunol 366: 123–37. doi:10.1007/82_2012_253.

23. Sharken Simon J (1999) How to conduct a focus group. Fieldstone Alliance. Available: http://www.tgci.com/podcasts/how-conduct-focus-group-judith-sharken-simon. Accessed 2013 Jan 5.

24. Guidelines for conducting a focus group (2005). Eliot and Associates. Available: http://assessment.aas.duke.edu/resources.php. Accessed 2013 Jan 5.

25. Saaty TL (2008) Decision making with the analytic hierarchy process. Int J Services Sci 1(1): 83–98.

26. Toloie-Eshlaghy A, Nazari Farokhi E (2011) Measuring the importance and the weight of decision makers in the criteria weighting activities of group decision making process. American Journal of Scientific Research 24: 6–12.

27. Gilsdorf A, Krause G (2011) Prioritisation of infectious diseases in public health: feedback on the prioritisation methodology, 15 July 2008 to 15 January 2009. Euro Surveill 16(18). Available: http://www.eurosurveillance.org/ViewArticle.aspx?ArticleId=19861. Accessed 2013 Dec 15.

28. Hsu C-C, Sandford BA (2007) The Delphi technique: Making sense of consensus. Practical Assessment Research and Evaluation. Available: http://pareonline.net/pdf/v12n10.pdf. Accessed 2013 Jan 5.

29. Gore SM (1987) Biostatistics and the Medical Research Council. MRC News 35: 19–20.

30. Skinner DC (2009) Developing a decision model. In: Introduction to Decision Analysis. Gainesville, FL: Probabilistic Publishing. 150–153.

31. Jones J, Hunter D (1995) Consensus methods for medical and health services research. BMJ 311: 376–380.

32. Krause G, Working Group on Prioritization at the Robert Koch Institute (2008) Prioritization of infectious diseases in public health-call for comments. Euro Surveill 13(40). Available: http://www.eurosurveillance.org/ViewArticle.aspx?ArticleId=18996. Accessed 2013 Dec 12.

33. Ryan M, Farrar S (2000) Using conjoint analysis to elicit preferences for health care. BMJ 320: 1530–1533.

13

Prediction and Control of Brucellosis Transmission of Dairy Cattle in Zhejiang Province, China

Juan Zhang[1,2◊], Gui-Quan Sun[2,3◊], Xiang-Dong Sun[4], Qiang Hou[5], Mingtao Li[2], Baoxu Huang[4], Haiyan Wang[6], Zhen Jin[2]*

1 School of Mechatronic Engineering, North University of China, Taiyuan, Shan'xi, People's Republic of China, 2 Complex Systems Research Center, Shanxi University, Taiyuan, Shan'xi, People's Republic of China, 3 School of Mathematical Science, Fudan University, Shanghai, People's Republic of China, 4 The Laboratory of Animal Epidemiological Surveillance, China Animal Health & Epidemiology Center, Qingdao, Shandong, People's Republic of China, 5 Department of Mathematics, North University of China, Taiyuan, Shan'xi, People's Republic of China, 6 School of Mathematical & Natural Sciences, Arizona State University, Phoenix, AZ, United States of America

Abstract

Brucellosis is a bacterial disease caused by brucella; mainly spread by direct contact transmission through the brucella carriers, or indirect contact transmission by the environment containing large quantities of bacteria discharged by the infected individuals. At the beginning of 21st century, the epidemic among dairy cows in Zhejiang province, began to come back and has become a localized prevalent epidemic. Combining the pathology of brucellosis, the reported positive data characteristics, and the feeding method in Zhejiang province, this paper establishes an *SEIV* dynamic model to excavate the internal transmission dynamics, fit the real disease situation, predict brucellosis tendency and assess control measures in dairy cows. By careful analysis, we give some quantitative results as follows. (1) The external input of dairy cows from northern areas may lead to high fluctuation of the number of the infectious cows in Zhejiang province that can reach several hundreds. In this case, the disease cannot be controlled and the infection situation cannot easily be predicted. Thus, this paper encourages cows farms to insist on self-supplying production of the dairy cows. (2) The effect of transmission rate of brucella in environment to dairy cattle on brucellosis spreading is greater than transmission rate of the infectious dairy cattle to susceptible cattle. The prevalence of the epidemic is mainly aroused by environment transmission. (3) Under certain circumstances, the epidemic will become a periodic phenomenon. (4) For Zhejiang province, besides measures that have already been adopted, sterilization times of the infected regions is suggested as twice a week, and should be combined with management of the birth rate of dairy cows to control brucellosis spread.

Editor: Caroline Colijn, Imperial College London, United Kingdom

Funding: This research is supported by the National Natural Science Foundation of China under grants (11171314, 11147015, and 11301490), Natural Science Foundation of Shan'Xi Province grant no. 2012021002-1, The specialized research fund for the doctoral program of higher education (preferential development) no. 20121420130001, China Postdoctoral Science Foundation under grant no. 2012M520814, and Shanghai Postdoctoral Science Foundation under grant no. 13R21410100 and IDRC104519-010. The funders had no role in study design, data collection and analysis, decision to publish, or preparation of the manuscript.

Competing Interests: The authors have declared that no competing interests exist.

* Email: jinzhn@263.net

◊ These authors contributed equally to this work.

Introduction

Brucellosis, also called Bang's disease, Crimean fever, Gibraltar fever, Malta fever, Maltese fever, Mediterranean fever, Rock fever, or Undulant fever, is a highly contagious zoonosis caused by brucella. In China, it is usually called "Lazybones disease". It is listed in Class B animal epidemics by the World Organisation for Animal Health (OIE) and Class II as one of the notifiable diseases by the Law on Prevention and Control of Infectious Diseases of the People's Republic of China [1]. In 1985, according to the characteristics of brucella and host specificity, the committee of WHO divided Brucella into 6 species, that is *B. melitensis* (goats and sheep), *B. suis* (pigs), *B. abortus* (cows and bison), *B. ovis* (sheep), *and B. canis* (dogs) [2]. For cows, *B. melitensis*, *B. suis*, *B. abortus* are found, and *B. abortus* is the dominant species [3]. *B. abortus*, *B. melitensis*, *B. suis*, and *B. canis* are pathogens to invade human. Brucella is highly contagious, and can be spread by direct contact transmission through the brucella carriers or indirect contact transmission when animals ingest contaminated forages or the excrement containing large quantities of bacteria, generally discharged by infected animals. The brucella can survive 20-120 days in soil, 70–150 days in water, and 2 months in food such as milk and meat [4]. However, the brucella can be killed easily by direct sunlight within a few hours or by high temperatures within a few minutes. Once infected by brucellosis, animals should go through 14–180 days incubation [4] until they show symptoms.

The finding of brucella carriers, for dairy cows, mainly depends on regular detection. Diagnosis methods during the detection process are based on bacteriology or serology, which generally includes screening tests and supplemental tests. Screening tests are used to locate infected population, but there is a high percentage of false positive results. So, supplemental tests, which include complement fixation, rivanol precipitation and milk samples test, are used to clarify the results of screening tests [5]. However, there also exist some false negative herds not to be detected by tests. It follows that these diagnosis are not completely effective and only about 84%–98% of infected dairy herds can be detectable [6]. However, whether the dairy herd in incubation can be detectable is an outstanding issue.

Zhejiang province is located on the southern part of China, in which there are hills, mountains, basins, islands and the Qiantang river. It belongs to subtropical monsoon climate area with four entirely different seasons, plentiful sunshine and rainfall. Thus, the farming there has experienced extensive development. In 1950s, that Hangzhou, Ningbo, Huzhou city in Zhejiang province imported infected dairy cows from north provinces made the Zhejiang province develop a brucellosis prevalence among dairy cows. From 1983 to 1995, Zhejiang province carried out brucellosis general census and culled all the detected positive reactors of livestock [7]. Consequently, in 1995, the brucellosis epidemic in Zhejiang province reached control standards of government regulations. However, at the beginning of the 21st century, the epidemic situation between livestock, especially dairy cows, began to come back, even increased year by year and has lead to the local prevalence of brucellosis [8]. In 2001, there was only 14 infected dairy cows. Quickly, it increased to 248 in 2005 and 527 in 2009, respectively. In 2010, the accumulative number of the infected dairy cows arrived 1808. Simultaneously, the diagnosis methods taken in Zhejiang province were serological examination: tube agglutination test (SAT) and complement fixation test (CFT) [8]. Though culling the reactors and regular detection are taken powerfully, the positive data of dairy cows in Zhejiang are rising year by year, which has negatively influenced the local economy, even leads to the local prevalence of human brucellosis. By the full-survey and analysis for brucellosis in Zhejiang province, some crucial factors are found to interpret the spread of brucellosis. Firstly, during the past ten years, the livestock breeding, dairy, and the leather processing industry had experienced great development. A mass of dairy cows, beefs, row furs and other animal by-products were imported from the northern pastoral areas annually. When the brucellosis in the northern pastoral area began to return, and the imported cows from northern areas cannot get effective quarantine inspection and were directly mixed with local cows in Zhejiang [8], brucellosis was brought into Zhejiang province. Secondly, culling measure cannot be carried out completely and effectively, so the sources of infection are not removed thoroughly [8]. Lastly, the sensitivities of the surveillance and confirmation tests were not 100%, collected from the literature as follows: 84% for the SAT [9,10] and 89% for the CFT [9,11–13]. Moreover, there exists improper handling in practical culling and test processes. So, some infected dairy cows cannot be detectable and will become hidden dangers to cause the spread of brucellosis. It is thus clear that the recent reemergence of brucellosis in dairy cows poses a serious threat on the economy and public health in Zhejiang province and we need resort to dynamical modeling to explore the inherent factors of brucellosis transmission and assess prevention and control measures.

Mathematical models which are applied to investigate epidemic spreading have various forms, such as dynamical systems, statistical models, game theoretic models and so on, where the dynamical system is a very important method, whose main idea is to build evolution rule that describes how future states follow from the current states. Therefore, the dynamical system shows inherent link and internal change pattern of sub-populations, and can be applied to forecast future states of disease in considered populations. So far, dynamical models have been adopted to explore the transmission dynamics of brucellosis. In 1994, Gonzalez-Guzman and Naulin [14] built a model about bovine brucellosis, used singular perturbations method to analyse the dynamical behavior, and

obtained a threshold parameter for the outbreak of the disease. In 2009, Xie and Horan [15] built a simple dynamical model, including the susceptible, the infected, and the resistant subclass, to discuss brucellosis in elk and cow populations. They mainly investigated private responses and ecological impacts of policies, and found feedbacks between jointly determined disease dynamics and decentralized economic behavior matter, whose novel point is to combine disease with the economic factor. Because hosts can also be infected by a contaminated environment, Ainseba et al. [16] considered two transmission modes about the ovine brucellosis: direct mode caused by contact with infected individuals, and indirect mode related to the presence of virulent organisms including brucella in the environment, which we think is a dominant and important factor for brucellosis transmission. They obtained the reproduction number, and investigated the effect of a slaughtering policy. Xie and Horan [15] and Ainseba et al. [16] only investigated the transmission dynamics of brucellosis between animals. In 2005, besides transmission within sheep and cow populations, Zinsstag et al. [17] considered the transmission to humans to fit demographic and seroprevalence data from livestock and annually reported new human brucellosis cases in Mongolia from 1991 to 1999. The livestocks are classified into three subclasses: the susceptible, the seropositive, and the immunized. They mainly showed that average effective reproductive ratios were 1.2 for sheep and 1.7 for cows. However, there is very few research to study the brucellosis in China which is more serious. Hou et al. [18] investigated the transmission dynamics of sheep brucellosis in Inner Mongolia Autonomous Region of China and discussed the effects of vaccination, disinfection and eliminating strategies between young and adult sheep.

In 2011, while in collaboration with China Animal Health & Epidemiology Center in Qingdao, we went to Zhejiang province to carry out field research. We mainly visited dairy cow raising areas and communicated with local farmers and government, by which the detailed information about dairy cow breeding was obtained. The breeding mode for dairy cows is mainly large-scale raising zone construction. Zhejiang province imported some fine varieties of dairy cows from northern areas every year. As a result, the input of dairy cows has brought brucellosis into Zhejiang province. According to the breeding mode, control measures in Zhejiang province, the model established in this paper has five characteristics. Firstly, since the breeding mode for dairy cows in Zhejiang province is mainly large-scale raising zone construction, so standard incidence rate is adopted. Secondly, for dairy cattle in Zhejiang province, taking safety of milk products into consideration, vaccination for cattle is not carried out. So, it is not included in our model. Thirdly, since there are 14–180 days incubation period for cattle brucellosis, the exposed subclass is considered. Individuals in the period of incubation are hardly detectable, but can infect the healthy dairy cows by direct contact or by discharging brucella to environment, thus the consideration for incubation period is necessary. Moreover, the import of cattle from north areas is considered, since it is the main reason of prevalence of brucellosis in Zhejiang. Finally, there exist two transmission modes for brucellosis: direct transmission between individuals and the transmission of infected environment. Since dairy cows are infected mainly through ingesting contaminated forages or the excrement discharged by infected animals, the infection through environment is vital and indispensable, even more important than the direct contact transmission between the individuals. For previous models, [15–18] adopted bilinear incidence rate and considered immunized groups. Environment transmission did not be considered in [14,15,17]. The import of individual from other areas was not considered by [14,15,17,18]. Based on these literatures, this paper builds an SEIV model with external input of dairy cows to fit the real situation, reveal the transmission mechanism, predict the spread situation and assess control measures of dairy cattle brucellosis in Zhejiang province in China. After 2000, there is more relatively regular and standard management in Zhejiang province: large-scale raising zone construction, regular inspection and positive-cull. The detailed data and information can be obtained. Studying the situation in Zhejiang province can provide suggestion and revelations for whole cattle management and epidemic control in China.

In addition, there are three points that need to supplement. Firstly, for brucellosis, prevention and control measures, that is detection twice a year and 100% culling of the detected positive cows that have already been adopted in the Zhejiang province are, are all considered in our model. Moreover, the discharge rates of amount of brucella between the exposed and infectious is assumed to be the same. In fact, the amount of brucella discharged by the exposed and infectious should be different. In order to distinguish the difference between the exposed and infectious, a supplementary parameter should be introduced. As we know, the discharge rate is hard to quantify and the supplementary parameter is also uncertain. So, it makes little sense to distinguish the difference of amount of brucella discharged by the exposed and infectious that can increase the number of uncertain parameter and has little effect on analysis result. Finally, we obtain the positive data of dairy cows in Zhejiang province which are reliable and sufficient, and can use them to confirm the validity of the dynamical model.

Methods

Dynamical model

The populations we consider in the model are the dairy cows and the brucella contained in excreta discharged by infected dairy cows into environment. Let $N(t)$ be the total number of dairy cows in Zhejiang province under consideration at any time t, which are classified into three subclasses: the susceptible, exposed and infectious denoted by $S(t), E(t)$ and $I(t)$, respectively. The quantity of brucella in environment is denoted by $V(t)$. With regard to $V(t)$, it is very difficult to determine the quantity in environment and the quantity that is enough to infect an individual. Hence, in this paper, we define that the average number of bacteria that are needed to infect a host with brucellosis is called *an infectious unit* [18]. Thus the unit of $V(t)$ is *the infectious unit*, shortly "*IU*". The mathematical model to be discussed is to study the rate of change of the all populations, especially the infectious dairy cows. Our assumptions on the transmission process of brucellosis among dairy cows are demonstrated in the following flowchart (Fig. 1). According to Fig. 1, the deterministic dynamic model is given as follows, where parameters are described in Table 1. The detailed description of model is given in Appendix S1.

$$\begin{cases} \dfrac{dS(t)}{dt} = (1-c_1-c_2)A + bS(t) - \epsilon\beta\dfrac{S(t)E(t)}{N(t)} - \beta\dfrac{S(t)I(t)}{N(t)} \\ \qquad\qquad - \alpha S(t)V(t) - mS(t), \\[2mm] \dfrac{dE(t)}{dt} = c_1A + \epsilon\beta\dfrac{S(t)E(t)}{N(t)} + \beta\dfrac{S(t)I(t)}{N(t)} + \alpha S(t)V(t) \\ \qquad\qquad - mE(t) - \delta E(t), \\[2mm] \dfrac{dI(t)}{dt} = c_2A + \delta E(t) - mI(t) - \sigma\mu I(t), \\[2mm] \dfrac{dV(t)}{dt} = r(E(t)+I(t)) - wV(t) - klV(t). \end{cases} \qquad (1)$$

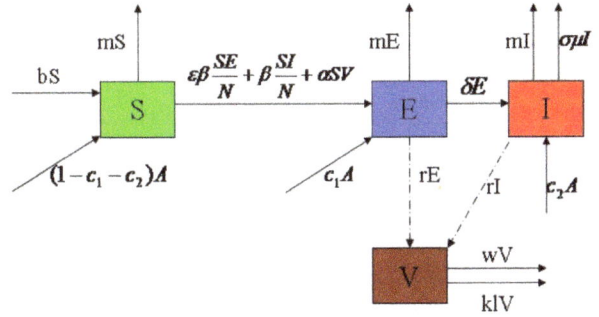

Figure 1. Flow diagram on the dynamical transmission of brucellosis among dairy cattle. Solid arrows represent transfer orientation of population (the department from one subclass and incoming to another subclass). For a subclass, the incoming solid arrows (point to the subclass) represent the recruitment of cattle to this subclass, and the outgoing solid arrows (point to other subclass) represent the runoff of cattle or brucella from this subclass. Dash arrows only represent incoming of brucella to environment discharged by E and I.

Due to the complexity of system, we just give limited results about dynamical behaviors in Table 2, whose related theorems and proofs can be seen in Appendix S1, and related Figures are given as Figs S1, S2, S3 and S4, where P^0 is the disease-free equilibrium, O is zero equilibrium, P^* is endemic equilibrium, and R_0 is the basic reproduction number [20,21].

The Interpretation of Parameter Values

Now, we interpret the parameter values as follows. Due to limited data, we have to make assumptions about c_1, c_2, ϵ, b, k, r, l, $E(0)$, and $V(0)$, where c_1, c_2, b, k, r and l are taken as random numbers from certain reasonable intervals. Recently, the number of cattle in Zhejiang province is between 40000 and 80000 and the number of infected cattle is from 100 to 600, so the infected rate is about 0.00125 to 0.015. So, we assume that c_1 is between 0.001 and 0.003 and the value of c_2 is less a little than c_1. For b and r, we give the corresponding reasonable intervals by fitting real data. k is disinfection effective rate and should be between 0 and 1. 100% is impossible and the disinfection measure is taken well in Zhejiang province, so we assume the interval is from 0.5 to 0.9. l is the disinfection frequency. According to personal communication, breeding field is disinfected about once a week. There are 52 weeks in one year. So, l is taken random number between 40 and 60. A, β and α are obtained by parameter estimation. D_1 and D_2 are obtained during fitting data by stochastic model to make the perturbation amplitude of solution consistency with the actual data. σ is assumed according to the personal communication of authors during field research. In Zhejiang province, government carries out surveillance tests twice a year, and the unit of time taken in the model (1) is one year, so $\sigma = 2$. Because the sensitivities of tube agglutination test (SAT) and complement fixation test (CFT) adopted as the diagnosis methods are 84% and 89%, we assume the average sensitivity is 85%. Moreover, Zhejiang province culls all the discovered positive reactors, so the culling rate for the infected herd is 85%, that is $\mu = 0.85$. The detailed introduction of basic knowledge about dairy cows can be seen in [6]. A heifer(dairy cow) reaches sexual maturity within 18 months of age and it will have no reproduction value after the third pregnancy [6]. So, the dairy cow is removed from the herd at four

Table 1. Description of parameters in the model (1) and (2).

Parameters	Value	Unit	Comments	resource
A		$year^{-1}$	Annual introduction number of dairy cow.	estimating
c_1	[0.001,0.003]	none	The proportion of the exposed on A.	assuming
c_2	[0.0005,0.0025]	none	The proportion of the infective ion A.	assuming
b	[0.05,0.15]	$year^{-1}$	Annual birth rate of S(t).	assuming
ϵ	0.5	none	Auxiliary parameter.	assuming
β		none	I(t)-to-S(t) transmission rate.	estimating
α		none	V(t)-to-S(t) transmission rate.	estimating
m	0.25	$year^{-1}$	Dairy cow natural elimination rate.	[6]
δ	6	$year^{-1}$	Clinical outcome rate of exposed cows.	[4]
σ	2	none	The frequency of annual quarantine.	[a]
μ	0.85	$year^{-1}$	The culling rate of I(t) after quarantining.	[9–13]
r	[3,7]	IU	The discharging quantity of brucella by E and I.	assuming
w	6	$year^{-1}$	The natural death rate of V(t).	[4]
k	[0.5,0.9]	none	The effective disinfection rate each time.	assuming
l	[40,60]	$year^{-1}$	The frequency of disinfection annually.	assuming
D_1	0.002	none	The intensity of white noise.	fitting
D_2	0.0015	none	The intensity of white noise.	fitting
$S(0)$	40000	individual	The initial number of the susceptible cows.	[19]
$E(0)$	7	individual	The initial number of the exposed cows.	assuming
$I(0)$	14	individual	The initial number of the infective cows.	[b]
$V(0)$	100	IU	The initial quantity of brucella.	assuming

[a] Field research and personal communication. [b] The Laboratory of Animal Epidemiological Surveillance, China Animal Health & Epidemiology Center.

years of age on average, that is $m = \frac{1}{4} = 0.25$. According to [4], for dairy herds, the brucella has a 14–180 day incubation period. Here we take 2 months, so $\delta = 1/\frac{2}{12} = 6$. Besides, the brucella can survive 20–120 days in soil, 70–150 days in water, 2 months in food such as milk and meat. So, we take the mean value 2 months, that is $w = 1/\frac{2}{12} = 6$. The initial number of dairy cows $N(0)$ in Zhejiang province is taken from [19], which can be viewed as the initial number of the susceptible cows $S(0)$ for the numbers of $E(0)$ and $I(0)$ are very few relatively. The data of $I(t)$ from 2001 to 2010 is provided by China Animal Health and Epidemiology Center in Qingdao city.

The least-square estimated method

We apply the least-square method to carry out parameter estimation, which is implemented by the command *fminsearch*, a part of the optimization toolbox in MATLAB. Let $\hat{I}(t)$ be the real data and $I(t)$ is the theoretical result of model. The estimation method is to find parameter values such that the value of

$$f(\theta,n) = \sum_{i=1}^{n} (I(t) - \hat{I}(t))^2$$ is the least, where θ is the parameter vector and n is the number of real data.

Results

Numerical Fitting and Prediction

The real new data about infected dairy cattle and cattle population are listed in Tables S1 and S2 in Appendix S1,

respectively. By running 100 times, the estimated parameter values are listed in Table 3 and corresponding fitting results by deterministic model are given in Fig. 2, where the red dots is the real number of annual new infectious cattle in Zhejiang province and the boxplots is drawn by applying 100 times of simulation results by deterministic model. It is obvious that real data have certain fluctuation and the theoretic fitting result of deterministic model is general trend of the epidemic.

Recently, the government in Zhejiang province has intensely taken powerful quarantine inspection and slaughter of the positive reactors to control brucellosis. However, there still remains the positive dairy herds in the process of the quarantine inspection. Based on the literatures and full-survey in Zhejiang province, it is known that the most crucial factor which leads to the prevalence of brucellosis is the import of infected dairy cows from the the the northern pastoral areas, which are the high-prevalence areas. However, the import does not get effective detection, which leads to the input of the infected dairy cows [8]. Moreover, the positive data in several cities in Zhejiang province had randomness, which can be seen in Fig. 3. Particularly, in Fig. 3(c), Huzhou city always was exempt from brucellosis before 2004. However, in 2005, suddenly 25 cows tested positive, then all of them were culled and disposed of. During the following three years, Huzhou city was free of brucellosis infection in dairy cows and had no infection source. However, in 2009, the positive cases reappeared. The interpretation of this ruleless phenomenon can be the randomness of input of the infectious dairy cows from the outsides.

Thus, in order to more precisely fit the data of positive cases in Zhejiang province, we need to resort to the stochastic dynamic model, which can be obtained by adding stochastic perturbations to some parameters in model (1). Because the randomness is caused by the input of the brucellosis carriers. So, we add stochastic perturbations to c_1 and c_2. So, the model (1) is rewritten as the following form to fit the real data:

$$
\begin{cases}
\dfrac{dS(t)}{dt} = (1-c_1-c_2)A + bS(t) - \epsilon\beta\dfrac{S(t)E(t)}{N(t)} - \beta\dfrac{S(t)I(t)}{N(t)} \\
\qquad - \alpha S(t)V(t) - mS(t), \\[2mm]
\dfrac{dE(t)}{dt} = (c_1 + D_1\zeta(t))A + \epsilon\beta\dfrac{S(t)E(t)}{N(t)} + \beta\dfrac{S(t)I(t)}{N(t)} \\
\qquad + \alpha S(t)V(t) - mE(t) - \delta E(t), \\[2mm]
\dfrac{dI(t)}{dt} = (c_2 + D_2\zeta(t))A + \delta E(t) - mI(t) - \sigma\mu I(t), \\[2mm]
\dfrac{dV(t)}{dt} = r(E(t)+I(t)) - wV(t) - klV(t),
\end{cases}
\tag{2}
$$

where, $\zeta(t)$ is a time series of random deviates derived from the normal distribution with mean zero and unit variance; $D_i(i=1,2)$ represents the intensity of $\zeta(t)$. In this case, $D_1\zeta(t)$ and $D_2\zeta(t)$ also can be reviewed as stochastic perturbations to A if adding the first three equations together. Next, we use this stochastic dynamic model to fit the positive data of the infective dairy cows in Zhejiang provinc. The parameter values and the initial values adopted in fitting are listed in Table 1 and some parameter values $(c_1, c_2, b, k, r$ and $l)$ are fixed to be cosntant. During the simulation, what is difference with deterministic model is to add perturbations(white noise) $D_1\zeta(t), D_2\zeta(t)$ to the parameters c_1 and c_2, respectively, where $\zeta(t) \sim N(0,1)$. Due to the stochastic perturbations, the fitting result is different when we run the program about the stochastic dynamic model every time. 100 times of fitting result are given in Fig. 4, where one of the best fitting result is given in Fig. 5. The good fitting result demonstrates our mathematical model has certain rationality, so we can use it to predict the disease situation and assess the prevention and control measures. The prediction trend of brucellosis in Zhejiang province by deterministic model and stochastic model are shown in Fig. 6 (a) and (b), respectively. From Fig. 6(a), with randomness of import of infected dairy cows, the prediction situations can have large differences that can reach up to several hundreds. When the system attains steady state, the number of positive cattle will be between 1500 and 2000. From Fig. 6(b), we can see that brucellosis cases of the dairy cows will steadily increase in the next 17 years and arrive a peak(about 2700), then decrease to 1500

and lastly tend to a steady state about 1700, which is mean value in Fig. 6(a). By applying deterministic model, we can obtain the general and mean trend of epidemic. By applying stochastic model, although ruleless perturbation are added, the cases range of dairy cattle can be obtained. From Fig. 6, it can be seen that if not to take more efficient measures, the disease in dairy cows cannot be controlled. With the randomness of import of brucellosis carriers, the situation in Zhejiang province cannot be precisely predicted. So, firstly we encourage Zhejiang province to take self-supplying of dairy cows, rather than the importation of dairy cows from north areas, which is the first conclusion in this paper.

Control Measures Assessment

A is the number of import cattle and its effect on disease is effect of the import number. μ is the culling rate of positive cattle and its effect on disease is effect of culling measure. l is the frequency of disinfection and its effect on disease is effect of disinfection measure. β is the cattle-to-cattle transmission rate and its effect on disease is effect of direct contact rate. α is the brucella-to-cattle transmission rate and its effect on disease is effect of indirect contact rate (environment contact rate). b is the birth rate and its effect on disease is effect of the birth number. c1 and c2 are the proportions of exposed and infectious cattle on the whole import cattle, respectively. c1 and c2 are related with the detection strength for the import cattle. When detection rate is larger, c1, c2 may be smaller.

The influences of c_1 and c_2 on disease spread are relatively large, whose effects on the accumulated number of infectious cattle during ten years (2011-2020) are given in Fig. 7. Compared Fig. 7(a) with Fig. 7(b), it is easily to know that the effect of c_1 is larger. When c_1 varies from 0.0005 to 0.02, the accumulated number of the infectious cattle will rise to 9000 from less than 1000. If the same changes are taken for c_2, the accumulated number of the infectious cattle will rise to 8000 from more than 1000. Therefore, firstly and the most important, the detection strength should be enhanced and the import of the brucella carriers must be completely eradicated, or the disease cannot be removed and predicted precisely. Let c_1 and c_2 equal to zero, we can calculate the basic reproduction number $R_0 = 1.37$, whose calculation can be seen in Appendix S1. At the same time, we can carry out sensitivity analysis of some crucial parameters, see Fig. 8. From the five figures, we can see that R_0 is linear in term of A, β and α, concave function in term of μ and l. Observing the shape of curves and the ordinate axes, it can be easily known that when μ and l is smaller, their influences are bigger than A, β and α. When they increase, the influences become smaller and smaller, especially, when $\mu > 0.8$ and $l > 100$. In addition, according to the current situation, μ cannot make $R_0 < 1$, even $\mu = 1$, that is all

Table 2. Equilibria and stability.

Cases	Conditions	Equilibria	Stability	Possible steady state
$A\neq 0, c_1\neq 0, c_2\neq 0$		P^*	Not proved	P^* or limit cycle
$A\neq 0, c_1 = 0, c_2 = 0$	$m > b, R_0 < 1$	P^0	G.A.S.	P^0
	$m > b, R_0 > 1$	P^0, P^*	uniformly persistent	P^* or limit cycle
	$m \leq b$	P^*	Not proved	P^* or limit cycle
$A = 0, c_1 = 0, c_2 = 0$	$m > b$	O	G.A.S.	O
	$m = b$	O, P^0	P^0 is stable	P^0.
	$m < b$	O, P^*	Not proved	O or P^* or limit cycle

Table 3. Values of estimated parameters.

β		α		A	
mean value	CI	mean value	CI	mean value	CI
5.3899×10^{-5}	$[4.4286 \times 10^{-5}, 6.3513 \times 10^{-5}]$	2.1216×10^{-4}	$[1.9459 \times 10^{-4}, 2.2973 \times 10^{-4}]$	15807	$[13905, 17708]$

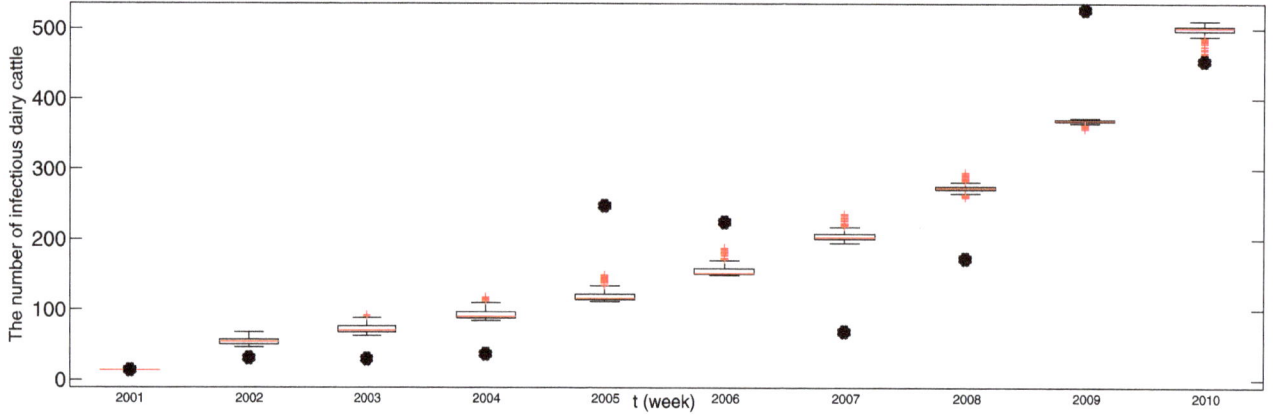

Figure 2. 100 times of fitting results of positive data in Zhejiang province by deterministic model, where blue dotes are real data and the boxplot is the result of model (1). The parameter values taken in simulation are given in Table 1 and the estimated parameter values are given in Table 3.

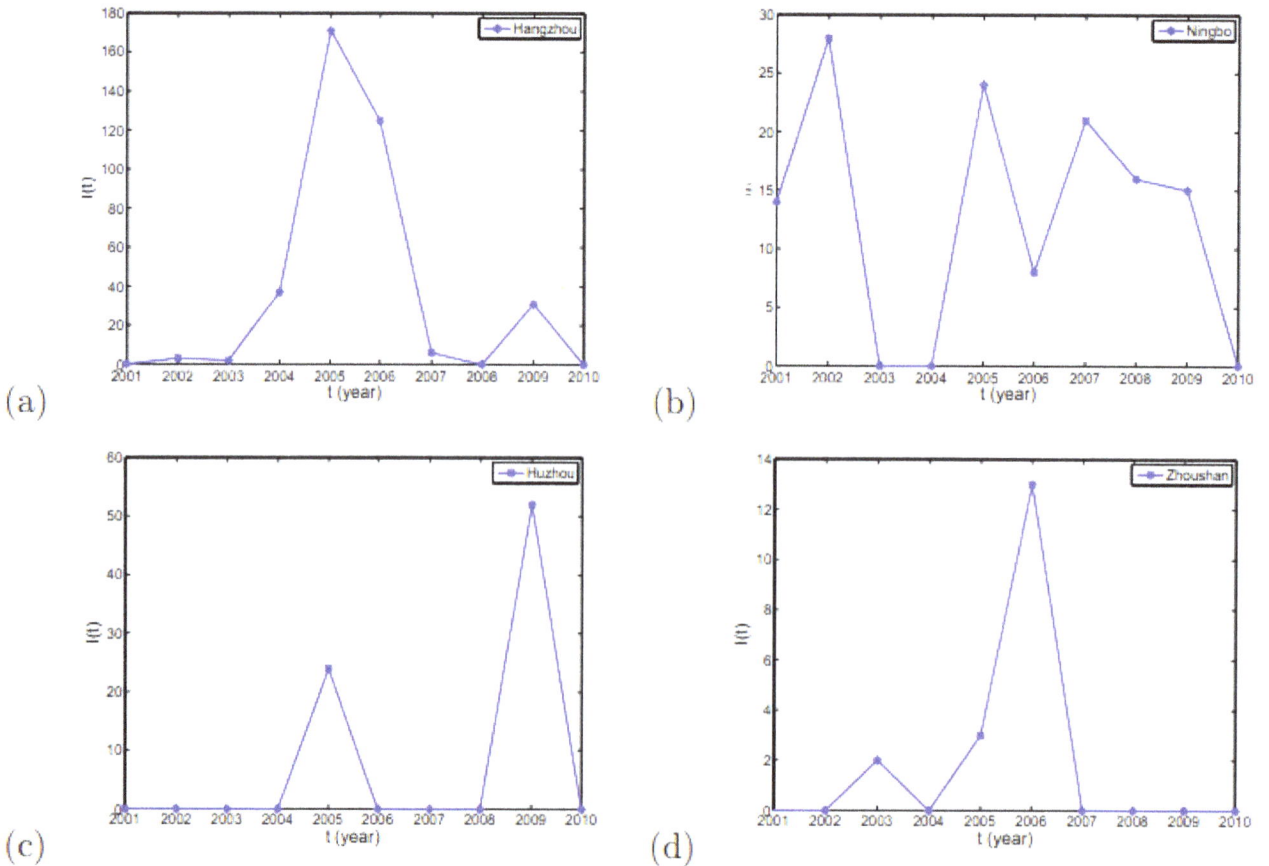

Figure 3. The real positive data of cows infected with brucellosis in Hangzhou city, Ningbo city, Huzhou city and Zhoushan city in Zhenjiang province. (a) Hangzhou city. (b) Ningbo city. (c) Huzhou city. (d) Zhoushan city. These data are listed in Table S1 in Appendix S1.

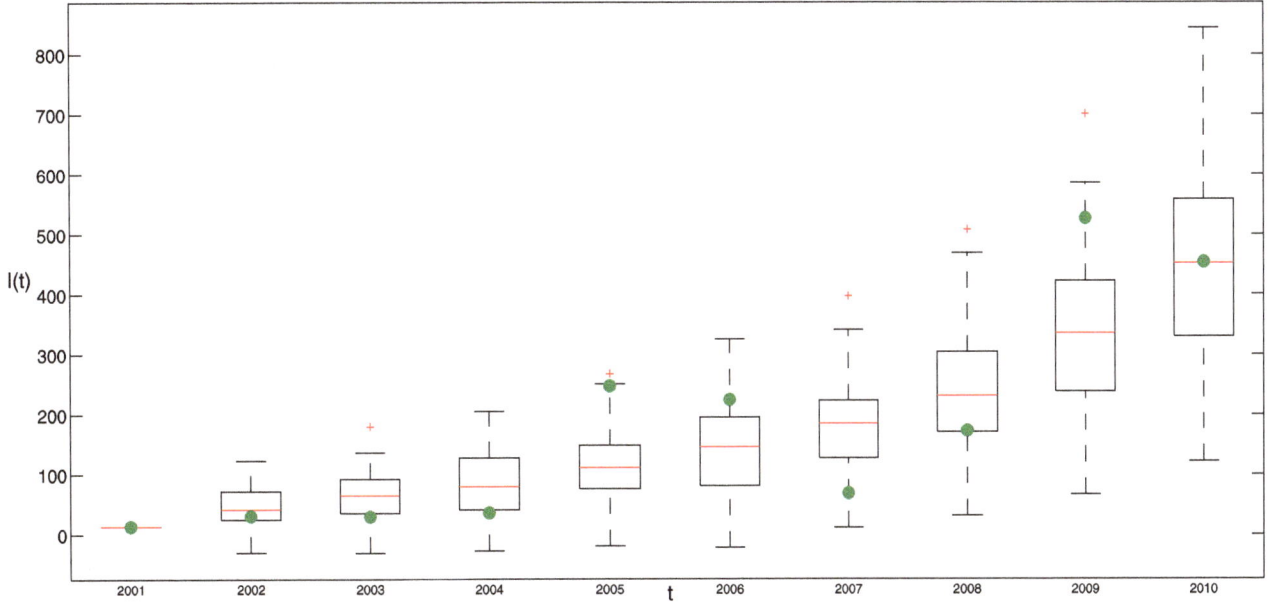

Figure 4. 100 times of fitting result of positive data in Zhejiang province by stochastic model (2), where green dotes are real data and the boxplot is the result of model (2). Here $A=13000, c_1=0.002, c_2=0.0015, b=0.1, \beta=2.1\times10^{-5}, \alpha=2.06\times10^{-4}, r=5, k=0.7$ and $l=52$. Other parameter values and initial values of variables taken in simulation are given in Table 1.

the infected dairy cows are culled, which is because of the existence of and the exposed subclass and environment transmission. The culling measure, that is $\mu=0.85$, adopted by Zhejiang province is enough. With regards to Fig. 8(c), sterilization once a week, that is $l=52$, can be changed into twice a week, that is

$l=104$, which is enough. However, the two measures cannot remove the brucellosis in dairy cows. So, the influence of A should be considered. If $A<9500$, $R_0<1$, which can make the disease disappear. Otherwise, the disease will be persistent. Next, it is necessary to compare the influence of β and α. The decreasing of α

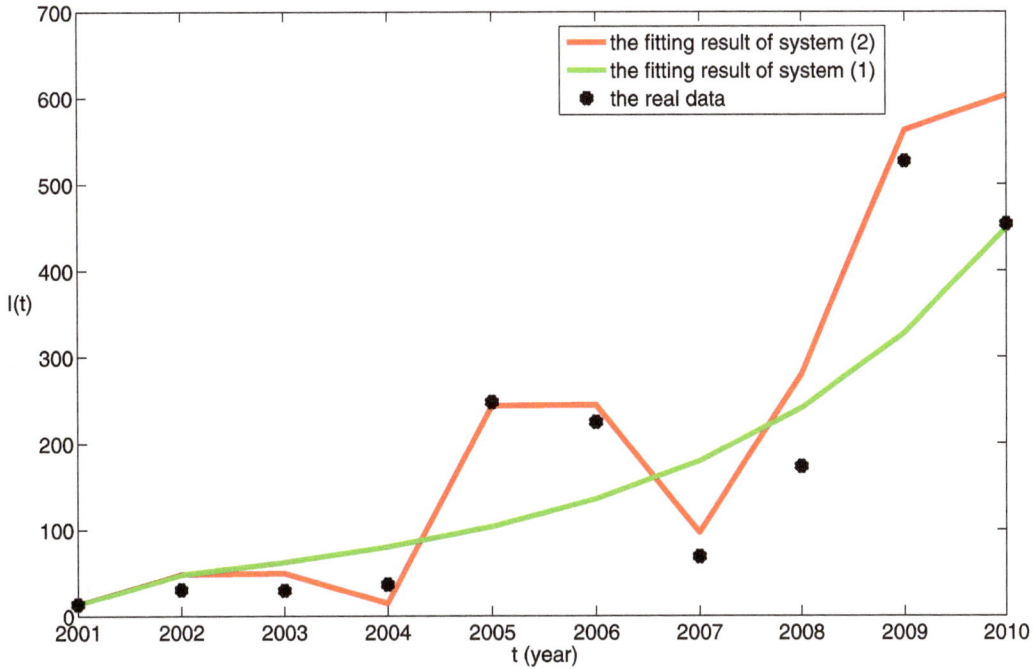

Figure 5. The comparison between the reported positive dairy cows in Zhejiang province in China from 2001 to 2010 and the simulation results of $I(t)$ in models (1) and (2), which is one of the best fitting results. The blue dots represent the reported data. The green curve is the solution of system (1) and the red curve is an example of a simulation of system(2). Here $A=13000, c_1=0.002, c_2=0.0015, b=0.1, \beta=2.1\times10^{-5}, \alpha=2.06\times10^{-4}, r=5, k=0.7$ and $l=52$.

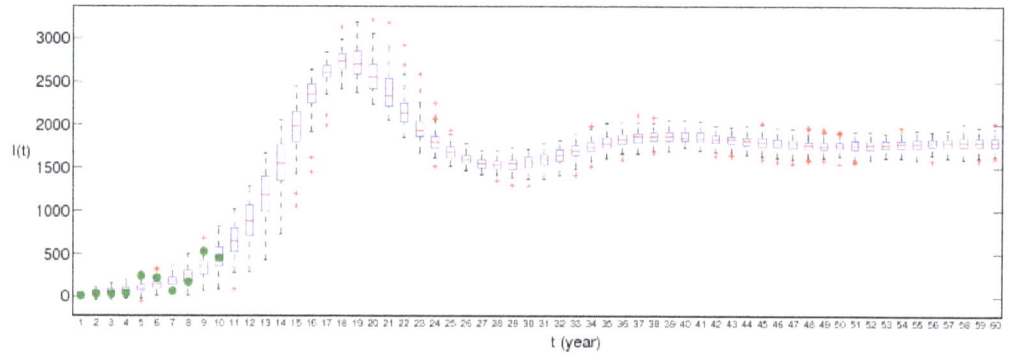

(a)

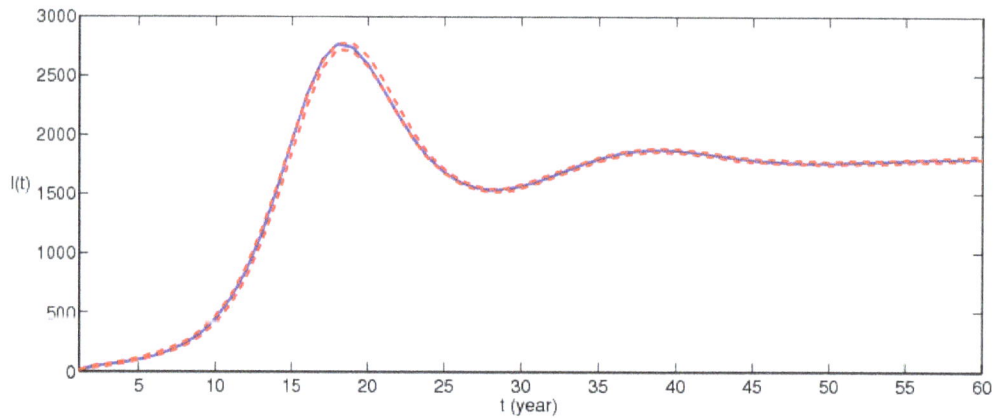

(b)

Figure 6. 100 times of prediction results of $I(t)$ in models (1) and (2) during 50 years. (a) in model (2); (b) in model (1), where blue curve is the mean values and the two red dotted curves represent 95% confidence interval.

and β can both reduce R_0. When $\alpha < 1.5 \times 10^{-4}$, R_0 will be less than 1. Sensitivity of β is less than α and Even $\beta = 0$ cannot make $R_0 < 1$, so the prevalence of brucellosis is mainly aroused by the environment transmission, and it should arouse more attention of government and farmers. Thus, that the effect of infection of brucella in environment on brucellosis spread is greater the infection during individuals is the second result obtained in this paper.

As we know, due to constraint of sensibility of detection methods, as long as there are dairy cows to import, the input of infected dairy cows is unavoidable. When $A = 0$, that is insisting on self-support, the disease situations under different conditions are shown in Fig. 9. Because the positive rates of dairy cows is more concerned, we give the solution curves of $I(t)/N(t)$ with t, not $I(t)$. From Fig. 9, we can know that under some conditions, there must appear periodic cycles, which is interesting result of this paper. Firstly, let us look at the prediction of the positive rate under different b. If Zhejiang province insists on self-support, b must be not less than m, 0.25, or the total number of dairy cows will go to zero. When $b = 0.25$, from the second result of Theorem 4, there is only one disease-free equilibrium. So, the brucellosis in Zhejiang province will disappear in 20 years, see Fig. 9(a). From the Fig. 9, when $b > 0.25$, the disease cannot disappear. If $b = 0.3$, the disease is prevalent and will be periodic with period of 20 years. Meanwhile, its positive rate circulates between 0.005 and 0.065. With increasing b, the positive rate will increase and the period will be shortened. From Fig. 9(b), we know that μ has large effect on disease control. When $\mu = 0.85$, the disease is also prevalent

with period of 20. When $\mu = 0.5$, the period becomes 30 and the positive rate can reach up to 0.25. So, with the increase of μ, the positive rate will decrease, however the period will be shortened. On the contrary, to increase l can shorten the period, which can reduce the disease situation temporarily. In 60 years, the positive rate is very low. However, once the disease outbreaks, the peak of wave becomes very high. From Fig. 9(d) and (e), it is easy to see that the influence of β on positive rate is less than α. When α increases, the period will enlarge, and the positive rate will rise. When $\alpha = 2 \times 10^{-6}$, the disease can be controlled temporarily. In conclusion, in order to eliminate disease thoroughly under insisting on self-support, government of Zhejiang province should control the birth rate b to be 0.25. If keeping the birth rate b be more than 0.25, it is necessary to control disinfection frequency l. It must be important to notice the influence of l. According to the common sense, the increasing of l can lead to relief of the disease, which can give us more time to find more effective measures. However, the peak of wave will increase with the growth of l, which should draw our attention as well. So, from Fig. 8(c), we suggest that twice a week is enough, which is another interesting and important result of this paper.

Uncertainty Analysis

Due to the lack of information, some initial value and parameter value are assumed and given roughly. Now, the effect of initial values $E(0), I(0)$ and parameter ε on the epidemic situation are given in Fig. 10. From Fig. 10, it can been easily to see that $E(0)$ and $I(0)$ have little influence on the epidemic situation. ε has no

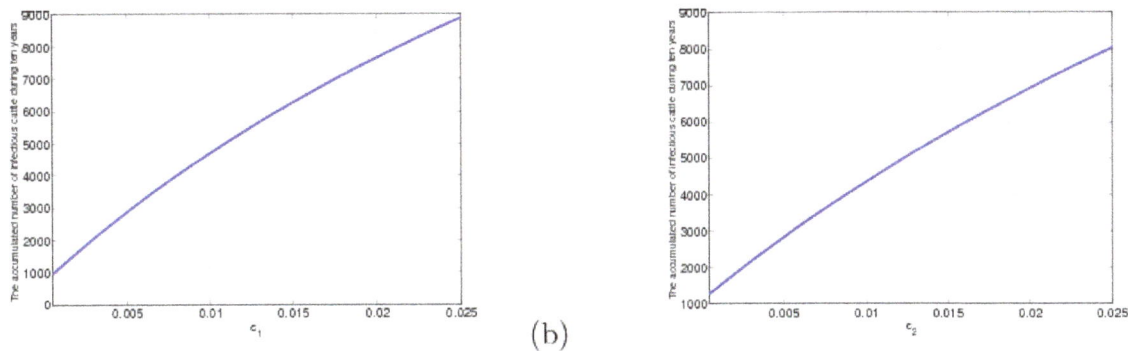

Figure 7. $\sum_{t=1}^{10} I(t)$ **in term of** c_1 **and** c_2. **(a)** c_1. **(b)** c_2. Here $A=13000$, $b=0.1$, $\beta=2.1 \times 10^{-5}$, $\alpha=2.06 \times 10^{-4}$, $r=5$, $k=0.7$ and $l=52$.

influence on epidemic spread, since the effect of direct transmission between individuals on epidemic spread is little.

In addition, if we only add stochastic perturbations to c_1 and c_2 and the number of import is constant. So, the model (2) is rewritten as the following form, whose fitting result is given in Fig. 11 and has little difference with Fig. 4. Thus, the model (2) and the model (3) are all right and both cases can be adopted to study cattle brucellosis in Zhejiang province.

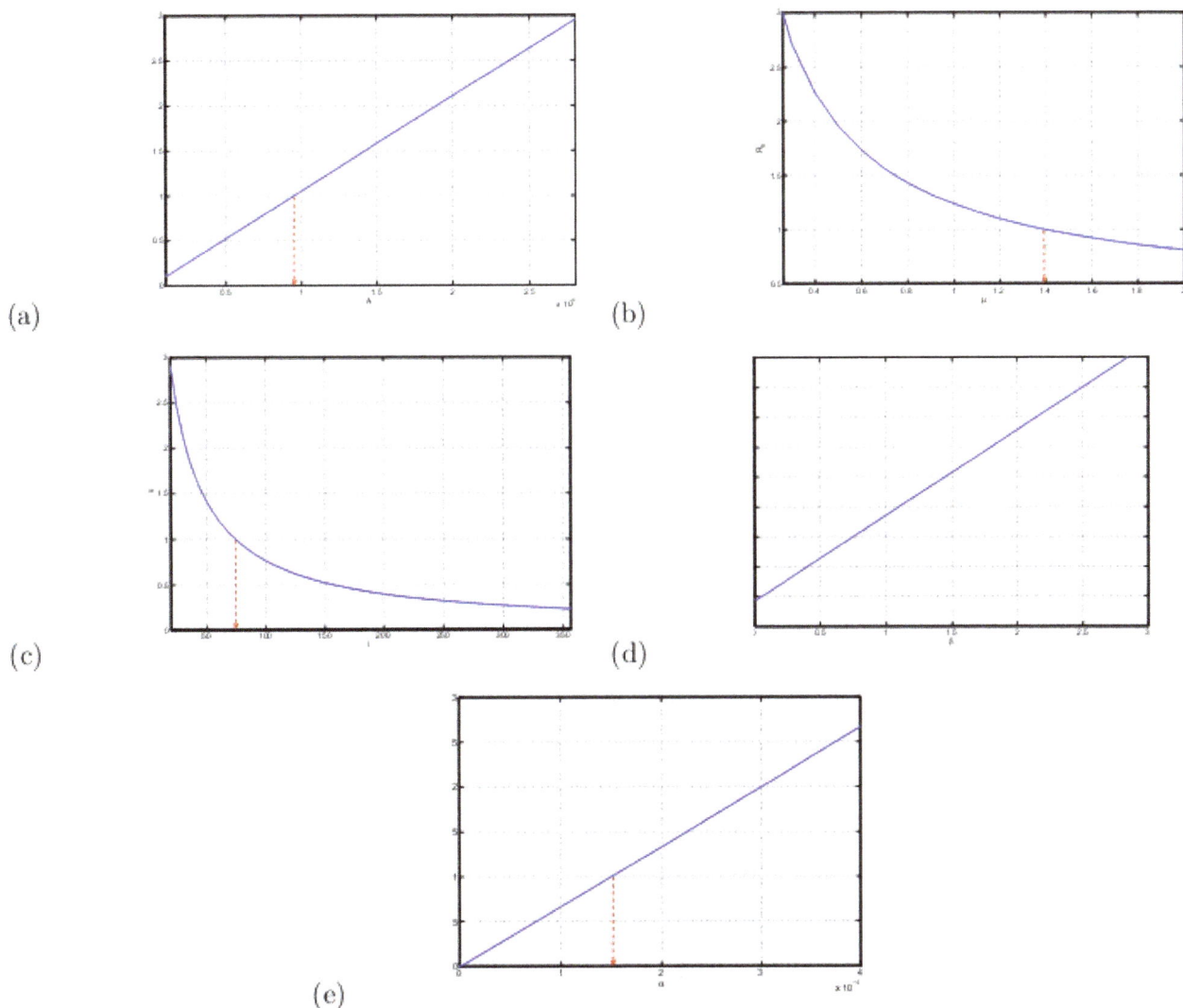

Figure 8. R_0 **in terms of** A, μ, l, β **and** α. (a) A. (b) μ. (c) l. (d) β. (e) α.

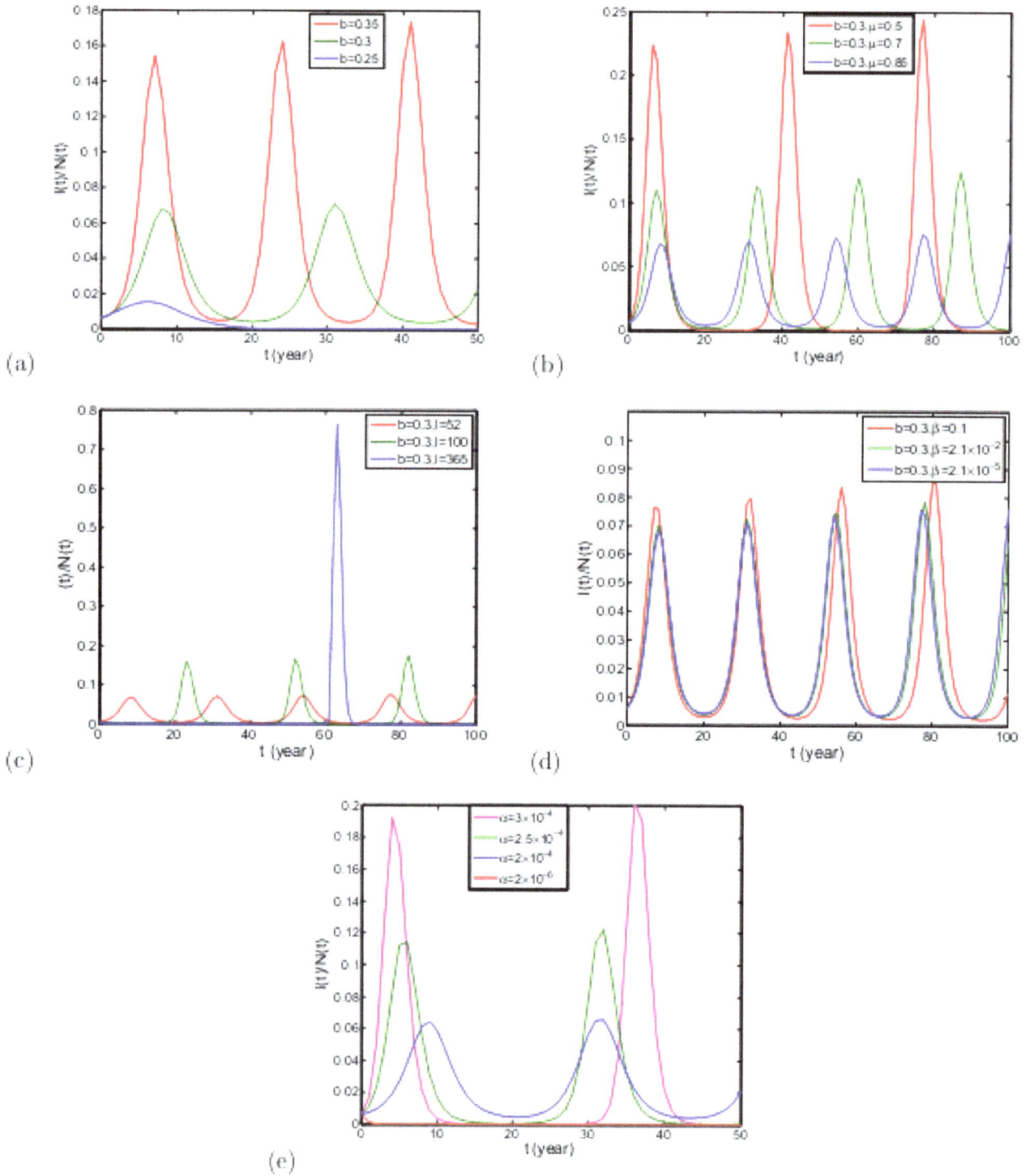

Figure 9. $I(t)/N(t)$ **with** t **under different** $b,\mu,l,\beta,\alpha.$ (a) b. (b) μ. (c) l. (d) β. (e) α. The initial values of variables can be seen in Table 1.

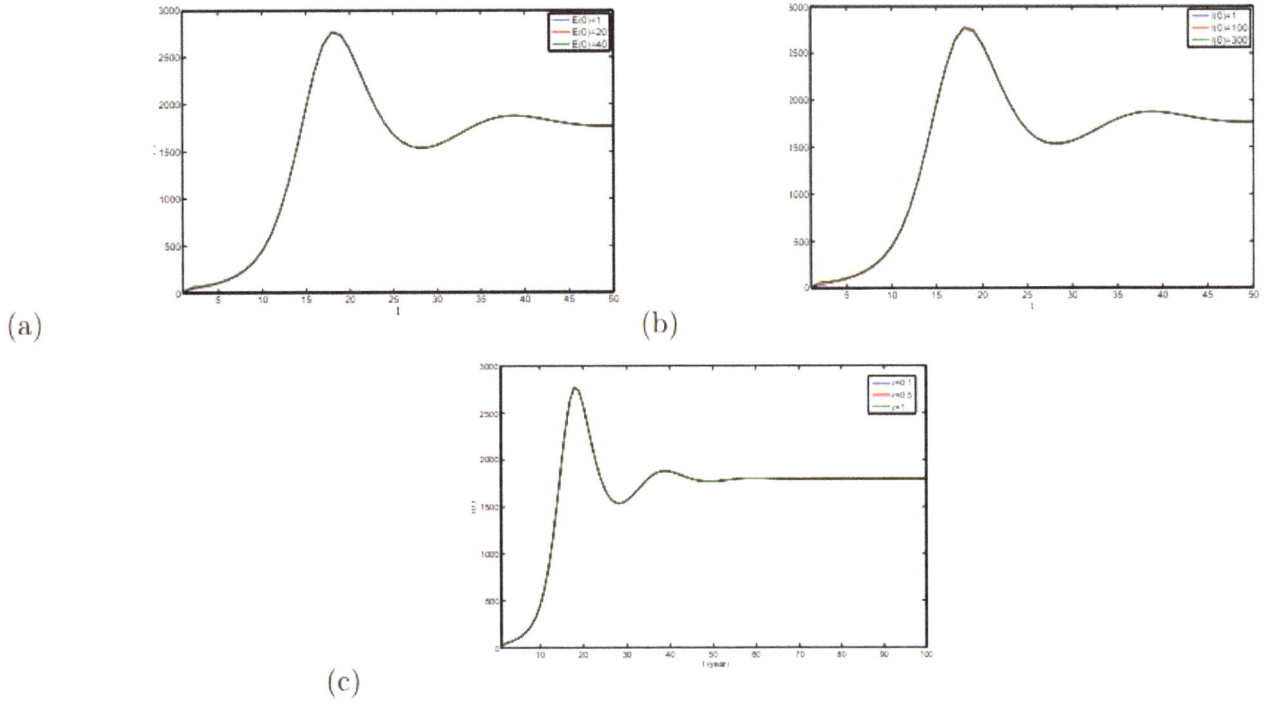

(a)

(b)

(c)

Figure 10. $I(t)$ **with** t **under different initial values and parameter** ε. (a) under different $E(0)$. (b) under different $I(0)$. (c) under different ϵ. The initial values of variables can be seen in Table 1.

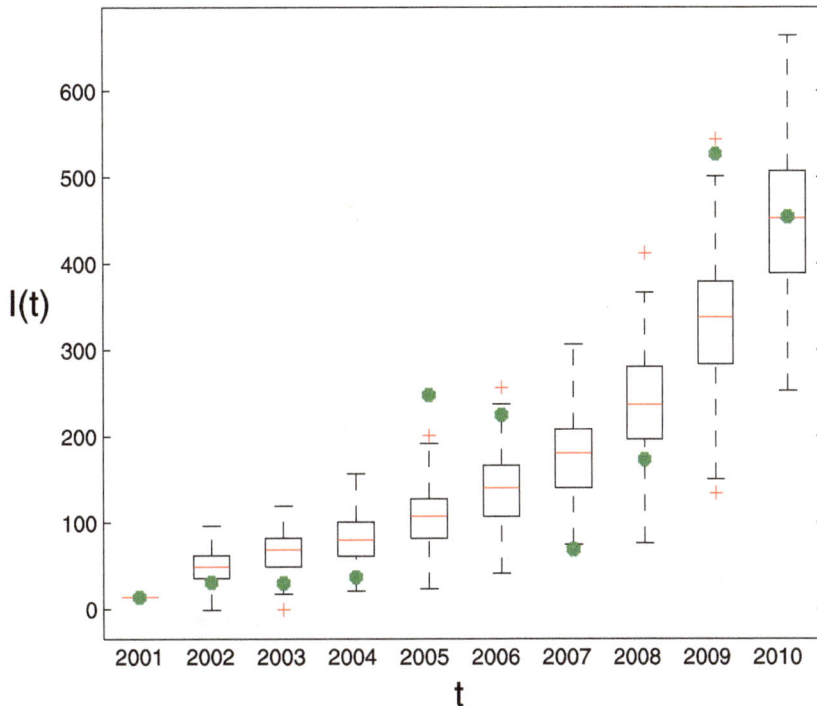

Figure 11. 100 times of fitting result of positive data in Zhejiang province by stochastic model (3), where green dotes are real data and the boxplot is the result of model (3). The parameter values and initial values of variables taken in simulation are the same as Fig. 4.

$$
\begin{cases}
\dfrac{dS(t)}{dt} = (1 - c_1 - D_1\zeta(t) - c_2 - D_2\zeta(t))A + bS(t) \\
\qquad\quad - \epsilon\beta\dfrac{S(t)E(t)}{N(t)} - \beta\dfrac{S(t)I(t)}{N(t)} - \alpha S(t)V(t) - mS(t), \\[2mm]
\dfrac{dE(t)}{dt} = (c_1 + D_1\zeta(t))A + \epsilon\beta\dfrac{S(t)E(t)}{N(t)} \\
\qquad\quad + \beta\dfrac{S(t)I(t)}{N(t)} + \alpha S(t)V(t) - mE(t) - \delta E(t), \\[2mm]
\dfrac{dI(t)}{dt} = (c_2 + D_2\zeta(t))A + \delta E(t) - mI(t) - \sigma\mu I(t), \\[2mm]
\dfrac{dV(t)}{dt} = r(E(t) + I(t)) - wV(t) - klV(t),
\end{cases} \tag{3}
$$

Discussion

Brucellosis is a notifiable disease that can infect cows, swine, goats, sheep, dogs and humans. In the Zhejiang province, brucellosis between dairy cows has attracted significant attraction of the public and government for it is a major public-health and economically devastating zoonosis. Although recently, the Zhejiang province has taken strict regulations to control brucellosis. the detection twice a year and culling all the infectious cows, however it is still a threat to the health of milk products and the development of breeding businesses. So, according to the transmission mechanism of brucellosis in dairy herd and the breeding business characteristic of Zhejiang province, this paper builds an *SEIV* dynamical model to investigate the internal transmission dynamics, predict the infection situation, and assess prevention and control measures. Currently, efforts are suggested to direct at regular detection and eliminating reactors [22–24], prevention(vaccination) [23,25] and sterilization [23]. Applying the dynamical model, this paper analyzes and forecasts the disease's behaviors with the quantitative point of view. After obtaining the corresponding precise parameter values, we can give the strength of measures to be needed to control the disease transmission.

For Zhejiang, the greatest danger comes from imported animals. With regulation, they should import dairy cows from brucellosis-free areas, and herds should be isolated for 30 days and retested to be seronegative before being blended with the local herd. However, in practice these are not well carried out. Moreover, the effective rate of test cannot reach up to 100%. It is concluded that import of cattle can make that the prediction situations can have large differences that can reach up to several hundred. So, firstly we encourage Zhejiang province to take self-supplying of dairy cows, rather than the importation of dairy cows from north areas. During intervention measures, elimination of seropositives is more discussed by [14,16,17], since it is more effective to reduce brucellosis prevalence in cattle. Gonzalez-Guzman and Naulin [14] gave the necessary rate of elimination of seropositives to control disease. [17] drew a conclusion that the test-and-slaughter intervention appeared more effective to reduce brucellosis prevalence in cattle than the vaccination scenarios. For Zhejiang province, the regular detection, eliminating reactors, and disinfection of environment in local herds have been implemented well: testing twice a year and 100% culling. Generally, herds must be tested at regular intervals until 2 or 3 successive tests are negative. To increase the frequency of tests annually will cost too much time and money, and it is strenuous. Though the frequency

of detection for dairy herds has better results at once a month [6], twice a year that is taken by Zhejiang province is enough. Slaughtering policy has been carried very well and is not considered and discussed in this paper. Ainseba et al. [16] concluded that the contamination of the environment can play an important role in the persistence of disease. In this paper, by simulation analysis, sterilization is a measures we should use carefully to control brucellosis in Zhejiang province. When l is larger, although brucellosis can be controlled temporarily, once the brucellosis appears, the disease must be a large outbreak. Since the complexity of the disinfection times, this measure should always be adjusted with regards to real circumstance. [17] gave simulated vaccination scenarios. However, vaccination of dairy herds can increase resistance to infection, however resistance may not be complete, and some vaccinated individual may become infected, depending on severity of exposure. Therefore, vaccination has many indeterminacies and needs more discussion [5], here it is not proposed. From Table 2, according to the current breeding model in Zhejiang province, we can know that under certain condition cattle brucellosis may be periodic and the cycle can be from 15 to 20 years long (Fig. 9), which was not found and discussed in previous literatures. According to the period, related government should not let their guard down and can propose corresponding prevention measure. In addition, by dynamical and sensitivity analysis, we suggest government to control brucellosis by managing the birth number of calf. All these control measures can reduce economic loss caused by brucellosis. Furthermore, Xie and Horan [15] investigates private responses and ecological impact of policies, which is our future research context. In summation, the brucellosis control and eradication program is multi-faceted and needs to combine several methods.

There are some limitation in our paper. Firstly, the amount of brucella discharged by the exposed and infectious should be different and an auxiliary parameter should be introduced. However, this difference between the discharge rates is hard to quantify and is also uncertain, so this paper assume that the exposed and infectious discharge the same amount of brucellosis into the environment.

In future work, we can investigate brucellosis from the following aspects: to begin with, managing the birth rate has larger influence in brucellosis spreading, but it has a close relationship with the economy. Hence, in order to discuss brucellosis comprehensively and fully, we should combine with economic factors and statistical methods. Secondly, vaccination of brucella for cows has many indeterminacies. After vaccination, resistance of herds may not be complete, and some vaccinated individual may become infected. Moreover, for dairy herds, vaccine may have some influence on milk. So, the vaccination measures need more discussion in our future work.

Supporting Information

Appendix S1. Table S1, The positive data of dairy cattle from 2001 to 2010 year in some cities of Zhejiang province and the whole province. **Table S2**, The dairy cattle population from 2000 to 2009 year in Zhejiang province.

Figure S1 (a) β **in term of** b. (b) l **in term of** b, **where** $\beta = 1.8$. The other parameter values are the same as in Fig. 5 of the main article.

Figure S2 $Re(\lambda_1)$ **in term of** μ **and** α. (a) μ. (b) α. $\beta = 1$ and other parameter values are the same as in Fig. 5 of the main article.

Figure S3 $I(t)$ and $S(t)$ with t under different b and β. (a) $\lambda_{1,2} = 0.0004 \pm 0.1324i$, $\lambda_3 = -6.7203$, $\lambda_4 = -43.8805$. (b)$\lambda_{1,2} = -0.0059 \pm 0.2188i$, $\lambda_3 = -7.2417$, $\lambda_4 = -42.5727$. (c) $\lambda_{1,2} = \pm 0.6216i$, $\lambda_3 = -7.1271$, $\lambda_4 = -42.8672$. (d) $\lambda_{1,2} = 0.0028 \pm 0.6967i$, $\lambda_3 = -7.1118$, $\lambda_4 = -42.9147$. The initial values $(S(0), E(0), I(0), V(0)) = (S^* + 2000, E^* + 10, I^* + 10, V^* + 10)$.

Figure S4 $I(t)$ with t under different parameters, where $b = 0.994913458$, $\beta = 1.8$. $\lambda_{1,2} = \pm 0.6216i$, $\lambda_3 = -7.1271$, $\lambda_4 = -42.8672$.

Acknowledgments

The authors would like to thank the two reviewers for their helpful comments and valuable suggestions.

Author Contributions

Conceived and designed the experiments: ZJ JZ GQS. Performed the experiments: MTL JZ. Analyzed the data: QH MTL. Contributed reagents/materials/analysis tools: GQS JZ. Wrote the paper: JZ ZJ GQS HYW. Provided data: XDS BXH.

References

1. Shang DQ, Xiao DL, Yin JM (2002) Epidemiology and control of brucellosis in China. Veterinary Microbiology 90: 165–182.
2. Liu JP, Yang ZQ, Ma J, Wang JW, Wang ZZ, et al. (2009) The Comprehensive Control Measures for Brucellosis. Progress in Veterinary Medicine 30(10): 121–124.
3. Smits HL, Kadri SM (2005) Brucellosis in India: a deceptive infectious disease. Indian J Med Res 122(5): 375–384.
4. Jiao JB, Yang JW, Yang XS (2009) The dairy cattle brucellosis and prevention and control(Nainiu bulujunbing jiqi fangkong). Animal Husbandry and Feed Science 30(3): 170–171.
5. Merck Sharp & Dohme Corp (2011) The Merck Veterinary Manual, Brucellosis in cattle (Contagious abortion, Bangs disease). Available: http://www.merckvetmanual.com/mvm/index.jsp? cfile = htm/bc/110502.htm.
6. England T, Kelly L, Jones RD, MacMillan A, Wooldridge M (2004) A simulation model of brucellosis spread in British cattle under several testing regimes. Preventive Veterinary Medicine 63: 63–73.
7. Xu WM, Shi SF, Yang Y, Jin HY, Wang H (2007) Epidemic situation and exploration of the prevention and control strategies on Brucellosis in Zhejiang Province. Chinese Rural Health Service Administration 27(3): 209–211.
8. Xu WM, Wang H, Zhu SJ, Yang Y, Wang J, et al. (2009) 2000–2007 the human and livestock brucellosis situation and control measure in Zhejiang province(2000–2007nian zhejiang sheng renchu bulujunbing yiqing yu kongzhicuoshi). Chinese Journal of Preventive Medicine 43(8): 746–747.
9. MacMillan A (1990) Conventional Serological Tests. Animal Brucellosis. Boca Raton, FL, USA:CRC Press.pp131–151.
10. Bercovich Z (1998) Maintenance of brucella abortus-free herds: a review with emphasis on the epidemiology and the problems in diagnosing Brucellosis in areas of low prevalence. Vet Quart 20: 81–88.
11. Stemshorn BW, Forbes LB, Eaglesome MD, Nielsen KH, Robertson FJ, et al. (1985) A comparison of standard serological tests for the diagnosis of bovine brucellosis in Canada. Can J Comp Med 49: 391–394.
12. MacMillan A (1994) Brucellosis: freedom but the risk remains. Cattle Pract 2: 469–474.
13. Bercovich Z, ter Laak EA, van Lipzig JHH (1992) Detection of brucellosis in dairy herds after an outbreak of the disease using delayed-type hypersensitivity test. Prev Vet Med 13: 277–285.
14. Gonzalez-Guzman J, Naulin R (1994) Analysis of a model of bovine brucellosis using singular perturbations. J Math Biol 33: 211–223.
15. Fang X, Richard DH (2009) Disease and behavioral dynamics for brucellosis control in greater yellowstone area. Journal of Agricultural and Resource Economics 34(1): 11–33.
16. Ainseba B, Benosman C, Magal P (2010) A model for ovine brucellosis incorporating direct and indirect transmission. Journal of Biological Dynamics 4(1): 2–11.
17. Zinsstag J, Roth F, Orkhon D, Chimed-Ochir G, Nansalmaa M, et al. (2005) A model of animal-human brucellosis transmission in Mongolia. Preventive Veterinary Medicine 69: 77–95.
18. Hou Q, Sun XD, Zhang J, Liu YJ, Wang YM, et al. (2013) Modeling the transmission dynamics of sheep brucellosis in Inner Mongolia Autonomous Region, China. Mathematical Biosciences 242: 51–58.
19. The Chinese Ministry of Agriculture (2001-2010) China animal industry yearbook(Zhongguo xumuye nianjian). China Agriculture Press.
20. Diekmann O, Heesterbeek JAP (2000) Mathematical epidemiology of infectious diseases: Modeling building, analysis and interpretation. Hoboken, NJ:Wiley.
21. Keeling MJ, Rohani P (2008) Modeling infectious diseases in human and animals. Princeton, NJ: Princeton University Press.
22. Renukaradhya GJ, Isloor S, Rajasekhar M(2002) Epidemiology, zoonotic aspects, vaccination and control/eradication of brucellosis in India. Veterinary Microbiology 90: 183–195.
23. Sandip R, Terry FM, Yan W (2011) A network control theory approach to modeling and optimal control of zoonoses: case study of brucellosis transmission in Sub-Saharan Africa. PloS neglected tropical disease 5(10): e1259.
24. Benkirane A (2006) Ovine and caprine brucellosis: World distribution and control/eradication strategies in West Asia/North Africa region, prevention. Small Ruminant Research 62: 19–25.
25. Alton GG (1987) Control of brucella melitensis infection in sheep and goats-a review. Trop Anita Hlth Prod 19: 65–74.

14

Modeling Tuberculosis Dynamics, Detection and Control in Cattle Herds

Mohammed El Amine Bekara[1], Aurélie Courcoul[1], Jean-Jacques Bénet[2], Benoit Durand[1]*

1 University Paris Est, Anses, Laboratory of Animal Health, Epidemiology Unit, Maisons-Alfort, France, 2 University Paris Est, National Veterinary School of Alfort (ENVA), EpiMAI Unit, Maisons-Alfort, France

Abstract

Epidemiological models are key tools for designing and evaluating detection and control strategies against animal infectious diseases. In France, after decades of decrease of bovine tuberculosis (bTB) incidence, the disease keeps circulating. Increasing prevalence levels are observed in several areas, where the detection and control strategy could be adapted. The objective of this work was to design and calibrate a model of the within-herd transmission of bTB. The proposed model is a stochastic model operating in discrete-time. Three health states were distinguished: susceptible, latent and infected. Dairy and beef herd dynamics and bTB detection and control programs were explicitly represented. Approximate Bayesian computation was used to estimate three model parameters from field data: the transmission parameter when animals are inside (β_{inside}) and outside ($\beta_{outside}$) buildings, and the duration of the latent phase. An independent dataset was used for model validation. The estimated median was 0.43 [0.16–0.84] month^{-1} for β_{inside} and 0.08 [0.01–0.32] month^{-1} for $\beta_{outside}$. The median duration of the latent period was estimated 3.5 [2–8] months. The sensitivity analysis showed only minor influences of fixed parameter values on these posterior estimates. Validation based on an independent dataset showed that in more than 80% of herds, the observed proportion of animals with detected lesions was between the 2.5% and 97.5% percentiles of the simulated distribution. In the absence of control program and once bTB has become enzootic within a herd, the median effective reproductive ratio was estimated to be 2.2 in beef herds and 1.7 in dairy herds. These low estimates are consistent with field observations of a low prevalence level in French bTB-infected herds.

Editor: Caroline Colijn, Imperial College London, United Kingdom

Funding: This work was supported by the French Ministry of Agriculture. The funder had no role in study design, data collection and analysis, decision to publish, or preparation of the manuscript.

Competing Interests: The authors have declared that no competing interests exist.

* Email: benoit.durand@anses.fr

Introduction

Bovine tuberculosis (bTB) is a chronic animal disease most often caused by *Mycobacterium bovis*, that mainly affects the respiratory system [1]. The main route of transmission of the infection between cattle is the respiratory route [2]. In France, a control program for bTB became mandatory in 1965. Detection of infected herds was based on an annual screening of animals using skin tests, and on routine inspection of carcasses at slaughter for bTB-like lesions (with subsequent isolation of *M. bovis* at the laboratory). Since 1990, the control program was reinforced by the compulsory screening (using skin tests) of animals introduced in bTB-free herds, these animals always originating from other bTB-free herds. In 1999, herd prevalence fell below 0.1% and the slaughter of all cattle in infected herds (termed below "total slaughter") was introduced in the control program. In 2001, France was declared officially free of bTB by the European Union. However, in recent years, an increase in bTB incidence has been observed in some departments. Similar trends have been observed in other European countries. In Great Britain and Ireland, the control programs became mandatory in 1950 and 1957, respectively. They were also based on an annual screening by skin test,

the slaughter of positive animals and the inspection of carcasses at the slaughterhouse [3]. bTB incidence decreased in both countries, but the epidemiological situation began to deteriorate gradually from the 1980s, partly because of the existence of a wildlife reservoir in badger populations [4]. In France, such a wildlife reservoir has not been identified, although wild boars, red deer and badgers with *M. bovis* lesions have been found in several departments. Unlike France, Great Britain or Ireland, there are countries where "test and slaughter" control programs were successful in eradicating bTB: Sweden was considered bTB-free in 1958, after 40 years of this type of control program [5] (sporadic cases have been reported afterwards, the last one in 1978 [6]).

In France, data collected over 35 years, between 1965 and 2000, have shown parallel evolutions of herd management practices (with a disappearance of family farms and a professionalization of breeders) and of herd structures (with changes in herd types with a switch from dairy to beef and increasing herd sizes). Besides the effectiveness of control programs, the decrease of bTB incidence between 1965 and 2000 could be partly attributable to these changes in herd management practices and in herd structures [7].

Table 1. Description of the four datasets.

Id	Data type	Number of herds (animals)		Period (geographic origin)	Control program
		Dairy	**Beef**		
A	Aggregated	5 (134)		1981–1983 (Nord)	Annual screening by SITT, slaughter of all cattle if>40% of SITT-positive animals, otherwise slaughter of SITT-positive only
B	Individual	1 (60)	12 (625)	2004–2006 (Dordogne)	Biennial screening by SITT confirmed by SICCT, slaughter of SICCT-positive animals, slaughter of all cattle in case of lesions and *M. bovis* isolation
	Aggregated	9 (684)	16 (1,011)		
C	Individual	3 (142)	11 (596)	2007–2010 (Dordogne)	Annual screening by SITT with second control by γIFN[1] and confirmation by SICCT, slaughter of SICCT-positive, slaughter of all cattle in case of lesions and *M. bovis* isolation
	Aggregated	7 (530)	22 (1,344)		
D	Aggregated		29 (6,317)	2005–2009 (Côte d'Or)	Biennial screening by SICCT, slaughter of SICCT-positive animals, slaughter of all cattle in case of lesions and *M. bovis* isolation

[1]To improve the specificity of the control program C, the γIFN assay used in this control program is a combination of two tests: the PPD γIFN and the ESAT-6 γIFN. The modified γIFN test can be positive (both tests are positive), negative (both tests are negative) or divergent (the results of the two tests are discordant).

Neither ante-mortem tests [8] nor post-mortem tests [6,9] used in bTB control programs have perfect sensitivity and specificity. With the decrease of infection prevalence and because of the increase of herd sizes (multiplied on average by 3.5 between 1965 and 2000 in France [7]), ante-mortem false-positive reactions became a major problem for the surveillance and control program and its acceptability by breeders. This led to an increasing complexity of testing procedures over the past fifteen years, with combinations of several tests: single intradermal tuberculin test (SITT), single intradermal comparative cervical tuberculin test (SICCT) and gamma interferon test (γIFN). Additionally, total slaughter has been replaced in some areas by the slaughter of reactive animals only. All these adaptations allowed reducing the number of animals slaughtered due to false-positive tests, the counterpart being the burdensomeness of control programs due to prolonged restriction of cattle movements.

The failure of the eradication of bTB in France and other European countries seems therefore the result of a complex interaction between the evolution of herd management practices and herd structures, the evolution of control programs, and the implication of wildlife as a reservoir for infection in cattle.

Mathematical modelling is used for the study of complex phenomena such as the dynamics of infectious agents [10]. Diseases with a long incubation period, such as bTB, are difficult to study experimentally or in the field because of prolonged waiting times for obtaining results and the high costs of conducting experimental studies [2]. Mathematical simulation models offer the possibility to test a range of control programs in a short time and to identify the most effective one [2].

A number of mathematical models have been developed to represent the spread of bTB and assess the effectiveness of control measures, especially for wildlife (badgers, opossums and white-tailed deer) [11]. Several models have been built to simulate the dynamics of bTB within cattle herds, to quantify the importance of within-farm bTB transmission by estimating the within-herd transmission coefficient of infection [2,12–14] or to evaluate detection and control strategies against bTB [2,13,15,16].

Each of these models incorporates three processes that shape the within-herd bTB infection dynamics: (i) the natural history of the disease, (ii) husbandry practices and (iii) the surveillance and control program [15]. Because points (ii) and (iii) are specific to a

particular context (geographical area and time period), the models mentioned above are difficult to extrapolate to other countries.

The aim of this study was to design, calibrate and validate a model of spread of *M. bovis* within a cattle herd. Parameter definition was designed to allow simulating various herd management practices as well as control programs of arbitrary complexity.

Materials and Methods

Ethical statement

bTB is a notifiable disease for which there are control and surveillance campaigns in France. Official methods for diagnosis of this disease are culture, PCR and histopathology. Therefore, all the datasets included in this study are issued from animals analyzed within an official context. No purpose killing of animals was performed for this study. All datasets were in complete agreement with national and European regulations. No ethical approval was necessary.

Data

Four datasets denoted A, B, C and D were used, which had been collected at different periods (between 1980 and 2010) in 3 French departments (Nord, Dordogne, and Côte d'Or). At that time and in these departments, four specific control programs were applied, also denoted A, B, C and D (Table 1).

The total number of herds in the four datasets was 115. All were submitted to a total slaughter. Out of all these 115 farms, detailed data for each animal (individual data) were available for 27 herds, namely the year of birth, the screening tests used, the date and results of these tests, the date of slaughter and the result of carcass inspection at the slaughterhouse (presence or absence of lesions). For the 88 remaining farms, we obtained a single data point aggregated at the herd level: the within-herd proportion of animals with detected lesions at total slaughter (Table 1). Dataset A was obtained from a case study conducted by Carnon [17]. The median percentage of animals with lesions per herd was 34.6% (min: 20.8%, max: 86.4%). Dataset B and C were obtained from the official veterinary services of Dordogne department. In dataset B, the median percentage of animals with lesions per herd was 6.4% (min: 0.1%, max 52%). In dataset C, it was 3.1% (min: 0.6%, max 43%). Data set D was obtained from the Alfort

National Veterinary School. The median percentage of animals with lesions per herd was 1% (min: 0.3%, max: 5%).

Model

The within-herd spread of bTB was modelled using a compartmental stochastic model operating in discrete time (Figure 1). The time step was one month. Hereafter, t represents the current time step and m the current month. Each cattle was represented by its age in years $i \in A = \{0,...,A\_max\}$ and its health state $j \in H = \{S,E,I\}$, with: S (susceptible): the animal is not infected, E (latent): the animal is infected but does not have lesions and does not excrete bacteria, and I (infectious): the animal is infected, has lesions and excretes bacteria. Animals were assumed to be grouped into batches according to their age class. To each age class i ($i \in A$) was assigned a batch denoted $L(i)$ (with $L(i) \subset A$). A given batch thus contained animals of one or several age classes. In practice, these batches are often placed by farmers on distant pastures and sometimes in separate buildings, animals from distinct batches having little contact with each other.

The control program was represented by a succession of steps numbered from 1 to D_{max}. During each of these steps, biological tests were performed on the entire or part of the herd; the results of these tests determined the following step. For example, in the control program B which was applied between 2004 and 2006 in the department of Dordogne (Figure 2), the first step is the yearly screening of all animals by SITT. If one animal is positive, the second step of control program is performed two months later: positive animals of step 1 are tested by SICCT, as well as a group of randomly selected negative animals. If one animal is positive in step 2, step 3 is performed 3 months later: positive animals of step 2 are slaughtered and, when lesions are observed, bacterial cultures are performed. If one animal is positive to the bacterial culture, the total slaughter (step 4) is performed 1 month later. The status of each animal with respect to the step of the control program was represented by an integer $k \in D = \{0,...,D\_max\}$, with: $k = 0$ if the animal has never been tested or always had negative test results, and $k > 0$ if the animal had positive results to tests performed in step k of the control program, and negative tests thereafter.

The state of a herd at time step t was represented by a triplet $\langle X_t, y_t, z_t \rangle$, where y_t is the number of the current step of the control program ($1 \leq y_t \leq D_{max}$), z_t is the date on which the biological tests associated with this step must be performed ($z_t \geq t$), and X_t is a state variable structured on age class, health status and step of the control program, which represents the state of the animals at time step t: $X_t (i,j,k)$ represents the number of animals in age class i ($i \in A$), health state j ($j \in H$), which have the status k ($k \in D$) with respect to the control program.

The dynamic of infection in the herd resulted from the implementation of three sequential processes (Figure 1): the demographic process (ageing and renewal of animals), the infectious process (transmission of infection and evolution of infected animals) and the process of detection and control. A full description of the model is given in Appendix S1.

The size of the herd was assumed constant over time and the herd was assumed closed. Slaughtered animals (routine slaughter or implementation of the control program) being replaced by susceptible young animals (0–1 years old) born in the same herd. The culling rate $k \in D$ was assumed to vary according to the month and to the age class.

We made the simplifying assumption that transmission can occur only between animals of the same batch. However, because of the ageing of animals, the composition of the batch changes every year. Animal transfers between batches then allowed the

between-batch infection spread. The within-herd transmission of bTB was modelled by a frequency-dependent function. Because $M. bovis$ transmission intensity was assumed to vary according to whether the animals are housed inside a stable (where the intensity of within-batch transmission is assumed to be high) or allowed to graze (where the intensity of within-batch transmission is assumed to be low), the transmission parameter (β_m) was assumed to vary according to the month. The transition from the latent (E) to the infectious (I) state was based on the transition rate α, where $1/\alpha$ is the duration of the latency period in months.

A step of the control program represented the implementation of one or more biological tests, some of which potentially requiring the slaughter of the animal (for detecting lesions). Tests implemented in the context of a control program could be performed on the entire or part of the herd; the sample of tested animals depending on the results of previous steps of the control program. A step k of the control program was then represented by the quadruplet $\langle Se_k, Sp_k, M_k, Q_k \rangle$, where:

- Se_k and Sp_k are the joint sensitivity and specificity of tests (assumed independent of age and identical for animals in health states E and I)
- m_k equals 1 if the tests require the slaughter of the animal and 0 otherwise
- Q_k is a parameter structured according to age class and to the status of animals with respect to the step of the control program, which defines the sampling plan for testing animals: $Q_k (i,k)$ is the probability that an animal is tested if it has age i and status k for the control program. This parameter verifies: $\sum_{(i,k) \in A \times D} Q_k (i,k) = 1$.

The step $k = 1$ of the control program corresponded to a screening in a bTB-free herd. The steps $k > 1$ corresponded to detection and control measures conducted in a herd known or suspected to be infected.

At each time step, it was further assumed that slaughterhouse surveillance allowed the detection of lesions in culled animals. This slaughterhouse surveillance combined the visual inspection of carcasses with the isolation of $M. bovis$ from lesions (Figures 2 and 3).

Parameterisation

Fixed parameters. Consistent estimates of the sensitivity and specificity of diagnostic tests are found in the literature, and herd management practices were assumed homogeneous in a given region. The values of the corresponding parameters were thus fixed according to literature or based on expert opinion.

Three batches were distinguished in beef herds: young heifers (1–2 years), heifers of reproductive age (2–3 years), and cows (after the first calving at 4 years) with calves and heifers fed by their mothers (<1year). In dairy herds, animals were also separated into three batches: young heifers (<1 year), heifers of reproductive age (1–2 years), and cows (after the first calving, at 3 years).

For both types of herds, the stabling period was between November and March. Renewal and routine cull of animals was assumed to occur between January and March, animals being culled from the age of 3 years in dairy herds and from the age of 4 years in beef herds. The maximum age of the cattle (A_{max}) was set to 15 years. Other fixed parameters (culling rate, sensitivity and specificity of screening and diagnostic tests) are given in Table 2.

Month-specific transmission parameters allowed representing the difference between the stabling and grazing period, with $\beta_m = \beta_{inside}$ during the stabling period (between November and March) and $\beta_m = \beta_{outside}$ for the remainder of the year. Because of

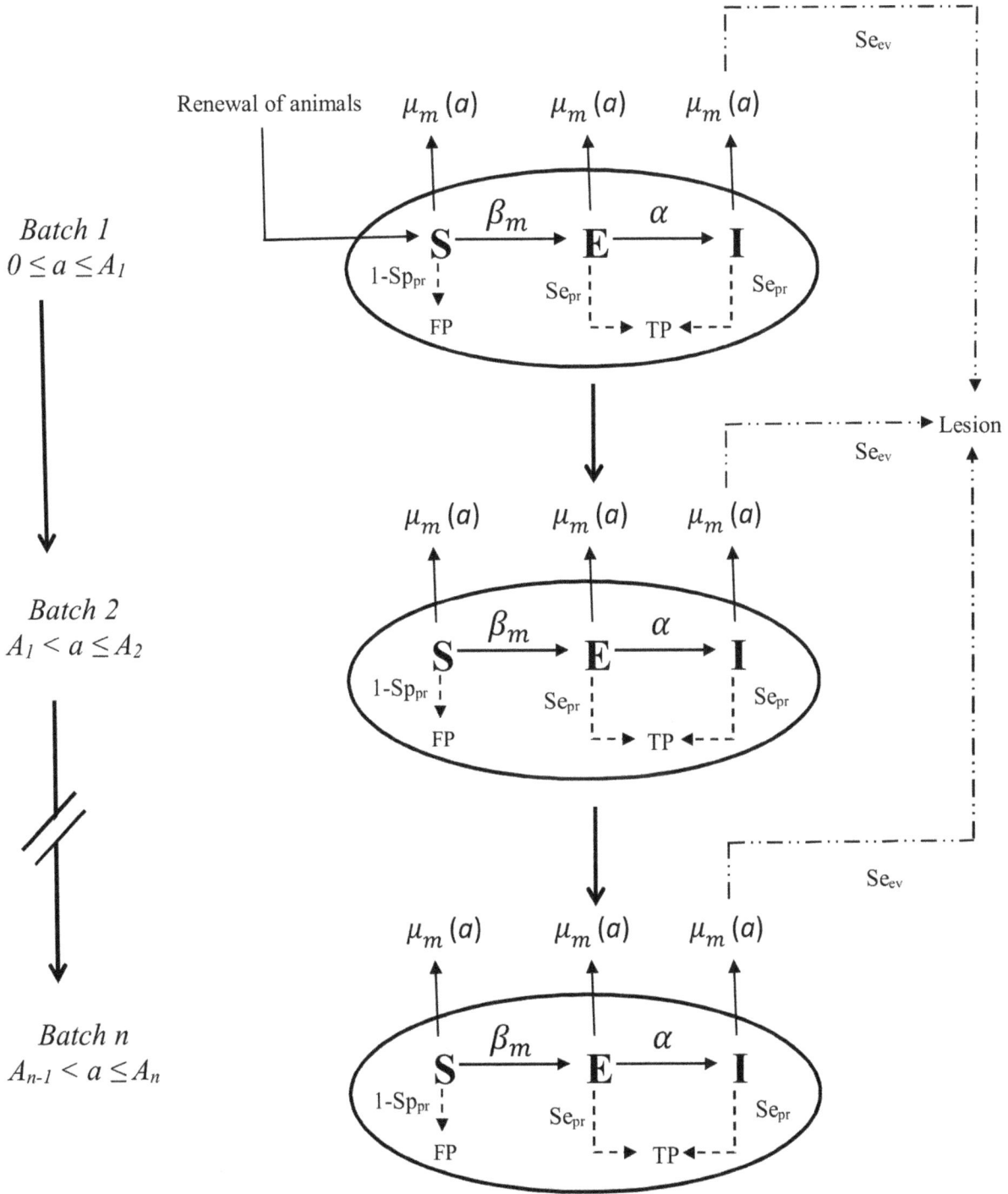

Batch 1
$0 \leq a \leq A_1$

Batch 2
$A_1 < a \leq A_2$

Batch n
$A_{n-1} < a \leq A_n$

Renewal of animals

$\mu_m(a)$ $\mu_m(a)$ $\mu_m(a)$

S $\xrightarrow{\beta_m}$ E $\xrightarrow{\alpha}$ I

$1-Sp_{pr}$ Se_{pr} Se_{pr}

FP TP

Se_{ev}

Lesion

Disease and demographic dynamics

Programmed surveillance (control program)

Slaughterhouse surveillance

Figure 1. Schematic representation of the model of within-herd transmission of bTB by three processes: the demographic process (renewal of cattle, reform and change of batches), the infectious process (transitions between health states S: susceptible, E: latent, I: infectious) and the process of detection and control. a: age class in years; Batch: group of animals; m: month; μ_m (a): culling rate for month m and age class a; β_m: month-specific transmission coefficient; Se_{pr}: test sensitivity of step k of programmed surveillance (control program); Sp_{pr}: test specificity of step k of programmed surveillance (control program); FP: false positive; TP: true positive; Se_{ev}: sensitivity of passive surveillance at the slaughterhouse.

the close contact between dairy cows that occurs twice per day in the milking parlour, β_{inside} was used throughout the year in dairy herds for the cows' batch.

Initial conditions assumed the presence of a single infected animal in the state E. To represent the introduction of infection through contact during grazing, this animal was randomly selected among animals that had access to pasture (all batches for beef herds and the first two batches in dairy herds). Simulations were stopped when there were no more infected animals (thanks to routine cull and/or to the control program), the current step of the control program being 1 (i.e. screening in a bTB-free herd).

Parameter estimation. As estimates available in the literature are divergent or uncertain, and because many aspects of bTB pathogenesis are yet to be elucidated, three parameters were estimated from field data: α (transition rate between the health states E and I), β_{inside} (transmission parameter when animals are inside the stable) and $\beta_{outside}$ (transmission parameter when animals are grazing). Individual-level data from datasets B and C were used, corresponding to 27 herds and 1423 animals (Table 1). Control programs B (Figure 2) and C (Figure 3) were modelled according to memos of the French Ministry of Agriculture, Food and Forestry.

The ABC (Approximate Bayesian Computation) method was used to estimate the parameters (α, β_{inside} and $\beta_{outside}$). This method aims at estimating the posterior distributions of the parameters where the calculation of the likelihood is difficult or burdensome [18].

The generic form of the ABC method's "rejection algorithm" is [18]:

1- Sample parameter values θ^* from the prior distribution $\pi(\theta)$.

2- Simulate a dataset χ^* using parameter values θ^*.

3- Calculate the summary statistics for the observed data $S(\chi o)$ and simulated data $S(\chi^*)$.

4- Compare the simulated data, $S(\chi^*)$, and the observed data, $S(\chi o)$, using the distance function, d, and the tolerance ε; if d $(S(\chi o), S(\chi^*)) \leq \varepsilon$, the value of θ^* is accepted. When $\varepsilon = 0$, the posterior distribution is exactly $\pi(\theta/S (\chi o))$, whereas when $\varepsilon \rightarrow +\infty$, the posterior distribution is equal to the prior distribution [19].

Other algorithms have been proposed for the ABC method (e.g. Markov Chain Monte Carlo or Sequential Monte Carlo). We used the rejection algorithm followed by a step of local linear regression as proposed by Beaumont et al. [19]. This step aims at reducing the variance of the posterior estimation in order to try to correct errors that are due to a non-zero value of the tolerance ε. A total of 100,000 simulations were performed for parameter estimation.

Prior distributions were uniform distributions U[0.027– 0.50]month^{-1} for α and U [0–2]month^{-1} for β_{inside} and $\beta_{outside}$. For α, these values correspond to a period of latency between 2 and 36 months. The lower bound (2 months) is the rounded value of the lower bound (87 days) of the estimation obtained by Neill et al. in an experimental study [20], while the upper bound (36 months) is a rounded value of the upper bound (34 months) of the estimated duration of latency in Perez et al. [2]. For β_{inside} and $\beta_{outside}$, the upper bound of the prior distribution was chosen arbitrarily after having verified by simulation that, using this value, the median simulated percentage of animals with lesions at total slaughter (22% and 17% for dairy and beef farms, respectively) was significantly higher than the observed value in dataset B (6.4%).

The choice of summary statistics is a crucial step in the ABC method. This choice involves a compromise between information loss and size of the statistic [21]. Using a poorly chosen set of summary statistics can often lead to an overestimation of credible

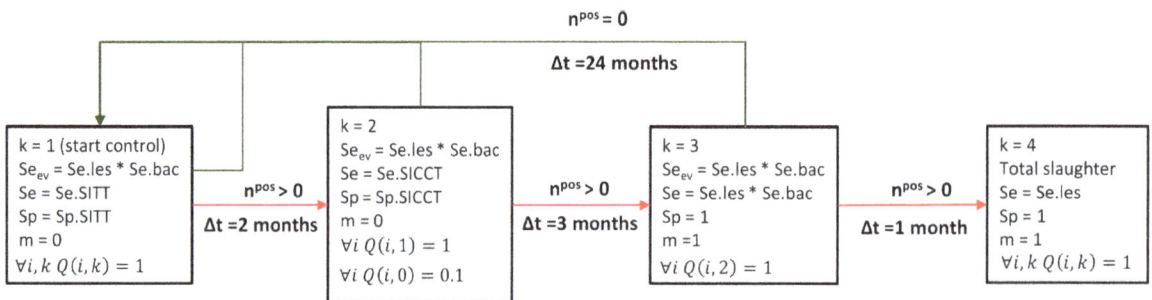

Figure 2. Control program B applied in the Dordogne department between 2004 and 2006. Step 1: biennial bTB screening using SITT (the herd being considered disease-free). All animals are tested ($\forall i,k Q(i,k)=1$). Sensitivity (Se) and specificity (Sp): those of SITT. Transition to step 2 if an animal is positive ($n^{pos}>0$), two months later ($\Delta t=2$ months). Step 2: confirmation of SITT positive results using SICCT. All the positive animals of step 1 are tested (μ i Q(i,1) = 1), as well as 10% of the negative animals (μ i Q(i,1) = 1). Sensitivity (Se) and specificity (Sp): those of SICCT. Transition to step 3 if an animal is positive, three months later. Step 3: slaughter of SICCT-positive animals and isolation of *M. bovis* from lesions. All the positive animals of step 2 (μ i Q(i,2) = 1) are slaughtered (m = 1) and bacterial culture is performed from observed lesions. Sensitivity (Se): sequential combination of a visual inspection at the slaughterhouse and of a bacterial culture. Transition to step 4 if an animal is positive, 1 month later. Step 4: total slaughter. All the animals ($\forall i,k Q(i,k)=1$) are slaughtered (m = 1). Routine detection of lesions at slaughterhouse. Sensitivity (Se_{ev}): sequential combination of a visual inspection at the slaughterhouse and of a bacterial culture. If a positive animal is thus detected, regardless of the current stage of control program, transition to step 4. See table 2 for the definition of the other parameters.

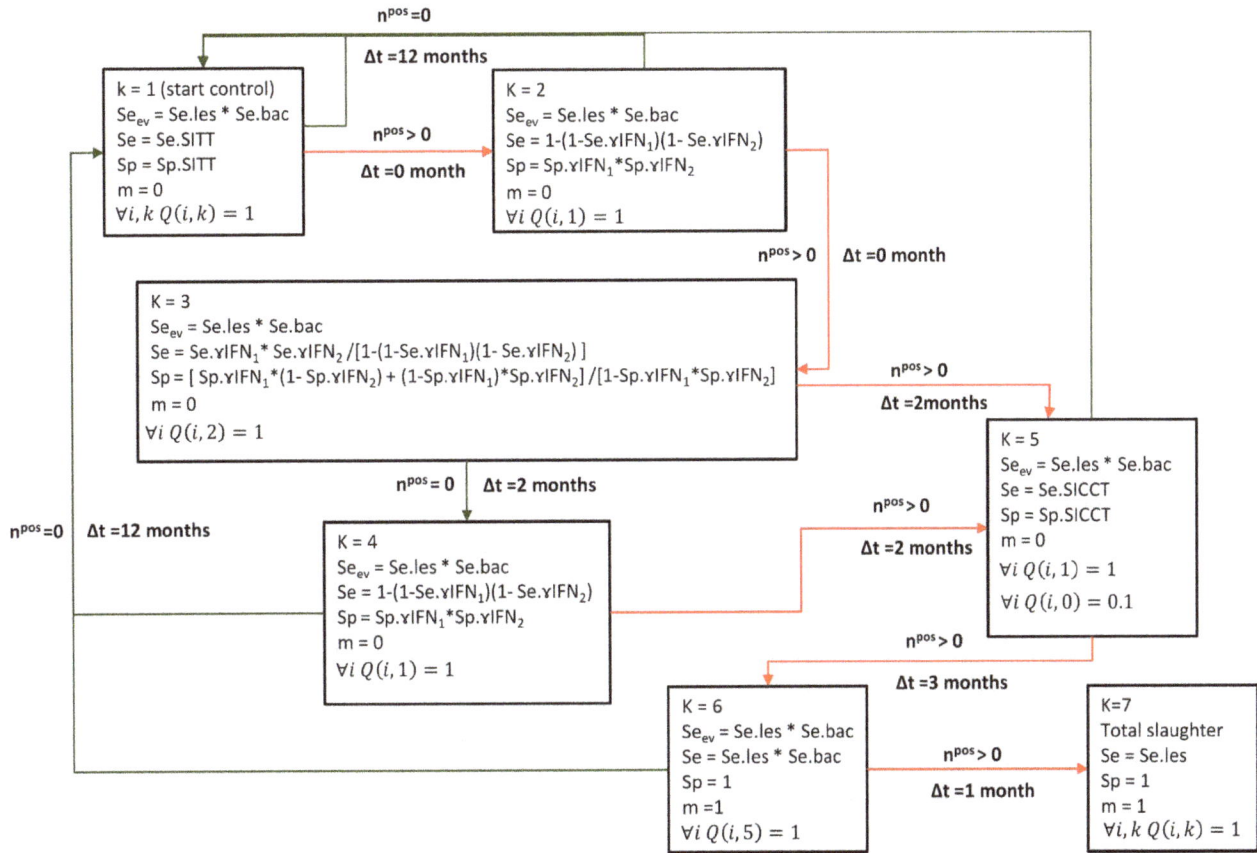

Figure 3. Control program C applied in the Dordogne department between 2007 and 2010. Step 1: yearly bTB screening using SITT (the herd being considered disease-free). All animals are tested (μ i,k Q(i,k) = 1). Sensitivity (Se) and specificity (Sp): those of SITT. Immediate transition to step 2 if an animal is positive ($n^{pos} > 0$). Step 2: confirmation of SITT positive results using PDD γIFN (γIFN1) and ESAT-6 γIFN (γIFN2). All the positive animals of step 1 are tested (μ i Q(i,1) = 1. Sensitivity (Se) and specificity (Sp): parallel combination of both tests (positivity to any of both tests). Immediate transition to step 3 if an animal is positive; otherwise: transition to step 1. Step 3: interpretation of the positive results of step 2 as convergent (both γIFN tests are positive) or not (only one of both tests is positive). All the positive animals of step 2 (μ i Q(i,2) = 1) are concerned. Sensitivity (Se) and Specificity (Sp): sequential combination of both tests in positive animals of step 2. Transition to step 5 if an animal is positive, and to step 4 otherwise, two months later. Step 4: second confirmation of SITT positive results using PDD γIFN (γIFN1) and ESAT-6 γIFN (γIFN2). All the positive animals of step 1 are tested (μ i Q(i,1) = 1). Sensitivity (Se) and specificity (Sp): same as for step 2. Transition to step 5 if an animal is positive, two months later; otherwise: transition to step 1, 12 months later. Step 5: confirmation of SITT positive results using SICCT. All the positive animals of step 1 are tested (μ i Q(i,1) = 1), as well as 10% of the negative animals (μ i Q(i,0) = 0.1). Sensitivity (Se) and specificity (Sp): those of SICCT. Transition to step 6 if an animal is positive, three months later. Step 6: slaughter of SICCT-positive animals and isolation of *M. bovis* from lesions. All the positive animals of step 5 (μ i Q(i,5) = 1) are slaughtered (m = 1) and bacterial culture is performed from observed lesions. Sensitivity (Se): sequential combination of a visual inspection at the slaughterhouse and of a bacterial culture. Transition to step 7 if an animal is positive, 1 month later ($\Delta t = 1$ month). Step 7: total slaughter. All the animals (μ i,k Q(i,k) = 1) are slaughtered (m = 1). Routine detection of lesions at slaughterhouse. Sensitivity (Se_{ev}): sequential combination of a visual inspection at the slaughterhouse and of a bacterial culture. If a positive animal is thus detected, regardless of the current stage of control program, transition to step 7. See table 2 for the definition of the other parameters.

intervals due to the loss of information [22]. One way to capture most of the information present in the data would be to use many statistics, but the accuracy and stability of the ABC method decrease rapidly with an increasing number of summary statistics [22,23]. In order to choose the best combination of summary statistics, eight combinations (Table 3) were tested on simulated data obtained using arbitrarily fixed parameter values. The tested summary statistics combined two types of variables, the time between the last negative control and the detection of infection and the percentage of animals with detected lesions, taking into account or not the batch, the type of herd and the year. The procedure used to select the best summary statistics among the eight tested combinations is described in Appendix S2. Briefly, parameter values were set to arbitrarily chosen values and used to generate 100 simulated datasets. In a first step, one of these

datasets was chosen and considered a pseudo-observation. Each set of summary statistics was then successively used to estimate the posterior distribution of the parameters, and we kept for further analysis the set of summary statistics for which the arbitrarily chosen parameter values were inside the corresponding 95% credibility interval. In a second step, the preceding procedure was successively applied to the 100 simulated datasets and we selected the set of summary statistics that maximized the proportion of cases for which the arbitrarily chosen parameter values were inside the 95% credibility interval of the posterior distribution of parameters.

The tolerance threshold ε was determined by choosing the proportion of retained simulations p_ε. A leave-one-out procedure was applied to a set of 100 datasets simulated using parameters (α, β_{inside}, $\beta_{outside}$) sampled from the prior distributions, to evaluate the

Table 2. Definitions and values of fixed parameters in the model.

Parameters	Description	Value	Range[1]	Reference
μ_m (i)	Culling rate			(Prof. Coureau, Alfort National Veterinary School, pers. Comm.)
	Dairy herd, 2000's	0.35	0.25; 0.45	
	Beef herd, 2000's	0.25	0.15; 0.35	
	All herds, 1980's	0.25		
Se.SITT	Sensitivity of single intradermal tuberculin test		0.635; 1	[8]
	1980's	0.72		
	2000's	0.839		
Sp.SITT	Specificity of single intradermal tuberculin test		0.755; 0.99	[8]
	1980's	0.988		
	2000's	0.968		
Se.SICCT	Sensitivity of single intra dermal comparative cervical tuberculin test	0.80	0.52; 1	[8]
Sp.SICCT	Specificity of single intra dermal comparative cervical tuberculin test	0.995	0.788; 1	[8]
Se.PPD γIFN	Sensitivity of gamma interferon test (PPD)	0.876	0.73; 1	[8]
Sp.PPD γIFN	Specificity of gamma interferon test (PPD)	0.966	0.850; 0.996	[8]
Se.ESAT-6 γIFN	Sensitivity of gamma interferon test (ESAT-6)	0.763	0.690; 0.836	[51]
Sp.ESAT-6 γIFN	Specificity of gamma interferon test (ESAT-6)	0.992	0.976; 1	[51]
qSICCT	Proportion of animals non-reactors to SITT tested six weeks later by SICCT	0.10	0.05; 0.15	(French Ministry of agriculture, Food and Forestry)
Se.bac	Sensitivity of bacterial culture	0.78	0.729; 0.828	[52]
Se.les	Sensitivity of visual inspection of carcass	0.50	0.255; 0.755	[6]

[1]Values used in the sensitivity analysis.

Table 3. Selection of the set of summary statistics based on simulated datasets generated using arbitrarily fixed parameter values: $\alpha = 0.083$ months, $\beta_{inside} = 0.5$, and $\beta_{inside} = 0.1$.

Id	Summary statistics	Dimension	Median [95% credible interval]			p[1]
			α	β_{inside}	$\beta_{outside}$	
A	Average percentage of animals with detected lesions[2]	1	0.72 [0.60–0.78]	0.79 [0.44–1.27]	0.61 [0,03–1,92]	–
B	Average percentage of animals with detected lesions in each batch	3	0.42 [0.00–2.43]	0.33 [0.28–0.70]	0.29 [0.00–3.9]	73%
C	Percentage of animals with detected lesions in each batch (n = 3) of each herd (n = 27)	81	0.13 [0.06–0.67]	0.35 [0.02–1.97]	0.44 [0.01–2.21]	49%
D	Same as C+percentage of herds submitted to total slaughter	82	0.97 [0.48–2.04]	0.05 [0.01–0.15]	0.03 [0.00–0.12]	–
E	Same as C+time between the last negative test and the detection of infection for each herd	108	0.29 [0.07–0.69]	0.35 [0.00–0.77]	0.07 [0.00–0.84]	32%
F	Same as E+percentage of herds submitted to total slaughter	109	0.33 [0.12–0.65]	0.29 [0.08–0.57]	0.08 [0.00–0.79]	–
G	Average percentage of animals with detected lesion for each batch, period[3] and herd type[4]; average time between the last negative test and the detection of infection for each period and herd type	16	0.26 [0.07–0.74]	0.27 [0.04–0.75]	0.07 [0.00–0.52]	71%
H	Same as G+percentage of herds submitted to total slaughter for each period and herd type	20	0.073 [0.05–0.54]	0.48 [0.03–0.76]	0.12 [0.00–0.59]	88%

[1]Proportion of cases for which each of the three arbitrarily fixed parameter values were inside the 95% credible interval of the posterior distributions (100 repetitions).
[2]For herds submitted to a total slaughter.
[3]Before 2007 (control program B) and after 2007 (control program C).
[4]Dairy of beef.

robustness of the estimates to the tolerance rate. Each of the 100 simulated datasets was successively considered a pseudo-observation and parameter values were estimated using the above procedure. A prediction error coefficient was calculated for each estimated parameter, for values of p_ε ranging from 0.1% to 5% [24]. The smallest value of p_ε for which the prediction error coefficient was stable for the three parameters (α, β_{inside}, $\beta_{outside}$) was thus selected.

We used the "abc" package of software R [25]. The function cv4abc was used to select the value for the proportion of retained simulations p_ε.

A sensitivity analysis was performed to evaluate the effect of changing the fixed parameter values (Table 2) on the estimated values of the transition rate (α) and of the transmission parameters (β_{inside} and $\beta_{outside}$). Two different values were selected for each fixed parameter (Table 2) according to literature (SITT, SICCT, γIFN and bacterial culture) or using fixed deviations ($\pm10\%$ or $\pm5\%$). Only first-order effects were analyzed and, for each scenario, α, β_{inside} and $\beta_{outside}$ were estimated by the ABC method, as described above. This operation was repeated 24 times (12 fixed parameters and 2 points per parameter) resulting in 24 posterior distributions for α, β_{inside} and $\beta_{outside}$. These were analysed using three generalised linear model (GLMs) (one per estimated parameter). The explanatory variables were the fixed parameters values (their deviation from their default values).

The GLMs were used to predict the effect of an increase of 5% of each fixed parameter on the average values of α, β_{inside} and $\beta_{outside}$. To identify the most influential fixed parameters, we compared the coefficient of variation of the posterior distributions (obtained using the default values of fixed parameters) with the relative error induced by a 5% change of fixed parameters, as predicted by the GLMs.

Validation

An internal validation was first performed using a leave-one-out cross-validation procedure. One hundred triples of parameter values (α, β_{inside} and $\beta_{outside}$) were randomly chosen among the 100,000 used for parameter estimation. Each was successively used to generate a dataset considered a pseudo-observation, and posterior distributions were estimated using the above procedure (without using the pseudo-observation). The reliability of the estimation procedure was quantified by the proportion of cases for which the triple (α, β_{inside} and $\beta_{outside}$) used to generate the dataset was within the 95% credible interval.

An external validation was performed to test the ability of the model to reproduce the observational data of bTB in France between 1980 and 2010, using the data that were not used for parameter estimation: dataset A, aggregated data from datasets B and C, and dataset D (Table 1). Each herd of these datasets was successively used to parameterize the model (herd size and type, control program - Figures 2, 3, S1 and S2), and the posterior distributions of parameters (α, β_{inside} and $\beta_{outside}$) were sampled to perform 1000 simulations. Those ending by a total slaughter were kept to compute the distribution of the proportion of animals with detected lesions. For each herd of the above datasets, the observed proportion was compared with the simulated distribution thus obtained. Furthermore, for dataset A, the predicted proportion of simulations ending by a total slaughter was compared with the percentage observed in the corresponding department in the 1980s: 5%.

Model exploitation

The basic reproduction ratio (R0) is used to measure the transmission potential of a disease. It is the number of secondary

infections produced by an infectious animal in a fully susceptible population that is totally susceptible. This indictor is of great importance in infectious disease modelling as, when R0<1, the disease tends to vanish, whereas when R0>1, the disease tends to spread and a large epidemic may occur [26]. However, in real situations, the population is rarely entirely susceptible, mainly because of the spread of infection (and the corresponding decrease in the number of susceptible individuals). We computed the effective reproductive ratio R(t): the average number of cases secondary to an infectious case in a population consisting of susceptible and infected individuals. Two average herds, respectively representative of a French dairy herd (81 cattle) and a French beef herd (70 cattle) in the 2000s, were considered. Disease dynamics was simulated in these herds without a control program, and the distribution of the effective reproductive ratio R(t) was calculated each month after the introduction of *M. bovis*, during 360 months (twice the maximal age of cows in the model: 15 years). Details of R(t) calculation are given in Appendix S3.

Results

Parameter estimation

The procedure used to choose the set of summary statistics first led to select B, C, E, G and H, for which, when using one simulated dataset as a pseudo-observation, the arbitrarily chosen parameter values were all inside the 95% credible interval of posterior distributions of parameters (Table 3). Their dimensions varied between 3 for B and 109 for F (Table 3). Among these five sets of summary statistics, H maximized the proportion of cases (88%) where the arbitrarily fixed parameters (α, β_{inside} and $\beta_{outside}$) were all within the credible interval of 95% of posterior distributions when using the 100 simulated datasets as pseudo-observations (Table 3). This set of summary statistics was thus chosen: a combination of statistics describing the percentage of animals with detected lesions per batch and the percentage of herds with total slaughter per herd type (dairy/beef) and per period (periods where control program B and C were applied). The evolution of the values of the prediction error coefficient according to the proportion of retained simulations led to select $p_\varepsilon = 2\%$.

The median of the posterior distribution of α was 0.28 (95% credible interval [CI]: [0.13–0.56]), which corresponds to a median latency period for bTB of 3.5 months (95% CI: [2–8] months) (Figure 4). The median value of bTB transmission coefficients were 0.43 month^{-1} (95% CI [0.16–0.84] month^{-1}) inside the stable (β_{inside}) and 0.08 month^{-1} (95% CI [0.01–0.32] month^{-1}) outside the stable ($\beta_{outside}$) (Figure 4). The median of the ratio $\beta_{inside}/\beta_{outside}$ was 5 (95% CI [0.8–100]). It was>1 in 95.6% of cases (Figure 4). Negative values of Spearman's rank correlation coefficient were observed between α and β_{inside} (−0.47, p< 0.0001), between α and $\beta_{outside}$ (−0.31, p<0.0001), and between β_{inside} and $\beta_{outside}$ (−0.35, p<0.0001). These negative correlations were expected, as the summary statistics (such as the proportion of animals showing lesions) may remain approximately the same if a higher value of α (i.e. a shorter latency period) is compensated by smaller values of β_{inside} and $\beta_{outside}$, or if a higher value of β_{inside} is compensated by a lower value of $\beta_{outside}$. The results of the sensitivity analysis of parameter estimates to variations of fixed parameter values are summarised in a tornado chart (Figure 5). A 5% increase in the values of the fixed parameters had limited effects on the estimation of α and $\beta_{outside}$ (Figure 5). For β_{inside}, the relative difference of the average posterior estimate greater than the coefficient of variation computed from the posterior distribution of for a single parameter: the specificity of the ESAT-6 γIFN

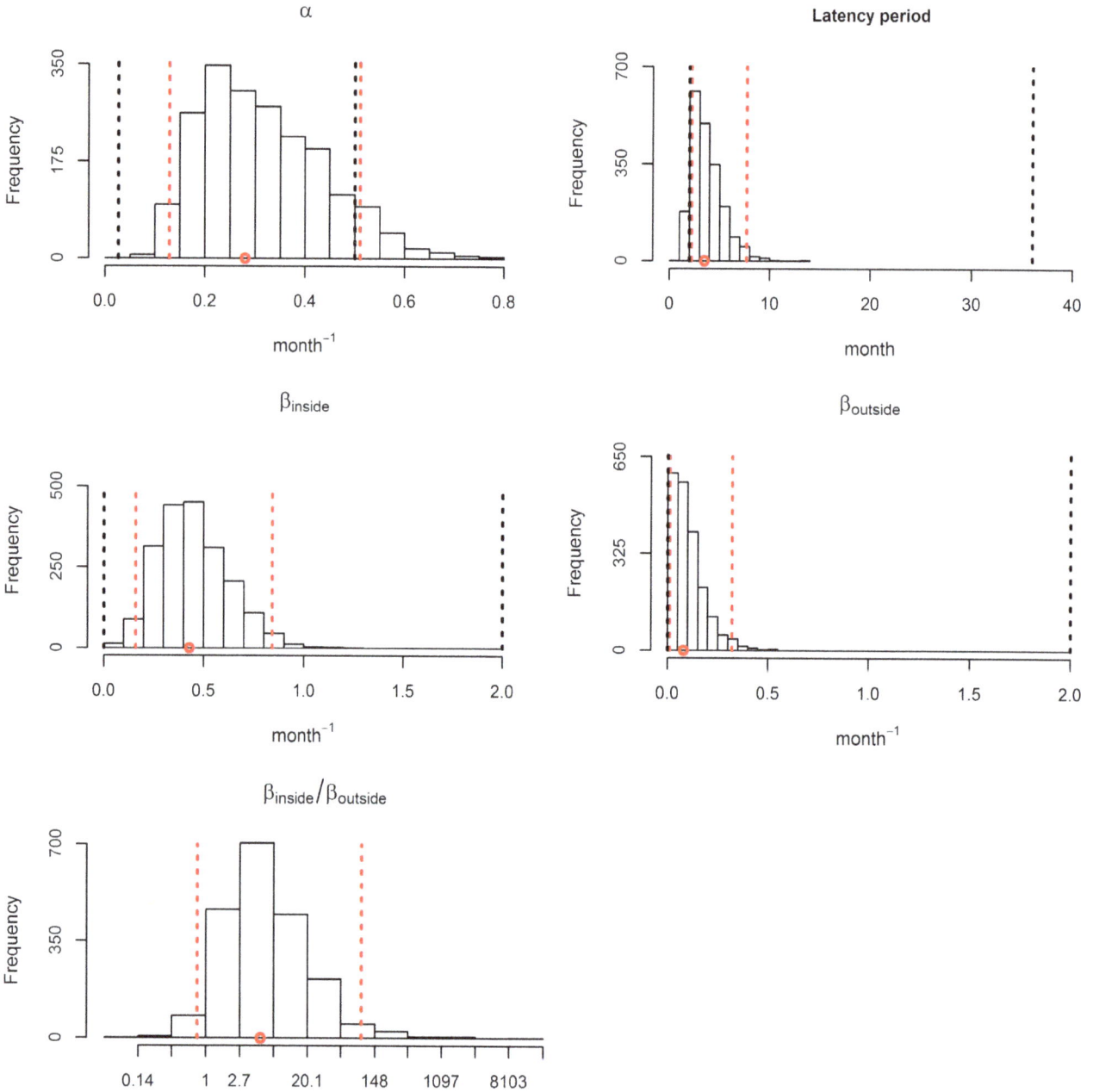

Figure 4. Posterior distribution of parameters α, β_{inside} **and** $\beta_{outside}$. Red dots: median value of parameter estimates; black dotted lines: lower and higher bounds of parameter prior distributions; red dotted lines: 95% credible intervals of the parameter posterior distributions. Histogram $\beta_{inside}/\beta_{outside}$ represents the value of log ratio $\beta_{inside}/\beta_{outside}$ but the x-axis values are not expressed in log.

test. A 5% increase of the specificity of the ESAT-6 γIFN test led to a 48.5% decrease of the average posterior estimate of β_{inside}.

Predicted bTB dynamics

Figure 6 and Table 4 represents the predicted bTB dynamics in two herds representing dairy farms (average size in 2000:81 animals) and beef herds (average size in 2000:70 animals) in France, with and without a control program (control program B, Table 1 and Figure 2). When the control program was simulated, after its introduction in a susceptible herd, bTB was predicted to disappear in 22% of cases in beef herds and in 17% of cases in dairy farms, thanks to routine cull: the median time from disease

introduction and disease extinction was less than 10 months, in both types of herds, with or without a control program (Table 4). In most cases, *M. bovis* did not disappear from the simulated herds and the disease was predicted to be detected through passive surveillance (at slaughterhouse) (13% for beef herds and 21% for dairy farms) or through active surveillance (screening using skin tests) (65% for beef herds and 62% for dairy farms). In both cases, the median time period between the introduction of infection and total slaughter was less than 3 years in the two types of herds (Table 4). In the absence of a control program (Figure 6a and 6b), the median proportion of infected animals was predicted to increase until reaching a plateau at 61 months in beef herds and

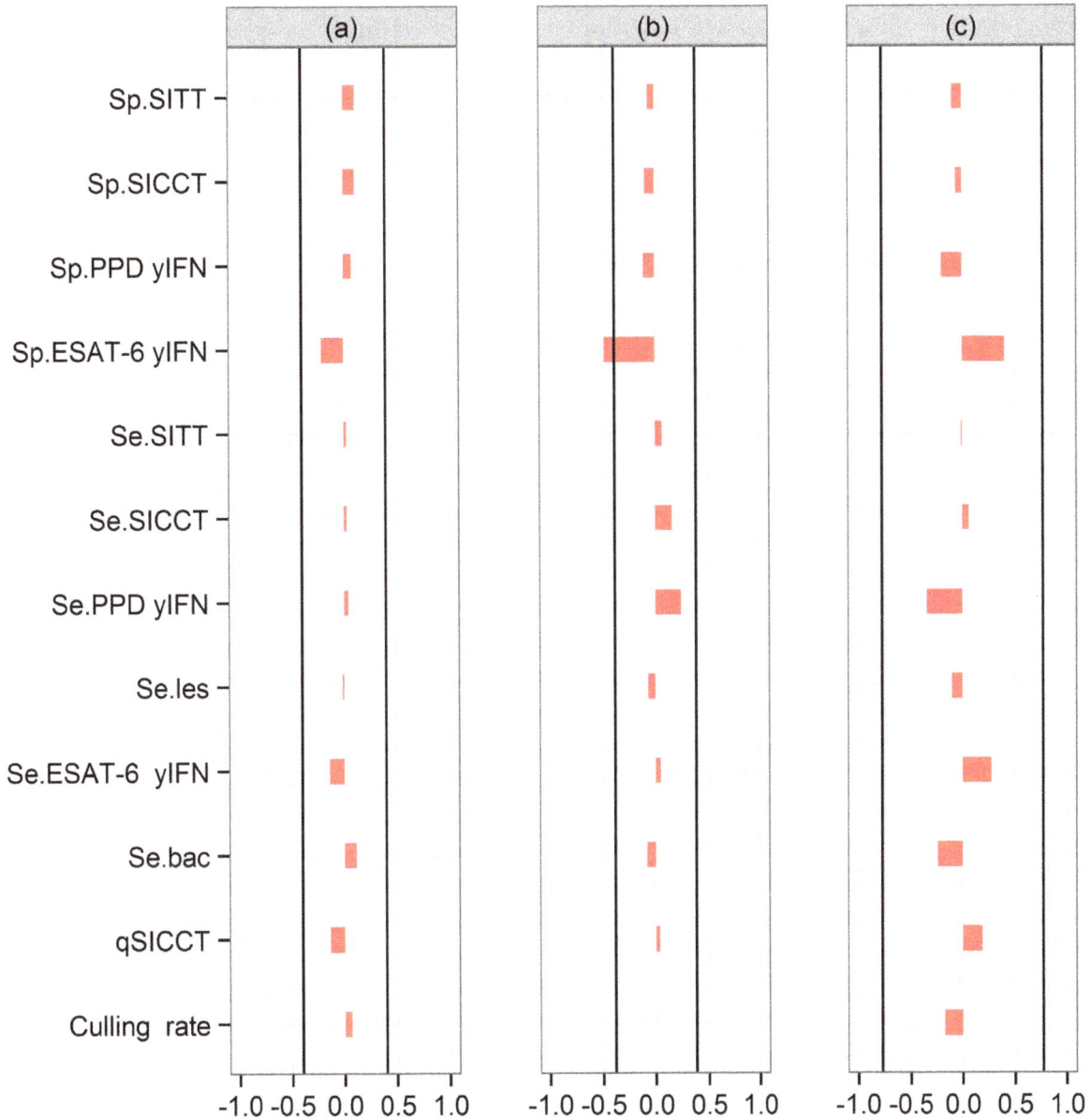

Figure 5. Impact of changes of fixed parameter values on the estimates of α, β_{inside} **and** $\beta_{outside}$. (a): relative error for α; (b): relative error for β_{inside}; (c): relative error for $\beta_{outside}$; black line: value of the coefficient of variation of the posterior distributions obtained when we using the default values of fixed parameters; if the relative error value is within the two black lines, the effect of fixed parameters values on parameter estimates in the model is considered limited; qSICCT: percentage of SITT-negative animals tested 6 weeks after by SICCT; see table 2 for the definition of the other parameters.

40 months in dairy herds (Figure 6a and 6b). The corresponding level of infection prevalence was predicted to be higher in beef herds (Figure 6a) than in dairy herds (Figure 6b): once reached the enzootic infection level the median prevalence of infected animals was 93% in beef farms and 53% in dairy herds. As expected, when a control program was used, the maximum percentage of infected animals was predicted to be lower in both types of herds (Figure 6c and 7d).

Validation

Internal validation showed that, for 83 of the 100 randomly selected simulations, the fixed values of the three parameters α,

β_{inside} and $\beta_{outside}$, were inside the 95% credible interval of the posterior distributions.

Using dataset A, external validation showed that, in four of five herds (farms 1, 2, 3 and 4), the observed percentage of cattle with lesions was between the 2.5% and 97.5% percentiles of the simulated proportion of animals with lesions at total slaughter (Figure 7). In the fifth herd, the observed percentage of animals with lesions was very high (86.6%) and was above the 97.5% percentile of the simulated distribution (Figure 7). The proportion of simulations ending with a total slaughter varied between 3% and 7%, depending on the herd. These values are close to the proportion of 5% reported by the French Ministry of Agriculture, Food and Forestry for that department at that time.

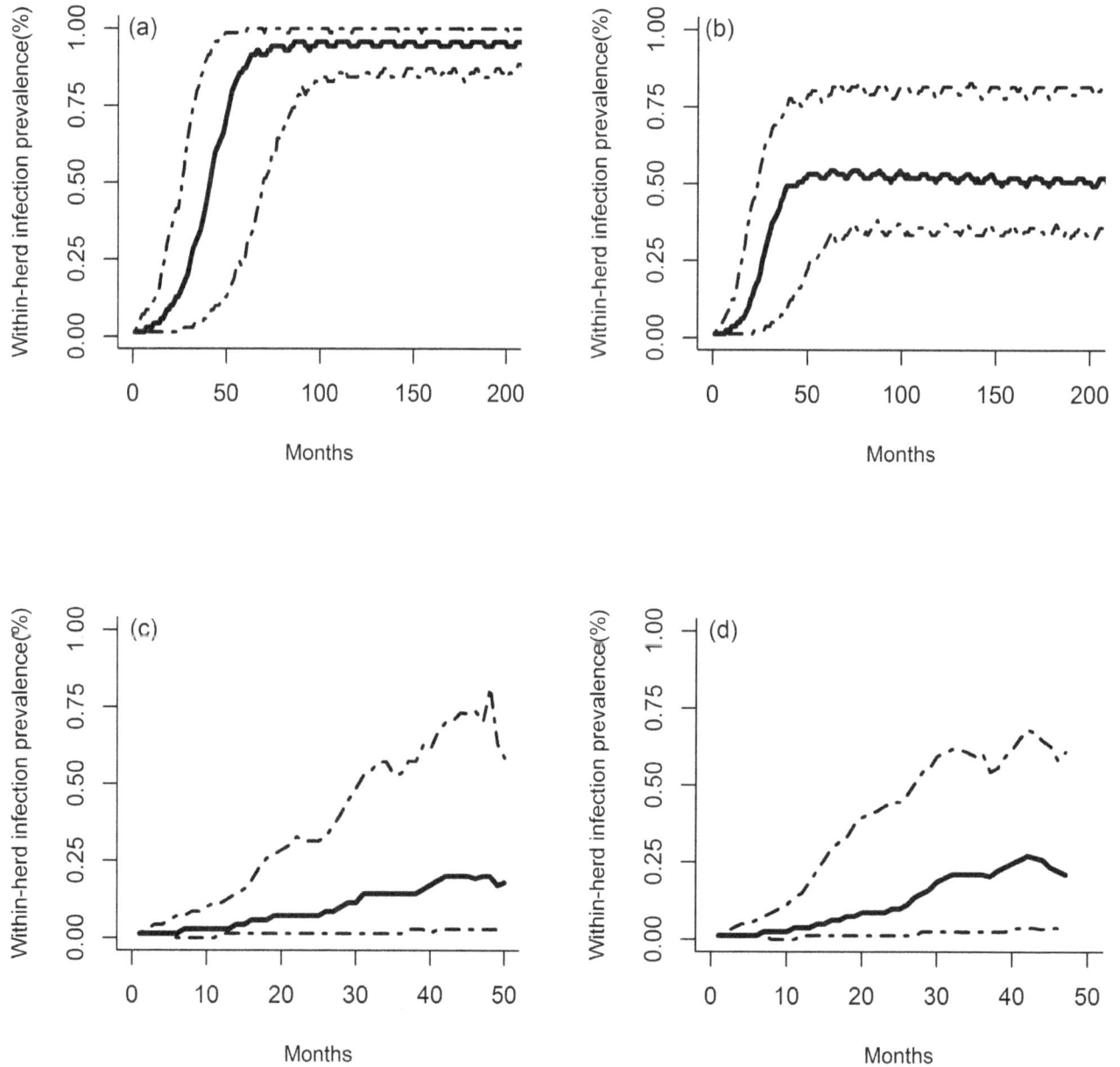

Figure 6. Monthly evolution of the simulated proportion of infected animals (animals in E or I health state; solid line: median, dashed: 2.5% and 97.5% percentiles) in standard French beef (a and c, 70 animals) and dairy (b and d, 81 animals) herds without (a and b) or with (c and d) implementation of control program B (1,000 simulations per scenario).

The observed percentage of animals with lesions was located between the 2.5% and 97.5% percentiles of the simulated proportion of animals with lesions in 92% (23 herds out of 25) and 83% (24 herds out of 29) of herds of datasets B and C, respectively. This percentage was 100% (29 herds out of 29) for dataset D.

Effective reproductive ratio

Figures 8a and 8b show the evolution of R(t) values over time. In both types of herds, the shape of the curve was similar, with an increase in the values of R(t) that reached a plateau 72 months after disease introduction in dairy herds and at 96 months after disease introduction in beef herds. After 30 simulated years, which corresponds to a situation of enzootic circulation of *M. bovis*

within the herd, the value of R(t) was slightly higher for beef herds than for dairy herds. The median value and the percentiles [2.5%–97.5%] of the predicted distribution of R(t) were 2.2 [1.8–2.8] for beef herds and 1.7 [1.5–2.2] for dairy herds (Figure 8a and Figure 8b). It was higher than 1 for each of the 1,000 simulations and higher than 2 for 11% of simulations in dairy herds and 79% in beef herds (Figure 8c and Figure 8d).

Discussion

In this work, we have built a stochastic discrete-time model to simulate bTB dynamics and control in cattle herds. The model accounts for interactions among the three processes that influence the within-herd evolution of bTB: (i) the natural history of the disease (infectious process), (ii) husbandry practices (demographic

Table 4. Predicted median and percentiles [2.5%–97.5%] of the distribution of outbreak duration (in months) in standard French beef herds (70 animals) and dairy herds (81 animals) without or with control programs (1,000 simulations per scenario).

		Beef herds	Dairy herds
Time to natural extinction of infection	Without a simulated control program	7 [3–30]	8 [4–32]
	With a simulated control program		
	No detection of infection	6 [3–11]	7 [4–16]
	Infection suspected but not confirmed[1]	8 [3–25]	8 [3–23]
Time to total slaughter of the herd after infection detection by routine skin testing		24 [9–50]	23 [9–48]
Time to total slaughter of the herd after infection detection by slaughterhouse surveillance		24 [8–50]	30 [9–47]

[1]No isolation of *M. bovis*, total slaughter is thus not applied.

process) and (iii) control programs (detection and control process). The model has been designed to allow simulating control programs of arbitrary degree of complexity. Parameterization allows representing various herd types and farming practices (in particular the differences between dairy herd and beef herd management). Epidemiological parameters of the within-herd transmission of bTB (duration of the latent state, transmission parameters) were estimated using a first set and the model was validated using a second set of field data collected between 1980 and 2010. Herd management practices and bTB control programs have evolved during this period and the model could be successfully adapted by changing parameter values, suggesting a good level of genericity and an ability to simulate various herd management systems and bTB detection and control programs of arbitrary complexity. The simulated effective reproductive ratio R(t) may allow assessing the effectiveness (*i.e.* whether R(t)<1) of different bTB control strategies or the effect of changes in herd management practices on the bTB within-herd dynamic.

Internal validation showed a good reliability of the estimation procedure of model parameters by the ABC method. External validation showed that the model was able to reproduce field data regarding bTB collected between 1980 and 2010 in several French departments. This suggests that the transmission coefficients (β_{inside} and $\beta_{outside}$) and the duration of the latent period ($1/\alpha$) have remained roughly constant between the 1980s and today, despite changes in parameters related to herd management practices such as the culling rate, the age at culling and the herd size.

Health states used in the proposed model (susceptible, latent and infectious) are consistent with the pathology of infection. However, published models often divide the latent state into two sub-states (latent, non-skin test-responsive and latent, skin test-responsive [13–15]) and use shorter time steps (day or week). Latent non-skin test-responsive animals spend an average of four weeks in this state before developing a positive skin test reaction [13,14,27]. Conlan et al. [28] estimated the median period of the latent non-skin test-responsive state at 28 days. As we used a monthly time step, it was thus not necessary to represent this health state. Infectious state *I* was defined by the presence of detectable lesions at slaughter. The type (open or stabilised) and the location of the lesions were not taken into account. This may induce an underestimation of within-herd transmission: an animal with so-called "open tuberculosis lesions" may infect the rest of the herd in a short period of time. However, much is unclear about open tuberculosis lesions, including the probability of developing this type of lesion, its duration and its infectivity [15]. Therefore we did not incorporate

the type of lesion in our model. This choice is in line with other epidemiological models of bTB [13–15].

Most of the models previously developed in the literature that simulated the within-herd spread of bTB used a single transmission parameter. In our model, we used two transmission parameters to distinguish transmission inside buildings and in pastures. Both transmission coefficients are related to herd practices, allowing to use the model for representing various farming systems by changing the grazing periods and the composition of batches. The within-herd transmission of bTB is considered higher in dairy herds than in beef herds [12]. This is attributed to a combination of several factors that contribute to the spread of infections in dairy herds such as the high contact rate, especially in the milking parlour [13], the high animal density and stress factors related to intense animal management [12,29–32]. The estimated value of β_{inside} was greater than that of $\beta_{outside}$ in 96% of cases, suggesting that the definition of two transmission coefficients allowed capturing the difference between dairy herds and beef herds in terms of within-herd transmission of bTB. Indeed, although the 95% credible intervals of the two within-herd transmission coefficients of bTB (β_{inside} and $\beta_{outside}$) overlapped, the median within-herd transmission coefficient inside the stable was 5 time as high as in the pasture: 0.43 month^{-1} [0,16–0.84] and 0.08 month^{-1} [0.01–0.32] for β_{inside} and $\beta_{outside}$, respectively. These estimated medians were consistent with the estimates of within-herd transmission of bTB in Spain proposed by Alvarez et al. [12], with higher transmission coefficients in dairy herds (median 0.39 month^{-1}) than in beef herds (0.19 month^{-1}). The estimated values of the transmission coefficients are also in the same range as values obtained by other studies: 0.22 month^{-1} in the study of Barlow et al. [13] and 0.18 months^{-1} in the study of Perez et al. in Argentina [2].

The only transmission route taken into account in our work is the direct transmission between animals of the same batch. Indirect transmission, the potential role of wildlife, contacts with cattle from other herds at pastures and contacts between cattle of different batches are not taken into account. In particular, between-batch disease transmission was not taken into account because we assumed that the probability of contact between animals of different batches was low: different batches of the same herd are often placed by the breeder on different and distant pastures and even sometimes in separate buildings. It should be noted that the transmission between batches does nevertheless occur in the model: as bTB is a chronic, slowly evolving disease, between-batch transmission occurs when animals are moved from one batch to another. However, the closed herd assumption would

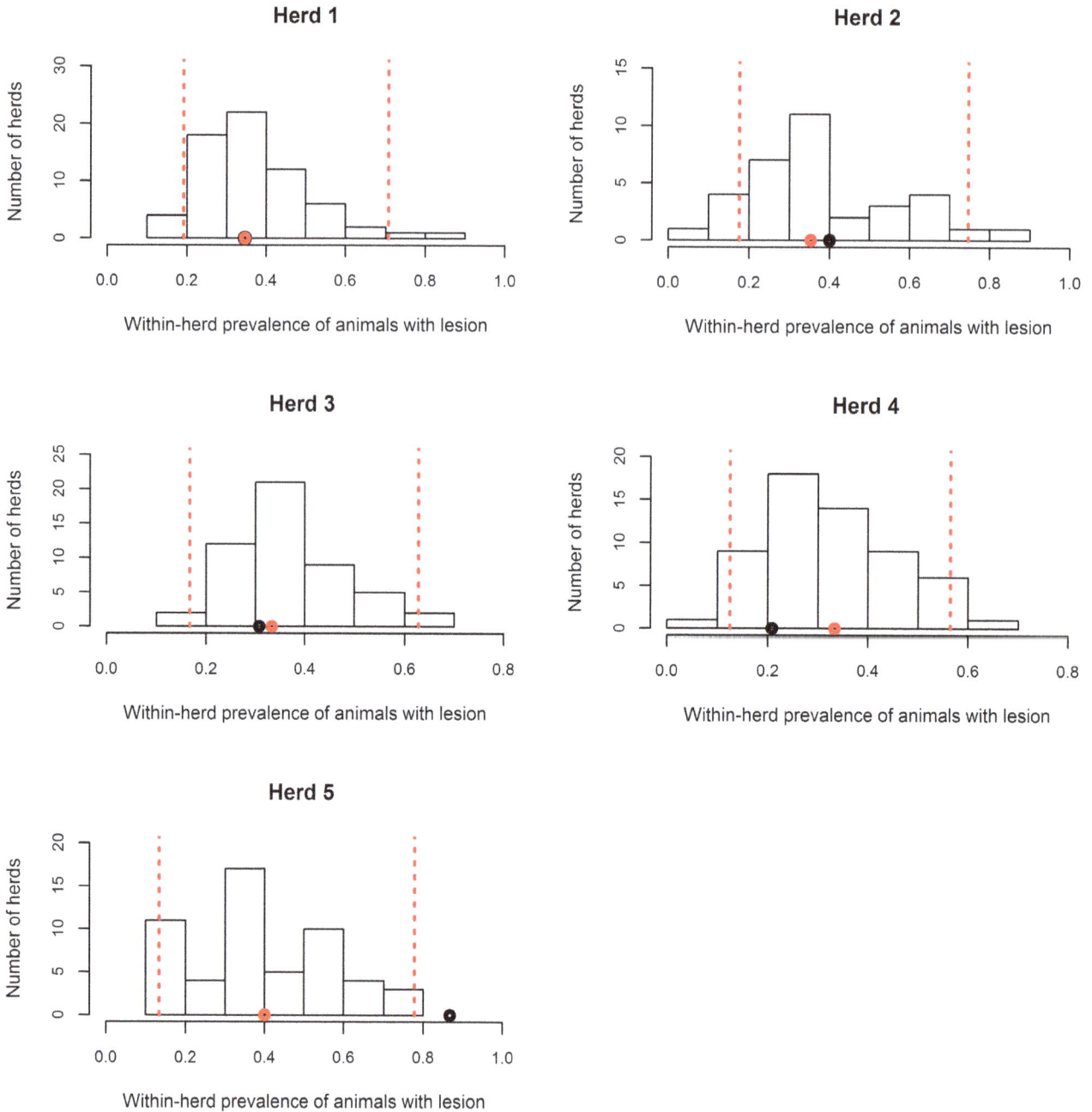

Figure 7. Observed and simulated proportions of animals with detected lesions when total slaughter is performed, for the 5 herds of dataset A. Black point: observed proportion of animals with bTB-like lesions in each herd; red point: simulated median proportion of animals with bTB-like lesions in each herd; dotted lines: 2.5% and 97.5% percentiles of the simulated distributions.

likely underestimate the persistence of *M. bovis* infection in herds, if wildlife or introduced animals can reintroduce infection [33].

The median duration of the estimated latency period (state *E*) was 3.5 months [2–8] months. This range of values is consistent with the chronic nature of bTB. However, our estimate of the latency duration was lower than the mean estimated duration of 24 months (95% confidence interval: 15–34 months) that was obtained by a simulation model of the within-herd transmission of bTB in Argentina [2]. This difference may be explained by differences among animals in the two countries, as the incubation period depends on the susceptibility of the host [34].

Model predictions for 2000 showed that the infected herds (dairy or beef) were in 15 to 20% of cases detected by slaughterhouse surveillance. This result was expected because the frequency of intradermal skin test applied in control program B was biennial. The percentage of spontaneous extinction of the disease (thanks to routine cull) was almost identical between dairy and beef herds.

When no control program was applied, simulated within-herd prevalence reached >50% in both types of farms. This simulated prevalence is high compared to the values observed in some parts of Africa and Asia (between 6% and 15%), where no control

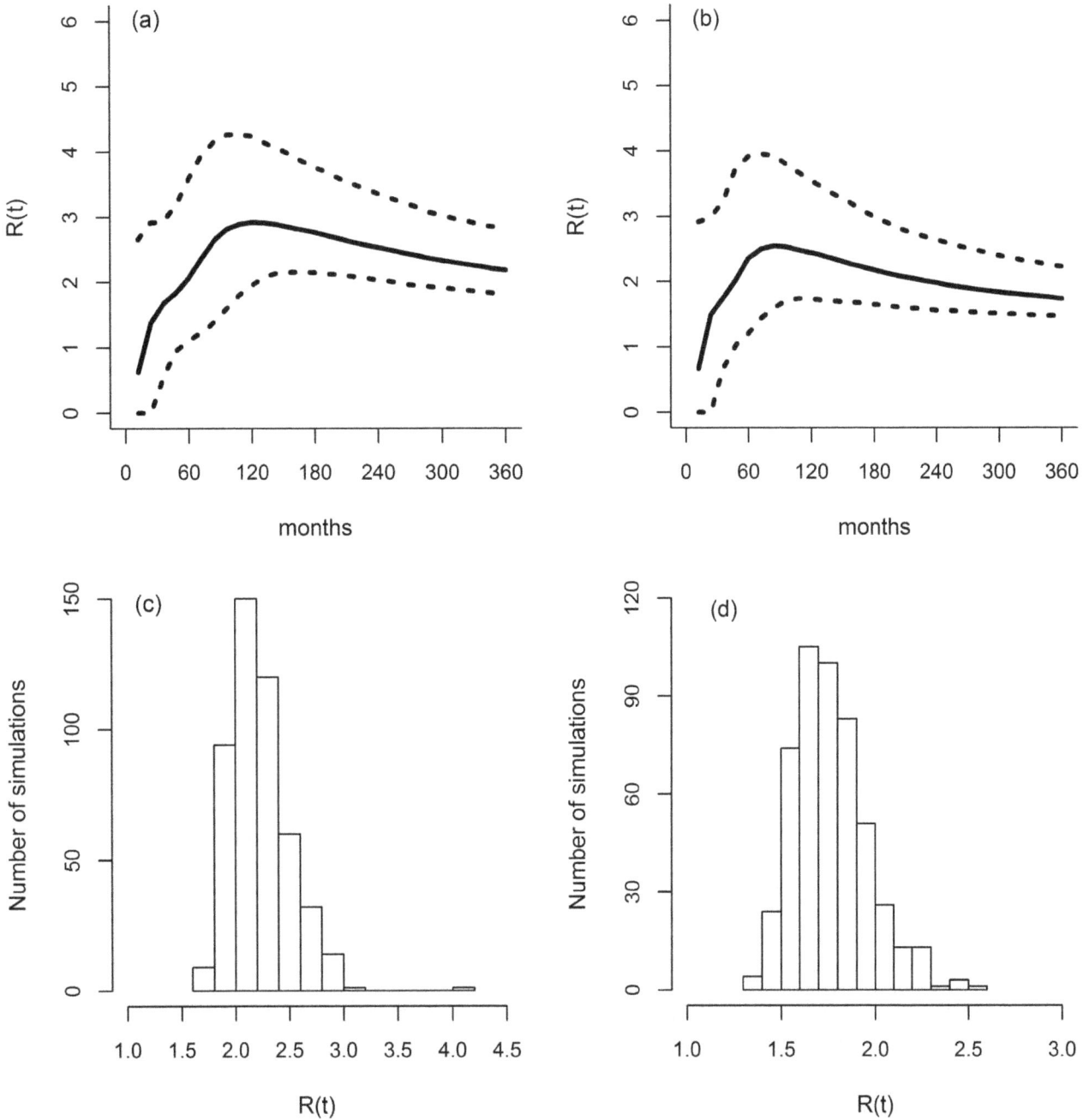

Figure 8. Monthly evolution of the simulated effective reproductive ratio R(t) (a and b), and distribution of this R(t) (c and d) when the disease has become enzootic (after 30 years) in standard French beef (a and c, 70 animals) and dairy (b and d, 81 animals) herds. Solid line: median; dashed: 2.5% and 97.5% percentiles.

program is applied [35,36]. In Africa and in Asia, most cattle are zebu (*B. indicus*) [37]. Ameni *et al.* [38] report that, under identical field husbandry conditions, a higher susceptibility to bTB was observed in Holstein cows than in zebus: (odds ratio: 2.32). In France dairy cattle are kept most of the time indoors, while beef cattle have stabling periods of approximately five months each year. Oppositely, in Africa and in Asia, cattle are most of the time kept outdoors, where contacts between animals are less intense than indoors, hence the lower observed within-herd prevalence in these regions.

The low predicted values of the effective reproductive ratio R(t) over time are consistent with field observations of a low bTB prevalence in French infected herds in the 2000s, and support the results of transmission trials indicating that cattle do not readily infect other cattle [39,40]. According to our estimation, when no control program is applied and once bTB has become enzootic within the herd, the median number of animals infected by an infectious animal is 2.2 in beef herds and 1.7 in dairy herds. This difference is due to a lower age at culling for dairy cows than for beef cows.

Several models have been proposed in the literature to simulate the dynamic of within-herd transmission of bTB: stochastic Reed-Frost model in discrete time [2,12], Reed-Frost model in continuous time [14], stochastic individual based model [15], compartmental stochastic model in continuous time [28] and compartmental stochastic model in discrete time [13,33,41]. We used a compartmental stochastic model operating in discrete time. Bovine TB health states are best represented using discrete health states (S-E-I), we thus chose to use a compartmental model. The scarcity and the discrete nature of the main simulated event which is the infection of animals (in a national survey in France between 2005 and 2007 in infected herds, the median of animals with lesion was 2), led us to use a stochastic approach rather than a deterministic approach. ABC methods are computationally cumbersome. Discrete time simulation was chosen as it appeared less computationally demanding than continuous time simulation. The duration of the time step (one month) was chosen because in literature the estimated duration of the latent state (in models with a single latent state [2] or with two states of latency [28]) was greater than one month. In addition, for the modeled screening, control and demographic processes, a one month time step also appeared satisfactory (frequency of tuberculin test, stabling period).

While this type of model is relatively easy to simulate, it is analytically difficult to manage when the number of states is high. In this case, numerical resolution by simulation is the only way to estimate the parameters [42]. The likelihood is difficult to calculate in our model, because the infection process is only partially observed (only a fraction of infectious animals is detected at the slaughterhouse, depending on the sensitivity of the visual inspection of carcasses). We thus chose to use the ABC method for the estimation of model parameters because this method does not require the calculation of the likelihood [43]. The choice of summary statistics and of the tolerance threshold are two sources of error in the ABC method [44]. To reduce errors linked to the choice of summary statistics, a preliminary step was performed in which several summary statistics were tested and compared using simulated data. Other methods have been proposed in the literature such as the algorithm developed by Barnes et al. [45] to choose a set of summary statistics from all possible summary statistics. This algorithm uses the mutual information as a selection tool [45]. Choosing a non-zero value for tolerance, ε, can bias the posterior estimation of the parameters [44]. To reduce errors due to non-zero values of ε, the local linear regression algorithm of the ABC method was used in our work for estimating the model parameters [19]. ABC-SMC (Sequential Monte Carlo) algorithm allows using specific methods to select the tolerance threshold [46,47]. But, according to Filippi et al. [48], more work needs to be done on the choice of tolerance threshold in the ABC-SMC algorithm. Besides, the use of the local linear regression algorithm is however not without problems, as the relationship between summary statistics and parameters is highly non-linear in most cases, which may bias the estimation of parameters [19].

The sensitivity analysis of a model is of great interest [42] because it helps to determine the most influential parameters. The sensitivity analysis performed here was used to independently assess the effect of fixed parameters values on the posterior parameter estimates. For practical reasons (of computation time required to perform this sensitivity analysis), the sensitivity analysis did not assess the effect of interactions among fixed parameters. Nevertheless, according to the literature, this method is the first step in exploring global associations (between the estimated and non-estimated parameters in the model), excluding interactions [49]. The results of the sensitivity analysis showed that fixed

parameters have only limited effects on the posterior parameter estimates, except for the effect of the specificity of ESAT-6 γIFN test on β_{inside}. The specificity of ESAT-6 γIFN test is used in control program C (Figure 3), which includes a 2-steps confirmation of positive SITT using γIFN test (steps 2 and 3 in Figure 3). When the specificity of ESAT-6 γIFN is increased to 100% (see Table 2), the overall specificity of the 3rd step of control program C also reaches 100% (see Figure 3). Because the overall sensitivity of both γIFN-based confirmation steps is low, the time required to detect bTB increases, which induces a decrease of β_{inside} estimate.

We assumed that the sensitivity and the specificity of the screening tests were independent of cattle age. Proaño-Perez et al. [50] reported a negative correlation between the age of cattle and the response to avian tuberculin. This result suggests that young animals are more likely to show false positive reactions to SITT than adult animals. The impact on our results is however likely to be limited, as the sensitivity analysis showed that the specificity of screening test had a little effect on the estimated values of the epidemiological model parameters (α, β_{inside} and $\beta_{outside}$).

In conclusion, the model proposed here has been designed to be generic enough to allow simulating various herd management systems and bTB detection and control programs. Its parameters have been estimated using field data and it has been validated using an independent dataset. In the future, this model will be used to analyse the impacts of changes of control programs and of herd management practices on the dynamics of bTB in France, between the beginning of the control program (in 1965) and obtaining the bTB-free status (in 2000). Besides, it will be used to assess the effectiveness of bTB control programs, in order to identify alternative strategies to the total slaughter protocol currently applied in infected herds.

Supporting Information

Figure S1 Control program A applied in the Nord department between 1981 and 1983. Step 1: yearly bTB screening using SITT (the herd being considered disease-free). All animals are tested (μ i,k Q(i,k) = 1). Sensitivity (Se) and specificity (Sp): those of SITT. Transition to step 2 if the proportion of positive animals exceeds a predefined threshold (n^{pos}/n^{test}>P.ab), one month later ($\Delta t = 1$ months). Transition to step 3 if positive results are observed, the proportion being below the threshold. Step 2: total slaughter. All the animals (μ i,k Q(i,k) = 1)are slaughtered (m = 1). Step 3: selective slaughter. Positive animals of step 1 (μ i Q(i,1) = 1)are slaughtered (m = 1). Transition to step 1, 6 months later. See table 2 for the definition of the other parameters.

Figure S2 Control program D applied in the Côte d'Or department between 2005 and 2009. Step 1: biennial bTB screening using SICCT (the herd being considered disease-free). All animals are tested (μ i,k Q(i,k) = 1). Sensitivity (Se) and specificity (Sp): those of SICCT. Immediate transition to step 2 if non-negative results are observed (n^{pos}>0). Step 2: interpretation of SICCT non-negative results. All the positive animals of step 1 (μ i Q(i,1) = 1) are concerned. Sensitivity: for an infected animal, probability that a non-negative positive result is not doubtful (pi: probability of a doubtful SICCT result for animals in health states E or I); specificity: for a susceptible animal, probability that a non-negative SICCT result is doubtful (ps: probability of a doubtful SICCT result for animals in health state S). Transition to step 3 if all the non-negative SICCT animals are doubtful, 2 months later; otherwise: transition to step 4, 3 months later. Step 3: confirmation of the positive results of step 1 using SICCT. All the positive animals of step 1 are tested (μ i Q(i,1) = 1), as well as 10% of the negative animals (i Q(i,0) = 0.1). Sensitivity (Se) and specificity (Sp): those of SICCT. Transition to step 5 if an animal is positive, three months later; otherwise: transition to step 1. Step 4: slaughter of the positive animals of step 2 and isolation of *M. bovis* from lesions. All the positive animals of step 2 (μ i Q(i,2) = 1) are slaughtered (m = 1) and bacterial culture is performed from observed lesions. Sensitivity (Se): sequential combination of a visual inspection at the slaughterhouse and of a bacterial culture. Transition to step 6 if an animal is positive, 1 month later (Δt = 1 month). Step 5: slaughter of the positive animals of step 3 and isolation of *M. bovis* from lesions. All the positive animals of step 3 (μ i Q(i,3) = 1) are slaughtered (m = 1) and bacterial culture is performed from observed lesions. Sensitivity (Se): sequential combination of a visual inspection at the slaughterhouse and of a bacterial culture. Transition to step 6 if an animal is positive, 1 month later (Δt = 1 month). Step 6: total slaughter. All the animals (μ i,k Q(i,k) = 1) are slaughtered (m = 1). Routine detection of lesions at slaughterhouse. Sensitivity (Se$_{ev}$): sequential combination of a visual inspection at the slaughterhouse and of a bacterial culture. If a positive animal is thus detected, regardless of the current stage of control program, transition to step 6. See table 2 for the definition of the other parameters.

Appendix S1 Model equations.

Appendix S2 Choice of summary statistics.

Appendix S3 Effective reproductive rate R(t).

Acknowledgments

The authors would like to thank the staff of the Departmental Director of Social Cohesion and Protection of Populations (DDCSPP) of Dordogne and the Departmental Director of Protection of Populations (DDPP) of Côte d'Or, for providing data. We would also like to thank Pr. Coureau from the Alfort National Veterinary School for giving us information on herd management practices in France.

Author Contributions

Conceived and designed the experiments: JJB AC BD MEAB. Performed the experiments: AC BD MEAB. Analyzed the data: BD MEAB. Contributed reagents/materials/analysis tools: JJB BD. Contributed to the writing of the manuscript: AC BD MEAB.

References

1. Radostits OM, Blood DC, Gay CC, Arundel JH, Ikede BO, et al. (1994) Veterinary Medicine: A Textbook of the Diseases of Cattle, Sheep, Pigs, Goats and Horses. London: Bailliere Tindall. 1763 p.
2. Perez AM, Ward MP, Charmandarian A, Ritacco V (2002) Simulation model of within-herd transmission of bovine tuberculosis in Argentine dairy herds. Prev Vet Med 54: 361–372.
3. Reynolds D (2006) A review of tuberculosis science and policy in Great Britain. Vet Microbiol 112: 119–126.
4. de la Rua-Domenech R (2006) Bovine Tuberculosis in the European Union and other countries: current status, control programmes and constrains to eradication. Gov Vet J 16: 19–45.
5. Wahlstrom H, Carpenter T, Giesecke J, Andersson M, Englund L, et al. (2000) Herd-based monitoring for tuberculosis in extensive swedish deer herds by culling and meat inspection rather than by intradermal tuberculin testing. Prev Vet Med 43: 103–116.
6. Cousins DV (2001) Mycobacterium bovis infection and control in domestic livestock. Rev Sci Tech 20: 71–85.
7. Bekara ME, Azizi L, Benet JJ, Durand B (2014) Spatial-temporal Variations of Bovine Tuberculosis Incidence in France between 1965 and 2000. Transbound Emerg Dis.
8. de la Rua-Domenech R, Goodchild AT, Vordermeier HM, Hewinson RG, Christiansen KH, et al. (2006) Ante mortem diagnosis of tuberculosis in cattle: a review of the tuberculin tests, gamma-interferon assay and other ancillary diagnostic techniques. Res Vet Sci 81: 190–210.
9. Corner LA (1994) Post mortem diagnosis of Mycobacterium bovis infection in cattle. Vet Microbiol 40: 53–63.
10. de Jong MCM (1995) Mathematical modelling in veterinary epidemiology: why model building is important. Prev Vet Med 25: 183–193.
11. Smith S, Anders B (1994) Mycobacterium mastoiditis caused by Mycobacterium bovis. Pediatr Infect Dis J 13: 538–539.
12. Alvarez J, Perez AM, Bezos J, Casal C, Romero B, et al. (2012) Eradication of bovine tuberculosis at a herd-level in Madrid, Spain: study of within-herd transmission dynamics over a 12 year period. BMC Vet Res 8: 100.
13. Barlow ND, Kean JM, Hickling G, Livingstone PG, Robson AB (1997) A simulation model for the spread of bovine tuberculosis within New Zealand cattle herds. Prev Vet Med 32: 57–75.
14. Griffin JM, Williams DH, Collins JD (1999) Tuberculosis Investigation Unit, University College Dublin. Selected papers: 55–58.
15. Fischer EA, van Roermund HJ, Hemerik L, van Asseldonk MA, de Jong MC (2005) Evaluation of surveillance strategies for bovine tuberculosis (Mycobacterium bovis) using an individual based epidemiological model. Prev Vet Med 67: 283–301.
16. Kao RR, Roberts MG, Ryan TJ (1997) A model of bovine tuberculosis control in domesticated cattle herds. Proc Biol Sci 264: 1069–1076.
17. Carnon F (1985) Contribution à l'étude épidémiologique de la tuberculose bovine dans le département du Nord. Maisons-Alfort: Ecole Nationale Vétérinaire d'Alfort. 210 p.
18. Toni T, Welch D, Strelkowa N, Ipsen A, Stumpf MP (2009) Approximate Bayesian computation scheme for parameter inference and model selection in dynamical systems. J R Soc Interface 6: 187–202.
19. Beaumont MA, Zhang W, Balding DJ (2002) Approximate Bayesian computation in population genetics. Genetics 162: 2025–2035.
20. Neill SD, Hanna J, Mackie DP, Bryson TG (1992) Isolation of Mycobacterium bovis from the respiratory tracts of skin test-negative cattle. Vet Rec 131: 45–47.
21. Aeschbacher S, Beaumont MA, Futschik A (2012) A novel approach for choosing summary statistics in approximate Bayesian computation. Genetics 192: 1027–1047.
22. Csillery K, Blum MG, Gaggiotti OE, Francois O (2010) Approximate Bayesian Computation (ABC) in practice. Trends Ecol Evol 25: 410–418.
23. Beaumont MA (2010) Approximate Bayesian computation in evolution and ecology. Annual Review of Ecology, Evolution, and Systematics 41: 379–406.
24. Csilléry K, François O, Blum MGB (2012) abc: an R package for approximate Bayesian computation (ABC). Methods in Ecology and Evolution 3: 475–479.
25. R Development Core Team (2013) R: A language and environment for statistical computing. Vienna, Austria: R Foundation for Statistical Computing.
26. Anderson RM, May RM (1991) Infectious diseases of humans: dynamics and control. Oxford and New York: Oxford University Press. 768 p.
27. Kleeberg HH (1960) The tuberculin test in cattle. J South African Vet Med Assoc 31: 213–225.
28. Conlan AJ, McKinley TJ, Karolemeas K, Pollock EB, Goodchild AV, et al. (2012) Estimating the hidden burden of bovine tuberculosis in Great Britain. PLoS Comput Biol 8: e1002730.
29. Karolemeas K, McKinley TJ, Clifton-Hadley RS, Goodchild AV, Mitchell A, et al. (2011) Recurrence of bovine tuberculosis breakdowns in Great Britain: risk factors and prediction. PrevVet Med 102: 22–29.
30. Porphyre T, Stevenson MA, McKenzie J (2008) Risk factors for bovine tuberculosis in New Zealand cattle farms and their relationship with possum control strategies. PrevVet Med 86: 93–106.
31. Ramirez-Villaescusa AM, Medley GF, Mason S, Green LE (2010) Risk factors for herd breakdown with bovine tuberculosis in 148 cattle herds in the south west of England. PrevVet Med 95: 224–230.
32. Vial F, Johnston WT, Donnelly CA (2011) Local cattle and badger populations affect the risk of confirmed tuberculosis in British cattle herds. PLoS One 6: e18058.
33. Smith RL, Schukken YH, Lu Z, Mitchell RM, Grohn YT (2013) Development of a model to simulate infection dynamics of Mycobacterium bovis in cattle herds in the United States. J Am Vet Med Assoc 243: 411–423.
34. Hagan WA, Bruner DW, Gillespie JH (1973) Hagan's Infectious diseases of domestic animals: with special reference to etiology, diagnosis, and biologic therapy. Californie: Comstock Pub. Associates. 1385 p.
35. Gumi B, Schelling E, Firdessa R, Aseffa A, Tschopp R, et al. (2011) Prevalence of bovine tuberculosis in pastoral cattle herds in the Oromia region, southern Ethiopia. Trop Anim Health Prod 43: 1081–1087.
36. Thakur A, Sharma M, Katoch VC, Dhar P, Katoch RC (2010) A study on the prevalence of Bovine Tuberculosis in farmed dairy cattle in Himachal Pradesh. Vet World 3: 408–413.
37. Ameni G, Aseffa A, Engers H, Young D, Hewinson G, et al. (2006) Cattle husbandry in Ethiopia is a predominant factor affecting the pathology of bovine tuberculosis and gamma interferon responses to mycobacterial antigens. Clin Vaccine Immunol 13: 1030–1036.

38. Ameni G, Aseffa A, Engers H, Young D, Gordon S, et al. (2007) High prevalence and increased severity of pathology of bovine tuberculosis in Holsteins compared to zebu breeds under field cattle husbandry in central Ethiopia. Clin Vaccine Immunol 14: 1356–1361.

39. Costello E, Doherty ML, Monaghan ML, Quigley FC, O'Reilly PF (1998) A study of cattle-to-cattle transmission of Mycobacterium bovis infection. Vet J 155: 245–250.

40. O'Reilly LM, Costello E (1988) Bovine tuberculosis with special reference to the epidemiological significance of pulmonary lesions. Irish Veterinary News: 11–21.

41. Brooks-Pollock E, Roberts GO, Keeling MJ (2014) A dynamic model of bovine tuberculosis spread and control in Great Britain. Nature 511: 228–231.

42. Pouillot R, Dufour B, Durand B (2004) A deterministic and stochastic simulation model for intra-herd paratuberculosis transmission. Vet Res 35: 53–68.

43. Tanaka MM, Francis AR, Luciani F, Sisson SA (2006) Using approximate Bayesian computation to estimate tuberculosis transmission parameters from genotype data. Genetics 173: 1511–1520.

44. Sunnaker M, Busetto AG, Numminen E, Corander J, Foll M, et al. (2013) Approximate Bayesian computation. PLoS Comput Biol 9: e1002803.

45. Barnes C, Filippi S, Stumpf MPH, Thorne T (2012) Considerate approaches to constructing summary statistics for ABC model selection. Statistics and Computing 22: 1181–1197.

46. Del Moral P, Doucet A, Jasra A (2012) An adaptive sequential Monte Carlo method for approximate Bayesian computation. Statistics and Computing 22: 1009–1020.

47. Drovandi CC, Pettitt AN (2011) Estimation of parameters for macroparasite population evolution using approximate bayesian computation. Biometrics 67: 225–233.

48. Filippi S, Barnes CP, Cornebise J, Stumpf MP (2013) On optimality of kernels for approximate Bayesian computation using sequential Monte Carlo. Stat Appl Genet Mol Biol 12: 87–107.

49. Vose D (2000) Risk Analysis, A quantitative guide. Chichester: Wiley and Sons. 752 p.

50. Proano-Perez F, Benitez-Ortiz W, Celi-Erazo M, Ron-Garrido L, Benitez-Capistros R, et al. (2009) Comparative intradermal tuberculin test in dairy cattle in the north of Ecuador and risk factors associated with bovine tuberculosis. Am J Trop Med Hyg 81: 1103–1109.

51. Pollock JM, Girvin RM, Lightbody KA, Clements RA, Neill SD, et al. (2000) Assessment of defined antigens for the diagnosis of bovine tuberculosis in skin test-reactor cattle. Vet Rec 146: 659–665.

52. Courcoul A, Moyen JL, Brugere L, Faye S, Henault S, et al. (2014) Estimation of sensitivity and specificity of bacteriology, histopathology and PCR for the confirmatory diagnosis of bovine tuberculosis using latent class analysis. PLoS One 9: e90334.

15

Demographic Model of the Swiss Cattle Population for the Years 2009-2011 Stratified by Gender, Age and Production Type

Sara Schärrer[1]*, Patrick Presi[1], Jan Hattendorf[2], Nakul Chitnis[2,3], Martin Reist[4], Jakob Zinsstag[2]

1 Veterinary Public Health Institute/University of Berne, Berne, Switzerland, 2 Swiss Tropical and Public Health Institute/University of Basel, Basel, Switzerland, 3 Fogarty International Center, National Institutes of Health, Bethesda, Maryland, United States of America, 4 Federal Food Safety and Veterinary Office, Bern, Switzerland

Abstract

Demographic composition and dynamics of animal and human populations are important determinants for the transmission dynamics of infectious disease and for the effect of infectious disease or environmental disasters on productivity. In many circumstances, demographic data are not available or of poor quality. Since 1999 Switzerland has been recording cattle movements, births, deaths and slaughter in an animal movement database (AMD). The data present in the AMD offers the opportunity for analysing and understanding the dynamic of the Swiss cattle population. A dynamic population model can serve as a building block for future disease transmission models and help policy makers in developing strategies regarding animal health, animal welfare, livestock management and productivity. The Swiss cattle population was therefore modelled using a system of ordinary differential equations. The model was stratified by production type (dairy or beef), age and gender (male and female calves: 0–1 year, heifers and young bulls: 1–2 years, cows and bulls: older than 2 years). The simulation of the Swiss cattle population reflects the observed pattern accurately. Parameters were optimized on the basis of the goodness-of-fit (using the Powell algorithm). The fitted rates were compared with calculated rates from the AMD and differed only marginally. This gives confidence in the fitted rates of parameters that are not directly deductible from the AMD (e.g. the proportion of calves that are moved from the dairy system to fattening plants).

Editor: Edna Hillmann, ETH Zurich, Switzerland

Funding: The study was funded as part of a PhD project by the Swiss Federal Veterinary Office. The funders had no role in study design, data collection and analysis, decision to publish, or preparation of the manuscript.

Competing Interests: The authors have declared that no competing interests exist.

* Email: sara.schaerrer@vetsuisse.unibe.ch

Introduction

Switzerland has been collecting data about cattle including date of birth, date of slaughter, date of death (other than slaughter for consumption) and information regarding movements on a mandatory basis since 1999. The purpose of a national database of animal movements was originally to restore consumer trust during the BSE crisis by assuring traceability and therefore a better food safety of beef products and to provide a tool for epizootic disease surveillance and control [1,2]. The AMD contains detailed and complete datasets about the Swiss cattle population for several years offering the opportunity to get an insight into the population dynamics. Understanding the demographic of the livestock population in turn provides accurate parameters needed to develop models of disease transmission and helps policy makers in developing strategies regarding animal health, animal welfare and livestock management [3].

Early detection of disease, monitoring of present agents and substantiation of freedom from disease are described as key tasks of modern public veterinary services in order to allow international trade with agricultural goods and to document a good sanitary status of domestic livestock [4–6].

To monitor the health status of the cattle population, the Swiss veterinary authorities invest substantial resources in yearly surveillance programmes that have to meet international standards. One way to maintain the standards while reducing the costs is the application of risk based targeted approaches (e.g. [7]). Other approaches comprise logistical improvements such as better exploiting infrastructures where already a lot of potential information carriers are available e.g. slaughterhouse or milk quality testing laboratories [8]. With the implementation of bulk milk testing in 2010 [9,10] the production type became an important criterion for shaping the sampling strategy of national surveillance programs. As beef and fattening cattle, correspond to one third of the population, they have to be handled separately. The two production types (dairy and beef) do not only differ with respect to purpose but also with respect to management practices. The resulting differences in age distribution and slaughter rates in the two sub populations are of interest for the planning of stratified surveillance programmes to assure the representativeness of the sample (e.g. for sampling at the slaughterhouse level).

The objective of this study was therefore to create an AMD data driven demographic model that simulates the age and gender specific dynamics of the Swiss cattle population according to the production type. The derived rates describing population dynamics can be used for livestock development planning and associated economic analyses, as a backbone for disease transmission models

Table 1. The Swiss cattle population 2009–2011.

Year	No of farms	No of cattle (January 1th)	No of dairy cows (January 1th)	No of slaughtered animals	No of births
2009	42'966	1'608'062	675'285	647'715	721'810
2010	42'233	1'610'277	671'874	648'313	719'004
2011	41'465	1'612'230	676'253	653'754	718'697

Numbers are extracted from the Swiss animal movement database (AMD).

or for the design of cost-effective disease control and monitoring programmes.

Here we present the first dynamic demographic model of the Swiss cattle population. It is based on over 30 million data points collected in the Swiss animal movement database (AMD) between 2009 and 2011.

Materials and Methods

2.1 The Swiss cattle population

The major livestock species in Switzerland is cattle. Although the number of farms decreases, for the years 2009–2011 the number of cattle in Switzerland is stable at roughly 1.6 million animals (table 1). Two thirds of the Swiss cattle industry is dedicated to dairy production. As a consequence, adult dairy cows (older than two years) make the largest demographic segment (figure 1). The average lifespan of a dairy cow in Switzerland is 6.2 years and the average number of calves in a lifetime is 3.7. The oldest cow that died between 2009 and 2011 was 25 years old.

Due to subsidies for ecological and behaviourally sound husbandry and strict animal protection legislation, small holdings with less than hundred animals are still the most common farm type. Over the summer month (May–October) one fourth of the livestock is moved to alpine pastures.

2.2 Data management

The Swiss animal movement database (AMD) contains information on farm level (e.g. location, production type), animal level (e.g. birthdate, gender, and breed), movement records (date, movement type) and stays (i.e. for every animal the start and end date of a stay on any holding is recorded). The data used for the models was an extract from the AMD, containing all recorded movements (25.5 million entries) and stays (15.8 million entries) from January 1999 until January 2012.

Birthdate, date of death (slaughter or natural) and gender are recorded on individual animal level, while the production type is available on farm level. The production type for each animal was consequently determined by the farm it stayed on at the given time step. Calf mortality consisted of notified stillbirths and mortality. As stays on alpine pastures are recorded only since 2008 and the quality of those recordings improved notably in 2009, only data from 2009 to 2011 was used for fitting of the population model.

2.3 The model

The Swiss cattle population was simulated using a system dynamic software [11]. The model is composed of a series of coupled difference equations. Compartments were defined by production type (dairy or beef), age class and gender. Calves were defined as animal being less than one year old, heifer and young bulls as one to two years old and cows and bulls as older than two years. We assumed that cows calve for the first time at the age of two and therefore the category "heifer" doesn't contribute to births. The beef and dairy system are connected through the transfer of calves from dairy farms to fattening plants, which is represented in the model as "fattening". The model is represented in figure 2.

The dynamic of the cattle population is simulated by month as time unit. Equations (1)–(12) show the number of animals per compartment (for parameter notation see table 2 and 3).

To represent the seasonal fluctuations in the number of births and death calves, we used a sinusodial-function with amplitude (a), phase (φ) and average (μ) as parameters to fit (equations (13)–(20)). The frequency (ω) was set to $\frac{2\pi}{12}$.

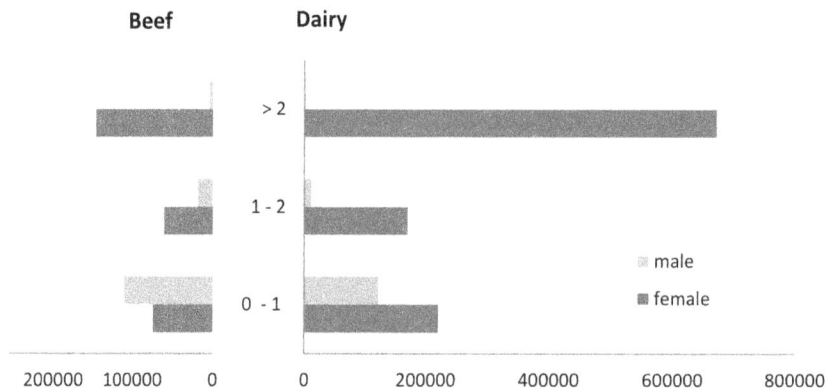

Figure 1. Demographic of the Swiss cattle population per age class and sex in number of animals.

$$\frac{dX_{DF}(t)}{dt} = b_{XDF}(t)*Z_{DF} - (m_{XDF}(t) \\ + s_{XDF} + f_{XDF} + tr_{XDF}) * X_{DF} \tag{1}$$

$$\frac{dY_{DM}(t)}{dt} = tr_{XDM} * X_{DM} - (m_{YDM} + s_{YDM} + tr_{YDM})*Y_{DM} \tag{6}$$

$$\frac{dY_{BF}(t)}{dt} = tr_{XBF} * X_{BF} - (m_{YBF} + s_{YBF} + tr_{YBF}) * Y_{BF} \tag{7}$$

$$\frac{dX_{DM}(t)}{dt} = b_{XDM}(t)*Z_{DF} - (m_{XDM}(t) \\ + s_{XDM} + f_{XDM} + tr_{XDM}) * X_{DM} \tag{2}$$

$$\frac{dY_{BM}(t)}{dt} = tr_{XBM} * X_{DF} - (m_{YBM} + s_{YBM} + tr_{YBM}) * Y_{BM} \tag{8}$$

$$\frac{dX_{BF}(t)}{dt} = b_{XBF}(t)*Z_{BF} + f_{XDF} * X_{DF} \\ - (m_{XBF}(t) + s_{XBF} + tr_{XBF}) * X_{BF} \tag{3}$$

$$\frac{dZ_{DF}(t)}{dt} = tr_{YDF} * Y_{DF} - (m_{ZDF} + s_{ZDF}) * Z_{DF} \tag{9}$$

$$\frac{dX_{BM}(t)}{dt} = b_{XBM}(t)*Z_{BF} + f_{XDM} * X_{DM} \\ - (m_{XBM}(t) + s_{XBM} + tr_{XBM}) * X_{BM} \tag{4}$$

$$\frac{dZ_{DM}(t)}{dt} = tr_{YDM} * Y_{DM} - (m_{ZDM} + s_{ZDM}) * Z_{DM} \tag{10}$$

$$\frac{dY_{DF}(t)}{dt} = tr_{XDF} * X_{DF} - (m_{YDF} + s_{YDF} + tr_{YDF}) * Y_{DF} \tag{5}$$

$$\frac{dZ_{BF}(t)}{dt} = tr_{YBF} * Y_{BF} - (m_{ZBF} + s_{ZBF}) * Z_{BF} \tag{11}$$

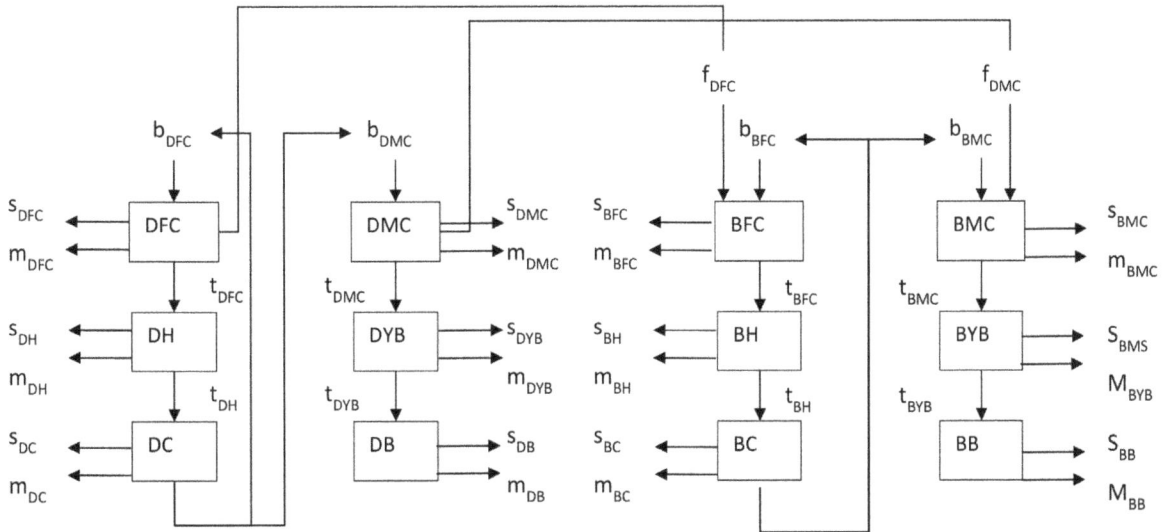

Figure 2. Schematic representation of the Vensim model. Arrows represent flows of animals into or out of a compound, boxes represents numbers of animals at a given time point in a category. s: slaughter; m: mortality; b: birth; tr: transition; f: fattening; D: dairy; B: beef; F: female; M: male; X: calves; Y: subadults; Z: adults.

Table 2. Nomenclature for subscripts in Equations 1–12.

	Description	type
X	Calves	age class
Y	Subadults	age class
Z	Adults	age class
D	Dairy	production type
B	Beef	production type
F	Female	gender
M	Male	gender

$$\frac{dZ_{BM}(t)}{dt} = tr_{YBM} * Y_{BM} - (m_{ZBM} + s_{ZBM}) * Z_{BM} \quad (12)$$

$$m_{XDM}(t) = \mu_{2XDM} + a_{2XDM} * \sin(t * \omega + \varphi_{2XDM}) \quad (16)$$

$$b_{XDF}(t) = \mu_{1XDF} + a_{1XDF} * \sin(t * \omega + \varphi_{1XDF}) \quad (13)$$

$$b_{XBF}(t) = \mu_{1XBF} + a_{1XBF} * \sin(t * \omega + \varphi_{1XBF}) \quad (17)$$

$$m_{XDF}(t) = \mu_{2XDF} + a_{2XDF} * \sin(t * \omega + \varphi_{2XDF}) \quad (14)$$

$$m_{XBF}(t) = \mu_{2XBF} + a_{2XBF} * \sin(t * \omega + \varphi_{2XBF}) \quad (18)$$

$$b_{XDM}(t) = \mu_{1XDM} + a_{1XDM} * \sin(t * \omega + \varphi_{1XDM}) \quad (15)$$

$$b_{XBM}(t) = \mu_{1XBM} + a_{1XBM} * \sin(t * \omega + \varphi_{1XBM}) \quad (19)$$

$$m_{XBM}(t) = \mu_{2XBM} + a_{2XBM} * \sin(t * \omega + \varphi_{2XBM}) \quad (20)$$

Table 3. Compartments and parameters in Equations 1–12.

	Description	Unit
X	No of calves	Animals
Y	No of subadults	Animals
Z	No of adults	Animals
s	slaughter rate	month^{-1}
m	mortality rate	month^{-1}
b	birth rate	month^{-1}
tr	transition rate	month^{-1}
f	fattening rate	month^{-1}
μ	Average	month^{-1}
a	Amplitude	month^{-1}
ω	Frequency	month^{-1}
φ	Phase	Dimensionless

Table 4. Monthly population parameters for the Swiss cattle population.

		Dairy			Beef		
			Month^{-1}	95%-CI		Month^{-1}	95%-CI
slaughter rates	Female calf	s_{XDF}	0.0197	[0.0192, 0.0201]	s_{XBF}	0.0396	[0.0389, 0.0403]
	Heifer	s_{YDF}	0.0065	[0.0062, 0.0069]	s_{YBF}	0.0261	[0.0253, 0.0269]
	Cow	s_{ZDF}	0.0190	[0.0189, 0.0191]	s_{ZBF}	0.0233	[0.0231, 0.0235]
	Male calf	s_{XDM}	0.1123	[0.1103, 0.1144]	s_{XBM}	0.0638	[0.0631, 0.0645]
	Young bull	s_{YDM}	0.1702	[0.1658, 0.1748]	s_{YBM}	0.2834	[0.2768, 0.2902]
	Bull	s_{ZDM}	0.1113	[0.1072, 0.1156]	s_{ZBM}	0.0606	[0.0590, 0.0623]
mortality rates	Female calf	μ_{2XDF}	0.0094	[0.0089, 0.0098]	μ_{2XBF}	0.0059	[0.0055, 0.0062]
	Heifer	m_{YDF}	0.0007	[0.0006, 0.0007]	m_{YBF}	0.0008	[0.0007, 0.0009]
	Cow	m_{ZDF}	0.0013	[0.0012, 0.0013]	m_{ZBF}	0.0013	[0.0013, 0.0014]
	Male calf	μ_{2XDM}	0.0255	[0.0241, 0.0269]	μ_{2XBM}	0.0074	[0.0071, 0.0078]
	Young bull	m_{YDM}	0.0017	[0.0015, 0.0019]	m_{YBM}	0.0017	[0.0015, 0.0019]
	Bull	m_{ZDM}	0.0022	[0.0016, 0.0028]	m_{ZBM}	0.0026	[0.0021, 0.0031]
transition rates	Female calf	tr_{XDF}	0.0684	[0.0678, 0.0689]	tr_{XBF}	0.0718	[0.0710, 0.0725]
	Heifer	tr_{YDF}	0.0804	[0.0797, 0.0812]	tr_{YBF}	0.0615	[0.0607, 0.0624]
	Male calf	tr_{XDM}	0.0207	[0.0203, 0.0212]	tr_{XBM}	0.0511	[0.0505, 0.0518]
	Young bull	tr_{YDM}	0.0234	[0.0226, 0.0243]	tr_{YBM}	0.0161	[0.0157, 0.0165]
fattening rates	Female calf	f_{XDF}	0.0172	[0.0170, 0.0175]			
	Male calf	f_{XDM}	0.0731	[0.0722, 0.0740]			
birth rates	Female calf	μ_{1XDF}	0.0374	[0.0373, 0.0376]	μ_{1XBF}	0.0335	[0.0332, 0.0339]
	Male calf	μ_{1XDM}	0.0392	[0.0389, 0.0396]	μ_{1XBM}	0.0352	[0.0347, 0.0357]

D: dairy; B: beef; F: female; M: male; X: calf, Y: subadult, Z: adult. Small letters indicate rates (s: slaughter, m: mortality, f: fattening, tr: transition to next age class). μ1: average birth rate; μ2: average mortality rate;

Table 5. Values for the amplitudes and phases in the trigonometric functions of the presented Swiss cattle population model.

	Dairy			Beef	
		95%-CI			95%-CI
a_{1XDF}	0.0031	[0.0022, 0.0041]	a_{1XBF}	0.0009	[0, 0.0023]
a_{1XDM}	0.0091	[0.0073, 0.0109]	a_{1XBM}	0.0040	[0.0024, 0.0056]
a_{2XDF}	0.0029	[0.0020, 0.0038]	a_{2XBF}	0.0013	[0.0008, 0.0018]
a_{2XDM}	0.0063	[0.0037, 0.0088]	a_{2XBM}	0.0016	[0.0010, 0.0022]
φ_{1XDF}	1.6799	[1.4046, 1.9574]	φ_{1XBF}	2.9510	[1.1437, 4.7768]
φ_{1XDM}	1.9245	[1.7428, 2.1096]	φ_{1XBM}	2.4772	[2.0699, 2.8935]
φ_{2XDF}	1.6576	[1.3443, 1.9727]	φ_{2XBF}	1.0713	[0.6834, 1.4582]
φ_{2XDM}	1.7900	[1.3820, 2.1969]	φ_{2XBM}	0.9218	[0.5575, 1.2856]

D: dairy; B: beef; F: female; M: male; X: calf, Y: subadult, Z: adult. a 1: amplitude for birth rate; a 2: amplitude for mortality rate; φ_1: phase for birth rate; φ_2: phase for mortality rate;

2.3.1 Model fitting. The number of living animals was extracted at the beginning of each month, number of birth, slaughter and death from the AMD per month, age class, production type and gender from January 2009 to December 2011. This data-set served to optimize the model parameters on the basis of the goodness-of-fit of the nonlinear maximum-likelihood optimization using the Powell algorithm [12]. Parameters were fitted stepwise, adding a variable at every step to the payoff values, using the outcome rates from the previous step as

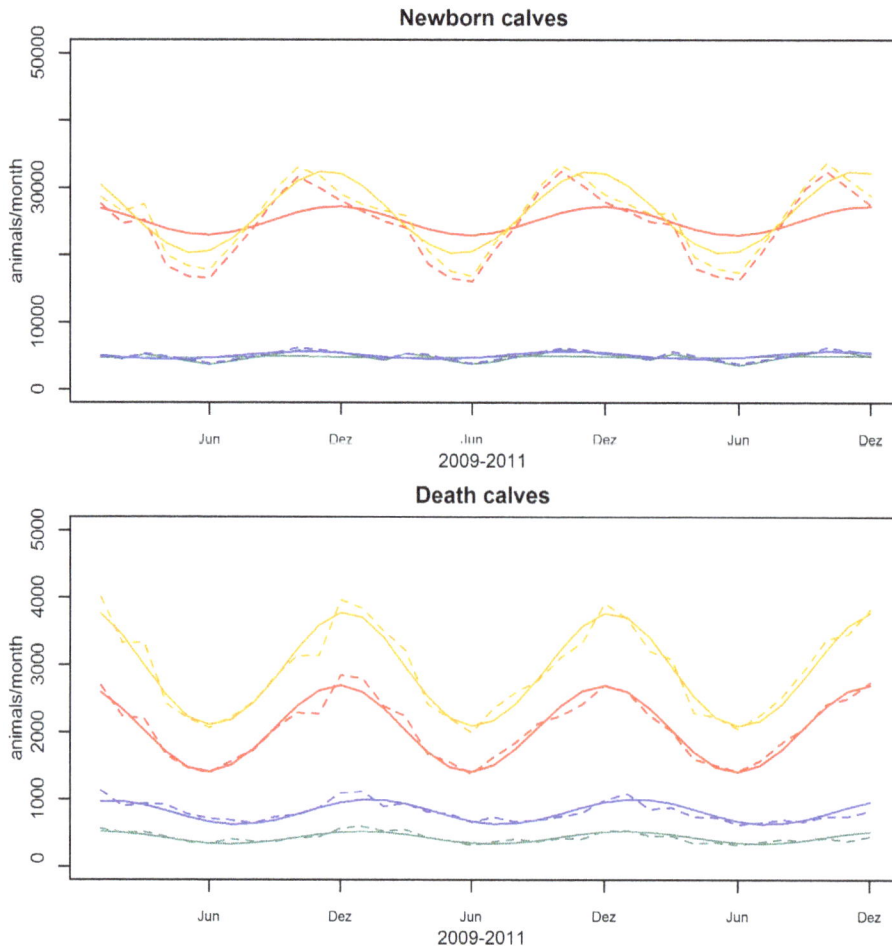

Figure 3. Seasonal pattern of birth and mortality in calves. Solid line: model data, dashed lines: AMD data. Orange: dairy male calf, red: dairy female calf, blue: beef male calf, green: beef female calf.

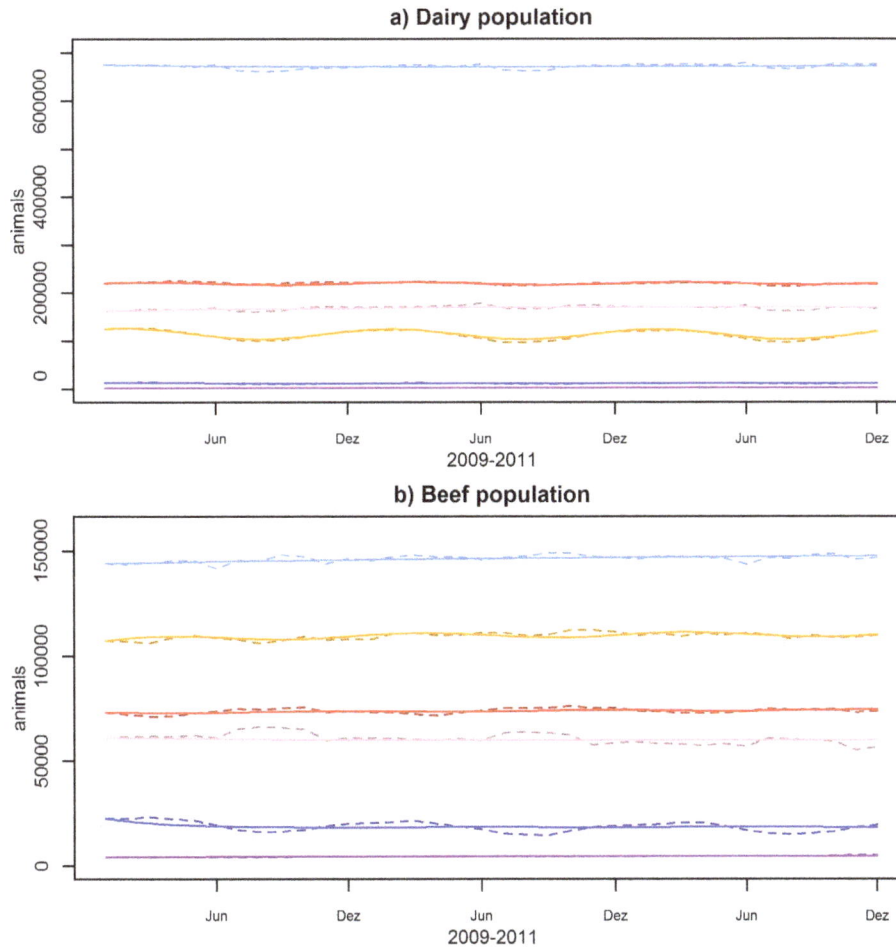

Figure 4. Animal numbers per age category. a) Dairy population. b) Beef population. Solid line: model data, dashed lines: AMD data. Light blue: cow, orange: male calf, red: female calf, pink: heifer, blue: young bull, purple: bull.

initial search point (maximum and minimum values set to +/− 10%).

2.3.2 Comparison of calculated and fitted rates. Birth, slaughter and mortality rates were calculated from the AMD data and compared to the fitted values from the model. Average birth rates were calculated as number of calves per month and category divided by the number of cows on the first of the months of the according production type and averaged over the 3 years period. Mortality and slaughter rates were calculated as number of death or slaughtered animals per month divided by the number of animals of the same age category and production type on the first of the month and averaged over the 3 years period. Model and empirical estimates were correlated in R [13].

2.3.3 Sensitivity analysis. The model was rebuilt with the statistical software R. To assess the sensitivity of the model, each parameter was varied separately using a range from −10% to +10% of the fitted value from the Vensim model (baseline), divided in 100 steps. For each value, the resulting absolute change in total numbers of animals compared to the baseline was represented graphically (Figures S1–S10, supplementary material).

Results

In table 4 the fitted parameter values from the demographic model are shown. The model allowed the calculation of parameters that are not directly deductible from the AMD (transition rates and fattening rates).

By introducing parameters (amplitude and phase, table 5) to describe calf mortality and birth rates as trigonometric functions, the seasonal dynamic of changes in the population can be described more accurately than with the corresponding linear parameters deducted from the monthly extracts of the AMD (figure 3).

The correlation of the empirical parameters from the AMD and the fitted values gives a correlation coefficient of 0.994. The good fit of the model to the empirical data is also illustrated in figure 4.

As expected, the beef and dairy sector show differences in the demographic composition. While the proportions of young female animals are comparable (18.5% dairy female calves, 17.8% beef female calves 14.2% dairy heifers and 14.6% beef heifers), dairy cows account for around 56.7% of the dairy population while beef cows account for 35.5% of the beef population. For male animals the differences are even more noticeable: beef male calves, young bulls and bulls make 26.5%, 4.6% and 1.1% of the beef population compared to 9.6%, 1.0% and 0.2% for dairy male calves, dairy young bulls and dairy bulls respectively (all proportions are means over the 36 month of data analysis).

As import and export of live cattle are negligible for Switzerland (6'787 imported animals from 2009 to 2011 and 3'318 exported animals over the same period), the beef population is maintained

Calf restocking in the beef sector

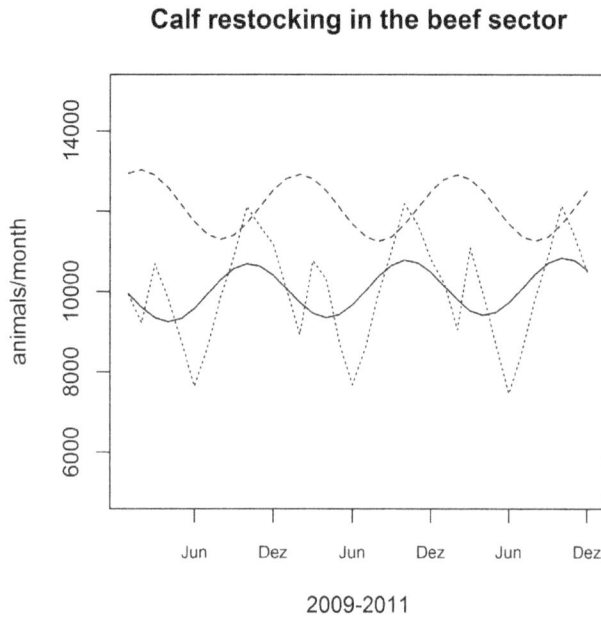

2009-2011

Figure 5. Restocking of calves in the beef sector. Dashed line: dairy calves transferred to fattening plants (VENSIM), solid line:born beef calves (VENSIM), dotted line: born beef calves (AMD).

to a considerable extend by calves from the dairy industry. Almost every month more dairy calves are transferred to fattening plants (i.e. to from the dairy to the beef industry) than were born within the beef industry (figure 5).

The number of slaughtered animals does not show a clear seasonal pattern (AMD data, figure 6) and the slaughter rate in the model is linear.

The sensitivity analysis shows, that the dairy female calf birth average and the dairy cow slaughter rate have the biggest influence on the total population with a change in animal numbers bigger than 50'000 after 3 years of simulation (figures S1–S10, supplementary material).

Discussion

4.1 The Swiss cattle population

The composition of the Swiss cattle population accentuates that the milk industry dominates the domestic production and shapes the population dynamic. Adult dairy cows account for over 40% of all animals (figure 4). The importance of dairy female animals for the total population is reflected in the high sensitivity of the beef population to changes in the dairy cow slaughter rate and the dairy female birth rate (figures S2, S6, supplementary material). The irregular slaughter pattern indicates that the farmers keep the population constant by management decisions.

The higher monthly average mortality of dairy male calves compared to their contemporaries (0.0255 compared to 0.0094 (XDF), 0.0074 (XBM) and 0.0059 (XBF)) is in line with findings of other authors. [14] and [15] found higher mortality rates in dairy breeds than in beef breeds and higher mortality rates in male calves than female calves. As they all defined calves as maximum 180 days of age, the broader categories in our model might explain why dairy male calves differ as much from the others as the effect of early perinatal mortality with higher risk of dystocia for male calves [14] is combined with management decisions, i.e. less care for the economically relatively uninteresting male dairy calves

[15]. As we also determined the production type on farm level and not according to the breed as in the above mentioned studies, effects of management decisions on the calve mortality might be even more manifest.

When deducting yearly rates roughly by multiplying the monthly age transition rates by 12, the difference in the management of beef and dairy animals becomes more obvious: while 82% of female dairy calves reach the next age class, only 25% of dairy male calves live through their first year. For beef calves 86% of the females and 61% of the males reach the next age class which reflects the interest of fattening beef breeds for more than 12 month. The most valued group of animals, dairy heifers, reach adulthood in 96% of the cases while more beef heifers are slaughtered and only 74% get two years old.

4.2 Model assumptions

In high productive agriculture systems of the developed world the population dynamics of livestock is controlled by the farmer and depends on policy and economics rather than on resource limitation or other external factors e.g. [16]. Bleul [14] states, that 80% of Swiss cows are inseminated artificially. For this reason we did not consider a resource constraint i.e. a carrying capacity in our model. The results may be of use for countries in similar economic situation but with less complete records but are to be applied carefully to cattle population that live under more resource dependent natural conditions.

The difference in the birth rates of dairy female and male calves in the model is an artefact presumably due to the difference in the dynamic of the two compartments. Dairy female calves are the most important segment to maintain the population which makes the model sensitive to any change in dairy female calf births. A conservative simulation gives a more stable overall result.

As alpine pastures usually use the gained milk directly for cheese production and it enters therefore not in commerce or they have young stock not yet lactating, they are mostly in the beef category regardless the provenience of the cattle. Therefore the data was corrected over the summer months, using the production type of the farm of origin from the movement records to alpine pastures. The visible seasonal bumps in beef heifers in figure 4 show, that the correction is imperfect due to an incomplete registration of the movements from and to alpine pastures. Since 2012 these are mandatory and improvement of the data quality can be expected.

To integrate the seasonality of birth and mortality in calves, we assumed a sinusoidal pattern and did not investigate other functions.

4.3 Future applications of the model

This is the first dynamic population model for Swiss cattle. As the data source is the complete record of the cattle population, a very good fit could be expected. Nonetheless the fitted population parameters allow a close to reality simulation of the population for future development planning scenario analysis, serve as a backbone to disease transmission models and for the simulation of disease surveillance and control (e.g. [17]).

The fitted population parameters allow building age and sex structured transmission models to simulate disease dynamics with different prevalences in different age classes (e.g. infectious bovine rhinotracheitis IBR, Brucellosis).

Furthermore the transmission rates of different age and production type categories to the slaughterhouse give precise information, which proportions of populations and subpopulations would be basically available for testing at the slaughterhouse in which time period. The slaughterhouse is a very convenient spot for sampling, because it allows taking samples from many animals

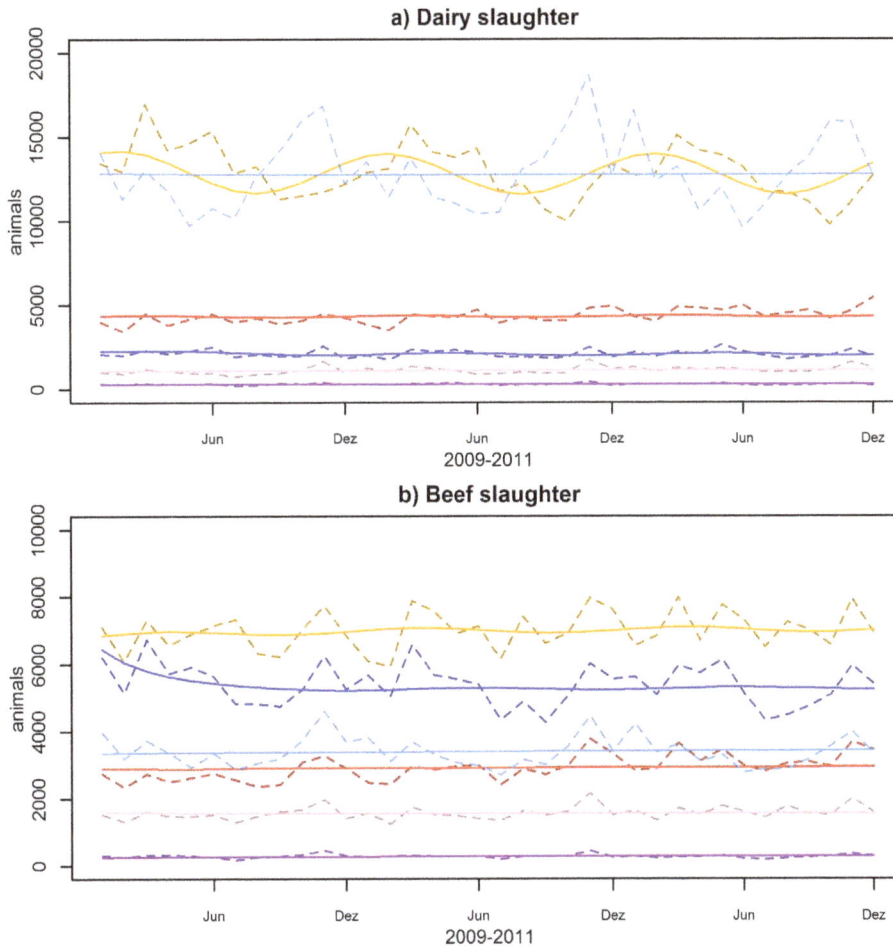

Figure 6. Slaughter numbers per age category. a) Dairy population. b) Beef population. Solid line: model data, dashed lines: AMD data. Light blue: cow, orange: male calf, red: female calf, pink: heifer, blue: young bull, purple: bull.

from different farms of origin within a short time period. Furthermore, there are diseases such as bovine spongiform encephalopathy (BSE) that can only be diagnosed in tissue matrices accessible at slaughter, e.g. brainstem.

As the outcome parameters in the model are calculated for the dairy and beef sector separately, surveillance systems with different components for the different production types can be simulated (e.g. IBR, Brucellosis). For example the efficacy of combining bulk tank milk sampling with slaughterhouse or on farm sampling can be evaluated. As the transfer from calves from the dairy sector to the beef sector is included, the model allows a realistic simulation of disease transmission in the overall population and of the effect of different surveillance strategies on the system sensitivity for different production types.

The fitted population parameters can also be interpreted as baseline parameters for the healthy Swiss cattle population. As seasonal effects are included in the parameter fitting, they can be used to search for aberrations in present data (e.g. increased mortality) to detect health events in an early stage.

In the healthy population most female calves are kept to restock the dairy population, as can be inferred from the relatively low transmission rates of female dairy calves to slaughter. If that segment is affected by an epidemic leading to increased abortions, calf mortality or decreased fertility, consequences on population structure and management are to be expected. Achievement of

breeding objectives might be delayed or even out of reach. Impacts on the milk and meat markets are to be expected. The impact on population structure such as decrease of adult dairy cows in the slaughter population can be estimated by model derived transmission factors.

Conclusions

The Swiss animal movement database is a reliable source of information about the Swiss cattle population and can provide stakeholders and decision makers with important knowledge without expensive and laborious field work. The presented demographic model allows a simulation of Swiss cattle production and economics under different policy scenarios and can be used as the demographic backbone for disease transmission models.

Supporting Information

Figure S1 Influence of varying slaughter rates on the number of animals in the dairy population.

Figure S2 Influence of varying slaughter rates on the number of animals in the beef population.

Figure S3   Influence of varying mortality rates on the number of animals in the dairy population.

Figure S4   Influence of varying mortality rates on the number of animals in the beef population.

Figure S5   Influence of varying average birth rates on the number of animals in the dairy population.

Figure S6   Influence of varying average birth rates on the number of animals in the beef population.

Figure S7   Influence of varying fattening rates (calves transferring from the dairy to the beef sector) on the number of animals in the dairy population.

Figure S8   Influence of varying fattening rates (calves transferring from the dairy to the beef sector) on the number of animals in the beef population.

Figure S9   legends for the colour scales for the dairy population.

Figure S10   legends for the colour scales for the beef population.

Author Contributions

Analyzed the data: SS JZ JH NC. Wrote the paper: SS JH NC MR JZ PP. Model design: SS JZ JH NC PP MR.

References

1. Golan E, Krissoff B, Kuchler F, Calvin L, Nelson K, et al. (2004) Traceability in the U. S. Food Supply: Economic Theory and Industry Studies. Agric Econ Rep 830.
2. Lüdi F (2004) Demographie, räumliche Verteilung und Dynamik der schweizerischen Rindviehpopulation in den Jahren 2002 und 2003.
3. O'Connor J, More S, Griffin J, O'Leary E (2009) Modelling the demographics of the Irish cattle population. Prev Vet Med 89: 249–254. Available: http://www.ncbi.nlm.nih.gov/pubmed/19327855. Accessed 13 June 2012.
4. Anonymous (2002) Agreement between the European Community and the Swiss Confederation on trade in agricultural products.
5. Anonymous (1995) Tierseuchenverordnung, SR 916.401. Bern. Available: http://www.admin.ch/opc/de/classified-compilation/19950206/index.html.
6. WTO (n.d.) The WTO Agreement on the Application of Sanitary and Phytosanitary Measures (SPS Agreement). Available: http://www.wto.org/english/tratop_e/sps_e/spsagr_e.htm.
7. Stärk K, Regula G, Hernandez J, Knopf L, Fuchs K, et al. (2006) Concepts for risk-based surveillance in the field of veterinary medicine and veterinary public health: Review of current approaches. BMC Health Serv Res 6: 20. doi:10.1186/1472-6963-6-20.
8. Hadorn D, Racloz V, Schwermer H, Stärk K (2009) Establishing a cost-effective national surveillance system for Bluetongue using scenario tree modelling. Vet Res 40: 57. doi:10.1051/vetres/2009040.
9. Reber A, Reist M, Schwermer H (2012) Cost-effectiveness of bulk-tank milk testing for surveys to demonstrate freedom from infectious bovine rhinotracheitis and bovine enzootic leucosis in Switzerland. SAT 154: 189–197. doi:10.1024/0036-7281/.
10. Reist M, Jemmi T, Stärk K (2012) Policy-driven development of cost-effective, risk-based surveillance strategies. Prev Vet Med 105: 176–184. Available: http://www.ncbi.nlm.nih.gov/pubmed/22265642. Accessed 4 April 2013.
11. Ventana Systems I (2008) Vensim: Simulator for Business.
12. Press W, Flannery B, Teukolsky S, Viatour P (1991) Numerical Recipies in C. Cambridge.
13. R Development Core Team (2008) R: A language and environment for statistical computing. Available: http://www.r-project.org.
14. Bleul U (2011) Risk factors and rates of perinatal and postnatal mortality in cattle in Switzerland. Livest Sci 135: 257–264. Available: http://linkinghub.elsevier.com/retrieve/pii/S1871141310004142. Accessed 21 August 2014.
15. Perrin J, Ducrot C, Vinard J, Hendrikx P, Calavas D (2011) Analyse de la mortalité bovine en France de 2003 à 2009. INRA Prod Anim 24: 235–244.
16. Rosen S, Murphy K, Scheinkman J (2012) Cattle Cycles. J Polit Econ 102: 468–492.
17. Riley S (2007) Large-scale spatial-transmission models of infectious disease. Science 316: 1298–1301. Available: http://www.ncbi.nlm.nih.gov/pubmed/17540894. Accessed 11 July 2014.

Underlying Mechanism of Antimicrobial Activity of Chitosan Microparticles and Implications for the Treatment of Infectious Diseases

Soo Jin Jeon[1,2], Manhwan Oh[1,2], Won-Sik Yeo[1,2], Klibs N. Galvão[3,4], Kwang Cheol Jeong[1,2]*

1 Emerging Pathogens Institute, University of Florida, Gainesville, Florida, United States of America, 2 Department of Animal Sciences, Institute of Food and Agricultural Sciences, University of Florida, Gainesville, Florida, United States of America, 3 Department of Large Animal Clinical Sciences, College of Veterinary Medicine, University of Florida, Gainesville, Florida, United States of America, 4 D. H. Barron Reproductive and Perinatal Biology Research Program, University of Florida, Gainesville, Florida, United States of America

Abstract

The emergence of antibiotic resistant microorganisms is a great public health concern and has triggered an urgent need to develop alternative antibiotics. Chitosan microparticles (CM), derived from chitosan, have been shown to reduce *E. coli* O157:H7 shedding in a cattle model, indicating potential use as an alternative antimicrobial agent. However, the underlying mechanism of CM on reducing the shedding of this pathogen remains unclear. To understand the mode of action, we studied molecular mechanisms of antimicrobial activity of CM using *in vitro* and *in vivo* methods. We report that CM are an effective bactericidal agent with capability to disrupt cell membranes. Binding assays and genetic studies with an *ompA* mutant strain demonstrated that outer membrane protein OmpA of *E. coli* O157:H7 is critical for CM binding, and this binding activity is coupled with a bactericidal effect of CM. This activity was also demonstrated in an animal model using cows with uterine diseases. CM treatment effectively reduced shedding of intrauterine pathogenic *E. coli* (IUPEC) in the uterus compared to antibiotic treatment. Since Shiga-toxins encoded in the genome of bacteriophage is often overexpressed during antibiotic treatment, antibiotic therapy is generally not recommended because of high risk of hemolytic uremic syndrome. However, CM treatment did not induce bacteriophage or Shiga-toxins in *E. coli* O157:H7; suggesting that CM can be a potential candidate to treat infections caused by this pathogen. This work establishes an underlying mechanism whereby CM exert antimicrobial activity *in vitro* and *in vivo*, providing significant insight for the treatment of diseases caused by a broad spectrum of pathogens including antibiotic resistant microorganisms.

Editor: Marie-Joelle Virolle, University Paris South, France

Funding: This work was supported by USDA-AFRI Grants program (Nanotechnology for Agricultural and Food Systems, 2014-67021-21597) to KCJ. This work was also supported in part by Milk Check-Off grants (F003431) and USDA-NIFA-CRIS program (FLA-VME-005176) to KNG and KCJ. The funders had not role in study design, data collection and analysis, decision to publish, or preparation of the manuscript.

Competing Interests: The authors have declared that no competing interests exist.

* E-mail: kcjeong@ufl.edu

Introduction

Chitosan has been highlighted as a potential candidate for targeting antibiotic resistant microorganisms due to a broad spectrum of antimicrobial activity and biocompatibility [1,2,3,4,5,6]. Chitosan, a deacetylated derivative of chitin, is a linear biopolymer composed of β-(1–4)-linked N-acetyl-D-glucos-amine [7]. Recently, chitosan derived from shrimp has been recognized as a Generally Recognized As Safe (GRAS) for general use in foods by the US Food and Drug Administration [8]. In addition, Japan and Korea have approved chitosan as a food additive since 1983 and 1995, respectively [9].

Various theories have been proposed to explain the mode of action leading to the antimicrobial activity of chitosan [1,10,11,12]. Though the exact mechanism has yet to be elucidated, the intracellular leakage hypothesis is widely accepted [1,10,11,12]. In this mechanism, positively charged chitosan binds to the negatively charged bacterial surface leading to altered membrane permeability, which results in leakage of intracellular constituents causing cell death [3,5,11]. However, it has been

reported that antimicrobial activity of chitosan is limited to acidic conditions due to the loss of positive charges on the amino group at neutral pH [3,5]. This restricts the use of chitosan as an antimicrobial agent at neutral pH.

Recently, we found that chitosan microparticles (CM), derived from chitosan by cross-linking, reduced pathogenic *Escherichia* coli O157:H7 shedding in cattle. This result was unexpected because the gastrointestinal (GI) tract normally maintains neutral pH where antimicrobial activity of chitosan is abolished [13]. In this earlier study, CM, administered orally with feeds, significantly shortened the duration of *E. coli* O157:H7 shedding from 13.8 days to 3.8 days and reduced the total number of this pathogen in cattle. We observed that the pathogen was completely removed from the GI tract in 60% of the calves, indicating that CM retain activity at neutral pH. These data suggest that CM can be a great candidate to intervene enteric pathogens. Although we suggested that reduction of *E. coli* O157:H7 by oral CM administration might be a result of the pathogen binding activity of CM, the previous study failed to differentiate whether the reduction of *E.*

coil O157:H7 was mediated by antimicrobial activity or detaching activity of CM in the GI tract [13].

This study was designed to address the mode of action of CM by identification of binding targets in *E. coli* O157:H7. In addition to the measurement of antimicrobial activity of CM *in vitro*, an *in vivo* assessment was conducted using cows with uterine diseases to evaluate the potential for clinical application. Here, we present our findings that CM specifically interact with a bacterial surface protein, Outer Membrane Protein A (OmpA), and this interaction is coupled with antimicrobial activity. *In vivo* CM efficacy evaluated in cows with uterine diseases confirmed that CM are effective in reducing the disease-causing agent, implying potential use of this agent for disease treatment.

Materials and Methods

Ethics statement

Standard practices of animal care and use were applied to animals used in this project. Research protocols were approved by the University of Florida Institutional Animal Care and Use Committee (IACUC Protocol #: 201207405).

Preparation of chitosan microparticles

CM were prepared as described previously [14]. Briefly, chitosan was purchased from Sigma-Aldrich (448869-250G, SIGMA-ALDRICH) and a 0.25% of chitosan solution (w/v) was prepared with 2% acetic acid (v/v) and 1% tween 80 (v/v). For cross-linking of chitosan, 10% of sodium sulfate (w/v) was added dropwise to the chitosan solution during stirring and sonication for 20 min. When the chitosan solution became cloudy, the chitosan microparticles were collected by centrifugation at 6000 rpm for 10 min and washed with MiliQ Water three times. The size and structure of CM were analyzed by scanning electron microscopy (EVO MA10 XVP, Carl Zeiss), and the distribution of particle size was determined by the diameter of 200 particles using image J 1.46r (National Institutes of Health, USA).

Bacterial strains

Antimicrobial activity of CM was assessed using various bacteria. *Escherichia coli* O157:H7 EDL933 (ATCC48935), Intra-uterine pathogenic *Escherichia coli*, *Salmonella enterica* CDC3041-1, and *Klebsiella pneumoniae* were grown in LB medium and tested; *Vibrio cholera* 395 classical O1, grown in LB medium supplemented with 1% NaCl, and *Streptococcus uberis*, grown in Brain Heart Infusion broth, were also tested. The wild-type strain and the mutants are listed in Table 1.

In vitro antimicrobial activity assay

A single colony of each strain was inoculated in 5 ml of appropriate broth medium and incubated at 37°C with shaking at 200 rpm overnight. The next day, bacterial cultures were diluted 1:100 in fresh medium and again incubated at 37°C until reaching a late-log phase. Approximately 5×10^4 CFU/ml of bacteria were inoculated into 2 ml of LB medium (pH 5–9) containing CM (0.05%–0.2%). After 6 h, bacteria diluted up to 10^{-8} were plated on appropriate agar and incubated at 37°C overnight to count colony-forming unit (CFU). Reduction in the number of CFU represented the antimicrobial activity.

Live/Dead viability assay

Bacterial viability was determined using a live/dead assay (Molecular Probes, Inc., Eugene) following manufacturer's in-structions. Briefly, 5×10^4 CFU/ml of *E. coli* O157:H7 was incubated with 0.2% CM at 37°C for 3 h and then incubated at

Table 1. Strains and plasmids.

Strains	Description	References
E. coli **EDL933**	*E. coli* **O157:H7, wild-type**	**ATCC48935**
KCJ688	EDL933 + pEYFP	This study
KCJ832	*Δeae*::kan + pEYFP	This study
KCJ846	*ΔecpA*::kan + pEYFP	This study
KCJ834	*ΔcsgA*::kan + pEYFP	This study
KCJ848	*ΔompA*::kan + pEYFP	This study
KCJ826	*ΔespA*::kan + pEYFP	This study
KCJ830	*ΔfimA*::kan + pEYFP	This study
KCJ838	*ΔfliA*::kan + pEYFP	This study
KCJ824	*ΔirgA*::kan + pEYFP	This study
KCJ844	*ΔlpfA*::kan + pEYFP	This study
KCJ828	*ΔnanA*::kan + pEYFP	This study
KCJ836	*ΔpgaA*::kan + pEYFP	This study
KCJ820	*ΔsfmA*::kan + pEYFP	This study
KCJ822	*Δtir*::kan + pEYFP	This study
KCJ840	*ΔyehD*::kan + pEYFP	This study
KCJ842	*ΔyfcV*::kan + pEYFP	This study
KCJ850	*ΔwaaL*::kan + pEYFP	This study
KCJ806	*ΔompA*	This study
KCJ1449	*ΔompA*+pOmpA	This study
KCJ852	IUPEC	Laboratory collection
KCJ855	*V. cholera*	Laboratory collection
KCJ165	*S. enterica*	CDC3041-1
KCJ1332	*K. pneumoniae*	Laboratory collection
KCJ145	*S. uberis*	Laboratory collection
pEYFP	Yellow Fluorescence Protein	Clontech
pKD4	Used as *kan* template	[15]
pKD46	Red recombinase expression plasmid	[15]

room temperature in the dark with SYTO 9 and propidium iodide. After a 15 min incubation, bacteria were observed using the fluorescence microscope (Leica Microsystems Wetzlar GmbH, Germany). Viability was determined by fluorescence colors that bacteria emit (i.e. dead bacteria present red fluorescence, and live bacteria present green fluorescence). As controls, bacteria were treated with 70% isopropyl alcohol for dead bacteria or untreated for live bacteria.

Gene deletion and complementation

Genes of interest were deleted in the chromosomal DNA of *E. coli* O157:H7 by the PCR one-step λ Red recombinase method [15]. Briefly, the kanamycin resistance gene was amplified using a template plasmid pKD4 and primers with 50-nt extensions that are homologous to regions adjacent to a targeted gene (Table 2). The PCR product was electrophorated into the *E. coli* O157:H7 with the Red system expression plasmid pKD46. The electro-phorated *E. coli* O157:H7 was added to 1 ml of LB, incubated at 37°C for 1 h, and then plated onto LB agar with kanamycin for selection.

A *ΔompA* strain was transformed with a pUC18 carrying the *ompA* gene to create a complement strain (*ΔompA*+pOmpA) using

Table 2. Oligonucleotides.

Names	Genes	Sequences
KCP021	ompA-F[m]	ATAAGTACCGCATAAAACCTACTATTGCTCCGCGTTTTTTACTGTAGGCTGGAGCTGCTTCG
KCP022	ompA-R[m]	GGGGCGTCGTCGCCCCAAAAAGATGGTCTGCTCTTGAATTCGCATATGAATATCCTCCTTAGTTCC
KCP023	ecpA-F[m]	CCCTGTAGTGCAGGAGTTAAGTTGAGCCCTTCTTTATGTTACTGTAGGCTGGAGCTGCTTCG
KCP024	ecpA-R[m]	TCGACCCCCCGATGGGGACGACCATGTAGTCTCTCTAATTGACATATGAATATCCTCCTTAGTTCC
KCP025	fimA-F[m]	CATGTCGATTTAGAAATAGTTTTTTGAAAGGAAAGCAGCATGTGTAGGCTGGAGCTGCTTCG
KCP026	fimA-R[m]	GTCGCATCCGCATTAGCAGCACCCGGGGTTGCCTCGCCCATATGAATATCCTCCTTAGTTCC
KCP027	pgaA-F[m]	ATGTCTCTCTCTAAAACCGTTATGTACCTCATTATGTCCTACTGTAGGCTGGAGCTGCTTCG
KCP028	pgaA-R[m]	CCTCTATAAATAAAGGTAATGCATTGTATAAATAGGAATTTTCATATGAATATCCTCCTTAGTTCC
KCP029	nanA-F[m]	TAGTCTGTTCGTAGTGAAGTCTCCATAAATACCGTTGCTTAATGTAGGCTGGAGCTGCTTCG
KCP030	nanA-R[m]	GGGGAGTGGGCCATCCCCGCTCGCTCCCCTTTGTTGAGTGGGCATATGAATATCCTCCTTAGTTCC
KCP031	csgA-F[m]	TTCCATTCGACTTTTAAATCAATCCGATGGGGGTTTTACATGTGTAGGCTGGAGCTGCTTCG
KCP032	csgA-R[m]	GGGCTTGCGCCCTGTTTCTTTAATACAGATGATGTATTAGTACATATGAATATCCTCCTTAGTTCC
KCP063	lpfA-F[m]	TAAAATTATGTAGTTCTAAAAGAAAAATTACATTAAAAAATTTGTAGGCTGGAGCTGCTTCG
KCP064	lpfA-R[m]	CTGATTACCGCCGTTAATGCGGCGGTAAACATTTTGCCTGCTCATATGAATATCCTCCTTAGTTCC
KCP065	eae-F[m]	ATTAAATAAAGAGTAAGATTGAGTAACACCACCTCGGTATTGTGTAGGCTGGAGCTGCTTCG
KCP066	eae-R[m]	GGCTGATTTTGTTATGTATAAAATCGGCCCCACCAATACCTTCATATGAATATCCTCCTTAGTTCC
KCP067	tir-F[m]	TTCCTAACAATAGATAAATGTATTTTATTTTTCCTCTATAAATGTAGGCTGGAGCTGCTTCG
KCP068	tir-R[m]	AAGGGGGGAGGGAGGGAGATTTATTTTACTAATACCTATATACATATGAATATCCTCCTTAGTTCC
KCP069	espA-F[m]	TAAAAAAACAAAAGGACTCTTTTTAATAGTTCTCCATATATCTGTAGGCTGGAGCTGCTTCG
KCP070	espA-R[m]	TCTGTCCCATAGCAATAAATGCAATTCGTATCAATAGAGGCCCATATGAATATCCTCCTTAGTTCC
KCP071	fliA-F[m]	CTATTAGTACGGCTATTGAGTATATTGCGTCCCGACAAATAGTGTAGGCTGGAGCTGCTTCG
KCP072	fliA-R[m]	CTTGAGGACCATCAGTTTCAATTTCACGCCGTAAATGACTGCCATATGAATATCCTCCTTAGTTCC
KCP073	yehD-F[m]	TCTGAGAATTGTTTTGTTTTATTTGAATAATTCCTTACGTAGTGTAGGCTGGAGCTGCTTCG
KCP074	yehD-R[m]	GTAAAATTGAATGACTTTTTTGTTCTACTAATAAAATTTATACATATGAATATCCTCCTTAGTTCC
KCP075	yraH-F[m]	ATTAAATATGATTATGTACTTGTTACAAGGATAAGGTTATAATGTAGGCTGGAGCTGCTTCG
KCP076	yraH-R[m]	GAAAAGGGCGTTATCTGAAAGGTCAGATAACGCCGTAACGTACATATGAATATCCTCCTTAGTTCC
KCP077	sfmA-F[m]	TACTATCAGTGTCTTAAATAAAGTAATCGGTTATATACGGATTGTAGGCTGGAGCTGCTTCG
KCP078	sfmA-R[m]	GTTATAAGACGTGATATATAATTCAAAACAACGTGGTTTTGACATATGAATATCCTCCTTAGTTCC
KCP079	yfcV-F[m]	GTTACAAATATAAAAATTAATAAATACCAAATTCCTGTTTATTGTAGGCTGGAGCTGCTTCG
KCP080	yfcV-R[m]	GGTAAATTTTTGGGGTATCGGGCTTTCGATACCCCCATAGTGCATATGAATATCCTCCTTAGTTCC
KCP708	ompA-F	ATGATAACGAGTCGACAAAAATGAAAAAGACAGCTATCGCGATTG
KCP709	ompA-R	CCCGGAATTCTTAAGCTTGCGGCTGAGTTACAAC

[m]Primers were designed for gene inactivation in chromosomal DNA of *E. coli* O157:H7.

primers PKC708 and PKC709 (Table 2). We confirmed the absence of the *ompA* gene in the *ΔompA* mutant and the restoration of *ompA* in the *ΔompA*+pOmpA strain by PCR. A growth curve was measured (OD_{600}) every 30 min for 12 h using a plate reader (Gen5, BioTek). The complementation was measured by an *in vitro* binding assay and an antibacterial activity assay. These strains were stained with the blue-fluorescent DAPI (Invitrogen) and observed by fluorescence microscopy (Leica Microsystems Wetzlar GmbH, Germany).

In vitro CM binding assay

E. coli O157:H7 was loaded on 6-mm wells of CM-coated, poly-Lysine-coated, or uncoated slides to examine cell attachment to CM (Electron Microscopy Sciences of Hatfield, PA). To prevent desiccation of bacteria, the glass was kept in a humid chamber during incubation. After incubation, the glass was washed 3 times with phosphate buffered saline (PBS) to remove unbound cells and added with antifade reagent (ProLong Gold, Invitrogen) to protect

fluorescent dyes from photobleaching. The mounted wells were observed by fluorescence microscopy (Leica Microsystems Wetzlar GmbH, Germany). To identify the molecular target of CM in the cell attachment, *E. coli* O157:H7 wild-type and 15 mutants carrying pEYFP (Clontech, Table 1) were grown in LB medium at 37°C for 3 h with isopropyl-β-D-thiogalactopyranoside (IPTG). These strains in late log phase were harvested at 4000 rpm for 1 min. Approximately 10^6 CFU/ml of each strain prepared in LB medium was incubated on a CM-coated glass. The CM-coated glass was prepared earlier by loading 20 μl of 0.1% CM on 6-mm wells of the glass. The following procedures for washing, mounting, and examination were the same as described above.

Phage induction analysis

Bacterial cell lysis was measured by spectrophotometer to monitor phage induction. *E. coli* O157:H7 was grown in LB medium until exponential phase (OD_{600} = 0.7). Different concentrations of CM, mitomycin C, and medium alone (as a control) were added in eight replicates. Optical density of cultures was measured by spectrophotometer (Gen5, BioTek) every 30 min during 7 h with moderate shaking. Phage induction was also evaluated by sodium dodecyl sulfate polyacrylamide gel electrophoresis (SDS-PAGE). *E. coli* O157:H7 was grown in LB medium until exponential phase (OD$_{600}$ = 0.7). CM (0.2%), mitomycin C (1 µg/ml, Fisher Scientific BP-2531-2), and medium alone were added in 10 ml of bacterial culture, respectively, followed by incubation for 18 h. To remove unlysed cells and debris, the bacterial culture was centrifuged at 4,000 rpm for 20 min at 4°C. The The supernatants were filtered through 0.22 µm-pore-size membrane filter (Fisher Scientific 09-719A) and phage particles expected to be induced by treatments were precipitated by the addition of 20% polyethylene glycol 8000 (PEG, Fluka 81268) and 2.5 M NaCl. The precipitated phage particles were incubated on ice for 30 min and then centrifuged at 14,000 rpm for 20 min. Centrifugation was repeated twice to remove all of the PEG solution. The pellets were resuspended in STE buffer (1 M Tris [pH 8], 0.5 M EDTA [pH 8], and 5 M NaCl), mixed with 5× SDS loading buffer, boiled for 5 min, and applied to an 12% polyacrylamide gel. The protein bands were visualized by staining with Coomassie blue.

Western blot analysis of Shiga-toxin II expression

E. coli O157:H7 was grown in LB medium until exponential phase (OD$_{600}$ = 0.7). CM (0.2%), mitomycin C (1 µg/ml), and medium alone were added in 10 ml of bacterial culture, respectively. The cultures of *E. coli* O157:H7 were incubated for 18 h, centrifuged at 4,000 rpm for 20 min at 4°C, and filtered through 0.22 µm-pore-size membrane filter to remove bacteria. For precipitation of proteins present in the supernatants, filtered cultures were mixed with 100% trichloroacetic acid (Fisher Scientific BP555-1) to create the final 20%. The mixtures were incubated on ice for 30 min and centrifuged at 14,000 rpm at 4°C for 30 min. The supernatant was carefully removed and the pellet was washed with cold acetone. The cold acetone needed to be aspirated following centrifugation at 14,000 rpm at 4°C for 15 min. The remaining pellets were suspended with sterile water and protein concentrations were measured by spectrophotometer (Nanodrop 1000, Thermo Scientific). Subsequently, the proteins were separated by 12% sodium dodecyl sulfate polyacrylamide gel and transferred to a polyvinylidene difluoride membrane (0.45 µm pores, Immobilon-P, Millipore) for western blot. The membrane was blocked in 5% skim milk in TBST (10 mM Tris-HCL [pH 7.4], 150 mM NaCl, and 0.05% Tween-20) for 1 h at RT and incubated with monoclonal Verotoxin II-α subunit antibody (Meridian, Life Science Inc.) overnight at 4°C. After washing with TBST, the membrane was incubated at RT for 45 min with HRP-conjugated secondary antibody (GE Healthcare) diluted 1:10000 in TBST. After washing with TBST, the membrane was incubated with a chemiluminescent substrate (ECL Plus, GE Healthcare), and exposed to Kodak BioMax film (Carestream Kodak X-Omat LS film, F1274 Sigma).

Animal management

Cows used in this experiment were housed in freestall barns equipped with fans and sprinklers that were activated when ambient temperature exceeded 18°C. Barns were cleaned twice daily and freestalls were bedded twice a week with sand. Cows were fed totally mixed ration twice daily formulated to meet or exceed the nutrient requirements of a lactation Holstein cow weighing 650 Kg of body weight and producing 45 Kg of 3.5% fat corrected milk per day. Fresh water was available ad libitum. Cows were vaccinated and treated for common diseases according to standard operating procedures (SOP) developed with participation of the veterinarians from the University of Florida, college of veterinary medicine, food animal reproduction and medicine service.

In vivo antimicrobial activity of CM in cows with uterine diseases

For *in vivo* animal experiments, Holstein cows (8–10/group) having metritis (inflammation of all layers of the uterus) were used for this study. Metritis was diagnosed by the presence of red-brownish fetid uterine discharge at either 4, 7, or 10 days postpartum. Cows (n = 18) were randomly assigned to one of 2 treatments as they were diagnosed with metritis: CM treatment, Cows (n = 8) were treated for 5 days with 8 g of CM dissolved in 10 ml of sterile water via intrauterine infusion; Ceftiofur treatment, cows (n = 10) were intramuscularly treated for 5 days with 2.2 mg/kg of Ceftiofur hydrochloride (Excenel, Zoetis, Zoetis Inc., Madison, NJ). The uterus of a cow with metritis has a volume of approximately 4 L; therefore, the dose of CM used was approximately 0.2%. For enumeration of *E. coli* in uterus, uterine swabs were daily collected for 7 days starting at day 0. Swab samples were suspended in 0.1% (w/v) peptone and serially diluted, and plated on CHROMagar (CHROMagar, Paris, France) in duplicates. Plates were incubated at 37°C overnight and the numbers of CFU/ml were counted.

Statistical analysis

All experiments were carried out in triplicate, and average values with standard error of the mean are reported. Data were compared with student's t test using the GraphPad Prism InStat 3.1. *P* values less than 0.05 were considered as statistically significant.

Results

Antimicrobial properties of CM

CM have been shown to reduce *E. coli* O157:H7 from in cattle when administered orally [13], but the mode of action was not clearly understood. To understand if the *E. coli* O157:H7 reduction was caused by either scrubbing or antimicrobial action, antimicrobial activity was determined by a standard plating method after incubation of *E. coli* O157:H7 with CM at various concentrations, ranging from 0% to 0.2%. CM showed a concentration dependent bactericidal activity against *E. coli* O157:H7 (Fig. 1A). Of all concentrations examined, 0.2% CM showed the most antimicrobial activity resulting in complete inhibition of *E. coli* O157:H7 during 6 h of incubation. Growth of *E. coli* O157:H7 was inhibited by 0.1% CM, showing steady level of *E. coli* O157:H7 numbers during 12 h of incubation. Although bacterial growth reached the level in controls (no CM treatment), 0.05% CM treatment showed decreased growth rate until 9 h post incubation.

Using the Live/Dead assay, live bacteria with intact membranes emit green fluorescence (stained with SYTO 9); whereas, bacteria with damaged membranes emit red fluorescence (stained with propidium iodide) due to the penetration of this dye into the cytosol through the damaged membranes. As shown in Fig 1B, dead *E. coli* O157:H7 cells, (permeabilized with 70% isopropanol as a positive control) emitted red fluorescence; whereas, live intact cells (no treatment) emitted green fluorescence. *E. coli* O157:H7 treated with 0.2% CM was stained in red fluorescence, indicating that the bacterial membranes were permeabilized by CM treatment. These data demonstrate the bactericidal activity of CM.

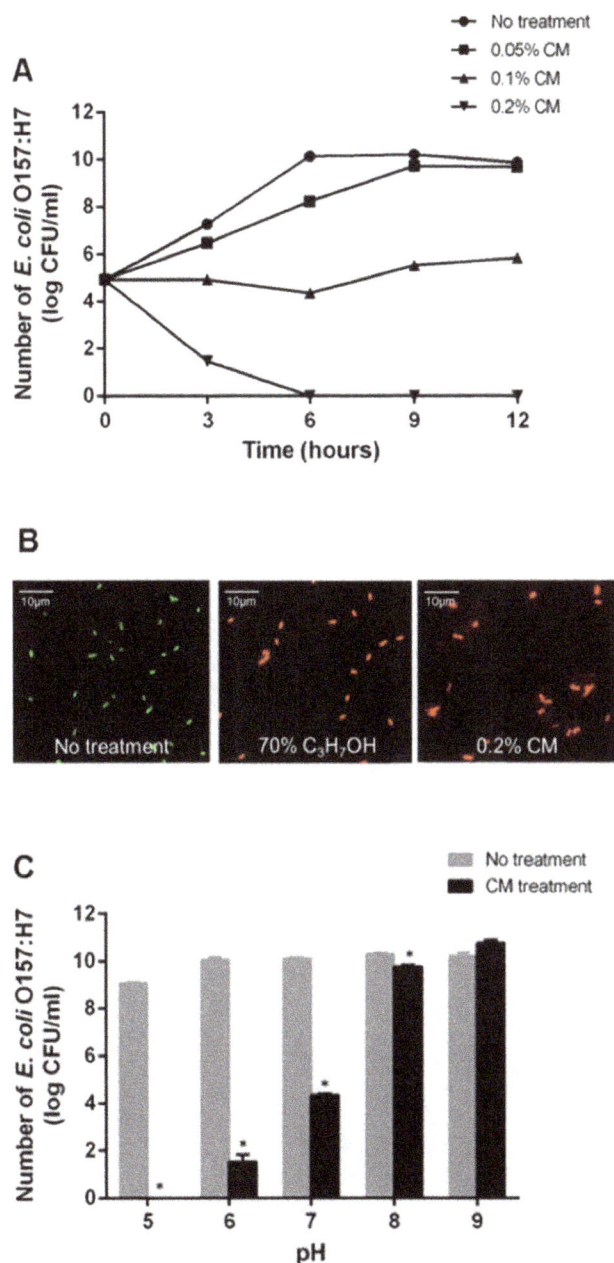

Figure 1. Antimicrobial activity of chitosan microparticles. (A) Survival curve of *E. coli* O157:H7 during CM treatment. *E. coli* O157:H7 was grown with CM at 0% (circle), 0.05% (square), 0.1% (triangle), or 0.2% (inverted triangle), and each time point represents the mean values and standard error of means (SEM) of colony forming units (CFU) recovered from triplicate test tubes. (B) LIVE/DEAD viability assay. *E. coli* O157:H7 was incubated with 0.2% CM at 37°C for 3 h and then incubated with SYTO 9 (green, live) and propidium iodide (red, dead) for 15 minutes, and then bacteria were observed using the fluorescence microscope (Leica Microsystems Wetzlar GmbH, Germany). Fluorescent micrograph of *E. coli* O157:H7 treated with either 0% CM (left), 70% isopropanol (middle), or 0.2% CM. Results shown are representative of three independent experiments. (C) pH effect on antimicrobial activity of CM. *E. coli* O157:H7 was incubated for 6 h in the presence of 0.1% CM in LB broth at various pH (ranging from pH 5 to pH 9) and viable cells were counted using direct plating method; Mean values ± SEM are plotted from three independent experiments; * *P*<0.05, *t*-test.

Previous studies have shown that antimicrobial activity of chitosan is abolished at neutral pH due to the pKa value of amino group in chitosan (pKa = 6.5) [11]. However, CM feeding to cows revealed a reduction of *E. coli* O157:H7 numbers in cattle [13], suggesting some antimicrobial activity at neutral pH. This led us to test antimicrobial activity at different pH, including the neutral pH. Although the strongest antimicrobial activity was observed at acidic pH (pH5), CM still had significant antimicrobial activity at pH7 (Fig. 1C). These data suggest that the bactericidal activity was likely the reason for the reduction of *E. coli* O157:H7 shedding in a previous study [13]. This unexpected antimicrobial activity of CM at pH7, where positively charged amino groups are unlikely, led us to speculate that CM may exert antimicrobial activity at neutral pH, which is distinct to the proposed charge dependent activity at acidic pH.

Identification of CM binding target in *E. coli* O157:H7

To test if CM binding to *E. coli* O157:H7 is necessary for antimicrobial activity, we used *in vitro* binding assay of CM. CM were generated by ion gelation with sodium sulfate [14,16], and we visualized and the measured particles using scanning electron microscopy analysis. The diameter of the prepared CM was 0.6±0.076 μm (mean ± SD, n = 200) with spherical shape and rough surface (inset) structure (Fig. 2A and 2B). Binding activity of CM to *E. coli* O157:H7 was measured using CM-coated glass slides (Fig. 2C). *E. coli* O157:H7 strain expressing enhanced yellow fluorescence protein (EYFP) attached to the CM and poly-lysine (positive control) coated wells, while no cells attached to the untreated wells (Fig. 2C), indicating that CM have significant binding capacity to *E. coli* O157:H7. These data suggest that a direct contact between CM and this pathogen may result in bactericidal effect. From these findings, we hypothesized that surface exposed molecules in *E. coli* O157:H7 might bind to CM. To determine if the observed binding was related to a specific bacterial gene, we constructed mutant strains lacking individual gene in *E. coli* O157:H7 using λ-Red homologous recombination [15]. Total of 15 genes, which are known to be important for bacterial adhesion during colonization, were selected to identify potential binding partners of CM. The target genes are summarized in Table 1. The constructed mutant strains were used for *in vitro* CM binding assay to identify potential binding partners. A total of 10^4 cells were loaded into the CM-coated wells, incubated, and then unattached cells were removed by washing before enumeration with a fluorescent microscope. As shown in figure 2D, the *ΔompA* mutant shows significantly reduced binding to CM compared to the wild-type strain and other mutant strains, suggesting OmpA is a target for CM binding.

Both OmpA and LPS are CM binding targets

The strains were tested to determine if the reduced CM binding activity of the *ompA* mutant was not caused by growth defect of the mutant strain. The *ΔompA* did not show any growth defect (Fig. 3A), indicating that deletion of this gene was not pleiotropic. Therefore, the reduction of CM binding (Fig. 2D) was solely caused by the *ΔompA* deletion. Functional complementation of the *ΔompA* mutant was evaluated with the CM binding assay. After CM binding and washing, the attached cells were stained with DAPI to visualize bacteria (Fig. 3B). A reduced number of the *ΔompA* mutant was observed but numbers were restored to the wild-type level by complementation (*ΔompA*+pOmpA). Taken together, these results indicate that OmpA protein specifically interacts with CM resulting in binding on the CM-coated slide.

It was noted that the *ΔompA* strain still had binding capacity to CM, suggesting that OmpA is not the only one interacting protein,

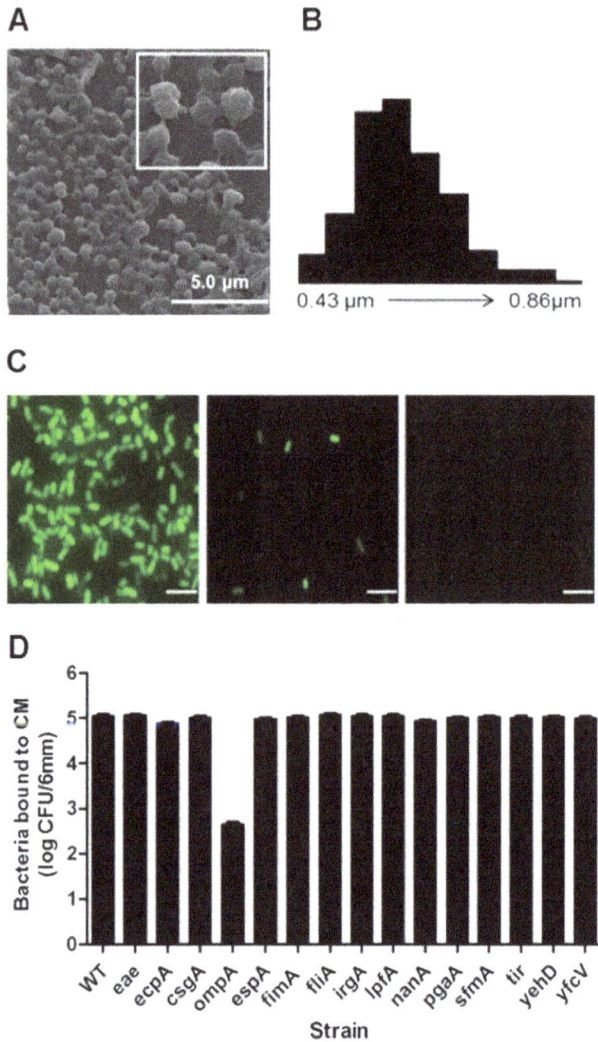

Figure 2. Identification of CM binding target using *in vitro* CM binding assay. (A) Scanning electron microscopy micrograph of CM. Inset is magnified image of CM. (B) The distribution of particle size was determined by measuring the diameter of 200 particles using image J software. (C) *In vitro* binding assay of *E. coli* O157:H7. Bacteria cells carrying pEYFP grown in the presence of IPTG were harvested and incubated on CM-coated (left), poly-lysine-coated (middle), or no-coated slides (right). Bacteria in 6-mm wells were observed by fluorescence microscopy. Scale bars represent 5 μm. (D) Identification of CM binding target. *E. coli* O157:H7 strains were grown in broth and cells were collected to incubate on CM-coated slides. Bound cells were enumerated by fluorescence microscopy. Strains used were: wild type plus vector (KCJ688), *Δeae* plus vector (KCJ832), *ΔecpA* plus vector (KCJ846), *ΔcsgA* plus vector (KCJ834), *ΔompA* plus vector (KCJ848), *ΔespA* plus vector (KCJ826), *ΔfimA* plus vector (KCJ830), *ΔfliA* plus vector (KCJ838), *ΔirgA* plus vector (KCJ824), *ΔlpfA* plus vector (KCJ844), *ΔnanA* plus vector (KCJ828), *ΔpgaA* plus vector (KCJ836), *ΔsfmA* plus vector (KCJ820), *Δtir* plus vector (KCJ822), *ΔyehD* plus vector (KCJ840), and *ΔyfcV* plus vector (KCJ842).

but other molecules are probably involved. To study this hypothesis, we tested if lipopolysaccharide (LPS) can be a binding target based on the previous finding that purified LPS bound to chitosan *in vitro* [17]. We generated a *ΔwaaL* mutant to remove O side chain in LPS. This mutant strain has more negative charges on cell surface compared to the wild-type strains because negatively charged lipid A and core components of LPS are

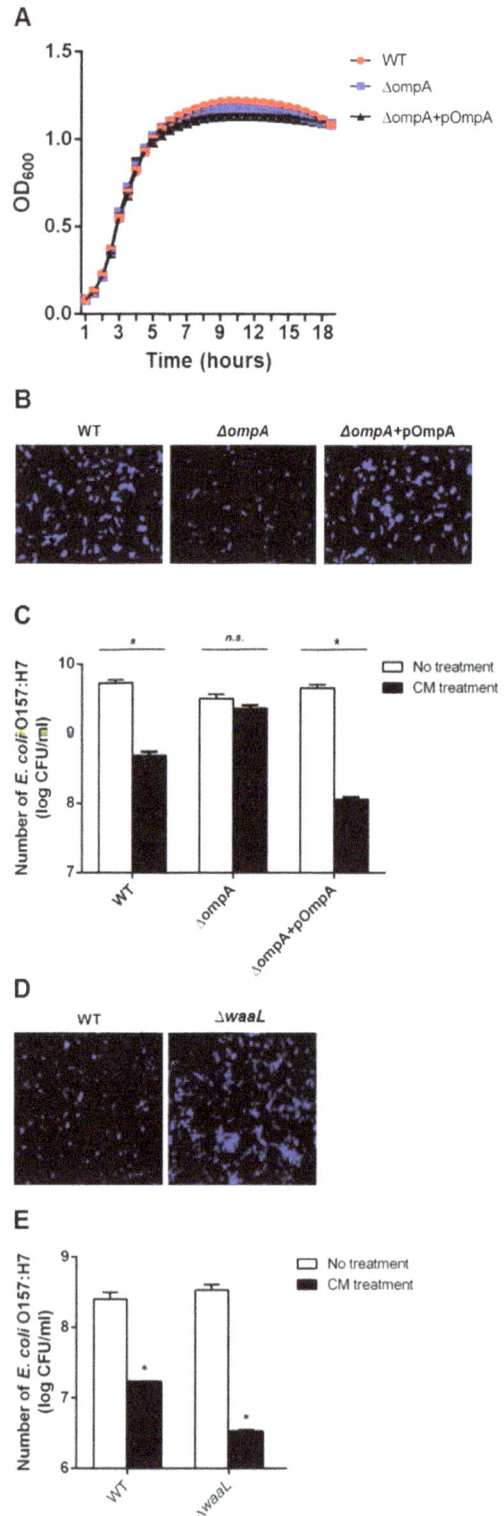

Figure 3. CM interaction with *E. coli* O157:H7 via OmpA and LPS is linked to antimicrobial activity. (A) Growth curve of wild-type (circle), *ΔompA* (KCJ806), and *ΔompA*+pOmpA (KCJ1449). (B) *In vitro* CM binding assay of the *ΔompA* strain. pOmpA complements the loss of binding activity of the *ΔompA* strain. Bound cells were stained with DAPI and enumerated with fluorescence microscopy. (C) Binding of CM to OmpA is linked to the antimicrobial activity of CM. Antibacterial activity of CM was attenuated in *ΔompA*, but restored with pOmpA. Strains used for antimicrobial assay were: wild-type (EDL933), *ΔompA*

(KCJ806), and $\Delta ompA$+pOmpA (KCJ1149). (D) *In vitro* binding assay of wild-type (left) and $\Delta waaL$ (right). Bound cells were stained with DAPI and enumerated with fluorescence microscopy. (E) Antimicrobial activity of CM increased in the $\Delta waaL$ mutant. Strains used for antimicrobial assay were: wild-type (EDL933) and $\Delta waaL$ (KCJ850). Mean values ± SEM are plotted from three independent experiments; * $P<0.05$, *t*-test.

exposed by the deletion of O side chain [18]. Therefore, we expected to increase the CM binding activity with the mutant strain. As shown in figure 3D, an increased number of $\Delta waaL$ mutant were observed on CM-coated slides compared to the wild-type strain, suggesting that LPS can bind to CM.

Association of CM binding with antimicrobial activity

To determine if CM binding to *E. coli* O157:H7 was coupled with antimicrobial activity, it was measured in the $\Delta ompA$ and $\Delta waaL$ strains. The wild-type, $\Delta ompA$, and the $\Delta ompA$ complement stains were grown to exponential phase and then incubated with CM (0.05%) for 6 h before enumeration. The growth of the wild-type and complemented strains was significantly inhibited compared to control cells; whereas, the $\Delta ompA$ strain was not affected by CM, indicating that OmpA was necessary for antimicrobial activity (Fig. 3C). However, the $\Delta ompA$ strain was sensitive at greater concentration at 0.1 and 0.2% (data not shown). In addition, the antimicrobial activity of CM was increased in the $\Delta waaL$ strain compared to the wild-type strain (Fig. 3E), suggesting that the enhanced binding activity in the strain (Fig. 3D) increased antimicrobial activity. Together, these data indicate that the bactericidal activity of CM is coupled with the binding activity to OmpA and LPS in *E. coli* O157:H7.

A broad-spectrum of antimicrobial activity

Antimicrobial activity of CM was tested using six important pathogens that cause disease in humans and animals. CM showed antimicrobial activity against all six pathogens with different efficacy depending on the pathogens (Fig. 4). Growth of *E. coli* O157:H7 and intrauterine pathogenic *E. coli* (IUPEC) were inhibited at 0.05%, and inactivated at 0.2%. In comparison to these *E. coli* species, *V. cholerae*, *S. enterica*, *K. pneumoniae*, and *S. uberis* were less sensitive to CM at 0.1 or 0.3%. *V. cholerae* was inactivated at 0.5%; whereas, *S. ubreis* was inactivated at 1%. Taken together, CM have a broad-spectrum of antimicrobial activity against important pathogens.

In vivo antimicrobial activity of CM

We evaluated *in vivo* antimicrobial activity of CM using cows with uterine diseases as a model animal. Uterine inflammatory diseases, such as metritis and endometritis, are highly prevalent in postpartum cows [19]. The cow uterus maintains its pH near neutral (pH 6.84–7.51) [20], thus it is an ideal *in vivo* model to test CM antimicrobial activity at neutral pH. Holstein cows with uterine diseases were administered with one of two treatments: one with ceftiofur (n = 10 cows), as positive reference, which is used normally to treat uterine infections and the other with CM (n = 8 cows). The number of IUPEC from uterine swab samples collected from the treated animals were enumerated by direct plating on CHROMagar *E. coli* (CHROMagar, Paris, France). *In vivo* antimicrobial activity was measured using cows actively shedding IUPEC prior to CM or ceftiofur treatment (day 0). Three and six cows were positive for IUPEC on day 0 in CM and ceftiofur treated cows, respectively (Fig. 5). Numbers of IUPEC were monitored in uterus for seven days. IUPEC numbers recovered

from CM treated cows were significantly reduced within five days in all treated animals (Fig. 5A). However, three out of five cows treated with ceftiofur still shed IUPEC on day five (Fig. 5B). Thus *in vivo* antimicrobial activity by CM was demonstrated, providing a great promise to treat infections as an alternative antimicrobial agent.

Effect of CM treatment on phage induction and Shiga-toxin production

We further investigated the possibility if CM can be used to treat *E. coli* O157:H7 infection. Shiga-toxin is an important virulence factor in *E. coli* O157:H7 and causes deadly hemolytic uremic syndrome in humans [21,22]. *stx* genes encoding Shiga-toxin are located in the prophage (BP-933W) in the *E. coli* O157:H7 EDL933 strain and induced when phage is triggered into the lytic cycle by antibiotic treatment [23]. Thus, antibiotic treatment is generally not recommended for patients infected with this pathogen [24].

To examine if CM have potential to treat patients infected with *E. coli* O157:H7, phage induction and Shiga-toxin production were monitored in CM treated cells. CM did not induce prophage or Shiga-toxin production (Fig. 6). Prophage induction was assessed by OD_{600} in the presence of CM at 0.05%, 0.1%, and 0.2%, along with a positive control (mitomycin C) and negative control (without treatment). Cell lysis was achieved with mitomycin C treatment (0.5 µg/ml), showing phage induction by antibiotic treatment (Fig. 6A). In the CM treated cells, cell lysis was not observed due to lack of cell growth with CM. Since it was unclear whether CM induced the phage in *E. coli* O157:H7, we detected phage particles as described previously [25]. Phage particles were collected and identified from the supernatants after CM or mitomycin C treatment. A protein profile associated with BP-933W induction was detected in supernatants from mitomycin C-treated cells as previously reported [25] but not in the supernatants of CM-treated and untreated cells (Fig 6B), indicating that CM kill bacteria prior to the phage induction. Western blot analysis for Shiga-toxin in the supernatant collected from CM-treated or mitomycin C-treated cells were conducted. Shiga-toxin was only detected in the mitomycin C-treated cells, but not in the CM-treated and untreated cells. Thus, CM exert antimicrobial activity before phage induction and Shiga-toxin production, implying CM may have potential in the treatment of infected humans.

Discussion

Our findings hold great promise of CM as an alternative antimicrobial agent for the treatment of bacterial infections, including antimicrobial resistant microorganisms. In this paper, we have shown the underlying mechanism of antimicrobial activity of CM, which disrupts bacterial cell membranes by interactions with the outer membrane protein OmpA at neutral pH, leading to cell death. Antimicrobial activity of CM was also confirmed using an animal model with uterine disease. Furthermore, CM did not induce phage or Shiga-toxin production in *E. coli* O157:H7.

Although the antimicrobial activity of chitosan has not been clearly understood, the hypothesis that ionic interactions between positively charged amino group in chitosan and negatively charged bacterial surface molecules such as LPS in acidic conditions [17] resulting in alteration of membrane permeability, has been widely accepted [12,26]. Based on the proposed antimicrobial mechanisms of chitosan, we assumed that CM might have the same antimicrobial mechanism as that of chitosan through the ionic interaction. However, we found that the antimicrobial activity of

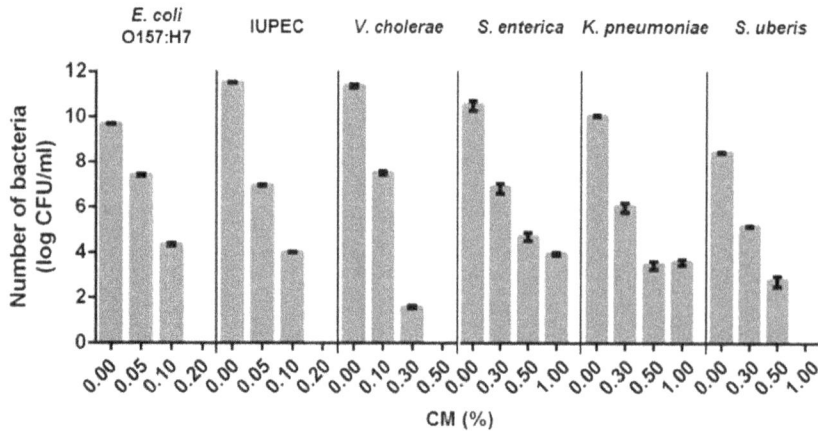

Figure 4. A broad antimicrobial activity of chitosan microparticles. Various strains including *E. coli* O157:H7, Intrauterine pathogenic *E. coli* (IUPEC), *V. cholerae, S. enterica, K. pneumoniae, S. uberis* were treated with CM at different concentrations and viable cells were measured after 6 h treatment; Mean values ± SEM are plotted from three independent experiments.

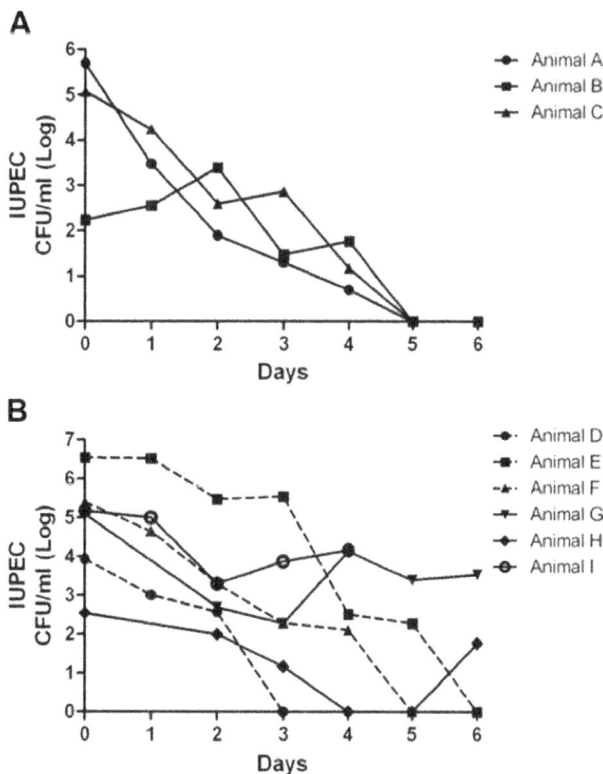

Figure 5. *In vivo* antimicrobial activity of chitosan microparticles. CM reduces number of intrauterine pathogenic E. coli (IUPEC) in the uterus. Dairy cattle with uterine disease were treated with either 0.2% CM (A), n=8, via intrauterine fusion or antibiotic Ceftiofur hydrochloride (B), n=10, systemically for five days. Swabs were collected from uterus for a seven days and IUPEC was enumerated on *E. coli* selective media CHROMagar. Plates were incubated at 37°C overnight, and the numbers of CFU/ml were counted. Numbers of IUPEC in the uterus are presented from individual animals shed this pathogen on Day 0. Solid lines represent animals without IUPEC after treatment; dashed lines represent animals with IUPEC after treatment.

CM was, in part, mediated through OmpA (Fig. 3C). OmpA is an integral bacterial outer membrane protein embedded as a β-barrel structure and it contributes to the structural integrity of the bacterial cell surface [27]. In addition, it contains four surface exposed loops [28] which are involved in the recognition of many ligands including small molecules such as iron-siderophore complexes or sugars [29,30]. Thus, we thought that the loops might be involved in the interaction with CM via ionic interaction. However, the surface-exposed loops of OmpA have a net negative charge of +1 [31], indicating that the ionic interaction between CM and the loops is unlikely.

We speculate that the CM-OmpA interaction is direct via hydrogen bond interaction. Multiple lines of evidence support our hypothesis. It has been shown that *E. coli* K1, which causes meningitis, especially in new-born babies [32], invades membranes via an interaction of OmpA with a D-glucosamine (monomer of chitosan) [33,34]. Recently, residues critical for the hydrogen bond interactions between OmpA with D-glucosamine were identified in the loops of OmpA by a computational simulation analysis [35]. In addition, N-acetylated D-glucosamine is a critical receptor for colonization of *V. cholea* in the GI tract. *V. cholera* secretes the GlcNAc-binding protein A (GbpA) to bind N-acetylated D-glucosamine [36]. The *gbpA* mutant strain failed to attach to HT-29 epithelial cells and to colonize in the GI tract in mice model, compared to the wild-type strain [36]. Although a detailed interaction for GbpA-N-acetylated D glucosamine was not proposed in the paper, the binding was probably mediated through hydrogen bond interactions, due to the absence of positive charges in N-acetylated D-glucosamine. Taken together, we conclude that OmpA is a direct target of CM binding, and the hydrogen bond interactions between the two molecules inhibit OmpA function, resulting in membrane disruption to cause cell death.

First, we speculated that it was unlikely that CM had positively charged free amino groups on the particle surface because i) CM were generated by cross-linking of the amino groups with sodium sulfate that would deplete free amino groups and ii) even if unoccupied amino groups remain after cross-linking, they must be deprotonated at neutral pH due to a pKa value around 6.5 [37]. However, our findings may suggest that ionic interaction is involved in the CM interaction with *E. coli* O157:H7 at neutral pH. As shown in figure 2D, the *ompA* mutant still binds to the CM-coated slides, suggesting that additional binding target(s) is

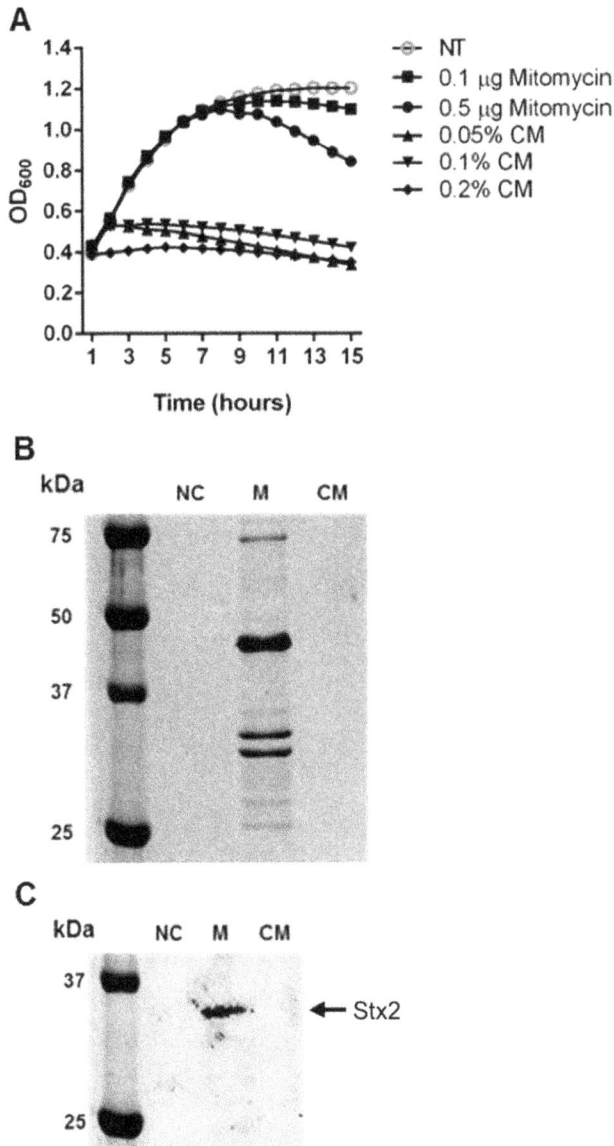

Figure 6. Chitosan microparticles do not induce bacterial phage and Shiga-toxin expression. (A) Phage induction was measured by a reduction of the OD_{600} of the bacterial culture with mitomicin C or CM at different concentrations. (B) SDS-PAGE analysis of phage proteins. Phage particles were obtained by PEG precipitation of cell lysate from mitomicin C-treated and CM-treated cultures. Phage proteins are visualized by Coomassie blue staining. (C) Shiga-toxin expression by CM treatment. E. coli O157:H7 strain was grown with CM and cell lysates were collected. Shiga-toxin expression was analyzed by Western blotting using antibody specific to Shiga-toxin. NC (negative control; without treatment), M (mitomicin C, 1 µg/ml), CM (chitosan microparticles, 0.2%).

involved in CM binding. One possible candidate is LPS because purified LPS is known to bind to chitosan in vitro [17], and we found that the ΔwaaL mutant, which exposes more negative charges on the cell surface, showed increased binding activity on CM-coated slides (Fig. 3D) and antimicrobial activity (Fig. 3E). In addition, antimicrobial activity increased at lower pH (pH 5)

compared to the neutral pH, suggesting CM have more positive charges at acidic pH that may bind to negatively charged bacterial surface molecules, such as LPS (Fig. 3D). Therefore, we hypothesize that CM bind to E. coli O157:H7 via two distinct mechanisms at neutral pH. First, a hydrogen bond interaction plays a key role in OmpA-mediated binding. Second, ionic interactions contribute to the binding activity. However, positively charged CM at acidic pH bind to negatively charged surface molecules such as LPS, resulting in magnified bacterial cell death.

In order to study if CM retain antimicrobial activity in vivo, cows with uterine diseases were used as an animal model. Uterine disease is one of the biggest challenges facing the dairy cattle industries. Economic and revenue losses are largely impacted by these diseases as a result of the infertility, increased culling, milk production decreases, and treatment cost from uterine diseases [38,39,40]. Because the causes of uterine diseases are often linked to a variety of different bacteria, including IUPEC, *Trueperella pyogenes*, *Fusobacterium necrophorum*, and *Prevotella melaninogenica*, treatment of these diseases are often challenging with 30% failure rate [41] using conventional antibiotic treatment. As shown in figure 5, animals treated with CM showed significantly reduced IUPEC numbers in the uterine samples and was even more effective than ceftiofur treatment, suggesting that CM can be used to treat animals with these diseases. In this initial CM treatment trial, we only focused on IUPEC in the uterus, thus additional studies are needed for other pathogens, including *Trueperella pyogenes*, *Fusobacterium necrophorum*, and *Prevotella melaninogenica*. However, CM have a broad-spectrum of antimicrobial activity including Gram negative and positive bacteria (Fig. 4), thus we speculate that CM may have antimicrobial activity against other etiological agents of uterine disease.

For the potential application of CM, it was evaluated that CM induce prophage and overexpress Shiga-toxin in E. coli O157:H7 (Fig. 6). Due to the expression of Shiga-toxins during phage induction, antibiotics are not generally recommended for treatment of E. coli O157:H7 [42,43]. Therefore, these results significantly emphasize the potential of CM as a therapeutic agent against this pathogen. Further studies regarding optimal CM treatment concentrations or pH effect on CM efficacy will be necessary to verify our initial findings. In addition, the broad-spectrum of antimicrobial activity of CM makes it possible to treat diseases caused by multiple pathogens such as uterine disease.

In this study, we have shown that underlying mechanisms of antimicrobial activity of CM. CM interact with OmpA protein at neutral pH, resulting in disruption of bacterial membranes and eventually leading to cell death. CM exert antimicrobial activity in an animal model with the uterine disease. Since CM treatment does not induce prophage and Shiga-toxin production, it holds promise as a treatment option for several pathogens.

Acknowledgments

We are grateful to Min Young Kang for technical support; Drs. Joseph Vogel, Wandy Beatty, Dong-Jin Park, and Charles Kaspar for helpful discussion.

Author Contributions

Conceived and designed the experiments: SJJ MO WY KNG KCJ. Performed the experiments: SJJ MO WY KNG KCJ. Analyzed the data: SJJ MO WY KNG KCJ. Wrote the paper: SJJ KNG KCJ.

References

1. Rabea EI, Badawy MET, Stevens CV, Smagghe G, Steurbaut W (2003) Chitosan as antimicrobial agent: applications and mode of action. Biomacromolecules 4: 1457–1465.

2. Chung YC, Wang HL, Chen YM, Li SL (2003) Effect of abiotic factors on the antibacterial activity of chitosan against waterborne pathogens. Bioresour Technol 88: 179–184.

3. Qi LF, Xu ZR, Jiang X, Hu CH, Zou XF (2004) Preparation and antibacterial activity of chitosan nanoparticles. Carbohydr Res 339: 2693–2700.

4. Darmadji P, Izumimoto M (1994) Effect of chitosan in meat preservation. Meat Sci 38: 243–254.

5. Liu H, Du YM, Wang XH, Sun LP (2004) Chitosan kills bacteria through cell membrane damage. Int J Food Microbiol 95: 147–155.

6. Papineau AM, Hoover DG, Knorr D, Farkas DF (1991) Antimicrobial effect of water-Soluble chitosans with high hydrostatic pressure. Food Biotechnol 5: 45–57.

7. Shahidi F, Arachchi JKV, Jeon YJ (1999) Food applications of chitin and chitosans. Trends Food Sci Technol 10: 37–51.

8. US Food and Drug Administration (2012) Shrimp-derived chitosan GRAS notification. Available: www.accessdata.fda.gov/scripts/fcn/gras_notices/GRN000443pdf. Accessed 2013 Dec 6.

9. Mahae N, Chalat C, Muhamud P (2011) Antioxidant and antimicrobial properties of chitosan-sugar complex. Int Food Res J 18: 1543–1551.

10. Sudarshan NR, Hoover DG, Knorr D (1992) Antibacterial action of chitosan. Food Biotechnol 6: 257–272.

11. Helander IM, Nurmiaho-Lassila EL, Ahvenainen R, Rhoades J, Roller S (2001) Chitosan disrupts the barrier properties of the outer membrane of Gram-negative bacteria. Int J Food Microbiol 71: 235–244.

12. Kong M, Chen XG, Xing K, Park HJ (2010) Antimicrobial properties of chitosan and mode of action: a state of the art review. Int J Food Microbiol 144: 51–63.

13. Jeong KC, Kang MY, Kang JH, Baumler DJ, Kaspar CW (2011) Reduction of Escherichia coli O157:H7 shedding in cattle by addition of chitosan microparticles to feed. Appl Environ Microbiol 77: 2011–2016.

14. van der Lubben IM, Verhoef JC, van Aelst AC, Borchard G, Junginger HE (2001) Chitosan microparticles for oral vaccination: preparation, characterization and preliminary in vivo uptake studies in murine Peyer's patches. Biomaterials 22: 687–694.

15. Datsenko KA, Wanner BL (2000) One-step inactivation of chromosomal genes in Escherichia coli K-12 using PCR products. Proc Natl Acad Sci USA 97: 6640–6645.

16. Shu XZ, Zhu KJ (2001) Chitosan/gelatin microspheres prepared by modified emulsification and ionotropic gelation. J Microencapsul 18: 237–245.

17. Davydova VN, Bratskaya SY, Gorbach VI, Solov'eva TF, Kaca W, et al. (2008) Comparative study of electrokinetic potentials and binding affinity of lipopolysaccharides-chitosan complexes. Biophys Chem 136: 1–6.

18. Raetz CRH, Whitfield C (2002) Lipopolysaccharide endotoxins. Annu Rev Biochem 71: 635–700.

19. Sheldon IM, Lewis GS, LeBlanc S, Gilbert RO (2006) Defining postpartum uterine disease in cattle. Theriogenology 65: 1516–1530.

20. Ozenc E, Seker E, Dogan N (2010) The effect of bacterial flora on uterine pH values, observed during the estrous cycle, gestation and in the cases of clinical metritis in cows. J Anim Vet Adv 9: 3000–3004.

21. Karmali MA (2004) Infection by shiga toxin-producing Escherichia coli - an overview. Mol Biotechnol 26: 117–122.

22. Rowe PC, Orrbine E, Lior H, Wells GA, Mclaine PN (1993) A prospective study of exposure to verotoxin-producing Escherichia coli among Canadian children with hemolytic uremic syndrome. Epidemiol Infect 110: 1–7.

23. Grif K, Dierich MP, Karch H, Allerberger F (1998) Strain-specific differences in the amount of shiga toxin released from enterohemorrhagic Escherichia coli O157 following exposure to subinhibitory concentrations of antimicrobial agents. Eur J Clin Microbiol Infect Dis 17: 761–766.

24. Serna A, Boedeker EC (2008) Pathogenesis and treatment of Shiga toxin-producing Escherichia coli infections. Curr Opin Gastroenterol 24: 38–47.

25. Park D, Stanton E, Ciezki K, Parrell D, Bozile M, et al. (2013) Evolution of the Stx2-encoding prophage in persistent bovine Escherichia coli O157:H7 strains. Appl Environ Microbiol 79: 1563–1572.

26. Xing K, Chen XG, Liu CS, Cha DS, Park HJ (2009) Oleoyl-chitosan nanoparticles inhibits Escherichia coli and Staphylococcus aureus by damaging the cell membrane and putative binding to extracellular or intracellular targets. Int J Food Microbiol 132: 127–133.

27. Koebnik R, Locher KP, Van Gelder P (2000) Structure and function of bacterial outer membrane proteins: barrels in a nutshell. Mol Microbiol 37: 239–253.

28. Pautsch A, Schulz GE (2000) High-resolution structure of the OmpA membrane domain. J Mol Biol 298: 273–282.

29. Killmann H, Benz R, Braun V (1993) Conversion of the Fhua transport protein into a diffusion channel through the outer membrane of Escherichia coli. Embo J 12: 3007–3016.

30. Klebba PE, Hofnung M, Charbit A (1994) A model of maltodextrin transport through the sugar-specific porin, LamB, based on deletion analysis. Embo J 13: 4670–4675.

31. Koebnik R (1999) Structural and functional roles of the surface-exposed loops of the beta-barrel membrane protein OmpA from Escherichia coli. J Bacteriol 181: 3688–3694.

32. Stoll BJ, Hansen N, Fanaroff AA, Wright LL, Carlo WA, et al. (2002) Changes in pathogens causing early-onset sepsis in very-low-birth-weight infants. N Engl J Med 347: 240–247.

33. Prasadarao NV (2002) Identification of Escherichia coli outer membrane protein A receptor on human brain microvascular endothelial cells. Infect Immun 70: 6513–6513.

34. Prasadarao NV, Srivastava PK, Rudrabhatla RS, Kim KS, Huang SH, et al. (2003) Cloning and expression of the Escherichia coli K1 outer membrane protein A receptor, a gp96 homologue. Infect Immun 71: 1680–1688.

35. Pascal TA, Abrol R, Mittal R, Wang Y, Prasadarao NV, et al. (2010) Experimental validation of the predicted binding site of Escherichia coli K1 outer membrane protein A to human brain microvascular endothelial Cells: identification of critical mutations that prevent E. coli meningitis. J Biol Chem 285: 37753–37761.

36. Kirn TJ, Jude BA, Taylor RK (2005) A colonization factor links Vibrio cholerae environmental survival and human infection. Nature 438: 863–866.

37. Lopez-Leon T, Carvalho ELS, Seijo B, Ortega-Vinuesa JL, Bastos-Gonzalez D (2005) Physicochemical characterization of chitosan nanoparticles: electrokinetic and stability behavior. J Colloid Interface Sci 283: 344–351.

38. Sheldon IM, Cronin J, Goetze L, Donofrio G, Schuberth HJ (2009) Defining postpartum uterine disease and the mechanisms of infection and immunity in the female reproductive tract in cattle. Biol Reprod 81: 1025–1032.

39. Galvao KN, Greco LF, Vilela JM, Sa MF, Santos JEP (2009) Effect of intrauterine infusion of ceftiofur on uterine health and fertility in dairy cows. J Dairy Sci 92: 1532–1542.

40. McDougall S, Macaulay R, Compton C (2007) Association between endometritis diagnosis using a novel intravaginal device and reproductive performance in dairy cattle. Anim Reprod Sci 99: 9–23.

41. McLaughlin CL, Stanisiewski E, Lucas MJ, Cornell CP, Watkins J, et al. (2012) Evaluation of two doses of ceftiofur crystalline free acid sterile suspension for treatment of metritis in lactating dairy cows. J dairy sci 95: 4363–4371.

42. Dundas S, Todd WTA, Stewart AI, Murdoch PS, Chaudhuri AK, et al. (2001) The central Scotland Escherichia coli O157:H7 outbreak: risk factors for the hemolytic uremic syndrome and death among hospitalized patients. Clin Infect Dis 33: 923–931.

43. Yoh M, Honda T (1997) The stimulating effect of fosfomycin, an antibiotic in common use in Japan, on the production/release of verotoxin-1 from enterohaemorrhagic Escherichia coli O157:H7 in vitro. Epidemiol Infect 119: 101–103.

17

Epizootic Pneumonia of Bighorn Sheep following Experimental Exposure to *Mycoplasma ovipneumoniae*

Thomas E. Besser[1,2]*, E. Frances Cassirer[3], Kathleen A. Potter[1,2], Kevin Lahmers[1], J. Lindsay Oaks[1,2], Sudarvili Shanthalingam[1], Subramaniam Srikumaran[1], William J. Foreyt[1]

1 Department of Veterinary Microbiology and Pathology, Washington State University, Pullman, Washington, United States of America, 2 Washington Animal Disease Diagnostic Laboratory, Washington State University, Pullman Washington, United States of America, 3 Idaho Department of Fish and Game, Lewiston, Idaho, United States of America

Abstract

Background: Bronchopneumonia is a population limiting disease of bighorn sheep (*Ovis canadensis*). The cause of this disease has been a subject of debate. Leukotoxin expressing *Mannheimia haemolytica* and *Bibersteinia trehalosi* produce acute pneumonia after experimental challenge but are infrequently isolated from animals in natural outbreaks. *Mycoplasma ovipneumoniae*, epidemiologically implicated in naturally occurring outbreaks, has received little experimental evaluation as a primary agent of bighorn sheep pneumonia.

Methodology/Principal Findings: In two experiments, bighorn sheep housed in multiple pens 7.6 to 12 m apart were exposed to *M. ovipneumoniae* by introduction of a single infected or challenged animal to a single pen. Respiratory disease was monitored by observation of clinical signs and confirmed by necropsy. Bacterial involvement in the pneumonic lungs was evaluated by conventional aerobic bacteriology and by culture-independent methods. In both experiments the challenge strain of *M. ovipneumoniae* was transmitted to all animals both within and between pens and all infected bighorn sheep developed bronchopneumonia. In six bighorn sheep in which the disease was allowed to run its course, three died with bronchopneumonia 34, 65, and 109 days after *M. ovipneumoniae* introduction. Diverse bacterial populations, predominantly including multiple obligate anaerobic species, were present in pneumonic lung tissues at necropsy.

Conclusions/Significance: Exposure to a single *M. ovipneumoniae* infected animal resulted in transmission of infection to all bighorn sheep both within the pen and in adjacent pens, and all infected sheep developed bronchopneumonia. The epidemiologic, pathologic and microbiologic findings in these experimental animals resembled those seen in naturally occurring pneumonia outbreaks in free ranging bighorn sheep.

Editor: Glenn F. Browning, The University of Melbourne, Australia

Funding: These studies were funded by grants from the Wyoming Wildlife/Livestock Disease Partnership (T. E. Besser, S. Srikumaran), the Washington Department of Fish and Wildlife (T. E. Besser), the Idaho Domestic Wildlife Research Oversight Committee (E. F. Cassirer), and the Oregon chapter of the Foundation for North American Wild Sheep (T. E. Besser) or the grant support that made these studies possible. The funders had no role in study design, data collection and analysis, decision to publish, or preparation of the manuscript.

Competing Interests: The authors have declared that no competing interests exist.

* Email: tbesser@vetmed.wsu.edu

Introduction

Bighorn sheep are a North American species that has failed to recover from steep declines at the turn of the 20th century despite strict protections and intensive management, and two populations (Sierra Nevada and Peninsular) are currently classified as endangered [1]. Epizootic pneumonia is limiting bighorn sheep population restoration and as such, the etiology is of considerable interest. The first appearance of the disease in a population is typically in the form of epizootics that affect animals of all ages and is sometimes accompanied by high (>50%) mortality rates. Subsequently, epizootics affecting primarily lambs may occur for decades [2]. Various causes have been proposed for this disease, including lungworms (*Protostrongylus* sp.) [3–6], Pasteurellaceae, especially *Mannheimia (Pasteurella) haemolytica,* [7–12] and more recently, *Mycoplasma ovipneumoniae* [13–16]. In a recent comparative review of the evidence supporting each of these possible etiologies we concluded that *M. ovipneumoniae* was most strongly supported as the primary epizootic agent of bighorn sheep pneumonia [14]. However, the only two previous experimental challenge studies with *M. ovipneumoniae* either did not reproduce disease [13] or were confounded by challenges with other agents [16]. The objective of this study was to improve upon previous investigations to better assess the outcome of experimental introduction of *M. ovipneumoniae* to naïve bighorn sheep.

Methods

Ethics statement

This study was carried out in accordance with the recommendations in the Guide for the Care and Use of Laboratory Animals of the National Institutes of Health and in conformance with

United States Department of Agriculture animal research guidelines, under protocols #03854 and #04482 approved by the Washington State University (WSU) Institutional Animal Care and Use Committee. As described in those protocols, euthanasia was performed by intravenous injection of sodium pentobarbital for animals observed to be in severe distress associated with pneumonia during the study and prior to necropsy examination for surviving animals at the end of each experiment.

Experimental aims

Experiment 1 was conducted to investigate the transmission of *M. ovipneumoniae* to bighorn sheep and their subsequent development of disease, using an infected domestic sheep source. Experiment 2 was conducted to investigate experimental direct *M. ovipneumoniae* infection of a single bighorn sheep and the subsequent transmission of this agent to conspecifics. Both experiments were conducted in multiple pens separated by short distances, which allowed investigation of transmission to both commingled and non-commingled animals.

Experimental animals

All experimental animals originated from herds and flocks unexposed to *M. ovipneumoniae* as determined by repeated testing with both serology on blood serum and PCR on enriched nasal swab cultures (using the methods described later in the 'Microbiological testing' section). In Experiment 1, three hand-reared bighorn sheep (yearling rams BHS #82 and #89 and yearling ewe BHS #07) that originated from a captive flock at WSU and three purchased domestic sheep (adult ewes DS #00 and #01 and yearling ewe DS #LA) were co-housed in three 46 m² pens, with one domestic and one bighorn sheep per pen. Pens were separated by 7.6–12 m. Experiment 1 animals had all been commingled in a single pen for 104 days immediately prior to the beginning of this experiment, as previously described [15]. One of the four bighorn sheep used in that prior study had died of *M. haemolytica* pneumonia, while the other three, which had demonstrated no signs of respiratory disease in that study, were used in experiment 1. In Experiment 2, wild bighorn sheep captured from the Asotin Creek population in Hells Canyon were housed in two 700 m² pens, 7.6 m apart, with three animals per pen (Pen #1: adult ewe BHS #40, yearling ewe BHS #38, and yearling ram BHS #39; Pen #2: adult ewes BHS #41 and #42 and adult ram BHS #C). The study pens had either never previously housed domestic or bighorn sheep (pen 1 in experiment 1; both pens in experiment 2) or had been rested for greater than one year since their previous occupancy by any *M. ovipneumoniae* infected sheep (pens 2 and 3 in experiment 1) prior to these experiments.

Experimental design

Experiment 1. A domestic ewe (DS #00) was placed in isolation and experimentally infected with *M. ovipneumoniae*. The inoculum consisted of ceftiofur-treated (100 ug/ml, 2 hrs, 37°C; Pfizer, Florham Park, NJ) nasal wash fluids from a domestic sheep naturally colonized with *M. ovipneumoniae* [16]. Following ceftiofur treatment, no aerobic bacterial growth was observed from the nasal wash fluids cultured under conditions expected to permit growth of *M. haemolytica, B. trehalosi,* or *P. multocida* (Columbia blood agar with 5% sheep blood, 35°C, overnight, 5% CO_2). DS #00 was then challenged with the treated nasal wash fluid by infusion of 15 ml in each nares, 10 ml orally and 5 ml into each conjunctival sac. Subsequent nasal swab samples obtained on days 1, 2, 4 and 7 post-challenge were all PCR positive for *M. ovipneumoniae* using the method described later in the 'Microbiological testing' section confirming that the experimental infection

had been successful. On post challenge day 7, DS #00 was introduced into pen #1 with BHS #82. Following commingling, DS #00 and BHS #82 were restrained for collection of nasal swab samples on days 1, 2, 4, 7, 14, 21, 28, and subsequently at 30 day intervals until the experiment was terminated. Rectal temperatures were recorded from both sheep approximately twice each week. Sheep in pens #2 (BHS #89 and DS #01) and #3 (BHS #07 and DS #LA) were restrained for rectal temperature determination and collection of nasal swabs for microbiology at approximately monthly intervals. All pens were observed daily for clinical signs of respiratory disease. The experiment was conducted October 2009–January 2010.

Experiment 2. BHS #39 was inoculated with *M. ovipneumoniae* just prior to its release into pen #1 with non-inoculated BHS #38 and #40. Non-inoculated BHS #C, #41, and #42 were housed in pen #2 on the same day. The inoculum for BHS #39 was prepared as described for that used in experiment 1 but originated from a different domestic sheep source. In lieu of computation of colony forming units, which is not possible for *M. ovipneumoniae* due to inconsistent growth on plated media, viable *M. ovipneumoniae* counts in the inoculum were determined using most probable number (MPN) using a custom 3×4 format: Triplicate enrichment broth tubes were inoculated at each of four decimal dilutions (10^{-2}–10^{-5}) of the treated nasal wash fluid [17], incubated (72 hrs, 35C) then PCR was used to detect growth of viable *M. ovipneumoniae*. The treated fluid was determined to contain 930 MPN/ml (95% confidence interval, 230 to 3800 MPN). Two of the bighorn sheep (BHS #38 and #39) in pen 1 were recaptured by drive net on day 21 of the experiment for nasal swab sampling to detect *M. ovipneumoniae* infection; otherwise, no live animal sampling was conducted in experiment #2 to reduce the risk of traumatic injury of the wild bighorn sheep involved. The experiment was conducted December 2011–June 2012.

Biosecurity. In both experiments, routine biosecurity measures included: 1) the pens containing the single *M. ovipneumoniae*-challenged animals (exposed pens) were located downwind of the prevailing wind direction from the pens containing no experimentally *M. ovipneumoniae* exposed animals (clean pens), 2) order of entry rules were established so that on any single day exposed pens were routinely entered by animal care staff for feeding and cleaning only after all work in clean pens had been completed, and 3) personal protective equipment (coveralls and boots) used in exposed pens were either not reused, or were sanitized prior to use in clean pens.

Clinical scores. Clinical score data were determined using the following cumulative point system: observed anorexia (1), nasal discharge (1), cough (2), dyspnea (1), head shaking (1), ear paresis (1) and weakness/incoordination (1).

Microbiological testing. Routine diagnostic testing performed by the Washington Animal Diagnostic Laboratory (fully accredited by the American Association of Veterinary Laboratory Diagnosticians) included detection of *M. ovipneumoniae*-specific and small ruminant lentivirus-specific antibodies in serum samples using competitive enzyme-linked immunosorbent assays (cELISA) [14,18,19], detection of *M. ovipneumoniae* colonization by broth enrichment of nasal swabs followed by *M. ovipneumoniae*-specific PCR testing of the broths [20,21], detection of Pasteurellaceae in pharyngeal swab samples by aerobic bacteriologic cultures, and detection of exposure to parainfluenza-3, border disease, and respiratory syncytial viruses by virus neutralization antibody assays applied to serum samples.

PCR tests specific for detection of *M. haemolytica, B. trehalosi,* and *P. multocida,* and *lktA* (the gene encoding the principal virulence factor of *M. haemolytica* and *B. trehalosi*) were applied to DNA extracted from pneumonic lung tissues using previously described primers (Table 1) and methods with minor modifications. All reactions were conducted individually in 20 μL volumes containing 80–300 ng of template DNA. For *M. haemolytica, B. trehalosi, lktA* and *P. multocida*, reactions contained 0.5 units of HotStar Taq DNA polymerase (Qiagen), 2 μL 10x PCR buffer (Qiagen), 4 μL Q-solution (Qiagen), 40 μM of each dNTP (Invitrogen). The *M. ovipneumoniae* reaction used QIAGEN Multiplex PCR mix. Primers were used at final concentrations of 0.2 μM (*M. haemolytica, B. trehalosi, P. multocida,* and *M. ovipneumoniae*) or 0.5 μM (leukotoxin A). Each reaction included an initial activation and denaturation step (95°C, 15 min) and a final 72°C extension step (10 min for Mhgcp-2, lktA, lktA set-1, and LM primers; 9 min for KMT primers; 5 min for Btsod and Mhgcp primers). Cycling conditions were as follows: *M. ovipneumoniae*, 30 cycles of 95°C for 30 s, 58°C for 30 s, 72°C for 30 s; *B. trehalosi* and *M. haemolytica* (Mhgcp and Btsod primers), 35 cycles of 95°C for 30 s, 55°C for 30 s, 72°C for 40 s; *P. multocida* and *lktA* (lktA primers), 30 cycles of 95°C for 60 s, 55°C for 60 s, 72°C for 60 s; *M. haemolytica* (Mhgcp-2 primers), 40 cycles of 95°C for 30 s, 54°C for 30 s, 72°C for 30 s; *lktA* (lktA set-1 primers), 40 cycles of 95°C for 30 s, 52°C for 30 s, 72°C for 40 s. Leukotoxin expression was detected in Pasteurellacae isolates by MTT dye reduction cytotoxicity assay as described previously [22].

The 16S–23S ribosomal operon intergenic spacer (IGS) regions of *M. ovipneumoniae* recovered from animals in these studies were PCR amplified (Table 1) and sequenced as previously described [23].

16S rDNA analyses to identify the predominant bacterial flora in pneumonic lung tissues. In previous studies, culture-independent evaluation of the microbial flora of lung tissues in naturally occurring bighorn sheep pneumonia revealed a polymicrobial flora late in the disease course [13,23]. For comparison, we applied the same methods to lung tissues of the experimentally challenged animals in this study. Note that more sensitive

detection of specific respiratory pathogens was provided by the PCR assays described earlier, whereas these 16S studies were designed instead to identify the numerically predominant bacteria in affected lungs. The library size used was based on the binary distribution to provide a 95% chance of detection of each taxon comprising 10% or more of the ribosomal operon frequency in the source tissue. Two 1 g samples of pneumonic lung tissues were aseptically collected from sites at least 10 cm apart, homogenized by stomaching, and DNA was extracted (DNeasy tissue kit; Qiagen, Valencia, CA) from 100 uL aliquots of each homogenate. 16S rDNA segments were PCR amplified and cloned as described [13]. Insert DNA was sequenced from 16 clones derived from each of the two homogenates from each animal, and each sequence was attributed to species (≥99% identity) or genus (≥97% identity) based on BLAST GenBank similarity [24].

Results

Experiment 1

M. ovipneumoniae infection of DS #00, introduced into pen 1 to start the experiment, was confirmed by positive nasal swab samples obtained on days 1, 4, and 7 after inoculation prior to its introduction into pen #1, and on days 1, 2, 4, 7, 14, 21, 28, 60 and 90 after its introduction into pen #1, confirming that the experimental colonization had been successful and maintained throughout experiment 1. *M. ovipneumoniae* was first detected in the bighorn sheep (BHS #82) commingled with DS #00 in pen #1 on day 28, and subsequent tests on days 60 and 90 were also positive. BHS #82 developed signs of respiratory disease including nasal discharge (onset day 37); coughing and fever (onset day 42); and lethargy and ear paresis (onset day 61) (Figure 1a). Signs of respiratory disease were observed in the bighorn sheep in pens #2 (BHS #89) and #3 (BHS #07) beginning on days 62 and 67, respectively; these signs also included fever, lethargy, paroxysmal coughing, nasal discharge, head shaking, and drooping ears. No signs of respiratory disease were observed in the commingled domestic sheep at any time during the experiment. *M.*

Table 1. Primers and PCR reaction targets used in these experiments.

Pathogen/Virulence gene	Target	Primer Name	Sequence (5' → 3')	Size (bp)	Reference
M. haemolytica	*gcp*	MhgcpF	AGA GGC CAA TCT GCA AAC CTC G	267	[33]
		MhgcpR	GTT CGT ATT GCC CAA CGC CG		
M. haemolytica	*gcp*	MhgcpF2	TGG GCA ATA CGA ACT ACT CGG G	227	[34]
		MhgcpR2	CTT TAA TCG TAT TCG CAG		
B. trehalosi	*sodA*	BtsodAF	GCC TGC GGA CAA ACG TGT TG	144	[33]
		BtsodAR	TTT CAA CAG AAC CAA AAT CAC GAA TG		
P. multocida	*kmt1*	KMT1T7	ATC CGC TAT TTA CCC AGT GG	460	[35]
		KMT1SP6	GCT GTA AAC GAA CTC GCC AC		
Pasteurellaceae leukotoxin	*lktA*	lktAF	TGT GGA TGC GTT TGA AGA AGG	1,145	[36]
		lktAR	ACT TGC TTT GAG GTG ATC CG		
M. haemolytica leukotoxin	*lktA*	lktAF set-1	CTT ACA TTT TAG CCC AAC GTG	497	[34]
		lktAR set-1	TAA ATT CGC AAG ATA ACG GG		
Mycoplasma ovipneumoniae	16s rDNA	LMF	TGA ACG GAA TAT GTT AGC TT	361	[20,21]
		LMR	GAC TTC ATC CTG CAC TCT GT		
Mycoplasma ovipneumoniae	16S–23S IGS	MoIGSF	GGA ACA CCT CCT TTC TAC GG	Variable~490	[23]
		MoIGSR	CCA AGG CAT CCA CCA AAT AC		

ovipneumoniae was detected in nasal swab samples from all bighorn and domestic sheep in pens #2 and #3 when sampled on day 70. The bighorn sheep were euthanized for necropsy on days 93 (BHS #89) and 99 (BHS #82 and #07). At necropsy, significant abnormal findings were limited to the respiratory tract. Bronchopneumonia affecting 25–50% of the lung volume was observed in all three bighorn sheep (Figure 2). Histopathological examination revealed peribronchiolitis with large lymphoid cuffs, bronchiectasis with purulent exudates, pulmonary atelectasis, and hyperplastic bronchial epithelia lacking visible cilia (Figure 2).

Experiment 2

On day 21 following release of the inoculated bighorn into pen #1, *M. ovipneumoniae* was detected in the inoculated animal and one pen mate (BHS #38 and #39); the third animal (BHS #40) evaded capture and sampling on that day. The first signs of respiratory disease were observed in pen #1 animals on day 21 during drive net capture for sampling, apparently triggered by exertion (Figure 2a). On day 34, inoculated BHS #39 died in pen

#1. On day 49, signs of respiratory disease were first observed in the bighorn sheep in pen #2 (Figure 2b). On days 65 and 109, #41, and #42 in pen #2 died or were euthanized *in extremis*. The surviving three bighorn sheep exhibited varying degrees of respiratory disease: BHS #38 showed persistent respiratory disease, while BHS #40 and #C showed decreasing respiratory disease over time, which became minimal after days 161 and 154, respectively. On day 204, the three surviving bighorn sheep were euthanized for necropsy. At necropsy, significant abnormal findings were limited to the respiratory tract. All six bighorn sheep had bronchopneumonia, with consolidation of lung tissue volumes ranging from an estimated 5% (BHS #40) to 80–100% (BHS #41) (Figure 2). Histopathological examination revealed severe peribronchiolitis with large lymphoid cuffs as seen in experiment 1. Animals that died or were euthanized in extremis had an overlying necrotizing bronchiolitis (#39) or abscessing bronchiolitis with bronchiectasis (BHS #41, #42) (Figure 2).

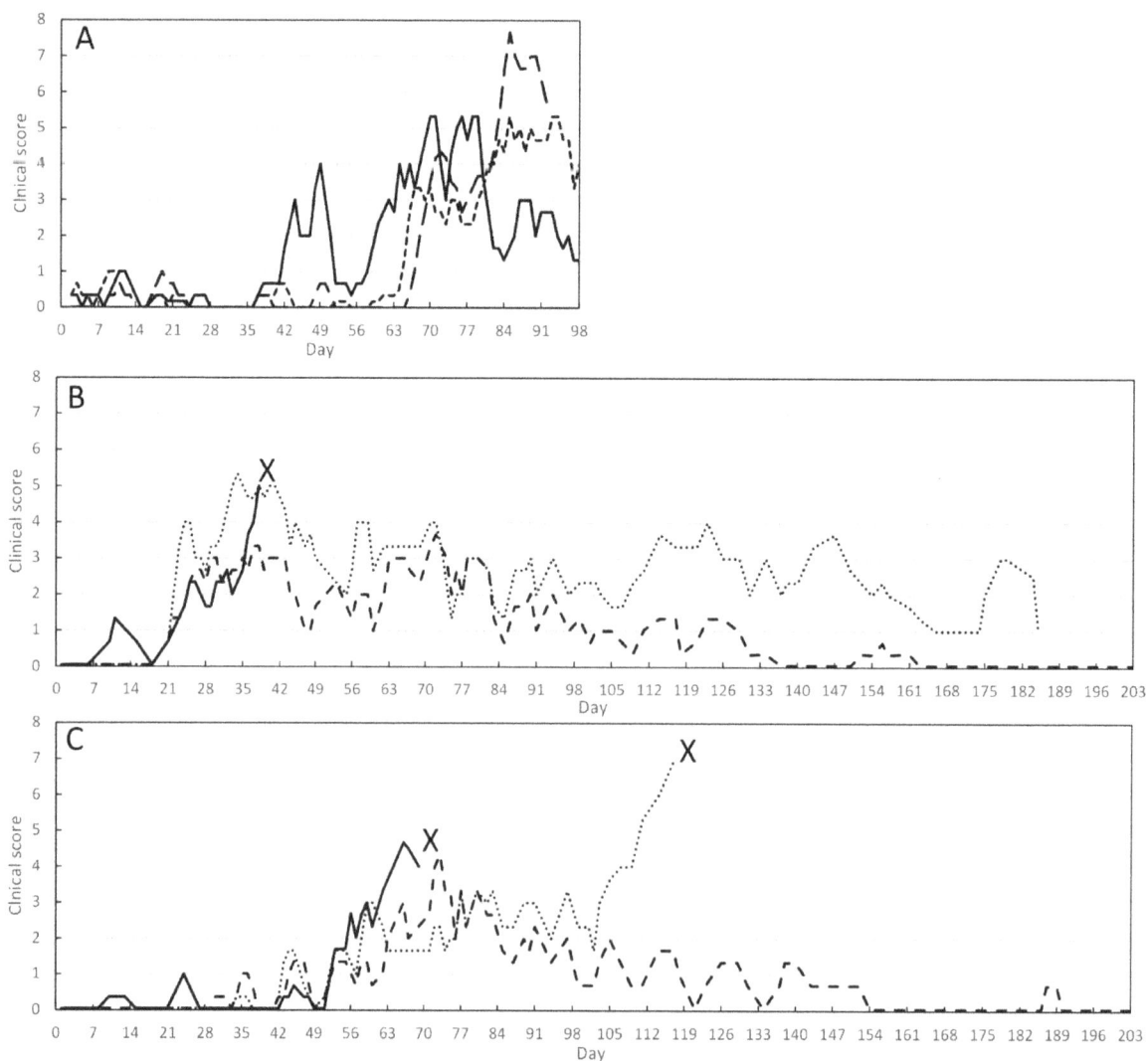

Figure 1. Clinical signs exhibited by *M. ovipneumoniae* infected bighorn sheep. Clinical scores (3-day moving averages) of bighorn sheep following introduction of *M. ovipneumoniae*: A) Experiment 1, 3 separate pens; solid line, Pen 1, BHS #82; dashed line, Pen 2, BHS #89; dotted line, Pen 3, BHS #07; B) Experiment 2, Pen 1: solid line, BHS #39 (died day 34); dashed line, BHS #40; dotted line; BHS #38.; C) Experiment 2, Pen 2: solid line, BHS #42 (euthanized day 109); dotted line, BHS #41 (died day 65); dashed line, BHS #C.

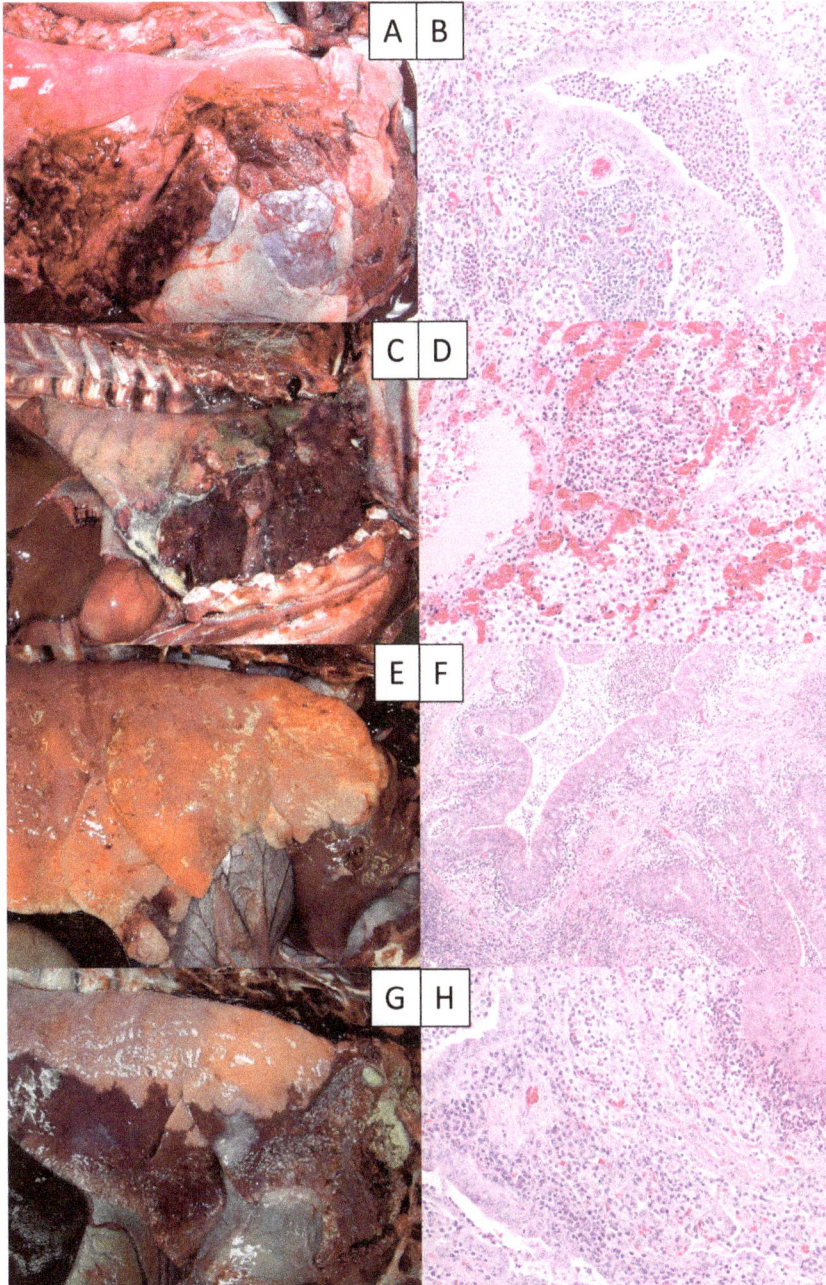

Figure 2. Gross and histologic lesions in lungs of bighorn sheep experimentally infected with *M. ovipneumoniae.* Images of BHS #82 (A, B), BHS #39 (C, D), BHS #C (E, F) and BHS #42 (G, H). Original magnification of histologic images was 200X (B, D, H) or 100X (F).

Microbiology

All bighorn sheep in both experiments seroconverted to *M. ovipneumoniae* (Table 2). Most experimental animals had neutralizing antibody to parainfluenza-3 virus, but no significant changes in antibody titers were observed during the experimental period. Detectable antibody to other ovine respiratory viruses, including border disease virus, ovine progressive pneumonia virus, and respiratory syncytial virus was occasionally observed in single samples.

M. ovipneumoniae was detected at necropsy in both upper and lower respiratory tracts of all bighorn sheep except BHS #40 whose lung tissues were PCR negative and whose upper

respiratory samples were PCR indeterminate (Table 3). Aerobic cultures and/or PCR tests identified *B. trehalosi* from pneumonic lung tissues from all bighorn sheep in both experiments (Table 3). *B. trehalosi* isolates from BHS #82 and #07 carried *lktA* and expressed leukotoxin activity (Table 3). *P. multocida* and *M. haemolytica* were not detected in these animals by either aerobic culture or PCR.

Culture independent survey of bacteria in pneumonic bighorn sheep lung tissues

DNA sequences of cloned 16S rDNA revealed that the predominant bacterial species in pneumonic sections of lung were

Table 2. Antibody responses to *M. ovipneumoniae* and parainfluenza-3 (PI-3) virus.

Experiment	ID	Pen	*M. ovipneumoniae*[1]		PI-3 virus[2]	
			Pre[3]	Post[3]	Pre[3]	Post[3]
1	82	1	−8%	93%	512	512
1	89	2	−7%	88%	128	128
1	07	3	−1%	92%	256	512
2	38	1	−6%	74%	Neg	64
2	39	1	−13%	67%	Neg	<32
2	40	1	−23%	75%	64	512
2	41	2	−19%	82%	512	NT
2	42	2	−11%	82%	256	NT
2	C	2	−4%	66%	256	512

[1]*M. ovipneumoniae* antibody detected by cELISA, expressed as percentage inhibition of the binding of an agent-specific monoclonal antibody [14,18].
[2]PI-3 virus neutralizing antibody detected by virus neutralization [37].
[3]Pre samples in experiment 1 were obtained on the day that the *M. ovipneumoniae* colonized domestic sheep was introduced to pen 1 and in experiment 2 were obtained on the day that BHS #39 was inoculated with *M. ovipneumoniae*. 'Post' samples in both experiments were obtained at necropsy. Neg = No titer detected. NT = Not tested, due to inadequate specimen volume.

diverse (Table 4). In experiment 1, *M. ovipneumoniae* was detected in the lung tissues of all animals. *B. trehalosi* also comprised substantial proportions of the pneumonic lung flora in two animals (BHS #82 and #07), while obligate anaerobic species, primarily *Fusobacterium* spp., predominated in the third animal (BHS #89). The flora identified in the pneumonic lungs of the animals in experiment 2 was also substantially comprised of mixed obligate anaerobes especially *Fusobacterium* spp. (Table 4).

Molecular epidemiology of respiratory pathogens. Consistent with epidemic transmission, *M. ovipneumoniae* strains recovered from all experimental sheep within each experiment shared identical IGS DNA sequences with the respective challenge inoculum (GenBank HQ615162 in experiment 1; KJ551511 in experiment 2).

Discussion

The most striking finding of these experiments was the high transmissibility of *M. ovipneumoniae* and the consistent development of pneumonia that followed infection of bighorn sheep. The bacterium was naturally transmitted from single experimentally inoculated animals (a domestic sheep in experiment 1 and a bighorn sheep in experiment 2) to all animals within and between pens up to 12 m distant. Eight of nine bighorn sheep exposed to *M. ovipneumoniae* developed severe bronchopneumonia and three died, while all the domestic sheep remained healthy.

Previous experimental challenge studies conducted with *M. haemolytica* or *B. trehalosi* in the absence of *M. ovipneumoniae* have not documented transmission. For example, Foreyt et al. [8]

Table 3. Microbiologic findings from pneumonic lung tissues, based on aerobic culture and species specific PCR.

Expt.	ID	Bacterial pathogens identified in pneumonic lung tissues				
		B. trehalosi	*M. haemolytica*	*lktA*	*M. ovipneumoniae*	Other[5]
1	82	Cult, *sodA*[1]	Neg[2]	Pos[3]	16S[4]	None
1	89	Cult, *sodA*	Neg	Neg[3]	16S	*Pasteurella* sp.[5]
1	07	Cult, *sodA*	Neg	Pos	16S	*Pasteurella* sp.
2	38	Cult, *sodA*	Neg	Neg	16S	*Pasteurella* sp.
2	39	NT, *sodA*	NT, Neg[2]	Neg	16S	NT[5]
2	40	Cult	Neg	Neg	Neg[4]	*Trueperella pyogenes*[5]
2	41	Cult, *sodA*	Neg	Neg	16S	None
2	42	Cult	Neg	Neg	16S	None
2	C	Cult	Neg	Neg	16S	*Pasteurella* sp.

[1]Cult = *B. trehalosi* detected by bacterial culture; *sodA* = *B. trehalosi* detected by *sodA* species-specific PCR (Table 1); NT = Unable to test by bacterial culture (overgrowth by *Proteus* sp.).
[2]Neg = *M. haemolytica* not detected by either bacterial culture or by PCR with either *gcp* primer set (Table 1); NT = Unable to test by bacterial culture (overgrowth by *Proteus* sp.).
[3]Neg = Pasteurellaceae *lktA* not detected in DNA extracts from pneumonic lung tissues by two different *lktA* PCRs (Table 1) [34,36]. Pos = *lktA* detected in *B. trehalosi* isolates obtained from BHS #82 and #07 [36].
[4]16S = *M. ovipneumoniae* detected by PCR (Table 1) [20]; Neg = *M. ovipneumoniae* not detected by PCR.
[5]*Pasteurella* sp., *Trueperella pyogenes* = Bacteria isolated and identified by aerobic culture; *Pasteurella* sp. were determined not to be *B. trehalosi*, *M. haemolytica*, or *P. multocida*; NT = Unable to test by bacterial culture due to overgrowth by *Proteus* sp.

Table 4. Microbiologic findings by 16S clone library (culture independent) method.

Expt.	ID	Bacterial species identified in pneumonic lung tissues					
		Btre[1]	Movi[1]	Fuso[1]	Prev[1]	Porphyro[1]	Other[1]
1	82	20 (62.5)[2]	8 (25)	0	3 (9.4)	0	1 (3.1)
1	89	1 (3.1)	7 (21.9)	21 (65.6)	1 (3.1)	0	2 (6.3)
1	07	16 (50.0)	12 (37.5)	0	0	0	4 (12.5)
2	38	4 (7.1)	2 (3.6)	8 (14.3)	20 (35.7)	9 (16.1)	13 (23.2)
2	C	0	0	17 (30.4)	5 (8.9)	19 (33.9)	15 (26.8)
2	39	2 (6.3)	0	24 (75.0)	0	0	6 (18.8)
2	40	0	0	0	0	0	56 (100.0)
2	41	1 (3.1)	0	21 (65.6)	5 (15.6)	0	5 (15.6)
2	42	0	0	31 (96.9)	0	0	1 (3.1)

[1]Btre = *B. trehalosi*; Movi = *M. ovipneumoniae*; Fuso = *Fusobacterium* sp.; Prev = *Prevotella* sp.; Porphyro = *Porphyromonas* sp.; Other = taxa other than those previously listed, each comprising <5% of sequenced clones.
[2]N (%) of the sequenced 16S clones from each animal whose DNA sequences were identical to those of the tabulated bacterial species in each column.

reported a series of three experiments in which commingled bighorn sheep were either challenged with intra-tracheal *M. haemolytica* or given sterile BHI as controls. Four of the five control bighorn sheep survived without evidence of disease while commingled with eight *M. haemolytica*-challenged bighorn sheep, of which seven died of pneumonia [8]. Commingled bighorn sheep also remained healthy in several other studies where individual bighorn sheep died with apparent *M. haemolytica* bronchopneumonia (confirmed by isolation of this bacterium from lung tissues) [15,25,26].

In addition to high transmissibility, the time course of disease development and the predominant microbiology of the pneumonic lung tissues following experimental introduction of *M. ovipneumoniae* differed from that seen in previous bighorn sheep challenge experiments with other respiratory pathogens. Bighorn sheep directly challenged with leukotoxin positive *M. haemolytica* or *B. trehalosi* develop peracute bronchopneumonia and >90% die within a week of challenges with 10^5 cfu or more [16,27–30]. In contrast, disease following experimental *M. ovipneumoniae* exposures was considerably slower in onset (14–21 days post infection) and development (deaths occurring 34 to 109 days post infection; respiratory disease persisted up to 6 months post-infection); this slow time course closely resembles that documented previously in bighorn lamb pneumonia outbreaks [13]. After lethal *M. haemolytica* challenge, the agent is typically isolated from lung tissues in high numbers and pure cultures [15,25]; in contrast in naturally occurring pneumonia outbreaks *M. ovipneumoniae* may be predominant early in the disease course but 16S library analyses have been used to document its overgrowth by diverse other bacteria later in the disease course [14,23]. Although the numbers of animals in the experimental *M. ovipneumoniae* infection studies reported here are small, the results are consistent with the trend for early predominance of *M. ovipneumoniae* followed by overgrowth by diverse other bacterial later in the disease course (Tables 3 and 4) [13,14,23].

Our results also differ from our previous attempt to experimentally reproduce respiratory disease by challenge inoculation of 1-week-old bighorn lambs with *M. ovipneumoniae*, which produced minor lesions and seroconversion but no clinically significant respiratory disease [13]. However, laboratory passage of *M. ovipneumoniae* (as was performed in that experiment) has been reported to attenuate virulence in *M. ovipneumoniae* [31]. Challenge of bighorn sheep with un-passaged *M. ovipneumoniae* produced different results, as observed here in experiment #2. In another study [16], nasal washings from domestic sheep naturally colonized with *M. ovipneumoniae* or lung homogenates from a *M. ovipneumoniae*-infected bighorn sheep were used for challenge of bighorn sheep after ceftiofur treatment to eliminate detectable Pasteurellaceae. Consistent with increased virulence of un-passaged *M. ovipneumoniae*, infection and respiratory disease signs were observed in all four bighorn sheep, one of which died 19 days following challenge. The three surviving animals continued to exhibit respiratory disease signs for 42 days, at which time the experiment was terminated by challenge with *M. haemolytica* (using a dose documented to be rapidly fatal to bighorn sheep even in the absence of *M. ovipneumoniae*) [16]. As a result, the longer term effects of the mycoplasma infection were not determined in that study. Therefore, the experiments reported here are the first in which naïve bighorn sheep were exposed to un-passaged *M. ovipneumoniae* and then followed over a time period comparable with the naturally occurring disease course.

The possibility of viral agents contributing to the disease observed in this study cannot be completely ruled out, since the inoculum was derived from nasal washings from domestic sheep and no virucidal treatments were applied. However, a previous study using ultrafiltrates of bighorn sheep pneumonic lung tissues or nasal washings from domestic sheep failed to reproduce any respiratory disease in inoculated susceptible bighorn sheep [16]. In addition, serologic monitoring for the predominant domestic sheep respiratory viruses did not demonstrate seroconversion of the experimental animals in this study, as described in the Results and in Table 2. Therefore, the most parsimonious interpretation of the data presented here is that the disease observed resulted from *M. ovipneumoniae* infection and the sequelae of that infection.

The transmission of *M. ovipneumoniae* from pen-to-pen in these experiments strongly suggests that direct contact is not necessary for epizootic spread of pneumonia in bighorn sheep. Feeding, watering and other procedures involving animal care or research staff were designed to minimize the risk of human or fomite-mediated transmission of the pathogen from pen to pen, although we recognize it is impossible to completely rule out this possibility. On the other hand, since aerosolized droplet transmission is recognized as a transmission route for the closely related bacterium, *Mycoplasma hyopneumoniae* (the cause of atypical pneumonia of swine) [32], it is plausible that a similar transmission mode occurs with *M. ovipneumoniae*. Infectious aerosols generated by coughing animals would likely contribute to the explosive nature of the pneumonia outbreaks observed following initial introduction of *M. ovipneumoniae* into naïve bighorn sheep populations.

In conclusion, we demonstrated that experimental *M. ovipneumoniae* infection of naïve bighorn sheep induces chronic, severe bronchopneumonia associated with multiple secondary bacterial infections and that this infection spread rapidly to animals both within the same pen and to animals in nearby pens. The significance of these findings would be clarified by parallel experiments specifically designed to determine transmissibility and associated disease outcomes in other agents associated with bighorn sheep pneumonia, particularly *M. haemolytica,* in the absence of *M. ovipneumoniae*. Furthermore, the case-fatality rates of *M. ovipneumoniae* infected animals described here contrasts

with the nearly 100% mortality that follows experimental commingling of bighorn sheep with presumptively or documented *M. ovipneumoniae*-positive domestic sheep and suggests an important role for polymicrobial secondary infections in determining mortality rates, which could be investigated in future studies. Finally, *M. ovipneumoniae* was still detected in nasal swab samples of several surviving bighorn sheep that were euthanized at the completion of these studies, suggesting that survivors of naturally occurring pneumonia outbreaks may continue to carry and shed this agent in nasal secretions. Such carriage may provide a mechanism for the post-invasion disease epizootics in lambs described in free-ranging populations. If so, this presumptive carrier state requires further study to characterize the factors that determine its occurrence and persistence, as these may be critical for the development of effective management control measures for this devastating disease.

Acknowledgments

We thank Donald P. Knowles for his contribution to the design of experiment 1 and manuscript editing, Margaret Highland for skillful technical assistance and for manuscript editing, Glen Weiser for providing custom selective media for Pasteurellaceae, Duane Chandler and Amy Hetrick for assistance with animal care, handling and restraint and sample collection, George Barrington for providing access to *M. ovipneumoniae* free domestic sheep, the Washington Department of Fish and Wildlife for wild bighorn sheep, Katie Baker for skillful technical assistance, and Shannon Lee Swist for serving as Principal Investigator of the Wyoming Wildlife/Livestock Disease Partnership grant.

Author Contributions

Conceived and designed the experiments: TEB EFC JLO S. Srikumaran WJF. Performed the experiments: TEB EFC JLO KAP KL S. Shanthalingam. Analyzed the data: TEB EFC KAP KL. Contributed reagents/materials/analysis tools: TEB EFC KAP KL S. Shanthalingam S. Srikumaran. Contributed to the writing of the manuscript: TEB EFC KAP S. Shanthalingam S. Srikumaran WJF.

References

1. Festa-Bianchet M (2008) *Ovis canadensis*. The IUCN Red List of Threatened Species. Available: http://www.iucnredlist.org/details/summary/15735/0. Accessed 2014 Jul 24.

2. Cassirer EF, Plowright RK, Manlove KR, Cross PC, Dobson AP, et al. (2012) Spatio-temporal dynamics of pneumonia in bighorn sheep (*Ovis canadensis*). J Animal Ecol 82: 518–528.

3. Marsh H (1938) Pneumonia in Rocky Mountain bighorn sheep. J Mammal 19: 214–219.

4. Buechner HK (1960) The bighorn sheep in the United States, its past, present, and future. Wildl Monog 4: 3–174.

5. Forrester DJ (1971) Bighorn sheep lungworm-pneumonia complex. In: Davis JW, Anderson RC, editors. Parasitic Diseases of Wild Mammals. Ames, IA: Iowa State University Press. 158–173.

6. Demartini JC, Davies RB (1977) An epizootic of pneumonia in captive bighorn sheep infected with *Muellerius* sp. J Wildl Dis 13: 117–124.

7. Miller MW (2001) Pasteurellosis. In: Williams ES, Barker, I K., editor. Infectious diseases of wild mammals. Ames IA USA: Iowa State University Press. 558.

8. Foreyt WJ, Snipes KP, Kasten RW (1994) Fatal pneumonia following inoculation of healthy bighorn sheep with *Pasteurella haemolytica* from healthy domestic sheep. J Wildl Dis 30: 137–145.

9. Kraabel BJ, Miller MW, Conlon JA, McNeil HJ (1998) Evaluation of a multivalent *Pasteurella haemolytica* vaccine in bighorn sheep: Protection from experimental challenge. J Wildl Dis 34: 325–333.

10. Rudolph KM, Hunter DL, Foreyt WJ, Cassirer EF, Rimler RB, et al. (2003) Sharing of *Pasteurella* spp. between free-ranging bighorn sheep and feral goats. J Wildl Dis 39: 897–903.

11. Rudolph KM, Hunter DL, Rimler RB, Cassirer EF, Foreyt WJ, et al. (2007) Microorganisms associated with a pneumonic epizootic in Rocky Mountain bighorn sheep (*Ovis canadensis canadensis*). J Zoo Wildl Med 38: 548–558.

12. Weiser GC, DeLong WJ, Paz JL, Shafii B, Price WJ, et al. (2003) Characterization of *Pasteurella multocida* associated with pneumonia in bighorn sheep. J Wildl Dis 39: 536–544.

13. Besser TE, Cassirer EF, Potter KA, VanderSchalie J, Fischer A, et al. (2008) Association of *Mycoplasma ovipneumoniae* infection with population-limiting respiratory disease in free-ranging rocky mountain bighorn sheep (*Ovis canadensis canadensis*). J Clin Microbiol 46: 423–430.

14. Besser TE, EF Cassirer, MA Highland, P Wolff, A Justice-Allen, et.al. (2012) Bighorn sheep pneumonia: Sorting out the cause of a polymicrobial disease. Prev Vet Med 108: 85–93.

15. Besser TE, Cassirer EF, Yamada C, Potter KA, Herndon C, et al. (2012) Survival of Bighorn Sheep (*Ovis canadensis*) Commingled with Domestic Sheep (*Ovis aries*) in the Absence of *Mycoplasma ovipneumoniae*. J Wildl Dis 48: 168–172.

16. Dassanayake RP, Shanthalingam S, Herndon CN, Subramaniam R, Lawrence PK, et al. (2010) *Mycoplasma ovipneumoniae* can predispose bighorn sheep to fatal *Mannheimia haemolytica* pneumonia. Vet Microbiol 145: 354–359.

17. Blodgett R (2010) Bacteriologic Analytical Manual Appendix 2: Most Probable Number from Serial Dilutions. Washington DC. Available: http://www.fda.gov/Food/FoodScience Research/LaboratoryMethods/ucm109656.htm. Accessed 2014 Jul 24.

18. Ziegler JC, Lahmers KK, Barrington GM, Parish SM, Kilzer K, et al. (2014) Safety and Immunogenicity of a Mycoplasma ovipneumoniae Bacterin for Domestic Sheep (*Ovis aries*). PLoS One 9(4): e95698.

19. Herrmann LM, Cheevers WP, Marshall KL, McGuire TC, Hutton MM, et al. (2003) Detection of serum antibodies to ovine progressive pneumonia virus in sheep by using a caprine arthritis-encephalitis virus competitive-inhibition enzyme-linked immunosorbent assay. Clin Diag Lab Immunol 10: 862–865.

20. Lawrence PK, Shanthalingam S, Dassanayake RP, Subramaniam R, Herndon CN, et al. (2010) Transmission of *Mannheimia haemolytica* from domestic sheep (*Ovis aries*) to bighorn sheep (*Ovis canadensis*): unequivocal demonstration with green fluorescent protein-tagged organisms. J Wildl Dis 46: 706–717; erratum, J Wildl Dis 46: 1346.

21. McAuliffe L, Hatchell FM, Ayling RD, King AI, Nicholas RA (2003) Detection of *Mycoplasma ovipneumoniae* in *Pasteurella*-vaccinated sheep flocks with respiratory disease in England. Vet Rec 153: 687–688.

22. Gentry MJ, Srikumaran S. (1991) Neutralizing monoclonal antibodies to *Pasteurella haemolytica* leukotoxin affinity purify the toxin from crude culture supernatants. Microb Pathog 10: 411–417.

23. Besser TE, Highland M, Baker K, Anderson NJ, Ramsey JM (2012) Causes of pneumonia epizootics among bighorn sheep, western United States, 2008–2010. Emerg Infect Dis 18: 406–414.

24. Petti CA (2007) Detection and identification of microorganisms by gene amplification and sequencing. Clin Infect Dis 44: 1108–1114.

25. Foreyt WJ, Jenkins EJ, Appleyard GD (2009) Transmission of lungworms (*Muellerius capillaris*) from domestic goats to bighorn sheep on common pasture. J Wildl Dis 45: 272–278.

26. Foreyt WJ, Lagerquist JE (1996) Experimental contact of bighorn sheep (*Ovis canadensis*) with horses and cattle, and comparison of neutrophil sensitivity to *Pasteurella haemolytica* cytotoxins. J Wildl Dis 32: 594–602.

27. Onderka DK, Rawluk SA, Wishart WD (1988) Susceptibility of Rocky Mountain bighorn sheep and domestic sheep to pneumonia induced by bighorn and domestic livestock strains of *Pasteurella haemolytica*. Can J Vet Res 52: 439–444.

28. Dassanayake RP, Shanthalingam S, Herndon CN, Lawrence PK, Cassirer EF, et al. (2009) *Mannheimia haemolytica* serotype A1 exhibits differential pathogenicity in two related species, *Ovis canadensis* and *Ovis aries*. Vet Microbiol 133: 366–371.

29. Subramaniam R, Shanthalingam S, Bavananthasivam J, Kugadas A, Potter KA, et al. (2011) A multivalent *Mannheimia-Bibersteinia* vaccine protects bighorn sheep against *Mannheimia haemolytica* challenge. Clin Vaccine Immunol 18: 1689–1694.

30. Foreyt WJ, Snipes KP, Kasten RW (1994) Fatal pneumonia following inoculation of healthy bighorn sheep with *Pasteurella haemolytica* from healthy domestic sheep. J Wildl Dis 30: 137–145.

31. Alley MR, Ionas G, Clarke JK (1999) Chronic non-progressive pneumonia of sheep in New Zealand - a review of the role of *Mycoplasma ovipneumoniae*. N Z Vet J 47: 155–160.

32. Desrosiers R (2011) Transmission of swine pathogens: different means, different needs. Anim Health Res Rev 12: 1–13.

33. Dassanayake RP, Call DR, Sawant AA, Casavant NC, Weiser GC, et al. (2010) *Bibersteinia trehalosi* inhibits the growth of *Mannheimia haemolytica* by a proximity-dependent mechanism. Appl Environ Microbiol 76: 1008–1013.

34. Shanthalingam S, Goldy A, Bavananthasivam J, Subramaniam R, Batra SA, et al. (2014) PCR assay detects *Mannheimia haemolytica* in culture-negative pneumonic lung tissues of bighorn sheep (*Ovis canadensis*) from outbreaks in the Western USA, 2009–2010. J Wildl Dis 50: 1–10.

35. Townsend KM, Frost AJ, Lee CW, Papadimitriou JM, Dawkins HJ (1998) Development of PCR assays for species- and type-specific identification of *Pasteurella multocida* isolates. J Clin Microbiol 36: 1096–1100.

36. Fisher MA, Weiser GC, Hunter DL, Ward ACS (1999) Use of a polymerase chain reaction method to detect the leukotoxin gene lktA in biogroup and biovariant isolates of *Pasteurella haemolytica* and *P. trehalosi*. Am J Vet Res 60: 1402–1406.

37. Rossi CR, Kiesel GK (1971) Microtiter tests for detecting antibody in bovine serum to parainfluenza 3 virus, infectious bovine rhinotracheitis virus, and bovine virus diarrhea virus. Appl Microbiol 22: 32–36.

18

NSFC Health Research Funding and Burden of Disease in China

Gelin Xu, Zhizhong Zhang, Qiushi Lv, Yun Li, Ruidong Ye, Yunyun Xiong, Yongjun Jiang, Xinfeng Liu*

Department of Neurology, Jinling Hospital, Nanjing University School of Medicine, Nanjing, Jiangsu Province, China

Abstract

Background: Allocation of health research funds among diseases has never been evaluated in China. This study aimed to examine the relationship between disease-specific funding levels of National Nature Science Foundation of China (NSFC), the main governmental resource for health research in China, and burden of disease.

Methods: Funding magnitudes for 53 diseases or conditions were obtained from the website of NSFC. Measures of disease burden, mortality, years of life lost (YLLs) and disability-adjusted life years (DALYs), were derived from the Global Burden of Disease Study 2010. The relationship between NSFC funding and disease burden was analyzed with univariate linear regression. For each measure associated with funding, regression-derived estimates were used to calculate the expected funds for each disease. The actual and expected funds were then compared. We also evaluated the impacts of changes of disease burden metrics since 1990, and differences from the world averages on NSFC funding.

Results: NSFC health research funding was associated with disease burden measured in mortality (R = 0.33, P = 0.02), YLLs (R = 0.39, P = 0.004), and DALYs (R = 0.40, P = 0.003). But none of the changes of mortality (R = 0.22, P = 0.12), YLLs (R = −0.04, P = 0.79) and DALYs (R = −0.003, P = 0.98) since 1990 was associated with the funding magnitudes. None of the differences of mortality (R = −0.11, P = 0.45), YLLs (R = −0.11, P = 0.43) and DALYs (R = −0.12, P = 0.38) from that of the concurrent world averages were associated with the funding magnitudes. Measured by DALY, stroke and COPD received the least funding compared to expected; while leukemia and diabetes received the most funding compared to expected.

Conclusion: Although NSFC funding were roughly associated with disease burden as measured in mortality, YLLs and DALYs. Some major diseases such as stroke were underfunded; while others such as leukaemia were overfunded. Change of disease burden during the last 20 years and country-specialized disease burden were not reflected in current allocation of NSFC funds.

Editor: Guangyuan He, Huazhong University of Science and Technology, China

Funding: This study was sponsored by Nature Science Foundation of Jiangsu (BE2013713) to GX. The funders had no role in study design, data collection and analysis, decision to publish, or preparation of the manuscript.

Competing Interests: The authors have declared that no competing interests exist.

* Email: xfliu2@vip.163.com

Introduction

In recent years, China is pouring cash into science and technology faster than its economy has expanded [1]. The total research and development (R&D) expenditure in China has increased by 23% annually on average over the past decade [2]. The central government's budget on science and technology reached 267.4 billion yuan renminbi (RMB), or US $43.6 billion, in 2014 [2]. Consistent with this trend, the governmental funding for health research is also increasing. Although still dwarfed by that of US (US $ 3.1 billion for National Natural Science Foundation of China (NSFC) against US $ 30 billion for US National Institute of Health (NIH) in 2014), China's governmental funds, principally NSFC, are becoming an important supporter for health research in the world [3].

However, the allocation of research funds among diseases, and its rationality has never been evaluated in China. The disburse-ment of grant money has been criticized for lack of transparency, and funding tends to go to eminent scientists and safe projects [4,5]. There are short-term (annual) and long-term (5 years) national priorities for health researches, but they are merely results of government decisions based on politic will, public opinions, extemporaneous expert comments and immediate experience from western countries, rather than on systematic analysis of China's own disease burden. Considering the limited resources, it is important for China to optimize the process for health fund allocation with disease burden as a reference, as did in USA and other countries [6–8].

NSFC is a centre goverment agency specialized in administrating basic research funds, and it is the main source for the health research funds. Utilizing the design and methods in previous studies for evaluating association of NIH funding level and disease burden in USA [6,7], this study evaluated the relationship between NSFC funding levels and measures of disease burden. We also

Table 1. Funding levels of NSFC and disease burden in China.

Condition or disease	NSFC research fund	Measure of disease burden in 2010					
		thousands (rank)					
	thousands in RMB (% of total)	Mortality	Mortality change since 1990	YLLs	YLLs change since 1990	DALYs	DALYs change since 1990
Leukaemia	327854 (12.8)	58 (17)	5 (25)	2390 (15)	−366 (40)	2418 (19)	−354 (42)
Diabetes	176635 (6.9)	160 (11)	90 (5)	3173 (13)	1251 (5)	7835 (9)	2989 (4)
Ischemic heart disease	169185 (6.6)	949 (2)	499 (1)	16084 (3)	7093 (1)	17886 (3)	7759 (1)
Dementia	115785 (4.5)	50 (20)	24 (11)	616 (30)	159 (17)	1593 (23)	636 (13)
Liver cancer	114225 (4.5)	370 (6)	131 (4)	10014 (6)	2684 (4)	10089 (7)	2718 (5)
Injury	103560 (4.0)	796 (4)	−56 (47)	31759 (1)	−12827 (51)	40804 (1)	−10386 (51)
Breast cancer	95360 (3.7)	53 (19)	23 (12)	1563 (17)	645 (8)	1671 (22)	716 (10)
Asthma	80060 (3.1)	20 (32)	−32 (45)	358 (37)	−173 (38)	1095 (30)	−143 (39)
Colorectal cancer	75990 (3.0)	150 (12)	57 (6)	3305 (11)	901 (7)	3423 (15)	975 (8)
Chronic kidney diseases	75389 (2.9)	82 (15)	28 (9)	2054 (16)	413 (11)	2782 (17)	696 (11)
Cirrhosis	68085 (2.7)	114 (13)	−61 (48)	3180 (12)	−2095 (47)	3316 (16)	−2088 (47)
Neonatal disorders	63730 (2.5)	83 (14)	−260 (52)	7173 (7)	−22334 (53)	8679 (8)	−22534 (53)
Lung cancer	63580 (2.5)	513 (5)	253 (3)	11197 (5)	4943 (2)	11318 (6)	5013 (3)
Hypertensive heart disease	61463 (2.4)	173 (10)	39 (7)	2734 (14)	458 (10)	2767 (18)	460 (15)
Stroke	55330 (2.2)	1727 (1)	387 (2)	29173 (2)	4829 (3)	30139 (2)	5262 (2)
Stomach cancer	53610 (2.1)	297 (7)	0 (38)	6523 (8)	−849 (43)	6616 (10)	−825 (43)
Hepatitis	53245 (2.1)	44 (23)	11 (16)	1319 (19)	−48 (34)	1443 (28)	−38 (37)
Brain cancers	52610 (2.1)	49 (21)	13 (14)	1473 (18)	232 (14)	1497 (26)	240 (19)
Depression	51335 (2.0)	0 (53)	0 (36)	0 (53)	0 (30)	11767 (5)	2297 (6)
Pneumonia	46600 (1.8)	195 (8)	−197 (51)	4771 (9)	−20173 (52)	5135 (11)	−20166 (52)
Schizophrenia	43260 (1.7)	9 (42)	−4 (40)	279 (39)	−171 (37)	3472 (14)	918 (9)
HIV-AIDS	40075 (1.6)	36 (24)	36 (8)	1111 (23)	1100 (6)	1752 (20)	1739 (7)
Peptic ulcer	39870 (1.6)	19 (33)	−36 (46)	382 (35)	−942 (45)	453 (41)	−958 (45)
Atrial fibrillation and flutter	39150 (1.5)	13 (37)	8 (18)	154 (47)	91 (22)	596 (39)	259 (18)
Prostate cancer	34530 (1.3)	11 (39)	7 (19)	165 (45)	97 (21)	178 (50)	109 (25)
Nasopharynx cancer	31250 (1.2)	34 (26)	12 (15)	1046 (24)	314 (13)	1060 (31)	320 (17)
Epilepsy	31240 (1.2)	12 (38)	−7 (42)	559 (32)	−424 (41)	1507 (25)	−216 (40)
Maternal disorders	30260 (1.2)	5 (49)	−16 (43)	272 (40)	−911 (44)	546 (40)	−855 (44)
COPD	29450 (1.2)	934 (3)	−493 (53)	12995 (4)	−10808 (50)	16724 (4)	−9746 (50)
Parkinson disease	29160 (1.1)	7 (47)	3 (30)	121 (49)	25 (28)	265 (44)	91 (28)
Tuberculosis	26710 (1.0)	45 (22)	−124 (50)	1172 (22)	−4059 (49)	1733 (21)	−4418 (49)
Cervical cancer	26245 (1.0)	25 (29)	5 (26)	727 (28)	180 (16)	742 (35)	185 (21)

Table 1. Cont.

Condition or disease	NSFC research fund thousands in RMB (% of total)	Measure of disease burden in 2010 thousands (rank)					
		Mortality	Mortality change since 1990	YLLs	YLLs change since 1990	DALYs	DALYs change since 1990
Pancreatic cancer	24051 (0.9)	58 (16)	26 (10)	1315 (20)	551 (9)	1322 (29)	555 (14)
Ovarian cancer	22270 (0.9)	21 (31)	6 (23)	594 (31)	141 (19)	603 (38)	145 (23)
Mouth cancer	19970 (0.8)	14 (36)	7 (21)	351 (38)	150 (18)	361 (43)	156 (22)
Oesophageal cancer	19480 (0.8)	176 (9)	7 (20)	3824 (10)	-15 (32)	3858 (12)	-10 (34)
Multiple sclerosis	18085 (0.7)	2 (51)	-2 (39)	50 (51)	-60 (35)	149 (52)	-26 (36)
Lymphoma	16400 (0.6)	29 (28)	6 (22)	835 (26)	40 (26)	854 (33)	50 (31)
Malaria	15050 (0.6)	0 (52)	0 (37)	2 (52)	-6 (31)	12 (53)	-4 (33)
Schistosomiasis	14650 (0.6)	9 (43)	0 (35)	222 (42)	-34 (33)	251 (45)	-23 (35)
Bladder cancer	13280 (0.5)	23 (30)	8 (17)	399 (34)	106 (20)	411 (42)	115 (24)
Pancreatitis	13110 (0.5)	8 (44)	2 (32)	188 (44)	25 (29)	205 (48)	27 (32)
Anaemias	12860 (0.5)	15 (35)	-5 (41)	420 (33)	-494 (42)	1513 (24)	-346 (41)
Cardiomyopathy and myocarditis	12710 (0.5)	35 (25)	3 (31)	985 (25)	-125 (36)	1013 (32)	-127 (38)
Alcohole Chinae disorders	10720 (0.4)	5 (50)	1 (33)	163 (46)	32 (27)	3489 (13)	688 (12)
Kidney cancer	10020 (0.4)	32 (27)	18 (13)	823 (27)	400 (12)	837 (34)	384 (16)
Melanoma	8330 (0.3)	7 (48)	4 (28)	153 (48)	75 (24)	156 (51)	77 (29)
Gallbladder cancer	7560 (0.3)	18 (34)	0 (34)	637 (29)	225 (15)	644 (37)	229 (20)
Peripheral vascular disease	6990 (0.3)	9 (41)	6 (24)	119 (51)	-346 (39)	182 (49)	100 (26)
Thyroid cancer	6660 (0.3)	8 (45)	3 (29)	201 (43)	67 (25)	213 (47)	76 (30)
Meningitis	5350 (0.2)	8 (46)	-23 (44)	358 (35)	-1488 (46)	675 (36)	-1555 (46)
Rheumatic heart disease	4470 (0.2)	57 (18)	-74 (49)	1270 (21)	-2581 (48)	1487 (27)	-2654 (48)
Multiple myeloma	1710 (0.1)	9 (40)	4 (27)	246 (41)	90 (23)	250 (46)	93 (27)
Association with NSFC research fund R		0.33	0.22	0.39	-0.04	0.40	-0.003
P		0.02	0.12	0.004	0.79	0.003	0.98

discussed the differences of health research system in China and USA and the possible factors influencing the health fund allocation among diseases.

Methods

The budgets for NSFC are determined at least one year before each fiscal year, and some major research plans are made even five years ago. To reflect this time lag, data of 2010 disease burden and 2012 NSFC funding were chosen to evaluate the relationship between disease burden and magnitude of research funding. Diseases were included in this study if 1) they were defined in *International Classification of Diseases, 9th revision, Clinical Modification (ICD-9-CM)*; 2) their funding levels of NSFC were available; and 3) their measures of the burden of disease were available in Global Burden of Disease (GBD) Study 2010 [9].

Data Sources

NSFC has eight departments responsible for funding researches in different scientific subjects: mathematics, chemistry, life science, geoscience, engineering and material science, information science, management science and health. Before 2010, health research was included in the life science department, which also involved specialties of biology, botany, ecology, zoology, forestry, microbiology, immunology, psychology, agronomy and veterinary medicine. In 2010, health research was separated from life science department as a separate department.

The health department of NSFC has a similar framework to NIH, but with fewer "institutes" (currently eight compared with 27 institutes and centers in NIH), and endued with less functions. Applicants submit their protocols to different institutes according to target disease. For example, No.1 institute is responsible for diseases in circulatory, respiratory, blood and digestive systems. No.2 institute is responsible for disease in urinary, genital and endocrine systems, and diseases of ophthalmology, otolaryngology and dentistry. No. 3 institute is responsible for diseases of neurology and psychology. No.4 institute is responsible for diseases of skin, locomotor system and injury. No. 5 institute is responsible for cancer. No. 6 institute is responsible for communicable diseases and occupational diseases. No. 7 institute is responsible for pharmacology and pharmaceutics. No. 8 institute is responsible for Traditional Chinese Medicine.

Data concerning the funding levels for specific diseases or conditions in 2012 fiscal year were obtained from the NSFC website (http://isisn.nsfc.gov.cn/egrantweb/). The funding data were updated annually by NSFC. Data concerning disease burden were derived from GBD Study 2010 [9].

Three measures were chosen to reflect disease burden from the GBD Study 2010: mortality, years of life lost (YLLs), and disability-adjusted life years (DALYs). In GBD Study, YLLs are calculated by multiplying the number of deaths in each age group by a reference life expectancy at that age. YLDs are calculated from the prevalence of a sequela multiplied by the disability weight for that sequela. Disability weights are based on surveys of general population. DALYs are the sum of YLLs and YLDs [10].

Due to the rapid population ageing and widespread westernized lifestyle changing, there is a remarkable change of disease

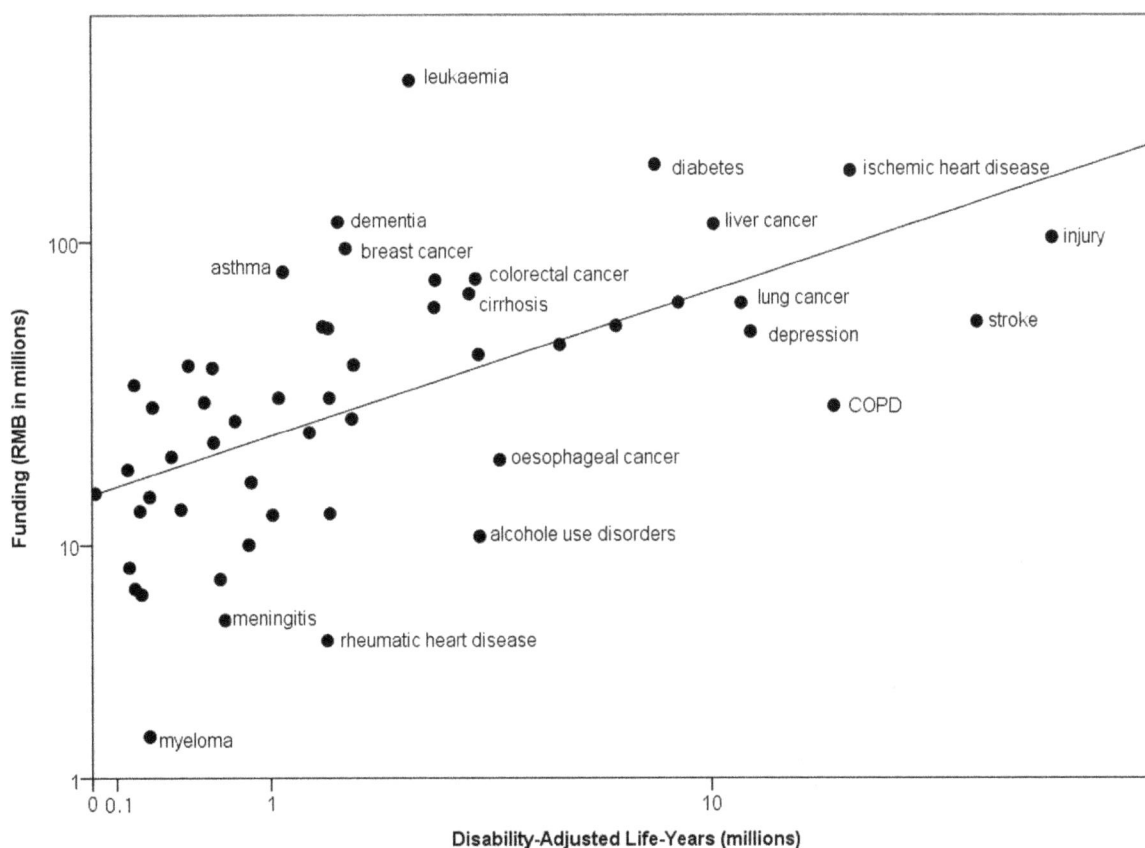

Figure 1. Relationship between NSFC disease-specific funding in 2012 and disability-adjusted life-years (DALYs) in 2012. Both X and Y axes are submitted to logarithmic scale. The line represents funding predicted on the basis of a linear regression with DALYs.

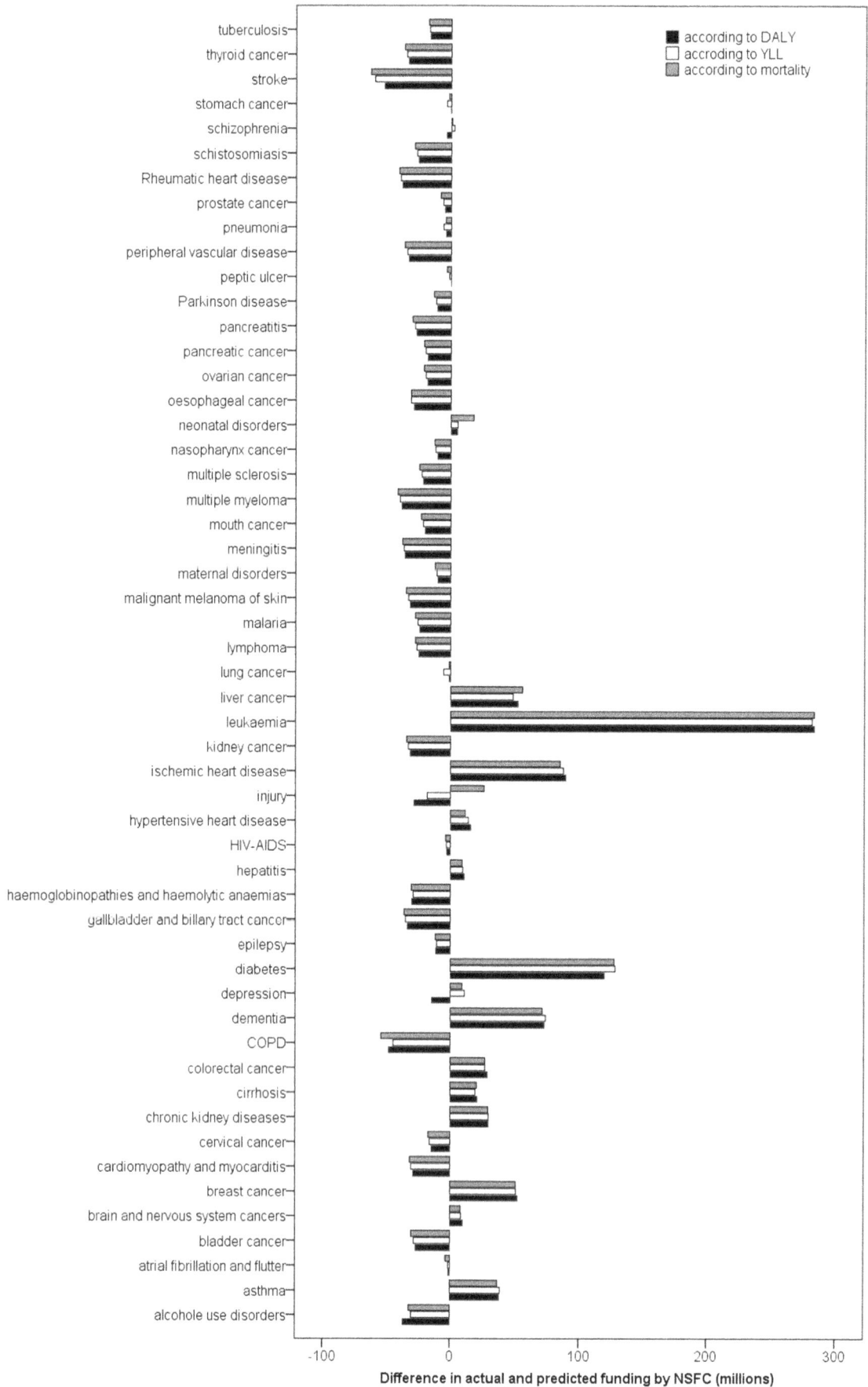

Difference in actual and predicted funding by NSFC (millions)

Figure 2. Differences between actual and expected disease-specific NSFC funding as predicted by mortality, YLLs and DALYs. Negative values indicates underfunded, and positive values indicates overfunded.

spectrum in China in recent 20 years. These trends may have influenced the allocation of research resources, because some disease may become more, while others less prevalent. We, therefore, evaluated the impacts of changes of mortality, YLLs, DALYs between 1990 and 2010 on disease funding. Data of disease burden, mortality, YLLs and DALYs for China in 1990, were also retrieved from GBD Study [9].

Some diseases are more prevalent, and pose an extra burden in China compared to the world average level. These diseases deserve extra research resource to accelerate improvements in prevention and management. Therefore, we evaluated the differences of mortality, YLLs and DALYs of each disease between China and the world average level. Data of mortality, YLLs and DALYs for the world average level in 2010 were retrieved from GBD Study [11–13].

Statistic Analysis

Univariate linear regression was performed to assess the relationship between funding levels and disease burden metrics. For each measure that had a significant association with funding, regression-derived estimates were used to calculate the expected NSFC funding for each disease. The expected and the actual funding magnitudes were then compared. In univarite regression analyses, we also evaluated the association of funding levels with changes of disease burden during 1990 and 2010, and with differences of disease burden between China and the worldwide average. The SPSS statistical package (Version 16, Chicago, Ill) was used for all statistic analyses.

Results

The total NSFC budget of 2012 fiscal year was 16.93 billion RMB (US $2.69 billion), with 4.12 billion RMB allocated to health research (disease targeted), of which 2.57 billion RMB (62.4%) was devoted to the 53 diseases included in this study. Disease funding ranged from about 2 million RMB for multiple myeloma, to 328 million for leukemia, with a median of 31 million RMB (4.8±5.5 million RMB, **Table 1**).

In the univariate regression analysis, NSFC health funding was associated with burden of disease measured in mortality (R = 0.33, P = 0.02), YLLs (R = 0.39, P = 0.004), and DALYs (R = 0.40, P = 0.003, **Table 1**).

Since 1990, the burdens decreased in some diseases, while increased in others in large extents (**Table 1**). The mortality of chronic obstructive pulmonary disorder (COPD) decreased from 1427 thousand in 1990 to 934 thousand in 2010, with a decrement of 493 thousand which ranked top among diseases. The mortality of neonatal disorders decreased from 343 thousand to 83 thousand, with a decrement of 260 thousand which ranked second among diseases. Progress in neonatal disorders contributed the largest reduction of DALYs (a decrement of 22534), followed by pneumonia (a decrement of 20166). On the other hand, ischemic heart disease induced the largest increment of mortality (499 thousand) during 1990 to 2010, followed by stroke (387 thousand). Ischemic heart disease also induced the largest increment of DALYs (7759 thousand), followed by stroke (5262 thousand). Because these transitional trends of disease burden may be a reflection of past research strength, and could have been used as indicators for allocating research resources, we analyzed the changes of disease burdens during 1990 to 2010. But none of the

changes of mortality (R = 0.22, P = 0.12), YLLs (R = −0.04, P = 0.79) and DALYs (R = −0.003, P = 0.98) was associated with NSFC funding magnitudes (**Table 1**).

Some diseases pose extra burden in China compare to the world averages, while others pose less burden. Of note, stroke demonstrated the largest extra mortality (126.1/100000 higher), YLLs (614/100000 higher) and DALYs (618/100000 higher) than the world averages. Ischemic heart disease induced the least extra mortality than the world average (35.6/100000 lower), and neonatal disorders induced the least extra YLLs (1985/100000 lower) and DALYs (2004/100000 lower) than the world averages. We analyzed differences of disease burden metrics in 2010 between China and world averages. But none of the differences of mortality (R = −0.11, P = 0.45), YLLs (R = −0.11, P = 0.43) and DALYs (R = −0.12, P = 0.38) to the world averages were associated with NFSC funding magnitudes (**Table 2**).

In standard multivariable analysis, DALYs became the only significant predictor for NSFC funding. The amount of predicted and actual NSFC funding as a function of DALYs is shown in **Figure 1**. The line represents the predicted funding levels if DALYs were the sole criterion for funding.

The difference between actual and predicted funding for each disease, with mortality, YLLs and DALYs as explanatory variables, is shown in **Figure 2**. Stroke, and COPD received the least funding compared to expected, while the leukemia and diabetes received the most funding compared to expected.

Discussion

In this study we analyzed the relationship between NSFC funding and burden of disease measured in mortality, YLLs and DALYs. Although the NSFC health funding was associated with disease burden, measured in mortality (R = 0.33, P = 0.02), YLLs (R = 0.39, P = 0.004), and DALYs (R = 0.40, P = 0.003), there exist significant differences between the actual and expected funding in some diseases according to these measures.

The relationship between disease research funding and burden of disease has been investigated in US National Institute of Health (NIH) system in several studies [6,7,14]. Disease incidence and prevalence were unrelated to funding, while mortality and YLLs weakly correlated with funding. DALYs were more strongly predictive [6,7]. In this study, mortality also weakly correlated with funding. Both YLLs and DALYs correlated significantly with NSFC funding. Although NSFC has a smaller total funding budget for health research, and is more inclusive and involves several subjects other than health, its organization is roughly similar to those of NIH. So it is not surprise that the overall profiles of NSFC funding distribution among diseases are similar to that of NIH.

The funding programs in NSFC can be classified as three types: free-applying, predetermined and investigator-targeted programs, which accounts for about 93%, 5% and 2% of the total budget respectively. For free-applying programs, there is no preset research scope, so applicants can choose any health research topics. For predetermined programs, every year one or two research topics were preset in each institute according to expertise and scientific needs. For the investigator-targeted programs, prominent investigators younger than 45 years were selected base on their previous academic achievements, and 1.5–3.0 million RMB was arranged to each awarder. With the money, they can choose any health research topics in five years. These arrange-

Table 2. Funding levels of NSFC and disease burden of world.

Condition or disease	NSFC research fund thousands in RMB (% of total)	Measure of disease burden in 2010 Age-standardized rate per 100000 (rank)					
		Mortality, World	Mortality, China-World	YLLs, World	YLLs, China-World	DALYs, World	DALYs, China-World
Leukaemia	327854 (12.8)	4.2(27)	0.0 (12)	137(23)	45 (7)	139(31)	46 (7)
Diabetes	176635 (6.9)	19.5(9)	−8.0 (46)	378(13)	−160 (43)	680(11)	−148 (41)
Ischemic heart disease	169185 (6.6)	105.7(1)	−35.6 (53)	1757(3)	−636 (48)	1884(3)	−642 (48)
Dementia	115785 (4.5)	7.1(18)	−3.2 (39)	66(34)	−20 (27)	165(28)	−46 (33)
Liver cancer	114225 (4.5)	11.5(14)	13.5 (4)	275(14)	379 (2)	277(17)	382 (2)
Injury	103560 (4.0)	74.3(3)	−17.6 (49)	3347(1)	−1024 (50)	4058(1)	−1118 (50)
Breast cancer	95360 (3.7)	6.6(19)	−3.1 (38)	161(21)	−62 (36)	174(27)	−67 (35)
Asthma	80060 (3.1)	5.2(23)	−3.7 (42)	125(27)	−100 (41)	326(15)	−242 (44)
Colorectal cancer	75990 (3.0)	10.8(17)	−0.2 (18)	201(19)	22 (9)	209(25)	21 (9)
Chronic kidney diseases	75389 (2.9)	11.1(16)	−5.3 (43)	249(15)	−108 (42)	307(16)	−116 (39)
Cirrhosis	68085 (2.7)	15.6(12)	−7.9 (45)	441(11)	−233 (45)	450(13)	−233 (43)
Neonatal disorders	63730 (2.5)	31.0(6)	−21.6 (51)	2794(2)	−1985 (53)	2931(2)	−2004 (53)
Lung cancer	63580 (2.5)	23.4(7)	12.4 (5)	465(10)	287 (3)	470(12)	290 (3)
Hypertensive heart disease	61463 (2.4)	13.1(13)	−0.3 (19)	216(17)	−23 (29)	222(23)	−28 (27)
Stroke	55330 (2.2)	88.4(2)	38.5 (1)	1421(5)	614 (1)	1484(5)	618 (1)
Stomach cancer	53610 (2.1)	11.5(15)	17.3 (3)	235(16)	204 (5)	238(20)	207 (4)
Hepatitis	53245 (2.1)	4.6(26)	−1.6 (33)	185(20)	−97 (40)	192(26)	−95 (37)
Brain cancers	52610 (2.1)	3(33)	0.3 (9)	87(32)	14 (10)	88(37)	14 (10)
Depression	51335 (2.0)	0(53)	0.0 (14)	0(53)	0 (16)	1078(9)	−260 (45)
Pneumonia	46600 (1.8)	41(5)	−25.1 (52)	1639(4)	−1204 (52)	1672(4)	−1208 (52)
Schizophrenia	43260 (1.7)	0.3(50)	0.3 (10)	9(49)	10 (12)	218(24)	8 (11)
HIV-AIDS	40075 (1.6)	21.4(8)	−19.0 (50)	1121(7)	−1010 (49)	1184(7)	−1065 (49)
Peptic ulcer	39870 (1.6)	3.7(29)	−2.3 (36)	93(28)	−67 (37)	98(33)	−67 (34)
Atrial fibrillation and flutter	39150 (1.5)	1.7(40)	−0.7 (25)	17(46)	−6 (21)	52(41)	−10 (21)
Prostate cancer	34530 (1.3)	3.8(28)	−2.9 (37)	48(38)	−36 (31)	55(39)	−42 (30)
Nasopharynx cancer	31250 (1.2)	1(46)	1.3 (7)	29(43)	39 (8)	29(47)	40 (8)
Epilepsy	31240 (1.2)	2.6(34)	−1.7 (35)	126(26)	−84 (39)	253(19)	−141 (40)
Maternal disorders	30260 (1.2)	3.7(30)	−3.4 (40)	208(18)	−189 (44)	234(21)	−196 (42)
COPD	29450 (1.2)	43.8(4)	26.8 (2)	687(8)	250 (4)	1114(8)	77 (6)
Parkinson disease	29160 (1.1)	1.7(41)	−1.2 (30)	19(45)	−11 (23)	28(48)	−9 (20)
Tuberculosis	26710 (1.0)	18(10)	−14.9 (47)	619(9)	−538 (47)	717(10)	−599 (47)

Table 2. Cont.

Condition or disease	NSFC research fund	Measure of disease burden in 2010					
	thousands in RMB (% of total)	Age-standardized rate per 100000 (rank)					
		Mortality, World	Mortality, China-World	YLLs, World	YLLs, China-World	DALYs, World	DALYs, China-World
Cervical cancer	26245 (1.0)	3.4(32)	−1.7 (34)	92(30)	−45 (34)	94(35)	−46 (31)
Pancreatic cancer	24051 (0.9)	4.7(25)	−0.7 (24)	89(31)	−1 (18)	89(36)	−1 (15)
Ovarian cancer	22270 (0.9)	2.4(37)	−1.0 (28)	59(35)	−20 (26)	60(38)	−21 (25)
Mouth cancer	19970 (0.8)	1.9(39)	−0.9 (27)	45(39)	−22 (28)	47(43)	−23 (26)
Oesophageal cancer	19480 (0.8)	6.1(20)	6.2 (6)	129(24)	128 (6)	130(32)	129 (5)
Multiple sclerosis	18085 (0.7)	0.3(51)	−0.2 (17)	8(50)	−5 (20)	16(51)	−6 (18)
Lymphoma	16400 (0.6)	3.5(31)	−1.4 (31)	93(29)	−33 (30)	94(34)	−34 (29)
Malaria	15050 (0.6)	16.7(11)	−16.7 (48)	1141(6)	−1141 (51)	1200(6)	−1199 (51)
Schistosomiasis	14650 (0.6)	0.2(52)	0.4 (8)	5(52)	10 (11)	48(42)	−31 (28)
Bladder cancer	13280 (0.5)	2.6(35)	−0.9 (26)	42(41)	−14 (24)	44(45)	−15 (22)
Pancreatitis	13110 (0.5)	1.2(44)	−0.6 (23)	31(42)	−19 (25)	34(46)	−20 (24)
Anaemias	12860 (0.5)	1.7(42)	−0.5 (22)	79(33)	−46 (35)	227(22)	−105 (38)
Cardiomyopathy/myocarditis	12710 (0.5)	6.1(21)	−3.6 (41)	156(22)	−84 (38)	162(29)	−87 (36)
Alcohole Chinae disorders	10720 (0.4)	1.7(43)	−1.4 (32)	55(36)	−45 (33)	256(18)	−20 (23)
Kidney cancer	10020 (0.4)	2.5(36)	−0.3 (20)	52(37)	5 (13)	53(40)	4 (12)
Melanoma	8330 (0.3)	0.7(47)	−0.2 (16)	16(47)	−6 (22)	17(50)	−6 (19)
Gallbladder cancer	7560 (0.3)	2.3(38)	−0.2 (15)	44(40)	0 (17)	44(44)	0 (14)
Peripheral vascular disease	6990 (0.3)	0.7(48)	0.0 (13)	8(51)	0 (15)	14(52)	−1 (16)
Thyroid cancer	6660 (0.3)	0.5(49)	0.1 (11)	11(48)	2 (14)	12(53)	2 (13)
Meningitis	5350 (0.2)	6.1(22)	−5.5 (44)	389(12)	−357 (46)	426(14)	−372 (46)
Rheumatic heart disease	4470 (0.2)	5.2(24)	−1.2 (29)	127(25)	−41 (32)	147(30)	−46 (32)
Multiple myeloma	1710 (0.1)	1.1(45)	−0.4 (21)	21(44)	−4 (19)	21(49)	−4 (17)
Association with NSFC research fund R		0.33	−0.11	0.24	−0.11	0.25	−0.12
P		0.02	0.45	0.09	0.43	0.07	0.38

ments made the distribution of NSFC health research fund among diseases largely determined by numbers of applications and applicants' interests in individual disease, which may be further influenced by international research trends, governmental policies and public opinions.

Based on the limited data of the present study, it is unlikely to determine why some diseases were underfunded, while others overfunded relative to disease burden. The over-funding of leukemia in China may be explained by the governmental reinforce of children health after the implementation of One-Child Policy in 1978. Successes in treating some types of leukemia in resent years, arsenic trioxide for acute promyelocytic leukemia as an example, which was originally discovered by Chinese researchers and they also contributed remarkably in the subsequent studies [15,16], may have further incited the enthusiasm for leukemia research in China. On the other hand, stroke and COPD remained as the most underfunded diseases. The limited data suggested that incidence, prevalence of stroke, COPD and several other chronic diseases are increasing rapidly in China in recent year due to population ageing, lifestyle transition and environment pollution [17,18]. These rapid changes in disease burdens have not reflected in the current NSFC funding assignment, possibly due to the unawareness of impact of these changes to public health or delayed responses to these changes. Furthermore, lack of major progress in managing stroke and COPD in recent years probably have depressed the interests for studying these chronic diseases.

Given the limited resource for health research, developing countries like China should allocate more research fund to their country-specific diseases–those with extra burden than other countries [19]. But in analyzing NCSF allocation, we failed to find this association. Measured by mortality, YLLs or DALYs, stroke poses the heaviest disease burden in China. The mortality, YLLs and DALYs of stroke in China is 38.5/100000, 614/100000 and 618/100000 higher than the world average level respectively, and all of these differences rank first among diseases. On the other hand, mortality, YLLs and DALYs of ischemic heart disease is 35.6/100000, 636/100000 and 642/100000 lower than the world average level respectively, which make it one of the least country-specific diseases in China. Although DALYs caused by stroke in 2010 (30139 thousand) is about two times of DALYs caused by ischemic heart disease (17886 thousand), the NSFC fund allocated for stroke is only one third of that for ischemic heart disease (55 vs 169 million RMB). This phenomenon of disproportionally underfunding of stroke and overfunding of ischemic heart disease in reference to disease burden was not observed in the recent NIH fund allocation [7].

The disease spectrum in China has changed significant in recent 20 years. Measured by DALYs, the disease burden of neonatal

disorders and pneumonia decreased with the largest extent (22534/100000 and 20166/100000) during 1990 to 2010; while DALYs due to ischemic heart disease and stroke increased with the largest extent (7759/100000 and 5262/100000) [9]. Theoretically, those with disease burden increased rapidly deserve more research resources to find approach for counteracting the trends. But we failed to find this association in NCSF allocation.

There are several limitations in this study which should be addressed when interpreting the results. First, we did not evaluate other sources, such as health research funds from government agencies other than NSFC. Other national funds, such as 863 projects, 973 projects, and National Supporting Programs administrated by Ministry of Science and Technology (MOST), account for about 10% of all governmental funds dedicated to health research in 2012 [20]. Funds from provincial government account for about 20% of all governmental funds dedicated to health research. Thus, contribution of resources other than NSFC for health research is unremarkable. Second, we did not include prevalence and incidence as measures for disease burden due to lack of recent data. In the previous studies, prevalence and incidence were not associated with NIH funding levels. We presume this is also the case in NSFC funding. Third, there may be fluctuation of funding magnitudes for a given diseases over years. The annual fluctuation of funding may be more predominant in less common diseases, for which the number of applicants is relatively small.

In conclusion, although the funding levels of NSFC were roughly associated with diseases burden as measured with mortality, YLLs and DALYs, some major diseases such as stroke were underfunded; with others such as leukemia were overfunded. Changes of disease burden during the past 20 years, and differences of disease burden from the world average have not been considered in allocating the current NSFC health funds.

Acknowledgments

This study was sponsored by Nature Science Foundation of Jiangsu (BE2013713) to GX. Authors thank Dr. Heqin Cao from NSFC for providing the annual funding data of NSFC, and for his suggestions in the study design and manuscript revision.

Author Contributions

Conceived and designed the experiments: GX ZZ QL YL RY YX YJ XL. Performed the experiments: GX ZZ QL YL. Analyzed the data: GX ZZ. Contributed reagents/materials/analysis tools: GX ZZ QL YJ XL. Wrote the paper: GX ZZ XL.

References

1. Van Noorden R (2014) China tops Europe in R&D intensity. Nature 505:144–145.
2. Qiu J (2014) China goes back to basics on research funding. Nature 507:148–149.
3. Morello L, Morrison J, Reardon S, Tollefson J, Witze A (2014) Obama's budget request falls flat. Nature 507:147–148.
4. Shi Y, Rao Y (2010) China's research culture. Science 329:1128.
5. Cao C, Li N, Li X, Liu L (2013) Science and Government. Reforming China's S&T system. Science 341:460–462.
6. Gross CP, Anderson GF, Powe NR (1999) The relation between funding by the National Institutes of Health and the burden of disease. N Engl J Med 340:1881–1887.
7. Gillum LA, Gouveia C, Dorsey ER, Pletcher M, Mathers CD, et al. (2011) NIH disease funding levels and burden of disease. PLoS One 6:e16837.
8. McCarthy M, Harvey G, Conceição C, la Torre G, Gulis G (2009) Comparing public-health research priorities in Europe. Health Res Policy Syst 7:17.

9. Yang G, Wang Y, Zeng Y, Gao GF, Liang X, et al. (2013) Rapid health transition in China, 1990–2010: findings from the Global Burden of Disease Study 2010. Lancet 381:1987–2015.
10. Murray CJ, Ezzati M, Flaxman AD, Lim S, Lozano R, et al. (2012) GBD 2010: design, definitions, and metrics. Lancet 380:2063–2066.
11. Lozano R, Naghavi M, Foreman K, Lim S, Shibuya K, et al. (2012) Global and regional mortality from 235 causes of death for 20 age groups in 1990 and 2010: a systematic analysis for the Global Burden of Disease Study 2010. Lancet 380:2095–2128.
12. Murray CJ, Vos T, Lozano R, Naghavi M, Flaxman AD, et al. (2012) Disability-adjusted life years (DALYs) for 291 diseases and injuries in 21 regions, 1990–2010: a systematic analysis for the Global Burden of Disease Study 2010. Lancet 380:2197–2223.
13. Vos T, Flaxman AD, Naghavi M, Lozano R, Michaud C, et al. (2012) Years lived with disability (YLDs) for 1160 sequelae of 289 diseases and injuries 1990–2010: a systematic analysis for the Global Burden of Disease Study 2010. Lancet 380:2163–2196.

14. Sampat BN, Buterbaugh K, Perl M (2013) New evidence on the allocation of NIH funds across diseases. Milbank Q 91:163–185.

15. Rao Y, Li R, Zhang D (2013) A drug from poison: how the therapeutic effect of arsenic trioxide on acute promyelocytic leukemia was discovered. Sci China Life Sci 56:495–502.

16. Wang ZY, Chen Z (2008) Acute promyelocytic leukemia: from highly fatal to highly curable. Blood 111:2505–2515.

17. Liu M, Wu B, Wang WZ, Lee LM, Zhang SH, et al. (2007) Stroke in China: epidemiology, prevention, and management strategies. Lancet Neurol 6:456–464.

18. Fang X, Wang X, Bai C (2011) COPD in China: the burden and importance of proper management. Chest 139:920–929.

19. Viergever RF, Olifson S, Ghaffar A, Terry RF (2010) A checklist for health research priority setting: nine common themes of good practice. Health Res Policy Syst 8:36.

20. National Bureau of Statistics Ministry of Science and Technology (2013) China Statistical Yearbook on Science and Technology. China Statistics Press. Beijing.

19

Poikilocytosis in Rabbits: Prevalence, Type, and Association with Disease

Mary M. Christopher[1]*, Michelle G. Hawkins[2], Andrew G. Burton[3]

1 Department of Pathology, Immunology and Microbiology, University of California Davis, Davis, CA, 95616, United States of America, 2 Department of Medicine and Epidemiology, University of California Davis, Davis, CA, 95616, United States of America, 3 William R. Pritchard Veterinary Medical Teaching Hospital, University of California Davis, Davis, CA, 95616, United States of America

Abstract

Rabbits (*Oryctolagus cuniculus*) are a popular companion animal, food animal, and animal model of human disease. Abnormal red cell shapes (poikilocytes) have been observed in rabbits, but their significance is unknown. The objective of this study was to investigate the prevalence and type of poikilocytosis in pet rabbits and its association with physiologic factors, clinical disease, and laboratory abnormalities. We retrospectively analyzed blood smears from 482 rabbits presented to the University of California-Davis Veterinary Medical Teaching Hospital from 1990 to 2010. Number and type of poikilocytes per 2000 red blood cells (RBCs) were counted and expressed as a percentage. Acanthocytes ($>$3% of RBCs) were found in 150/482 (31%) rabbits and echinocytes ($>$3% of RBCs) were found in 127/482 (27%) of rabbits, both healthy and diseased. Thirty-three of 482 (7%) rabbits had $>$30% acanthocytes and echinocytes combined. Mild to moderate ($>$0.5% of RBCs) fragmented red cells (schistocytes, microcytes, keratocytes, spherocytes) were found in 25/403 (6%) diseased and 0/79 (0%) healthy rabbits (P = 0.0240). Fragmentation and acanthocytosis were more severe in rabbits with inflammatory disease and malignant neoplasia compared with healthy rabbits (P$<$0.01). The % fragmented cells correlated with % polychromasia, RDW, and heterophil, monocyte, globulins, and fibrinogen concentrations (P$<$0.05). Echinocytosis was significantly associated with renal failure, azotemia, and acid-base/electrolyte abnormalities (P$<$0.05). Serum cholesterol concentration correlated significantly with % acanthocytes (P$<$0.0001), % echinocytes (P = 0.0069), and % fragmented cells (P = 0.0109), but correlations were weak (Spearman ρ $<$0.02). These findings provide important insights into underlying pathophysiologic mechanisms that appear to affect the prevalence and type of naturally-occurring poikilocytosis in rabbits. Our findings support the need to carefully document poikilocytes in research investigations and in clinical diagnosis and to determine their diagnostic and prognostic value.

Editor: Jan S. Suchodolski, GI Lab, United States of America

Funding: The authors have no support or funding to report.

Competing Interests: The authors have declared that no competing interests exist.

* Email: mmchristopher@ucdavis.edu

Introduction

Poikilocytosis is the presence of abnormally shaped erythrocytes in peripheral blood. Identification of poikilocytes is an important part of blood smear evaluation because shape changes often are associated with specific diseases, providing clues to underlying pathogenesis and facilitating diagnosis and treatment. Poikilocytes can result from biochemical changes, toxins, or physical damage to erythrocytes; regardless of cause, they can shorten erythrocyte survival and contribute to anemia [1,2]. In healthy pigs and young goats and calves, poikilocytes (acanthocytes, echninocytes, dacryo-cytes) are found normally in peripheral blood, without apparent pathologic consequence [1].

Rabbits are popular companion animals, are raised for meat, and are used extensively as animal models of human disease, including atherosclerosis, disorders of lipid metabolism, diabetes, and cardiovascular disease [3–5]. Acanthocytes have been observed in blood smears from healthy laboratory rabbits [6]. Described in 1967 as "thorn apple"-shaped red blood cells (RBCs), numerous acanthocytes (or acantho-echinocytes) were observed together with small microcytes about one-fourth the size

of a normal red cell [7]. Sanderson and Phillips [8] later described echinocytes, acanthocytes, and schistocytes in cardiac and arterial blood smears from healthy New Zealand White rabbits; they concluded that the poikilocytes were probably artifact and "indicative of a poorly prepared smear". However, while echinocytes can be the result of artifact (crenation), acanthocytes and schistocytes are pathologic cells that involve splenic remodeling and occur with in vivo fragmentation or membrane lipid abnormalities [1,9,10]. Acanthocytes, echinocytes, and occasionally schistocytes have been associated with liver disease and hypercholesterolemia in humans [2,10,11], dogs [12], and cats [13] and with disseminated intravascular coagulation and some types of neoplasia in dogs [12,14,15]. Red cell shape abnormalities (mainly acanthocytes) also are well described in laboratory rabbits [16,17] and dogs [18] fed atherogenic diets. In our hematology laboratory we have occasionally observed poikilocytes in companion rabbits presented to the University of California-Davis Veterinary Medical Teaching Hospital (VMTH). To the authors' knowledge, no studies have been done to quantify poikilocytes in healthy rabbits or to investigate possible links between poikilocytes and clinical or biochemical variables. A better understanding of red cell morphology in rabbits would be beneficial to researchers and clinicians alike.

The objectives of this study were to retrospectively characterize the prevalence, type, and severity of poikilocytes in a large cohort of rabbits and to investigate associations between poikilocytes and physiologic factors (age, sex, and breed), clinical disease, and CBC and biochemical findings. We hypothesized that poikilocytes in rabbits would be associated with specific diseases or laboratory abnormalities.

Materials and Methods

Study design and data collection

Electronic medical records from the University of California-Davis VMTH were searched retrospectively for rabbit visits between 1990 and 2010 at which a complete blood count (CBC) was done. Cases were excluded if a blood smear was not available or if a clinical diagnosis was not provided. Repeat visits by the same rabbit were excluded. Patient number, date, signalment (age, sex, breed), clinical and pathologic diagnoses, and CBC and biochemistry results were recorded. Age was reported in years and categorized as adult ($\geq$1 year old) or juvenile (<1 year). Clinical diagnoses were those reported in the visit summary by the clinician, and were based on the results of physical examination, laboratory tests, imaging, and occasionally, histopathology. Pathology results (biopsy and necropsy) were recorded if they were obtained within 6 months of the CBC and/or were relevant to the primary clinical disease. Healthy rabbits were those presented for routine physical examination or elective spay or neuter.

Hematology and biochemistry data

From January, 1990 to September, 2001 hematology results were obtained using a Baker Systems 9110 Plus hematology analyzer (BioChem ImmunoSystems Inc., Allentown, PA, USA). From September, 2001 to December, 2010 hematology results were obtained using an ADVIA 120 hematology system (Siemens Healthcare Diagnostics Inc., Tarrytown, NY, USA) with the rabbit setting in MultiSpecies System Software. Differential counts were obtained manually by counting 200 leukocytes in Wright-Giemsa-stained blood smears. Total plasma protein concentration was determined by refractometry and fibrinogen concentration was determined using the heat precipitation method. Hemolysis (pink plasma color) was qualitatively evaluated as mild, moderate, or marked. Biochemical results were obtained on a Roche Hitachi 917 analyzer (Roche Diagnostics Corporation, Indianapolis, IN, USA) from 2006 to 2010, Hitachi 717^c from 1997 to 2005, and Coulter Dacos analyzer (Coulter Electronics Inc, Hialeah, FL, USA) from 1990 to 1996. When instruments were upgraded, results were calibrated to retain consistency in results between analyzers.

Quantitation of poikilocytes

Original blood samples had been collected and processed according to our laboratory's standard operating procedure. Whole blood was placed into tubes containing EDTA and smears were prepared, air-dried, and stained by certified medical technologists within ~1 hour of collection. Poikilocytes were reported semiquantiatively (eg, few, moderate, many) by the technologists. Smears were coverslipped prior to storage in the laboratory slide archive.

On each original stained smear, 2000 RBCs were counted and characterized at 1000X magnification by a senior clinical

pathology resident (AGB) blinded to information about the rabbit. Poikilocytes were defined based on standard morphology and counting was limited to representative monolayer fields in which about half the erythrocytes were touching but did not overlap [1,19,20]. In severely anemic patients, counting was limited to areas where erythrocytes were separated by no more than one cell diameter. The number and type of poikilocytes were recorded and expressed as a percentage of RBCs. Poikilocytosis was subsequently classified as none (0%), rare (0.05–0.5%), mild (>0.5–3%), moderate (>3–10%), or marked (>10%). The number and percentage of polychromatophils were also recorded.

A board-certified clinical pathologist (MMC) independently determined % poikilocytes in a subset of the smears, also in a blinded manner; results from the two observers were averaged for analysis. The subset included a random sample consisting of every 10th slide (according to laboratory accession number) and all samples where the qualitative poikilocyte results in the original hematology report were widely discrepant from the quantitative results.

Statistical methods

Data were compiled in an Excel (Microsoft Corp, Redmond, WA, USA) spreadsheet and examined for aberrant entries. Statistical analyses were done using JMP 10.0.0 (SAS Institute Inc, Cary, NC, USA). Poikilocyte percentages were tested for normality by examination of histograms and Shapiro-Wilk tests. Differences in % poikilocytes between groups were evaluated using Wilcoxon/Kruskal-Wallis rank sums tests. Rabbits with none, rare, and mild (few) poikilocytes were combined and compared with those having moderate to marked poikilocytosis. Differences in age and hematologic and biochemical data were analyzed using Student's t test or ANOVA. Chi square analysis was used to compare nominal data. A multivariate model using Spearman's rank test was used to evaluate correlations among % poikilocytes and CBC and biochemistry variables. Principal component analysis was done using % poikilocytes and selected CBC and biochemistry variables. A P-value of.05 was used to indicate statistical significance.

Results

Nine-hundred-seventy-five rabbit visits with at least partial CBC results were identified during the 20-year period. Of these, 406 samples were excluded as repeat CBCs; 48 were excluded because smears were missing; 25 were excluded because they were native brush rabbits (*Sylvalagus bachmani*); and 14 were excluded because a clinical diagnosis was not reported. In total, 482 rabbits were included in the study.

Rabbits ranged from 3 months to 12 years of age (median 4 years), with 428 adults and 54 juveniles. Rabbits included 205 females (113 intact, 92 spayed) and 277 males (137 intact, 140 castrated). Rabbit breeds included Netherland Dwarf (n = 64), Lop (60), Mini-Lop (30), Mini-Rex (28), Holland Lop (20), New Zealand White (16), Dutch (13), Rex (10), Angora (8), French Lop (8), Flemish Giant (6), English Spot (5), English Lop (4), Dwarf (4), Dwarf Hotot (3), Lionhead (2), Chinchilla Rabbit (2), 1 each Dwarf Lionhead, Finnish Giant, Florida White, Havana, Hottot, Jersey Wooly, Lop-eared Angora, Norwegian Dwarf, and crossbred (21); breed was not specified for 170 rabbits.

Of the 482 rabbits, 79 were healthy and 403 were diseased. The mean ($\pm$ SD) age of healthy rabbits (1.6$\pm$1.9 years) was significantly lower than that of diseased rabbits (4.6$\pm$2.8 years) (P<0.0001, Student's t test). No difference was found in the proportion of females and males or in breed distribution between healthy and diseased rabbits.

Prevalence and type of poikilocytes

A total of 155/482 (32%) smears were quantified by two observers, with good agreement in % poikilocytes (average difference 0.05%±5% over a range of 0 to 70%). In the remaining smears, quantitative findings were similar to poikilocytes noted (or not) in the original laboratory report.

A majority of rabbits 251/482 (52%) had none, rare, or mild (<3%) poikilocytosis; 90/482 (19%) rabbits had moderate and 141 (29%) had marked poikilocytosis. Acanthocytes and echinocytes were the most frequently observed poikilocytes, with no significant difference between healthy and diseased rabbits (Figures 1–3). One-hundred-fifty of 482 (31%) rabbits had moderate to marked acanthocytosis and 127/482 (27%) had moderate to marked echinocytosis. Of these, 10 (2%) rabbits (including 1 healthy rabbit) had >30% acanthocytes and 11 (2%) rabbits (including 2 healthy rabbits) had >30% echinocytes. Acanthocytes and echinocytes often were observed together (Spearman ρ = 0.3896, P<0.0001) and overlapped in morphology; 33/482 (7%) rabbits had >30% acanthocytes and echinocytes combined. Acanthocyte morphology ranged from cells with one to two elongated blebs to multiple, smooth to sharply spiculated and irregularly-placed projections. Echinocytes had fine- to blunt-tipped, evenly spaced, short projections; those with blunt-tipped projections sometimes occurred together with irregularly-spiculated acanthocytes. No significant difference in the percentage of acanthocytes and echinocytes was observed between healthy and ill rabbits.

Schistocytes, microcytes, keratocytes, and spherocytes (subsequently combined as "fragmented" red cells) were observed in low numbers, with 457/482 (95%) rabbits having none to rare fragmented cells and 25/482 (5%) having mild to moderate

fragmentation (Figures 1–3). Only diseased rabbits had mild to moderate fragmentation (P = 0.0024, Chi square), and a higher percentage of fragmented cells was found in diseased compared with healthy rabbits (P = 0.0240, Wilcoxon) (Figure 2). Fragmented red cells usually were found together with acanthocytes, with or without echinocytes. Percent fragmented cells correlated significantly with % acanthocytes (Spearman's ρ = 0.4400, P<0.0001) and to a lesser extent with % echinocytes (Spearman's ρ = 0.2861, P<0.0001. Microcytes often were very small, less than one-fourth the diameter of a normal red cell. Ovalocytes, dacryocytes, blister cells, and knizocytes were observed in low numbers in a few rabbits, as were occasional stomatocytes, target cells and ghost cells; because of their low frequency, these poikilocytes were not analyzed further.

No significant difference in % poikilocytes was observed between samples with none (n = 374), slight (n = 101), or moderate (n = 7) sample hemolysis. Further, neither moderate to marked acanthocytosis or echinocytosis nor mild to moderate fragmentation were associated with the presence of sample hemolysis. None of the 7 samples with moderate hemolysis had increased fragmentation and only 3/98 samples with mild to moderate fragmentation had slight hemolysis.

Poikilocytes and physiologic factors

Associations between poikilocytes and physiologic factors were evaluated in clinically healthy rabbits (n = 79). Healthy rabbits included 47 adults and 32 juveniles ranging from 3 months to 8 years of age. No significant difference in % poikilocytes or in the proportion of samples with moderate to marked poikilocytosis was found between adult and juvenile rabbits; no correlation was found between age and % poikilocytes.

Healthy rabbits included 32 females (28 intact, 4 spayed) and 47 males (35 intact, 12 castrated). Female rabbits had a slightly higher

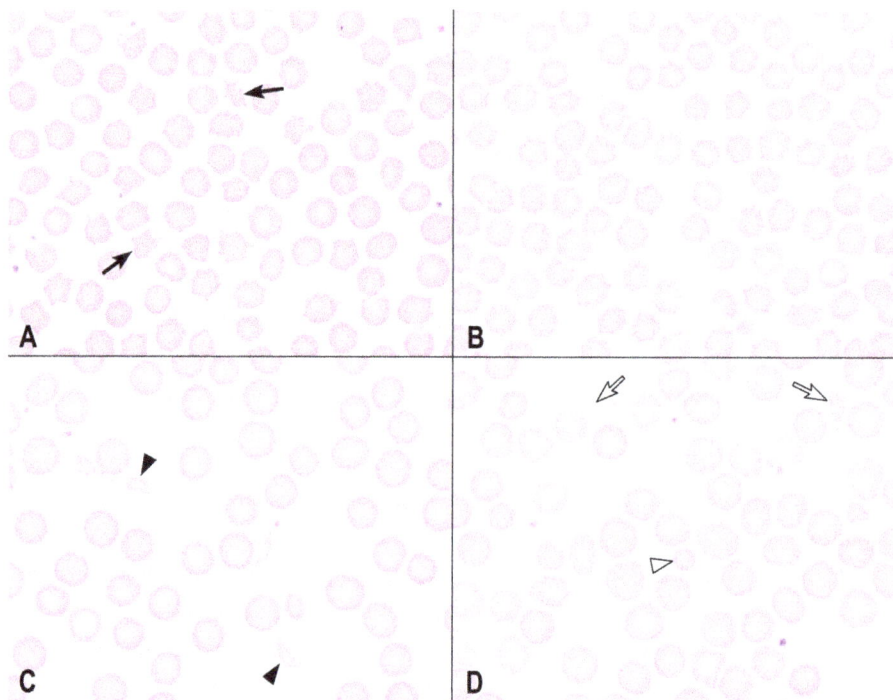

Figure 1. Poikilocytes in blood smears from rabbits. (A) Acanthocytes (arrows) in a healthy rabbit; (B) echinocytes in a rabbit with renal failure; (C) schistocytes (closed arrowheads) in a rabbit with a dental abscess; and (D) spherocytes (open arrowhead) and schistocytes (open arrows) in a rabbit with a mandibular abscess. Wright-Giemsa stain. Scale bar = 10 μm.

HEALTHY RABBITS (n = 79)

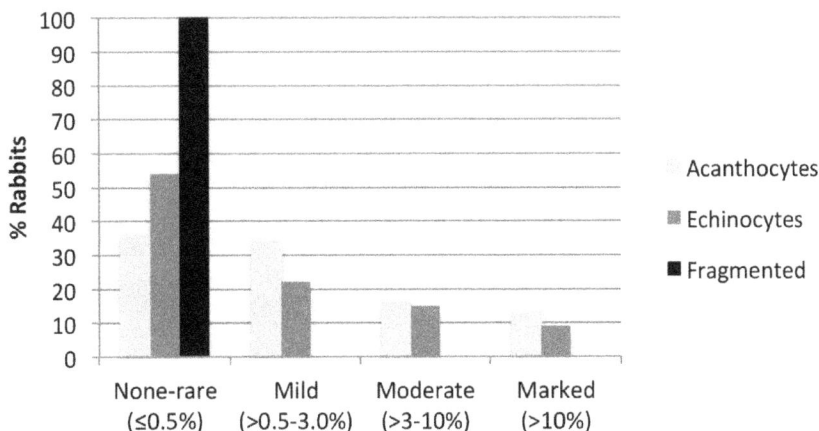

DISEASED RABBITS (n = 403)

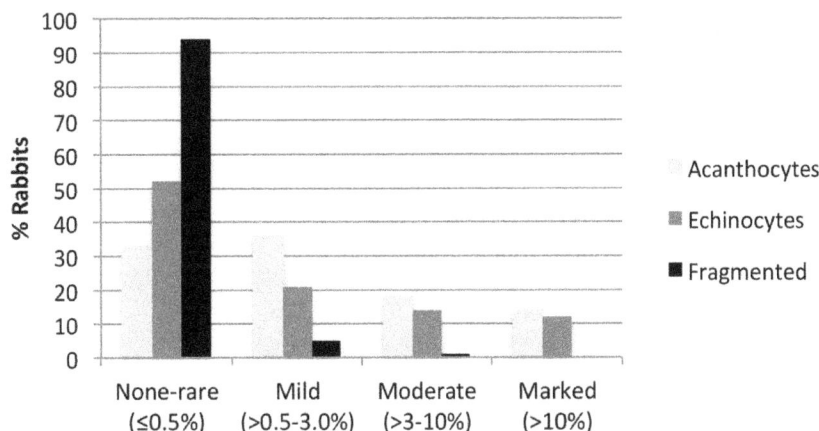

Figure 2. Prevalence of poikilocytes in 492 rabbits. Fragmented cells include schistocytes, keratocytes, microcytes, and spherocytes.

% echinocytes (median 0.8%, range 0–31.0%) than male rabbits (median 0.1%, range 0–28.8%) (P = 0.0309, Wilcoxon). A higher proportion of females than males had moderate to marked acanthocytosis (41/32, 44% vs 9/47, 15%) and echinocytosis (12/32, 84% vs 7/47, 15%) (P<0.05, Chi square).

Healthy rabbits included Netherland Dwarf (14), Mini-Rex (5), Dutch (4), Holland Lop (4), and Lop (4), New Zealand White (2), Mini-Lop (2), Lionhead (2), English Spot (2), 1 each of Angora, Dwarf, Dwarf Lionhead, English Lop, Flemish Giant, Hottot, and Rex; and cross-breed (5), breed was not reported for 28 rabbits. No significant breed difference was found in % poikilocytes or in the proportion of samples with moderate to marked poikilocytes, however samples sizes were small.

Poikilocytes and disease

Diseased rabbits were classified into 12 organ groups based on primary diagnosis (Table 1). Pathology results were available for 101/403 (25%) diseased rabbits, including 70 necropsy (with histopathology), 27 biopsy, and 4 cytology results. Rabbits also were grouped based on the specific disease process; groups with 10

or more rabbits were analyzed statistically for associations with poikilocytosis (Table 2).

No difference in the % or severity of acanthocytes and echinocytes was found on the basis of organ system, but a significantly lower % fragmented cells was found in healthy rabbits and in rabbits with ophthalmic disease compared with other organ systems (P<.05, Wilcoxon). Moderate to marked acanthocytosis and mild to moderate fragmentation were observed significantly more often in rabbits with septic and inflammatory disorders compared with healthy rabbits (Table 2). A significantly higher % of echinocytes (P = 0.0086) and moderate to marked echinocytosis (Table 2) were observed in rabbits with renal failure compared with healthy rabbits.

Poikilocytes and laboratory abnormalities

Significant differences were observed in laboratory values in rabbits with moderate to marked acanthocytosis or echinocytosis and with mild to moderate fragmentation (Table 3). Because few reticulocyte counts (n = 18) and band heterophils (n = 35) were reported, these analytes were not analyzed statistically.

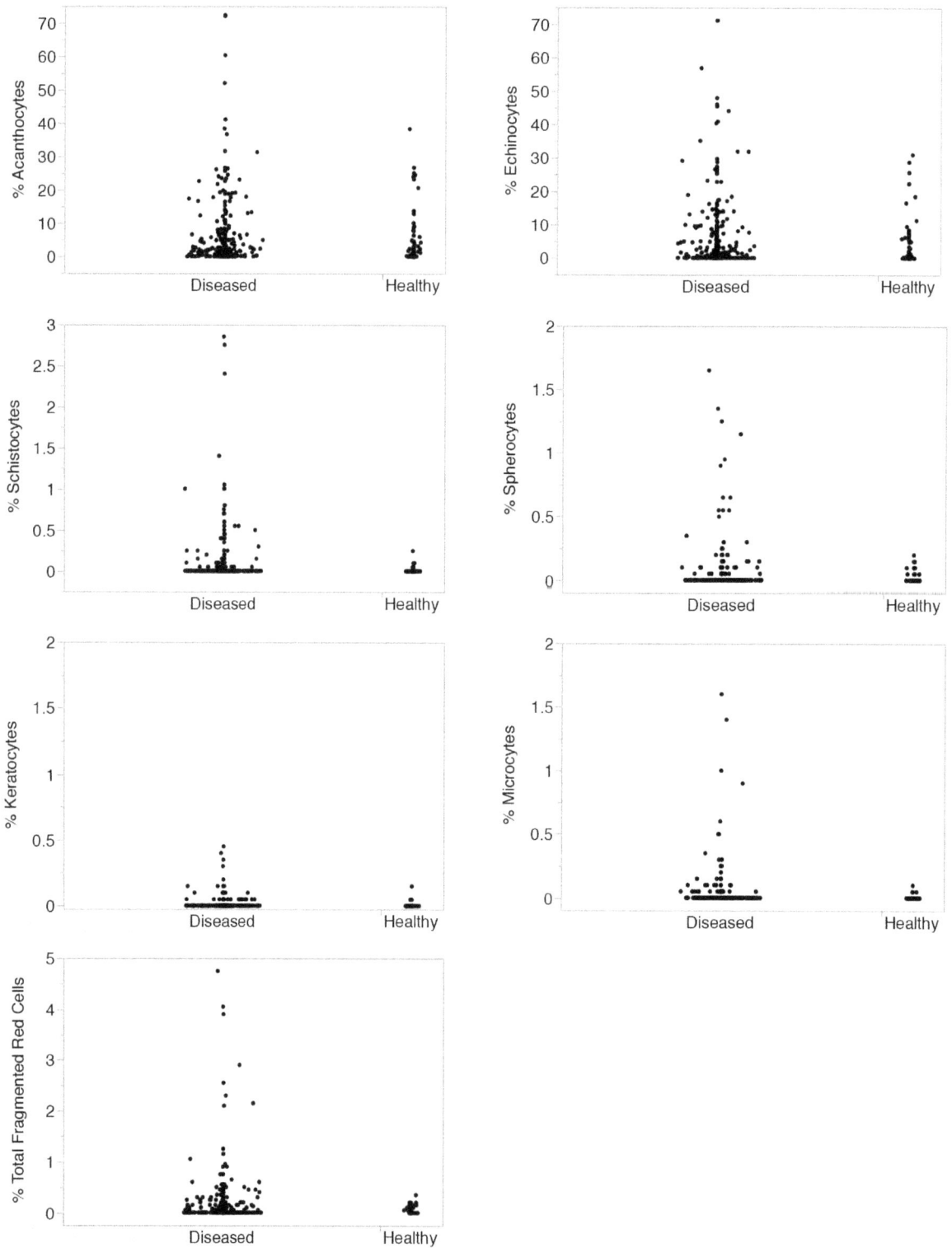

Figure 3. Dot plots of % poikilocytes in samples from healthy (n = 79) and diseased (n = 403) rabbits. Significant differences between healthy and diseased rabbits were observed for % schistocytes, % keratocytes, % microcytes, and % total fragmented cells (P<.05, Wilcoxon).

Based on Spearman rank correlation for all rabbits combined, % acanthocytes correlated positively with % polychromasia, red cell distribution width (RDW), and mean platelet volume (MPV) (P<0.02); % echinocytes correlated positively with RBC count, hematocrit (HCT), hemoglobin concentration (HGB), mean cell hemoglobin concentration (MCHC), MPV, anion gap, and sodium, potassium, chloride, and creatinine concentrations, and negatively with bicarbonate and glucose concentrations (P<0.01);

Table 1. Primary diagnosis by organ system for the 482 rabbits in the study (1990 to 2010).

Organ System	Disease	Clinical Diagnosis	Pathology Diagnosis	Total
Bone and joint	Fracture	14	0	14
	Degenerative joint disease	5	2	7
	Luxation	2	0	2
	Neoplasia (sarcoma, squamous cell carcinoma)	0	2	2
	Other (lameness, multifocal bony lesions)	2	0	2
Cardiovascular	Myxomatous valve degeneration	2	1	3
	Cardiomyopathy	1	1	2
	Arrythmia	1	0	1
Dental	Malocclusion/periodontitis	37	1	38
	Mandibular abscessation/osteomyelitis	29	9	38
Gastrointestinal	GI stasis	25	0	25
	Enteritis/gastritis/typhylitis/colitis	2	9	11
	Diarrhea	5	0	5
	Trichobezoar	0	3	3
	Abscess	1	1	2
	Neoplasia (papilloma, adenocarcinoma)	0	2	2
	Other (dysbiosis, cecal impaction)	4	0	4
Hemolymphatic	Mediastinal thymoma	2	2	4
	Lymphoma	0	3	3
	Regenerative anemia	1	0	1
Hepatic	Enzymopathy	4	0	4
	Hepatitis/cholangiohepatitis	0	3	3
	Torsion with necrosis	0	2	2
	Neoplasia (cystadenocarcinoma)	0	1	1
Neurologic	Encephalitozoonosis	0	6	6
	Ataxia/paresis/paralysis	6	0	6
	Myelopathy	5	0	5
	Vestibular disease	3	0	3
	CNS disease	3	0	3
	Neoplasia (pineocytoma)	0	1	1
	Bacterial meningoencephalitis	0	1	1
	Brain hemorrhage	0	1	1
	Other (lumbosacral disease, seizures, head trauma)	3	0	3
Ophthalmic	Keratitis/uveitis/ulcer	8	0	8
	Glaucoma/cataracts	5	0	5
	Chemosis/conjunctivitis	5	0	5
	Dacryocystitis	5	0	5
	Iris granuloma	3	0	3
	Other (corneal fibrosis, laceration, dystrichia, epicorneal membrane)	4	0	4
Reproductive	Uterine disease (endometritis, cysts, hydrometra, mass, varices)	4	1	5
	Neoplasia (testicular granular cell tumor)	0	1	1
Respiratory	Upper respiratory tract disease	20	3	23
	Bronchopneumonia	3	5	8
	Lung abscessation+pneumonia	0	4	4
	Neoplasia (carcinoma, granular cell tumor)	0	2	2
	Other (nasal mass, lung consolidation, stridor)	3	0	3
Skin/subcutis	Otitis	13	1	14
	Cellulitis (bite wounds, myiasis)	7	3	10
	Dermatitis, nonparasitic	9	5	14
	Dermatitis, parasitic	10	0	10

Table 1. Cont.

Organ System	Disease	Clinical Diagnosis	Pathology Diagnosis	Total
	Pododermatitis	6	0	6
	Abscess, soft tissue	3	3	6
	Laceration	6	0	6
	Neoplasia, malignant (sarcoma, squamous cell carcinoma)	0	7	7
	Neoplasia, benign (lipoma, polyp)	1	2	3
	Other (myositis/fibrosis, cutaneous mass)	3	0	3
Urinary	Renal failure	7	7	14
	Urolithiasis	8	0	8
	Urine sludge	7	0	7
	Cystitis	4	0	4
Other	Anorexia, weight loss	5	0	5
	Abdominal mass	1	0	1
	Hypercalcemia	1	0	1

% fragmented cells correlated positively with % polychromasia, MCHC, RDW, and heterophil, monocyte, and potassium concentrations, and negatively with bicarbonate and albumin concentrations (<0.02). Cholesterol correlated significantly with % acanthocytes ($P<0.0001$), % echinocytes ($P = 0.0069$), and % fragmented cells ($P = 0.0109$), but was not highly predictive (Spearman ρ <0.2).

We used principal component analysis to further visualize correlation patterns (Figure 4). In component 1, fragmented cells, and to a lesser extent acanthocytes, correlated positively with polychromasia, heterophils, monocytes, fibrinogen, globulins, and cholesterol; and negatively with albumin and HCT. In component 2, echinocytes correlated positively with azotemia, sodium, potassium, and anion gap; and negatively with bicarbonate.

Discussion

To our knowledge, this study is the first to quantify red cell morphology in a large population of rabbits. Acanthocytes and echinocytes comprised >3% of RBCs in about one-third of healthy and diseased rabbits and were slightly more frequent in healthy female than male rabbits. Fragmented red cells (schistocytes, microcytes, keratocytes, spherocytes) occurred in low numbers and were more frequently observed in diseased rabbits,

Table 2. The proportion of rabbits with specific diseases having moderate to marked acanthocytosis or echinocytosis and mild to moderate fragmentation as compared with healthy rabbits.

Disease†	Clinical Diagnosis	Pathologic Diagnosis	Acanthocytosis Mod-Mkd	Echinocytosis Mod-Mkd	Fragmentation Mild-Mod
Abscess	32	18	26/50 (52%)**	14/50 (28%)	7/50 (14%)***
Bronchopneumonia	3	9†	8/12 (67%)*	3/12 (25%)	1/12 (8%)**
Cellulitis§	7	3	7/10 (70%)**	4/10 (40%)	2/10 (20%)***
Dental (non-abscess)	37	1	11/38 (29%)	14/38 (36%)	2/38 (5%)*
Dermatitis	19	5	5/24 (21%)	6/24 (25%)	1/24 (4%)
Fracture	12	2	3/14 (21%)	2/14 (14%)	0/14 (0%)
GI inflammation§	2	9	4/11 (36%)	2/11 (18%)	1/11 (9%)**
GI stasis	25	0	5/25 (20%)	6/25 (24%)	0/25 (0%)
Neoplasia, malignant	0	22	5/22 (22%)	3/22 (14%)	2/22 (9%)**
Otitis	13	1	3/14 (21%)	3/14 (21%)	0/14 (0%)
Renal failure	7	7¶	4/14 (28%)	8/14 (57%)*	1/14 (7%)*
URTD	20	3	7/23 (30%)	7/23 (30%)	0/23 (0%)
Healthy	79	0	23/79 (29%)	19/79 (24%)	0/79 (0%)

*P<.05; **P<.01; ***P<.001.
†Four rabbits with bronchopneumonia also had lung abscessation; 4 had confirmed sepsis.
§Eight of 10 cases of cellulitis were septic (myiasis or bacterial); GI inflammation was septic in 7/11 cases (5 with intralesional bacteria, 1 with Coccidia, 1 with Coccidia and Giardia.
¶Two rabbits with renal failure also had pneumonia.
GI indicates gastrointestinal; URTD indicates upper respiratory tract disease.

Table 3. Hematologic and biochemical values (mean ± SEM) in 482 rabbits based on severity of poikilocytosis.

Analyte	Acanthocytosis			Echinocytosis			Fragmentation		
	Moderate-marked	None-mild	P value*	Moderate-marked	None-mild	P value*	Mild-moderate	None-rare	P value*
RBC (X10^6/µl)	5.8±0.1	5.8±0.1	–	6.0±0.1	5.7±0.1	0.0055	5.3±0.2	5.8±0.1	0.0241
HCT (%)	36.7±0.5	37.2±0.3	–	38.5±0.5	36.6±0.3	0.0012	34.3±1.1	37.2±0.2	0.0124
HGB (g/dl)	12.3±0.1	12.5±0.1	–	12.9±0.2	12.3±0.1	0.0055	11.1±0.4	12.5±0.1	0.0006
MCV (fl)	63.7±0.3	64.6±0.2	0.0454	64.6±0.3	64.2±0.2	–	65.3±0.8	64.3±0.2	–
MCH (pg)	21.4±0.1	21.7±0.1	–	21.5±0.1	21.6±0.1	–	20.9±0.3	21.6±0.1	0.0243
MCHC (g/dl)	33.6±0.1	33.6±0.1	–	33.4±0.1	33.7±0.1	–	32.1±0.3	33.7±0.1	<0.0001
RDW (%)	13.8±0.1	13.2±0.1	0.0008	13.4±0.1	13.4±0.1	–	16.1±0.3	13.3±0.1	<0.0001
POLY (%)	1.3±0.1	1.2±0.04	–	1.3±0.1	1.2±0.04	–	1.8±0.1	1.2±0.03	0.0002
WBC (/µl)	7677±264	7509±178	–	8036±287	7393±171	–	8493±646	7510±151	–
HET (/µl)	3780±211	3663±142	–	4022±230	3585±137	–	4914±515	3632±120	0.0159
LYM (/µl)	2940±143	2970±96	–	3008±156	2944±93	0.0116	2562±351	2983±82	–
MONO (/µl)	525±38	510±26	–	606±41	483±24	–	679±94	506±22	–
EOS (/µl)	89±8	84±5	–	80±8	88±5	–	81±19	86±4	–
BASO (/µl)	314±19	261±13	0.0226	278±21	277±12	–	238±47	280±11	–
PLT (X10^3/µl)	630±25	579±16	–	609±27	588±15	–	764±62	586±13	0.0057
MPV (fl)	7.4±0.2	7.2±0.1	–	7.7±0.2	7.1±0.1	0.0105	8.4±0.5	7.2±0.1	0.0228
TPP (g/dl)	7.2±0.1	7.1±0.04	–	7.3±0.1	7.1±0.1	–	7.1±0.1	7.2±0.04	–
FIB (mg/dl)	303±16	312±10	–	340±17	298±10	0.0377	408±38	304±9	0.0076
AG (mmol/L)	25.4±0.6	24.8±0.4	–	27.1±0.6	24.1±0.4	0.0001	26.3±1.7	25.0±0.3	–
Na (mmol/L)	144.0±0.4	143.6±0.2	–	144.6±0.4	143.4±0.2	0.0079	143.2±1.0	143.8±0.2	–
K (mmol/L)	4.6±0.1	4.4±0.1	0.0202	4.6±0.1	4.4±0.1	0.0271	5.0±0.2	4.4±0.04	0.0077
Cl (mmol/L)	102.9±0.4	102.5±0.3	–	103.6±0.5	102.3±0.3	0.0246	102.8±1.2	102.6±0.2	–
HCO3 (mmol/L)	20.3±0.5	20.9±0.3	–	18.5±0.4	21.6±0.3	<0.0001	19.1±1.2	20.8±0.2	–
CA (mg/dl)	14.7±0.1	14.4±0.1	–	14.5±0.1	14.5±0.1	–	14.2±0.3	14.5±0.1	–
PHOS (mg/dl)	3.6±0.2	3.7±0.1	–	4.0±0.2*	3.5±0.1	0.0331	3.5±0.5	3.7±0.1	–
BUN (mg/dl)	24.3±2.0	23.2±1.3	–	26.7±2.1	22.4±1.3	–	29.1±5.0	23.3±1.1	–
CREA (mg/dl)	1.3±0.1	1.4±0.1	–	1.7±0.1	1.3±0.1	0.0148	1.6±0.3	1.4±0.1	–
GLU (mg/dl)	164.7±4.0	166.4±2.7	–	158.3±4.3	168.6±2.6	0.0424	146.2±10.2	166.8±2.3	0.0482
T. PROT (g/dl)	7.3±0.2	6.9±0.1	–	7.0±0.2	7.1±0.1	–	6.9±0.5	7.1±0.1	–
ALB (g/dl)	5.3±0.1	5.2±0.1	–	5.1±0.1	5.2±0.1	–	4.4±0.2	5.3±0.04	<0.0001
GLOB (g/dl)	1.7±0.1	1.97±0.1	–	1.9±0.1	1.7±0.1	–	2.5±0.2	1.7±0.05	0.0010
CHOL (mg/dl)	58.1±3.9	43.5±2.6	0.0044	57.3±4.2	44.3±2.6	0.0094	93.5±9.9	45.6±2.2	<0.0001
T. BILI (mg/dl)	0.1±0.1	0.2±0.1	–	0.1±0.1	0.2±0.1	–	0.1±0.2	0.2±0.1	–
ALT (U/L)	50±17	81±11	–	57±18	77±11	–	66±44	71±10	–

Table 3. Cont.

Analyte	Acanthocytosis			Echinocytosis			Fragmentation		
	Moderate-marked	None-mild	P value*	Moderate-marked	None-mild	P value*	Mild-moderate	None-rare	P value*
AST (U/L)	44±62	129±42	–	64±67	116±41	–	63±159	104±36	–
ALP (U/L)	62±8	77±6	–	60±9	77±6	–	87±22	71±5	–
CK (U/L)	1244±430	2198±298	–	2429±465	1580±289	–	6567±1110	1658±246	<0.0001
GGT (U/L)	10±2	12±1	–	11±2	11±1	–	19±5	11±1	–
N	118-150	245-332	–	101-127	252-355	–	16-25	346-457	–

*Student's t test between rabbits having moderate-marked (>3% of RBCs) vs none-mild (≤3% of RBCs) acanthocytes or echinocytes, or mild-moderate (>0.5% of RBCs) vs none-rare (≤0.5% of RBCs) fragmented red cells.
– indicates no significant difference.

especially those with abscesses, bronchopneumonia, cellulitits, gastrointestinal inflammation, and malignant neoplasia. In addition, moderate to marked echinocytosis was associated with renal failure and electrolyte abnormalities. These findings suggest common pathophysiologic mechanisms of poikilocyte formation in sepsis (fragmentation) and uremia (echinocytes). Our findings warrant further investigation into the pathogenesis of red cell shape change in rabbits and assessment of the diagnostic or prognostic value of poikilocytes.

Acanthocytes and echinocytes were the most frequent poikilocytes observed in rabbits in this study; they often occurred together and formed a morphologic spectrum that sometimes made differentiation difficult [12]. Acanthocytes have irregularly spaced, blunt-tipped projections, an irreversible shape change that usually results from altered membrane cholesterol or phospholipids [1,10–12]. Echinocytes have evenly spaced, narrow-tipped, reversible projections that form in the presence of fatty acids, lysophospholipids, and a variety of chemical agents [1,9,11]. Although acanthocytes (and sometimes echinocytes) are a pathologic finding, echinocytes (crenation) can be an artifact of excess EDTA, prolonged blood storage, or slow drying of smears [1]. Acanthocytes (or acantho-echinocytes) were first reported in healthy laboratory rabbits nearly 50 years ago [7] and have been observed anecdotally in companion rabbits. However, because of the frequent attribution of echinocytes to artifact [8,9] and because, based on our results, only a small proportion of rabbits had many acanthocytes and/or echinocytes, these poikilocytes may be overlooked or considered as insignificant in the routine examination of rabbit blood. Our findings emphasize the importance of documenting all poikilocytes, including echinocytes.

Rabbits fed high cholesterol (atherogenic) diets routinely develop acanthocytes ("spur cells") or echinocytes [16,17,21–23]. Serum cholesterol concentrations in the rabbits in this study also were associated with poikilocytes, especially acanthocytes, but low correlation coefficients suggested other factors were also involved. Cholesterol and phospholipid abnormalities in hepatic disease are another cause of acanthocyte or echinocyte formation [1,2,10,13,24]; we found no correlation with hepatic disease in this study, but the sample size was small. Whether the result of diet or disease, high plasma cholesterol causes cholesterol-enrichment of red cell membranes, expanding the outer leaflet of the phospholipid bilayer (forming membrane projections) and increasing membrane rigidity [18]. Decreased deformability and increased fragility shorten red cell lifespan and contribute to regenerative anemia [25].

An important finding in this study was the association of fragmentation with inflammation (often septic) and with malignant neoplasia in rabbits. This could be the result of bacterial toxins or microangiopathy, with endothelial fibrin deposition and microthrombi causing physical damage to erythrocytes [12,14]. Fragmented erythrocytes usually occurred together with acanthocytes, which can undergo mechanical or "budding" fragmentation and which have been associated with fragmentation in dogs with hemangiosarcoma and glomerulonephritis [1,12,15]. Addition of Staphylococcal alpha toxin to suspensions of rabbit erythrocytes resulted in multiple, discrete surface blebs and finger-like protrusions (i.e., acanthocytes) that suggested separation of the cell membrane from the cell surface; human red cells were more resistant to this shape change [26]. In a murine model of bacterial sepsis, schistocytes (<1% of red cells) were observed 14 days post-infection and attributed to mild microangiopathic hemolysis [27].

Sepsis and inflammation-mediated oxidative damage and cytokines also alter red cell membranes, reducing deformability and increasing phagocytosis by macrophages [22,27,28]. Corre-

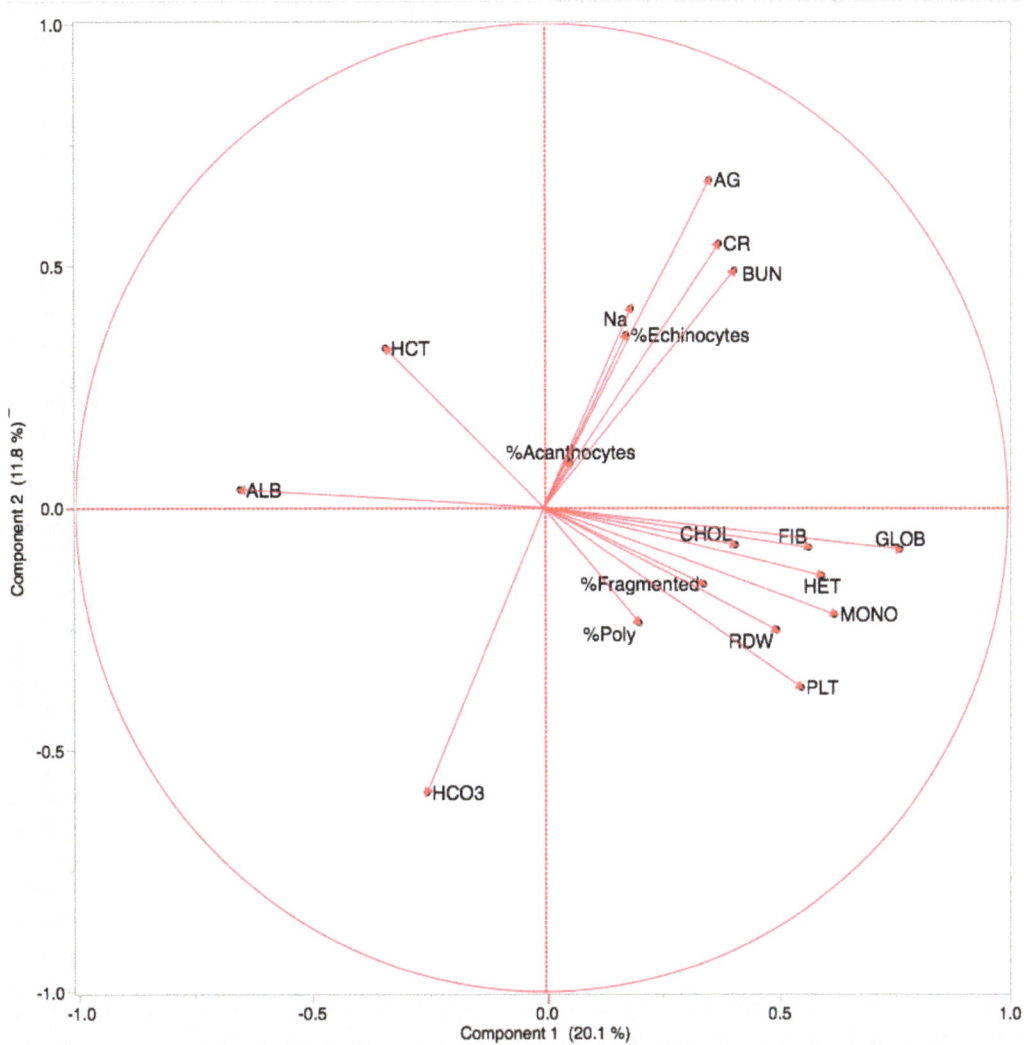

Figure 4. Principal component analysis of % poikilocytes and selected laboratory values. Two primary components were identified, in the right upper (component 2) and right lower (component 1) quadrants. The longer the arrow, the stronger the correlation. Analytes in left quadrants are negatively correlated with those in the diagonal quadrant.

lations between fragmentation and mild regenerative anemia and with heterophil, monocyte, fibrinogen, and globulins concentrations supported a relationship between bacterial infections, laboratory markers of inflammation, and red cell damage in the rabbits in our study. Lack of correlation of fragmented red cells with sample hemolysis was consistent with in vivo rather than in vitro fragment formation. Increased polychromatophils and fragments also contributed to high mean RDW and low MCH. High MPV and platelet counts supported reactive (inflammatory) thrombocytosis, in which IL-6-mediated thrombopoietin production stimulates platelet production [29]. False increases in MPV and platelet count from red cell fragments could have occurred in samples analyzed by the impedance analyzer in the first half of the study; however, the number of fragments was low.

Interestingly, high cholesterol diets can induce inflammation and oxidative stress together with acanthocyte formation in rabbits [30]. In one study [21] rabbits developed acanthocytes and fragments together with high concentrations of C-reactive protein, heterophils, and platelets, similar to our findings. The relationship between inflammation, hypercholesterolemia, and red cell mor-

phology in rabbits fed nonatherogenic diets is unclear, but warrants further study.

We combined spherocytes, keratocytes, microcytes, and schistocytes as fragmented red cells because they often appeared together and in low numbers [12]. No samples contained a predominance or high % of spherocytes, as in immune-mediated hemolytic anemia. Keratocytes form after rupture of "blister cells" (seen rarely in our rabbits) or due to mechanical trauma; they are considered schistocytes by the International Council for Standardization in Hematology [20] and are frequently observed in dogs with concurrent echinocytosis or acanthocytosis [1].

Strong associations between echinocytes, renal disease, and electrolyte abnormalities suggested uremia as one mechanism of moderate to marked echinocytosis in rabbits, as in other species [14,31–33]. Uremic toxins damage red cell membranes and lead to an influx of ionized calcium, externalization of phosphatidylserine in the lipid bilayer, and increased membrane rigidity concurrent with echinocyte formation [32–34]. In humans undergoing dialysis, % echinocytes correlated with intracellular calcium concentration and averaged 15–20% of RBCs [34]. The high anion gap in rabbits with echinocytosis and renal azotemia supported the presence of uremic acids. Increased echinocytes and red cell fragmentation in rabbits with renal disease also could have been associated with glomerulonephritis [1,9,12]. Increased plasma osmolality and hypernatremia (hypertonic dehydration) can also lead to echinocytosis, and may have been a factor in some rabbits in this study. Although smears in our laboratory are prepared soon after collection and dried rapidly, artifactual crenation likely contributed to echinocyte formation in some samples. Other disorders associated with echinocytosis in dogs (snakebite envenomation, lymphoma, cutaneous burns) [1,9], horses (total body cation depletion) [1,35], and rabbits (excess fluoride ingestion) [36] were not observed or associated with echinocytes in rabbits in this study.

A limitation of this retrospective study was the inability to verify underlying disease in all of the rabbits. In addition, we selected the primary disease process, but some rabbits had multiple problems. However, pathologic confirmation of disease was obtained in many of the rabbits, including diseases with potential relevance to poikilocyte formation. Further, many rabbits had diseases (such as fractures, dental malocclusion, and cystitis) that are readily diagnosed clinically or with imaging and laboratory tests. Despite

this limitation, the large size of the database and consistent relationships between poikilocytes and clinicopathologic abnormalities helped support the primary findings of our study.

In conclusion, acanthocytes and echinocytes comprised >3% of erythrocytes in about one-third of healthy and diseased rabbits; a small proportion of rabbits had >30% poikilocytes. Echinocytosis also was associated with renal disease and electrolyte abnormalities, consistent with the effect of uremia on red cells. Rabbits with abscesses, other inflammatory disorders, and malignant neoplasia had more red cell fragmentation, which was associated with mild regenerative anemia and hematologic and biochemical evidence of inflammation. Serum cholesterol concentration also correlated poikilocytosis, but was not strongly predictive. Future research is warranted to prospectively evaluate the pathophysiologic mechanisms of poikilocyte formation, the role of diet, and the diagnostic and prognostic value of poikilocytes in rabbits.

Author Contributions

Conceived and designed the experiments: MMC MGH. Performed the experiments: MMC AGB. Analyzed the data: MMC. Contributed to the writing of the manuscript: MMC AGB MGH.

References

1. Harvey JW (2012) Veterinary hematology: A diagnostic guide and color atlas. St. Louis, MO: Elsevier Inc. 360 p.
2. Marks PW (2013) Hematologic manifestations of liver disease. Semin Hematol 50: 216–221.
3. Duranthon V, Beaujean N, Brunner M, Odening KE, Navarrete Santos A, et al. (2012) On the emerging role of rabbit as human disease model and the instrumental role of novel transgenic tools. Transgenic Res 21: 699–713.
4. Russell JC, Proctor SD (2006) Small animal models of cardiovascular disease: tools for the study of the roles of metabolic syndrome. Cardiovasc Path 15: 318–330.
5. Yanni AE (2004) The laboratory rabbit: an animal model of atherosclerosis research. Lab Anim 38: 246–256.
6. Moore DM (1986) Hematology of rabbits. In: Feldman BF, Zinkl JG, Jain NC, editors. Schalm's veterinary hematology, 5th ed. Baltimore, MD: Lippincott, Williams, and Wilkins. pp. 1100–1106.
7. Schermer S (1967) The blood morphology of laboratory animals, 3rd ed. Philadelphia: FA Davis Co. 200 p.
8. Sanderson JH, Phillips CE (1981) An atlas of laboratory animal hematology. Oxford, UK: Clarendon Press. 473 p.
9. Weiss DJ, Kristensen A, Papenfuss N, McClay CB (1990) Quantitative evaluation of echinocytes in the dog. Vet Clin Pathol 19: 114–118.
10. Palek J (1994) Acanthocytosis, stomatocytosis, and related disorders. IN: Williams, WJ, Beutler E, Erslev AJ, and Lichtman MA, editors. Williams hematology. New York: McGraw-Hill, Inc. pp. 557–558.
11. Lange Y, Steck TL (1984) Mechanism of red blood cell acanthocytosis and echinocytosis in vivo. J Membr Biol 77: 153–159.
12. Weiss DJ, Kristensen A, Papenfuss N (1993) Quantitative evaluation of irregularly spiculated red blood cells in the dog. Vet Clin Pathol 22: 117–121.
13. Christopher MM, Lee SE (1994) Red cell morphologic alterations in cats with hepatic disease. Vet Clin Pathol 23: 7–12.
14. Rebar AH, Lewis HB, Denicola DB, Halliwell WH, Boon GD (1981) Red cell fragmentation in the dog: an editorial review. Vet Pathol 18: 415–426.
15. Warry E, Bohn A, Emanuelli M, Thamm D, Lana S (2013) Disease distribution in canine patients with acanthocytosis: 123 cases. Vet Clin Pathol 42: 465–470.
16. Pinter GG, Bailey RE (1961) Anemia of rabbits fed a cholesterol-containing diet. Am J Physiol 200: 292–296.
17. Pessina GP, Paulesu L, Bocci V (1981) Red cell modifications in cholesterol-fed rabbits. Int J Biochem 13: 805–810.
18. Cooper RA, Leslie MH, Knight D, Detweiler DK (1980) Red cell cholesterol enrichment and spur cell anemia in dogs fed a cholesterol-enriched, atherogenic diet. J Lipid Res 21: 1082–1089.
19. Weiss DJ (1984) Uniform evaluation and semi quantitative reporting of hematologic data in veterinary laboratories. Vet Clin Pathol 13: 27–31.
20. Zini G, D'Onofrio G, Briggs C, Erber W, Jou JM, et al. (2012) ICSH recommendations for identification, diagnostic value, and quantification of schistocytes. Int J Lab Hematol 34: 107–116.
21. Karbiner MS, Sierra L, Minahk C, Fonio MC, de Bruno MP, et al. (2013) The role of oxidative stress in alterations of hematological parameters and inflammatory markers induced by early hypercholesterolemia. Life Sci 93: 503–508.
22. López-Revuelta A, Sánchez-Gallego JI, García-Montero AC, Hernández-Hernández A, Sánchez-Yagüe J, et al. (2007) Membrane cholesterol in the regulation of aminophospholipid asymmetry and phagocytosis in oxidized erythrocytes. J Free Radic Biol Med 42: 1106–1118.
23. Kanakaraj P, Singh M (1989) Influence of hypercholesterolemia on morphological and rhelogical characteristics of erythrocytes. Atherosclerosis 76: 209–218.
24. Owen JS, Brown DJC, Harry DS, McIntyre N (1985) Erythrocyte echinocytosis in liver disease. J Clin Invest 76: 2275–2285.
25. Morse EE (1990) Mechanisms of hemolysis in liver disease. Ann Clin Lab Sci 20: 169–174.
26. Klainer AS, Chang T-W, Weinstein L (1972) Effects of purified Staphylococcal alpha toxin on the ultrastructure of human and rabbit erythrocytes. Infect Immunol 5: 808–813.
27. Kim A, Fung E, Parikh SG, Valore EV, Gabayan V, et al. (2014) A mouse model of anemia of inflammation: complex pathogenesis with partial dependence on hepcidin. Blood 123: 1129–1136.
28. Straat M, van Bruggen R, de Korte D, Juffermans NP (2012) Red blood cell clearance in inflammation. Transfus Med Hemother 39: 353–360.
29. Kaser A, Brandacher G, Steurer W, Kaser S, Offner FA, et al. (2001) Interleukin-6 stimulates thrombopoiesis through thrombopoietin: role in inflammatory thrombocytosis. Blood 98: 2720–2725.
30. Kuwai T, Hayashi J (2006) Nitric oxide pathway activation and impaired red blood cell deformability with hypercholesterolemia. J Atheroscler Thromb 13: 286–294.
31. Christopher MM (2008) Of human loss and erythrocyte survival: uremia and anemia in chronic renal disease. Israel Journal of Veterinary Medicine 63: 4–11.
32. Sakthivel R, Farooq SM, Kalaiselevi P, Varalakshmi P (2007) Investigation on the early events of apoptosis in senescent erythrocytes with special emphasis on intracellular free calcium and loss of phospholipid asymmetry in chronic renal failure. Clin Chim Acta 382: 1–7.
33. Lichtman MA, Beutler E, Kipps TJ, Seligsohn E, Kaushansky K, Prchal J (2006) Williams hematology, 7th ed. New York: McGraw-Hill Inc. 2296 p.
34. Agroyannis B, Kopelias I, Fourtounas C, Paraskevopoulos A, Tzanatos H, et al. (2001) Relation between echinocytosis and erythrocyte calcium content in hemodialyzed uremic patients. Artif Organs 25: 486–502.
35. Weiss DJ, Geor R, Smith II CM, McClay CB (1992) Furosemide-induced electrolyte depletion associated with echinocytosis in horses. Am J Vet Res 53: 1769–1772.
36. Susheela AK, Jain SK (1985) Fluoride toxicity: erythrocyte membrane abnormality and "echinocyte" formation. Fluoride Research, Studies in Environmental Science 27: 231–239.

20

Using Bayes' Rule to Define the Value of Evidence from Syndromic Surveillance

Mats Gunnar Andersson[1]*[◑], Céline Faverjon[2◑], Flavie Vial[3], Loïc Legrand[4,5], Agnès Leblond[5,6]

1 Department of Chemistry, Environment and Feed Hygiene, The National Veterinary Institute, Uppsala, Sweden, **2** INRA UR346 Animal Epidemiology, VetagroSup, Marcy L'Etoile, France, **3** Veterinary Public Health Institute, DCR-VPH, Vetsuisse Fakultät, Bern, Switzerland, **4** LABÉO - Frank Duncombe, Unité Risques Microbiens (U2RM), EA 4655, Normandie Universite, Caen, Normandy, France, **5** Réseau d'EpidémioSurveillance en Pathologie Equine (RESPE), Caen, France, **6** INRA UR346 Animal Epidemiology et Département Hippique, VetAgroSup, Marcy L'Etoile, France

Abstract

In this work we propose the adoption of a statistical framework used in the evaluation of forensic evidence as a tool for evaluating and presenting circumstantial "evidence" of a disease outbreak from syndromic surveillance. The basic idea is to exploit the predicted distributions of reported cases to calculate the ratio of the likelihood of observing n cases given an ongoing outbreak over the likelihood of observing n cases given no outbreak. The likelihood ratio defines the Value of Evidence (V). Using Bayes' rule, the prior odds for an ongoing outbreak are multiplied by V to obtain the posterior odds. This approach was applied to time series on the number of horses showing clinical respiratory symptoms or neurological symptoms. The separation between prior beliefs about the probability of an outbreak and the strength of evidence from syndromic surveillance offers a transparent reasoning process suitable for supporting decision makers. The value of evidence can be translated into a verbal statement, as often done in forensics or used for the production of risk maps. Furthermore, a Bayesian approach offers seamless integration of data from syndromic surveillance with results from predictive modeling and with information from other sources such as disease introduction risk assessments.

Editor: Simon Gubbins, The Pirbright Institute, United Kingdom

Funding: This work was funded by EMIDA ERA-NET through the Swedish research council Formas (http://www.formas.se/en/) (Contract no. 221-2011-2214) to MGA; EMIDA ERA-NET through Netherlands Food Consumer Product Safety Authority (www.nvwa.nl/english) and the Dutch Ministry of Economic Affairs (http://www.government.nl/ministries/ez) (project no. BO 20-009-009), and IFCE (Institut Français du Cheval et de l'Equitation) (http://www.ifce.fr/) to CF; INRA (Animal epidemiology Unit – EPIA) (http://www.inra.fr/en/Scientists-Students) and IFCE (Institut Français du Cheval et de l'Equitation) (http://www.ifce.fr/) to AL; 'Conseils Généraux du Calvados, de la Manche et de l'Orne' (County Councils) (http://www.calvados.fr/cms) to LL; Veterinary Public Health Institute, DCRVPH, Vetsuisse Fakultät, (http://www.vetsuisse.unibe.ch/vphi/content/index_ger.html) to FV. Labéo Frank Duncombe (http://www.labo-frank-duncombe.fr/) provided support in the form of a salary for author LL. The funders did not have any additional role in the study design, data collection and analysis, decision to publish, or preparation of the manuscript. The specific roles of these authors are articulated in the 'author contributions' section. The specific roles of these authors are articulated in the 'author contributions' section.

Competing Interests: LL is an employee of LABÉO. LABÉO was funded by the Conseils Généraux du Calvados, de la Manche et de l'Orne (County Councils). There are no patents, products in development or marketed products to declare.

* Email: gunnar.andersson@sva.se

◑ These authors contributed equally to this work.

Introduction

Syndromic surveillance appeared in the late 1990's and is becoming more and more popular in a wide range of human public health issues such as seasonal disease surveillance [1] and digital disease surveillance [2]. The wider acceptance of the relevance of the "One Health" concept [3] amongst public health practitioners has led to an increased exchange of methodologies and disease control knowledge between the human medicine and the veterinary sides. In the last 5 years, researchers in veterinary medicine have been investigating the application of syndromic surveillance methods for the early detection of zoonotic and non-zoonotic diseases [4].

There is no unique definition of "syndromic surveillance" but it is commonly accepted that it focuses on data collected prior to clinical diagnosis or laboratory confirmation [5,6]. It is therefore based on non-specific health indicators which result in a surveillance system with low specificity but allow the early detection of outbreaks without *a priori* considerations. This constitutes a major advantage over traditional approaches which focus on a disease, or a list of reportable diseases, and rely on the ability of clinicians to correctly diagnose cases, which may be difficult when faced with a rare or emerging disease [4]. Moreover, the systematic and continuous data collection and analysis processes reduce the impact of chronic under-reporting observed in classical passive surveillance systems and also increases the sensitivity of this method [4]. Syndromic surveillance does not replace traditional approaches to disease monitoring (e.g. risk-based, active etc…) but is seen as an interesting and complementary tool for outbreak detection with a low specificity but with better sensitivity and timeliness [7].

Current approaches used in syndromic surveillance first seek to define the normal properties of the syndrome time-series when no outbreak of disease is recorded [4,6] in order to be able to detect abnormal events overlaid on top of the background noise during an outbreak situation. In traditional aberration detection methods, an alarm goes off when the observed data exceed the expected values from the population [4,6]. Such algorithms have an epidemic threshold and provide a yes/no qualitative output: "No, there is no outbreak" or "Yes, something unusual is happening in the population".

This black or white vision of the health of the population of concern is simple but it may not always be adequate or useful for decision makers who may often find themselves in grey areas (indicator values close to the epidemic threshold). Moreover, binary result can also be difficult to combine with other epidemiological knowledge such as a probability of disease introduction or other complex parameters which influence decision making [8]. The development of syndromic surveillance quantitative outputs, which are more objective, flexible and easily interpretable, is a promising area of research.

The art of presenting scientific evidence to decision makers has been more extensively studied in forensic sciences in which legal certainty requires statements that clearly specify how strong the evidence for/against an hypothesis is and how the expert reached that conclusion. In recent years, the state of the art in forensic interpretation has been to evaluate forensic evidence using likelihood ratios in the framework of Bayesian hypothesis testing. Within this framework, it evaluates the extent to which results from forensic investigations speak in favor of the prosecutors or defendants hypotheses [9,10]. The Bayesian approach has been applied to a wide range of forensic problems including evidence based on DNA analysis [10], mass spectroscopy [11], transfer of glass, fibers and paint [10] and microbial counts [12]. However, although initially developed for the legal system, the approach has been identified as useful for supporting decision making in other situations such as the tracing of *Salmonella spp* [13].

The aim of this study is to test the applicability of the Bayesian likelihood ratio framework to the early detection of outbreaks in a syndromic surveillance system. Transferability of the method is demonstrated by using two examples based on real data coming from RESPE, the French surveillance network on equine diseases. The first example makes use of data on French horses presenting nervous symptoms (NeurSy) and aim to test the ability of our approach to detect simulated outbreaks of an exotic disease, West Nile Virus (WNV). West Nile disease is an important zoonotic disease and syndromic surveillance applied in horses could be used as an early warning system to protect the human population [14]. The second example focuses on data on French horses with respiratory symptoms (RespSy) and is used to detect outbreaks of divergent strains of equine influenza (New-Influenza), a non-zoonotic disease leading to vaccine failure [15–18].

Materials and Methods

Background theory and proposed framework

Forensic evaluation of evidence is based on Bayesian hypothesis testing. In a syndromic surveillance context, this would mean that, in a particular week, there are two mutually exclusive hypotheses that should be evaluated, for example: H_1 "There is an ongoing outbreak of disease x" and H_0 "There is NOT an ongoing outbreak of disease x". Without any extra information, the relative probability of the two hypotheses may be expressed as the *a priori* odds:

$$O_{pri} = \frac{P(H_1)}{P(H_0)} \qquad (Eq.1)$$

where

$P(H_1)$: The *a priori* probability for hypothesis H_1. Typically the probability of an ongoing outbreak of the disease of interest in a particular region.

$P(H_0)$: The *a priori* probability for hypothesis H_0 which is the complementary hypothesis to H_1. Typically the probability of an outbreak NOT going on.

In other words, the *a priori odds* define our *prior belief* about the disease status in the region. In a typical situation, the prior odds would be low (e.g. 1:1000) but under some circumstances, it might be higher (e.g. if an outbreak is ongoing in a neighboring country). When we are presented evidence (E) of some kind pointing in favor (or against) of H_1, this will make us update our belief. This posterior belief is expressed as the *a posteriori* odds.

$$O_{post} = \frac{P(H_1|E)}{P(H_0|E)} \qquad (Eq.2)$$

Where:

$P(H_1|E)$ is the probability of hypothesis H_1, given the evidence (E).

$P(H_0|E)$ is the probability of hypothesis H_0, given the evidence (E).

In syndromic surveillance, the evidence (E) is typically the number of reported suspected cases in a given time period. The degree to which the posterior belief differs from the prior belief will depend on the strength of the evidence. If the evidence is weak, the posterior odds will be similar to the prior odds whereas strong evidence in favor of H_1 would result in posterior odds being much higher than the prior odds. At this point, it is important to note that the hypotheses to evaluate (H_1) may differ and that the interpretation of the same piece of evidence would depend on the choice of H_1. For example 10 reported cases of syndromes in horses may be a strong evidence that there is something unusual going on if these are nervous cases $(H_1$ = "ongoing outbreak of some nervous disease (i.e. WNV)") but only weak evidence in favor of an equine influenza in the case of a respiratory syndrome $(H_1$ = "ongoing outbreak of equine influenza"), since in the latter case we might have expected far more reported cases.

This intuitive reasoning can be formalized by the application of Bayes' theorem:

$$O_{post} = V \times O_{pri} \equiv \frac{P(H_1|E)}{P(H_0|E)} = \frac{P(E|H_1)}{P(E|H_0)} \times \frac{P(H_1)}{P(H_0)} \qquad (Eq.3)$$

Where:

E is the number of reported cases of a syndrome in the particular week.

$P(E|H_1)$ is the probability of observing the evidence (E) given that H_1 is true.

$P(E|H_0)$ is the probability of observing the evidence (E) given that H_0 is true

In order to estimate $P(E|H_1)$ and $P(E|H_0)$ we need information on the probability distribution for the number of reported cases in a non-outbreak and outbreak situation. The probability of observing n cases given that H_1 is true can be estimated using statistical modeling of baseline data [19]. When the cases are independent (i.e. not clustered), the data can be modeled using a general dynamic Poisson model [19]. When cases are clustered (overdispersion), the Poisson model will underestimate the probability of observing very high or very low number of cases, and in such cases, the data can be modeled by continuous mixtures of the Poisson distribution including Negative Binomial (NB) distribution or Poisson-log-normal (PLN) distribution [19].

The probability of E (observation of n cases) during an outbreak is calculated as:

$$P(E|H_1) = \sum_{i=0}^{n} P_{base}(i) \times P_{out}(n-i) \qquad \text{(Eq.4)}$$

Where

$P_{base}(i)$ = Probability of drawing i cases from the baseline distribution (e.g. Poisson(λ) or NB(mu = mu$_{base}$, size = theta$_{base}$))

$P_{out}(i)$ = Probability of drawing i cases from the outbreak distribution (e.g. NB(mu = mu$_{out}$, size = theta$_{out}$))

The outbreak distribution may be estimated by fitting an appropriate probability distribution to data from historical outbreaks. In the absence of data, the outbreak distribution may be defined based on expert knowledge about the disease in question or assumptions about the distribution of a new disease. In most cases there would be a large uncertainty about the shape of the outbreak distribution.

The next estimate is the probability of observing the Evidence (E) that is the actual number of reported cases. In forensics, the value of evidence (V) is defined as the ratio between the posterior and prior odds for H_1 versus H_0. The value of evidence (Fig. 1, line Log(V)) can be calculated from the two distributions by dividing the probabilities for each number of observed cases using equation 5:

$$V = \frac{P(E|H_1)}{P(E|H_0)} \qquad \text{(Eq.5)}$$

As illustrated in Fig 1 the value of evidence will depend on the assumptions about the outbreak. In the examples A to D, 10 cases are reported from a region where the baseline prevalence is around 5 cases per week. If it is expected that an outbreak may be small, resulting in only a small number of extra cases, 10 reported cases would speak in favor of an outbreak (Fig. 1, A, C). If, on the other hand, the disease(s) of interest are expected to yield a relatively large number of cases the evidence would speak against an outbreak (Fig. 1, B, D).

In addition, the strength of the evidence will depend on the precision on the estimates for the number of outbreak-related cases. If the distributions are wide (low theta, Fig 1A, 1B), the absolute value of log(V) is smaller whereas more narrow distributions (high theta, Fig 1C, 1D) result in higher values of log(V). This is intuitive: the more we know about what we expect to see during an outbreak, the stronger conclusions we will make from the observed evidence.

Using the value of evidence for decision making

In contrast to traditional outbreak detection algorithms, the value of evidence approach does not have a built-in decision threshold. Typically a decision maker would not act upon syndromic surveillance data alone but rather combine it with other available knowledge. Cameron [20] proposed several approaches to disease freedom questions: (1) population or surveillance sensitivity, (2)

probability of freedom from disease, and (3) expected cost of error – i.e., consequences of false positive and false negative results. All approaches underline how the value of inspection findings will be augmented when interpreted in a broader context to complement other monitoring and surveillance systems (MOSS) activities. One option for a decision maker would be to set an action threshold for the posterior odds. We might, for example, want to initiate an epidemiological investigation if the odds that there is an ongoing outbreak are larger than 1:1 or 1:100. Ideally the decision maker would make a cost-benefit analysis taking into account the expected costs for taking action versus not taking action. For example the decision maker may initiate control measures (vaccination program *etc*) when the odds are such that, on average, the reduced loss from the early detection of the outbreak would exceed the extra costs from initiating control measures (or vaccination programs) in response to false alarms.

The combination of evidence evaluation and decision theory is discussed in [21]. The expected utility (ū) of action a_i is the average amount of loss that we expect to incur with this action. In the context of diseases surveillance, an action could be to implement movement restrictions, vaccination, sampling, control of vectors or to do nothing. The loss could be the direct financial losses (e.g. animal infection, disease and production losses) but also the indirect losses (e.g. surveillance and control costs, compensation costs, potential trade losses, social consequences). Since an unmanaged outbreak as well as actions will result in costs, the expected utility will always be zero or negative. In this framework the expected utility (ū) of action a_i is defined as:

$$\bar{u}(a_i|\cdot) = \sum_{j=0}^{1} u(C_{ij})p(H_j|\cdot) \qquad \text{(Eq.6)}$$

where

H_1 = Outbreak

H_0 = No outbreak

a_0 = No action

a_1 = Action

C_{ij} = Different scenarios with respect to hypothesis on outbreak status (H_0, H_1) and action (a_0, a_1) C_{00} represents the case with no disease and no action implemented. C_{01} is no disease but action implemented, C_{10} disease but no action and C_{11} is disease and action implemented)

$p(H_j|\cdot)$ = probability of hypothesis j given all available knowledge (Prior probability & evidence)

$u(C_{ij})$ = expected utility for each possible situation C_{ij}. Since gain is zero the utility is determined by economical and socio-economical loss.

According to this framework it is favorable to act when the expected utility of action ($\bar{u}(a_1|\cdot)$) is higher than the expected utility of no action ($\bar{u}(a_0|\cdot)$). The relation between posterior probability (P(Hi|E) and posterior odds (O$_{post}$) is defined by:

$$O_{post} = \frac{P(H_1|E)}{1 - P(H_1|E)} \qquad \text{(Eq.7)}$$

and

$$P(H_1|E) = \frac{O_{post}}{1 + O_{post}} \qquad \text{(Eq.8)}$$

Thus equation 6 can be reformulated as

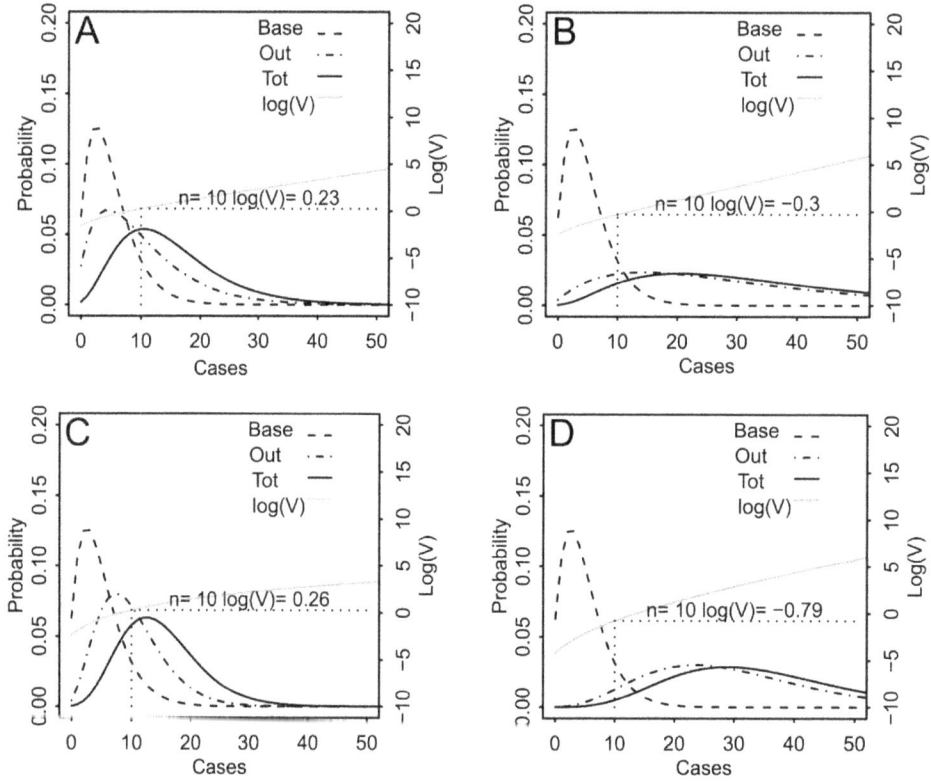

Figure 1. Value of evidence (V) and probability of observing 10 cases during a non-outbreak (Base) and outbreak situation (Out) with different assumptions about the magnitude of an outbreak. The baseline cases are distributed according to NB mu = 5, theta = 2.55. The value of evidence, log(V) is calculated as $log_{10}(p(n|outbreak)/p(n|baseline))$. The distribution during an outbreak (Tot) is the sum of baseline cases and outbreak cases. In the examples A to D outbreak related cases are distributed according to (A) NB(mu = 10, theta = 2), (B) NB(mu = 30, theta = 2), (C) NB(mu = 10, theta = 5), (D) NB(mu = 30, theta = 5).

$$\bar{u}(a_i|\cdot) = \sum_{j=0}^{1} u(C_{ij}) \times \frac{o_{post}}{(1 + O_{post})} \qquad (Eq.9)$$

For each value of O_{post} the expected utility for action a_1 and a_o is defined by eq. 9. The expected loss for each situation C_{ij} is based on expert opinion as indicated in table 1. An action threshold for posterior odds ($O_{post}*$) can be defined as the value of O_{post} where

$$\bar{u}(a_1|\cdot) = \bar{u}(a_0|\cdot)$$

In this work $O_{post}*$ was determined by numerical optimization. The derived action threshold for the value of evidence V* is calculated as:

$$V^* = \frac{O^*_{post}}{O_{pri}} \qquad (Eq.10)$$

where the prior odds for an ongoing outbreak $Log_{10}(O_{pri})$ is based on historical experience as well as knowledge about risk factors.

To make a decision, the risk manager would multiply the prior odds with the value of evidence using eq.3 to obtain the posterior odds for an outbreak $O_{post}(H_1 | E)$. If this odds goes over the action

threshold $Log_{10}(O_{post}*)$ where the expected utility from acting exceeds the utility for not acting, a decision would be taken to act.

Performance assessment

Sensitivity, specificity and predictive values of positive and negative tests are important concepts when planning animal health monitoring. In the syndromic surveillance context a true positive (TP) is when the system alerts when an outbreaks is ongoing. A true negative (TN) is no alert and no outbreak. A false negative (FN) is when the system does not alert when an outbreak is ongoing, and, false positive (FP) is when the system alerts in the absence of an outbreak.

Sensitivity (SE) is the probability that a true outbreak triggers an alert:

$$SE = {}^{TP}/_{(TP + FN)} \qquad (Eq.11)$$

Specificity (SP) is the probability the there is no alert when no outbreak is ongoing:

$$SP = {}^{TN}/_{(TN + FP)} \qquad (Eq.12)$$

The positive predictive value (PPV) is the probability of an indicated outbreak being a true outbreak:

Table 1. Expected utility associated with different actions and the derived decision threshold & decision.

	Scenario A		Scenario B		Scenario C Large	
	Small outbreak in Autumn		**Medium outbreak in Winter**		**outbreak in Spring**	
$u(C_{00})$ *Out− act−*	0		0		0	
$u(C_{10})$ *Out− act+*	−0. 5 M€		−0. 5 M€		−0. 5 M€	
$u(C_{01})$ *Out+ act−*	−5.1 M€		−5.3 M€		−10.1 M€	
$u(C_{11})$ *Out+ act+*	−3.9 M€		−4.1 M€		−6.3 M€	
Action threshold $Log_{10}(O_{post}*)$	−0.38		−0.38		−0.88	
$Log_{10}(O_{pri})$	−0.99		−3.03		−1.78	
Action Threshold $Log_{10}(V*)$	0.61		2.65		0.9	
Weeks	**w36**	**w39**	**w1**	**w4**	**w25**	**w28**
Cases observed per week	3	4	5	7	5	7
$Log_{10}(V)$	0.23	0.67	1.30	2.77	1.77	3.41
$Log_{10}(O_{post})$	−0.76	−0.34	−1.71	−0.34	−0.01	1.63
Action? V>V*	**No**	**Yes**	**No**	**Yes**	**Yes**	**Yes**

$$\text{PPV} = {TP}/{(TP+FP)} \qquad (Eq.13)$$

The Negative predictive value (NPV) is the probability that no signal of outbreak is true absence of an outbreak:

$$\text{NPV} = {TN}/{(TN+FN)} \qquad (Eq.14)$$

The PPV and NPV depend on the (prior) probability of an outbreak and in the performance assessment PPV was calculated as:

$$PPV = \frac{P_{pri} \times SE}{(1-P_{pri}) \times (1-SP) + SE \times P_{pri}} \qquad (Eq.15)$$

where:

P_{pri} = prior probability of ongoing outbreak in the week of interest

Implementation

Models were implemented in R×64 version 3.0.2 [22]. TheR-Scripts are included as part of the material (Script S1, S2, S3, S4).

Dynamic regression was performed with function *glm* (package {stats} [22] for Poisson regression and *glm.nb* (package {MASS}) [23]. The expected number of counts at time × were estimated with the *predict* function of the respective package. Alternative regression models were evaluated using the Akaike information criterion (AIC). In addition adjusted deviance (Deviance/df) was used as a measure of goodness of fit (GOF).

The receiver operating characteristic (ROC) curve was generated in R by simulation. Counts for negative weeks were sampled from a Poisson distribution (function *rpois* in package {stats}) with lambda equal to the predicted value for each week in 2011 and 2012 (n = 53000). Counts for positive weeks were generated by sampling values from the fitted outbreak distribution (function *rnbinom* in package {stats}) and adding to the baseline.

SE and SP were calculated for values of Log10(V) between -1 and +3 in steps of 0.01. The expected PPV for each value of V was calculated as above using the prior odds for outbreak from three scenarios.

Threshold values for posterior odds ($O_{post}*$) were estimated using the Solver function of Microsoft Excel 2007.

Sources of data

As a proof of principle the value of evidence framework was applied to neurological and respiratory syndromes in French horses. The associated time series are named NeurSy and RespSy, respectively. These data are collected through the passive surveillance system "RESPE", the French network for the surveillance of equine diseases (http://www.respe.net/). This system collects the declarations from veterinary practitioners registered as sentinels who fill online a standardized questionnaire depending on the syndrome concerned. Along with their declaration, veterinarians send standardized samples for the laboratory diagnosis. Tests for equine influenza, equine herpes 1 and 4 and equine arteritis viruses are implemented in the case of a respiratory syndrome, West Nile and equine herpes 1 viruses in the case of a nervous syndrome. In our study, we used these weekly time series.

Data from 2006 to 2010 were used to train our models and define the background noise of each time series when no outbreak occurs. We only used the data on the number of cases with no positive laboratory test result in order to remove the outbreaks from our datasets and obtain these outbreak free baselines. Then, different regression models were tested.

No real outbreak of West Nile disease and divergent strains of equine influenza (New-Influenza) occurred during this time. Instead fictive test data were used for demonstrating outbreak detection. The baselines in the test data were based on NeurSy and RespSy data from 2011 to 2012 where unexplained aberrations, not related to the diseases of interest, were filtered out and fictive outbreaks inserted based on historical data. The weekly counts from several real outbreaks were fitted together to model the outbreaks of each disease. The *prior odds* for each example are based on our knowledge on the epidemiology and risk factors for transmission of the disease. New-Influenza is supposed to have the same probability of occurrence over the year and the *prior odds* is thus considered as constant over time. West Nile disease transmission is linked to the vector's level of activity and is thus a seasonal disease. Different *prior odds* are set for each season for this disease.

Data Accessibility

The datasets supporting this article have been uploaded as part of the Material. The baseline data for NeurSy and RespSy are included in Table S1 and Table S2 respectively. The outbreak data for NeurSy and RespSy are included in Table S3 and Table S4 respectively.

The software R can be freely downloaded from the CRAN homepage (http://cran.r-project.org/).

Results

Case study – Neurological syndromes and WNV (NeurSy)

Non-outbreak situation. To define the background noise of the NeurSy time series when no outbreak occurred, we fitted alternative regression models based on Poisson and NB distributions from years 2006–2010 on data containing only cases with no positive laboratory results (figure S1). The models evaluated including sinod models with 1, 2 and 3 periods/year and season or month as factorial variables. To account for differences between years we dynamically calculate the average counts for 53 consecutive weeks (*histmean*). To ensure that an ongoing outbreak will not influence the estimate, we used a 10 week guard band [24] for calculation of *histmean*. For the Poisson as well as the NB regression the best fit were obtained with the simplest model:

$$counts \sim sin(2\pi t) + cos(2\pi t) + log(histmean)$$

where t is time in years. For the Poisson regression we obtained: AIC = 637.8, GOF(adjusted dev) = 1.156. For NB regression the corresponding parameters were: AIC: 639; GOF = 1.080. The inverse theta of the NB model was 10.45. Considering that the NB distribution converges to the Poisson distribution when inverse theta approaches infinity and that the GOF and AIC for the Poisson and NB models were very similar we conclude that the Poisson model adequately describes the random distribution in this data.

Outbreak definition. Three observed WNV outbreaks were used to simulated the outbreaks in our model: French outbreaks in horses in 2000 [25] and 2004 [14] where 76 and 32 confirmed cases were reported respectively among 131 and 72 horses presenting nervous symptoms, and the Italian outbreak in 1998 [26] where 14 cases of WNV in horses were investigated by week of onset.

The weekly counts from these three outbreaks were fitted to the NB distribution. The resulting outbreak distribution was NB(mu = 4.45, theta = 0.94). Based on this we predicted a median number of outbreak-related cases per week during an outbreak to be 3 with a 95% confidence interval of 0 to 18 cases.

Outbreak detection. Three scenarios were tested. The probability of an outbreak is not constant over the year, instead the relative probability of an outbreak occurring in spring (week 10 to 30), summer/autumn (week 31 to 46) and winter (week 47 to 9) is approximately 1:5:0.04. We chose to test one scenario per time period. i.e. the scenario A occurs in autumn, scenario B in winter and the scenario C in spring. For each scenario, the Poisson model was applied on the test set and one simulated peak/outbreak was inserted into the baseline (Figure 2). For each week the value of evidence was calculated using Eq5 where the probability of the observed number of cases during no outbreak $p(E|H_1)$ and during

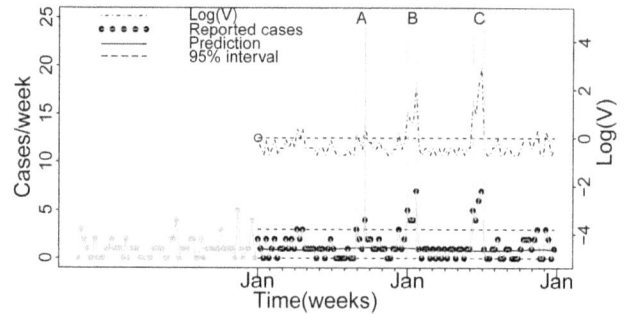

Figure 2. Application of NeurSy model on the test dataset. The vertical lines bounds peaks inserted during Year 1, week 36 to 39 (Scenario A), Year 2, week 1 to 4 (Scenario B) and Year 2, weeks 24 to 28 (Scenario C).

outbreak $p(E|H_0)$ were calculated using the fitted model. Examples of the calculation of V during a non outbreak (scenario A) and during outbreaks (scenarios B and C) are shown in Figure 3.

Decision scenarios

The decision making in the outbreak scenarios for both examples is summarized in table 1.

The expected utility $u(C_{ij})$ for each scenario considered are given together with the action thresholds for posterior odds (O_{post}*) and value of evidence (V*) in favor of an outbreak. That is the situation for which the decision to act and not act have the same expected utility.

The expected utility of taking action in response to false alert ($u(C_{01})$) represents the costs for increased surveillance and preventive actions such as mosquito control for WNV. The utility of not taking action when there is an outbreak ($u(C_{10})$) represents the costs for control and economical and socio-economical consequences of an outbreak when the response to the outbreak was delayed. The losses may depend on season and in the example we have assumed that a WNV outbreak in summer or spring in the south of France results in extra costs due to its impact on tourism. Finally the utility of taking action when there is an outbreak ($u(C_{11})$) represents the costs for surveillance plus the economical and socio-economical impact in case of a timely response to the outbreak.

For NeurSy (Scenarios A to C), the prior odds in the table are based on the assumption that an outbreak of WNV is likely to occur every 3 years over an averageof 5 weeks. The costs used are fictional but proportional to their expected relative contributions.

During the most at risk season regarding the probability of disease occurrence (Highest O_{pri}), the alarm threshold is low and 4 cases are sufficient to trigger an action (See Table 1. scenario A). For the season less at resk, the expected utilities are similar than during the most at risk season (O_{post}* are equal), but no action is implemented even if 7 cases are reported because they are unlikely due to WNV (Low O_{pri}) (See Table 1. scenario B).

Sensitivity, specificity and receiver operating characteristics

The sensitivity and specificity of a surveillance system is defined by the chosen action threshold. The tradeoff between sensitivity and specificity of a model may be summarized in a receiver operating characteristics (ROC) curve [27]. The ROC curve corresponding to the case WNV case study is shown in figure 4A.

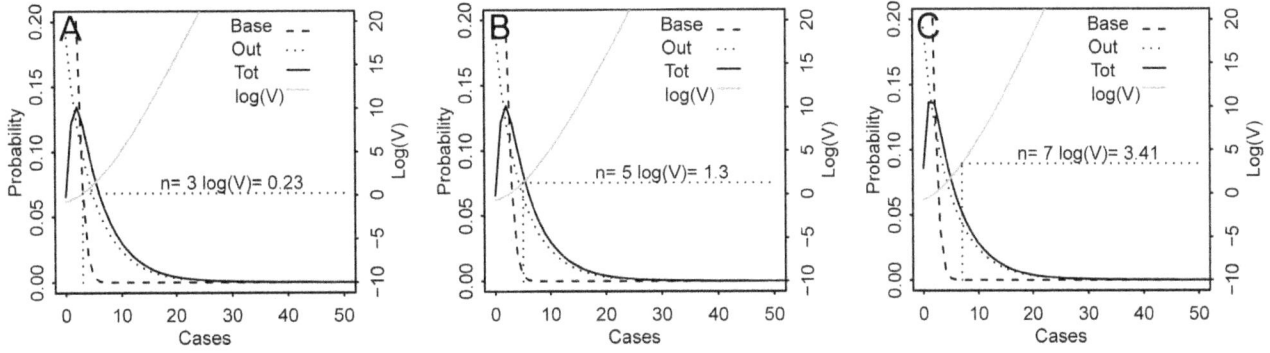

Figure 3. Value of evidence (V) and probability of observing _n_ cases of neurological syndromes in a week during a non-outbreak (Base) situation and during a WNV outbreak (Out). Out is the distribution of outbreak related cases and Tot is the total number of observed cases per week during an outbreak. (A) Scenario A, year 1 week 36, $\lambda = 1.08$, (B) Scenario B, year 2 week 1. $\lambda = 1.08$, (C) Scenario C, year 2 week 27, $\lambda = 0.81$.

The values of SE and SP arising from scenarios A to C are indicated by letters. The PPV i.e. the probability that an alarm corresponds to a real outbreak [28] depends not only on SE and SP but also on the prior probability of an outbreak as indicated in figure 4B.

Case study 2– Respiratory syndromes and equine influenza (RespSy)

The same approach was successfully applied to the RespSy dataset. However, in this case the analysis indicated a significant degree of overdispersion in the weekly counts. Using the same regression model (counts ~ $\sin(2\pi\ t) + \cos(2\pi t) + \log(\text{histmean})$) the NB model had lower AIC (1141 vs 1284) and GOF closer to one (1.14 vs 2.54) compared to the Poisson model. The theta parameter for the NB distribution was 1.78, and resulting in a much wider confidence interval for the expected number of cases in a non-outbreak situation (Figure S2) compared to the Poisson model (Figure S3). When the NB and Poisson models are applied to the same test dataset (Figure S4, S5) the latter will report a value of evidence for the inserted peaks (D, E) that is several orders of magnitude higher than does the NB model. The Poisson model also reports peaks with Log(V) close to 2 several times per year (Figure S5). An underlying assumption in the Poisson model is the

absence of overdispersion and, when this assumption does not hold, the Poisson model underestimates the probability of obtaining a large number of reported cases in the non-outbreak situation. Consequently it overestimates the value of evidence in favor of an outbreak. The overdispersion may be due to clustering in reporting. In the surveillance protocol veterinarians are encouraged not only to declare the diseased horse but also 1 to 3 additional horses (from the same stable), suspected to be in the incubation phase of influenza.

Discussion

In this work we have demonstrated how the value of evidence concept may be incorporated in a decision support system for syndromic surveillance and how the output may be used for risk assessment and informed decision making. According to the OIE - Terrestrial Animal Health Code [29] the decision to take action involves balancing costs for activities against economical and social consequences of a delayed response to an outbreak is the responsibility of the risk manager and should be separate from risk assessment.

Thus, although it is perfectly possible to build a system that outputs a best decision, the proposed approach is in concordance

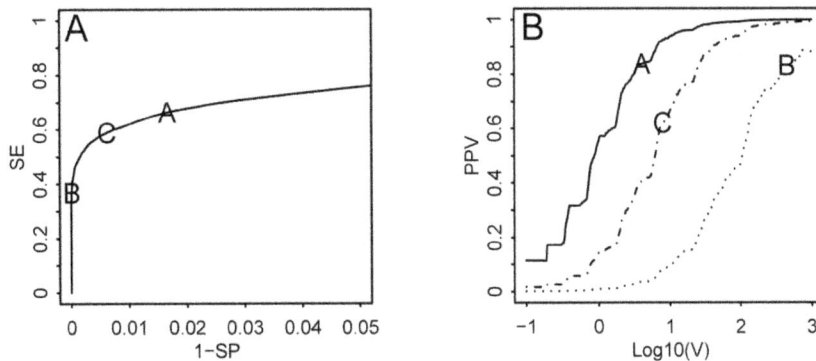

Figure 4. (A) ROC curve for outbreak detection of WNV based on neurological symptoms. Letters A–C indicate the decision threshold for Log(V*) in scenario A–C respectively (B). Positive Predictive Value (PPV) for different thresholds of $\text{Log}_{10}(V^*)$ given the prior probabilities of scenario A, B and C. The position of the letters indicate the action threshold for the respective scenario.

with the risk analysis framework [29] by offering explicit separation of assumptions (P_{prior}), scientific evidence (V) and criteria for decisions and a transparency of how the evidence is evaluated. In forensics, the value of evidence is typically presented to the court as a qualitative statement in which fixed verbal expressions correspond to specified intervals for V [10,30]. This approach may be useful also when presenting epidemiological results. For example a value of $Log_{10}(V)$ in the range 1–2 may be expressed as "results provide moderate evidence to support that an outbreak is ongoing". Alternatively intervals for V and/or O_{post} could be expressed using a color scale to produce maps representing the results from surveillance and risk of ongoing outbreaks of different diseases.

The model presented here is intended as a proof of concept and when setting up an operational syndromic surveillance system it will, as usual, be necessary to perform a careful evaluation of the baseline model to ensure that the regression model does not overfit to the baseline data. When designing the current model it was evident that high dimensional regression models were prone to find artefactual seasonal patterns that could severely bias the estimated probability of observing a number of counts in a particular week (results not shown). In the current implementation the model learns seasonal patterns and distribution of residuals (Inverse theta parameter of NB distribution) from manually curated data whereas the expected yearly average (*histmean*) is continuously updated from outbreak-filtered weekly data. Naturally the value of evidence concept may also be applied to a system where the baseline model is automatically retrained on new data. However, since the distribution parameter (theta) of the NB distribution would determine the cutoff in the filtering algorithm we argue that it is safer not to use the filtered data for estimation of the same parameter without prior inspection of the data. The same conclusion holds for seasonal patterns.

The overdispersion in the RespSy dataset is largely due to veterinarians sampling several horses in a stable upon suspicion. Thus, in this special case it might be possible to handle the overdispersion by pre-processing the data to remove redundant cases, provided that the same pre-processing is applied to new data on weekly basis. However, when the mechanism behind overdispersion in baseline counts is not so transparent that automatic filtering out redundant cases is possible the NB model will support a correct interpretation of the value of the peak in the count data.

As indicated in Figure 4 the tradeoff between SE and SP differs between seasons. This is natural since in case the (prior) probability of an outbreak differs between seasons the average sensitivity SE_{avr} and specificity SP_{avr} will be given by:

$$SE_{avr} = \frac{\sum_{i=1}^{n}(d_i \times SE_i \times P_i)}{\sum_{i=1}^{n}(d_i)} \quad \text{(Eq.16)}$$

$$SP_{avr} = \frac{\sum_{i=1}^{n}(d_i \times SP_i \times (1-P_i))}{\sum_{i=1}^{n}(d_i)} \quad \text{(Eq.17)}$$

where:

SE_i = sensitivity in season i
SP_i = specificity in season i
P_i = (prior) probability of outbreak in season i
d_i = (relative) duration of season i

Thus, by incorporating prior knowledge about the seasonality of the diseases of interest it is possible to achieve a high average sensitivity without sacrificing the PPV and SP. Another important attribute of outbreak detection is timeliness. Whereas there is no

general measure of timeliness [28] the number of cases are often small in the first week(s) of an outbreak, increasing the sensitivity (i.e. lowering the threshold for V and thus n) in the high risk season will result in improved timeliness as well as average sensitivity.

In this work we have introduced the framework using models that evaluate evidence from each week independently. Although this simple approach is suitable for presenting the framework and a reasonable choice for an early warning system, the evaluation of evidence from one week at a time is not a fundamental limitation of the approach. A model accounting for accumulation of evidence over several weeks may, for example, be constructed by considering, for each week in the interval [0…j] the conditional probability

$$P(E|H_{t-i})$$

Where
t is the week of interest
H_{t-i} is the hypothesis that an outbreak started i weeks before t
E_{t-n} is the number of reported cases in week [t-i… t]
The probability of observing n outbreak-related cases will not be uniform throughout the outbreak but depend on whether the outbreak is in its first, second or third week *etc*. When accounting for evidence from several weeks the value of evidence in favor of the hypothesis H_1 "An outbreak is going on" against H_0 "An outbreak is not going on" will be dependent on the prior probability of an outbreak starting in any of the preceding weeks. This is due to the fact that H_1 is composed of several sub-hypotheses:

$H_{1\ i=0}$: An outbreak started in week t
$H_{1\ i=1}$: An outbreak started in week t-1
..
$H_{1\ i=j}$: An outbreak started in week t-j
Consequently $p(H_1)$ depends on the relative probability of these sub-hypotheses. The value of evidence in favor of an outbreak going on in week of interest (V) can be calculated as the Bayes factor (B):

$$V = B = \frac{O_{post}}{O_{pri}} \quad \text{(Eq.18)}$$

where
O_{post} is the posterior odds of an outbreak going on in week of interest
O_{pri} is the prior odds of an outbreak going on in week of interest
Although in the more complex models the calculation of the value of evidence would depend on the prior probability of outbreak, the framework is still applicable for communicating the evidence to decision makers. Essentially any Markov Chain model could be applied in the evaluation of evidence framework and the choice of complexity is a tradeoff between on the one hand realism and on the other hand simplicity and transparency. However, we anticipate that in most situations there will not be sufficient data to support very complex models.

Supporting Information

Figure S1 Fitted baseline and one sided 95% confidence interval for weekly counts for case NeurSy Years 2006–2010. Poisson regression using model: counts ~ sin(2π t) + cos(2π t) + log(histmean).

Figure S2   Fitted baseline and one sided 95% confidence interval for weekly counts for case RespSy Years 2006–2010. NB regression using model: counts ~ sin(2π t) + cos(2π t) + log(histmean).

Figure S3   Fitted baseline and one sided 95% confidence interval for weekly counts for case RespSy Years 2006–2010. Poisson regression using model: counts ~ sin(2π t) + cos(2π t) + log(histmean).

Figure S4   Application of RespSy NB-model on the fictive test dataset. The vertical lines bounds peaks inserted during Year 1, week 36 to 39 (D), Year 2, week 24 to 28 (E). The gray points indicate historical data used to calculate the historical average (histmean).

Figure S5   Application of RespSy Poisson-model on the fictive test dataset. The vertical lines bounds peaks inserted during Year 1, week 36 to 39 (D), Year 2, week 24 to 28 (E). The gray points indicate historical data used to calculate the historical average (histmean).

Table S1   NeurSy baseline 2006–2012.

Table S2   RespSy baseline 2006–2012.

Table S3   NeurSy outbreak distribution.

Table S4   RespSy outbreak distribution.

Script S1   Script used to analyze time series data.

Script S2   Script used to illustrate the calculation of V in figures 1 and 3.

Script S3   Script used to prepare ROC and PPV plots.

Script S4   Script used to remove aberrations from baseline when preparing fictive test data.

Acknowledgments

Christel Marcillaud-Pitel for collecting and providing data from the RESPE (Réseau d'Epidémio-Surveillance en Pathologie Equine) and Fernanda Dórea for help with dynamic regression models.

Author Contributions

Conceived and designed the experiments: MGA. Analyzed the data: MGA CF. Contributed reagents/materials/analysis tools: AL LL. Wrote the paper: MGA CF FV AL. Organized baseline data collection: AL LL. Critical revision of manuscript: LL.

References

1. Hiller KM, Stoneking L, Min A, Rhodes SM (2013) Syndromic Surveillance for Influenza in the Emergency Department-A Systematic Review. PLoS One 8: e73832.
2. Gesualdo F, Stilo G, Agricola E, Gonfiantini MV, Pandolfi E, et al. (2013) Influenza-Like Illness Surveillance on Twitter through Automated Learning of Naïve Language. PLoS One 8: e82489.
3. Gibbs EP (2014) The evolution of One Health: a decade of progress and challenges for the future. Vet Rec 174: 85–91.
4. Dórea FC, Sanchez J, Revie CW (2011) Veterinary syndromic surveillance: Current initiatives and potential for development. Prev Vet Med 101: 1–17.
5. Katz R, May L, Baker J, Test E (2011) Redefining syndromic surveillance. Journal Epidemiol Global H 1: 21–31.
6. Shmueli G, Burkom H (2010) Statistical Challenges Facing Early Outbreak Detection in Biosurveillance. Technometrics 52: 39–51.
7. Buehler JW, Berkelman RL, Hartley DM, Peters CJ (2003) Syndromic Surveillance and Bioterrorism-related Epidemics. Emerg Infect Dis 9: 1197–1204.
8. Brownson RC, Fielding JE, Maylahn CM (2009) Evidence-Based Public Health: A Fundamental Concept for Public Health Practice. Annu Rev of Publ Health 30: 175–201.
9. Taroni F, Aitken C, Garbolino P, Biedermann A (2006) Bayesian Networks and Probabilistic Inference in Forensic Science. Chichester: John Wiley & Sons Ltd.
10. Aitken C, Roberts P, Jackson G (2010) Fundamentals of Probability and Statistical Evidence in Criminal Proceedings. Guidance for Judges, Lawyers, Forensic Scientists and Expert Witnesses. London: The Royal Statistical Society.
11. Jarman KH, Kreuzer-Martin HW, Wunschel DS, Valentine NB, Cliff JB, et al. (2008) Bayesian-integrated microbial forensics. Appl and Environ Microb 74: 3573–3582.
12. Keats A, FS L, Yee E (2006) Source Determination in Built-Up Environments Through Bayesian Inference With Validation Using the MUST Array and Joint Urban 2003 Tracer Experiments. Proc 14th Annual Conference of the Computational Fluid Dynamics Society of Canada, July 16–18,. Kingston, Canada.
13. Andersson G, Aspán A, Hultén C, Ågren E, Barker GC (2013) Application of forensic evaluation of evidence to the tracing of Salmonella. Symposium Salmonella and Salmonellosis I3S. Saint-Malo FRANCE.
14. Leblond A, Hendrikx P, Sabatier P (2007) West Nile Virus Outbreak Detection Using Syndromic Monitoring in Horses. Vector-Borne Zoonot 7: 403–410.
15. Legrand LJ, Pitel PH, Marcillaud-Pitel CJ, Cullinane AA, Courouce AM, et al. (2013) Surveillance of equine influenza viruses through the RESPE network in France from November 2005 to October 2010. Equine vet j 45: 776–783.
16. Martella V, Elia G, Decaro N, Di Trani L, Lorusso E, et al. (2007) An outbreak of equine influenza virus in vaccinated horses in Italy is due to an H3N8 strain closely related to recent North American representatives of the Florida sub-lineage. Vet Microbiol 121: 56–63.
17. Newton JR, Daly JM, Spencer L, Mumford JA (2006) Description of the outbreak of equine influenza (H3N8) in the United Kingdom in 2003, during which recently vaccinated horses in Newmarket developed respiratory disease. Vet Rec 158: 185–192.
18. Yamanaka T, Niwa H, Tsujimura K, Kondo T, Matsumura T (2008) Epidemic of equine influenza among vaccinated racehorses in Japan in 2007. J Vet Med Sci 70: 623–625.
19. Schmidt AM, Pereira JBM (2011) Modelling Time Series of Counts in Epidemiology. Int Stat Rev 79: 48–69.
20. Cameron AR (2012) The consequences of risk-based surveillance: Developing output-based standards for surveillance to demonstrate freedom from disease. Prev Vet Med 105: 280–286.
21. Gittelson SN (2013) Evolving from inferences to decisions in the in the interpretation of scientific evidence. Institute de Police Scientifique. Lausanne: Université de Lausanne.
22. R Core Team (2013) R: A language and environment for statistical computing. Vienna, Austria: R Foundation for Statistical Computing.
23. Venables WN, Ripley BD (2002) Modern Applied Statistics with S. New York: Springer.
24. Burkom HS, Elbert Y, Feldman A, Lin J (2004) Role of data aggregation in biosurveillance detection strategies with applications from ESSENCE. MMWR Morbidity and mortality weekly report 53 Suppl: 67–73.
25. Murgue B, Murri S, Zientara S, Durand B, Durand JP, et al. (2001) West Nile outbreak in horses in southern France, 2000: the return after 35 years. Emerg Infect Dis 7: 692–696.
26. Autorino GL, Battisti A, Deubel V, Ferrari G, Forletta R, et al. (2002) West Nile virus Epidemic in Horses, Tuscany Region, Italy. Emerg Infect Dis 8: 1372–1378.
27. Hastie T, Tibshirani R, Friedman J (2001) The elements of statistical learning, Data mining, inference and Prediction. New York: Springer Science + Business Media Inc.
28. Sosin DM (2003) Draft framework for evaluating syndromic surveillance systems. J Urban Health 80: i8–13.
29. OIE (2011) OIE - Terrestrial Animal Health Code. World Organization for Animal Health.
30. Nordgaard A, Ansell R, Drotz W, Jaeger L (2012) Scale of conclusions for the value of evidence. Law, probability & risk 11: 1–24.

21

Sympatric Woodland *Myotis* Bats Form Tight-Knit Social Groups with Exclusive Roost Home Ranges

Tom A. August[1,2], **Miles A. Nunn**[1], **Amy G. Fensome**[3], **Danielle M. Linton**[4], **Fiona Mathews**[5]*

1 Centre for Ecology and Hydrology, Wallingford, Oxfordshire, United Kingdom, 2 University of Exeter, Exeter, Devon, United Kingdom, 3 Biosciences, College of Life and Environmental Sciences, University of Exeter, Exeter, Devon, United Kingdom, 4 Wildlife Conservation Research Unit, Oxford University, Oxford, Oxfordshire, United Kingdom, 5 Biosciences, University of Exeter, Exeter, Devon, United Kingdom

Abstract

Background: The structuring of wild animal populations can influence population dynamics, disease spread, and information transfer. Social network analysis potentially offers insights into these processes but is rarely, if ever, used to investigate more than one species in a community. We therefore compared the social, temporal and spatial networks of sympatric *Myotis* bats (*M. nattereri* (Natterer's bats) and *M. daubentonii* (Daubenton's bats)), and asked: (1) are there long-lasting social associations within species? (2) do the ranges occupied by roosting social groups overlap within or between species? (3) are *M. daubentonii* bachelor colonies excluded from roosting in areas used by maternity groups?

Results: Using data on 490 ringed *M. nattereri* and 978 *M. daubentonii* from 379 colonies, we found that both species formed stable social groups encompassing multiple colonies. *M. nattereri* formed 11 mixed-sex social groups with few (4.3%) inter-group associations. Approximately half of all *M. nattereri* were associated with the same individuals when recaptured, with many associations being long-term (>100 days). In contrast, *M. daubentonii* were sexually segregated; only a quarter of pairs were associated at recapture after a few days, and inter-sex associations were not long-lasting. Social groups of *M. nattereri* and female *M. daubentonii* had small roost home ranges (mean 0.2 km^2 in each case). Intra specific overlap was low, but inter-specific overlap was high, suggesting territoriality within but not between species. *M. daubentonii* bachelor colonies did not appear to be excluded from roosting areas used by females.

Conclusions: Our data suggest marked species- and sex-specific patterns of disease and information transmission are likely between bats of the same genus despite sharing a common habitat. The clear partitioning of the woodland amongst social groups, and their apparent reliance on small patches of habitat for roosting, means that localised woodland management may be more important to bat conservation than previously recognised.

Editor: Brock Fenton, University of Western Ontario, Canada

Funding: This work is funded by the Natural Environment Research Council Grant no NE/G523571. The funders had no role in study design, data collection and analysis, decision to publish, or preparation of the manuscript.

Competing Interests: The authors have declared that no competing interests exist.

* Email: F.Mathews@exeter.ac.uk

Introduction

Approximately a third of all mammal species are bats, and the majority of these are long-lived and social for at least part of the year. Colonies, which can be mixed or single-sex, commonly contain tens to hundreds of individuals [1,2]. Previous studies of the spatial arrangement of social groups have found that whilst some bat species form social groups occupying exclusive roost home ranges [3,4] others have broadly overlapping roost home ranges [5]. Modern methods of social network analysis (SNA) offer considerable potential for understanding the behaviour of bats, but previous studies have considered only a single species at a single study site [4–11]. To our knowledge, there have been no previous studies on sympatric species, either amongst bats or in other orders, making this the first comparison of social networks between sympatric species within a genus (though see [12] for comparisons of populations without SNA). The present study tests predictions

about the social structure and spatial arrangement of two sympatric species based on their ecology and the potential for intra and inter-specific competition for roosting sites. The spatial distribution of bat social groups is important for wildlife conservation, whilst characterising the structures of social networks is fundamental to understanding disease transmission and information transfer.

Our study species were *M. daubentonii* and *M. nattereri*, sympatric medium sized insectivorous bats weighing 7–15 g and 6–12 g respectively [13]. *M. daubentonii* typically forages over water but frequently roosts in woodlands, whereas *M. nattereri* is a woodland specialist [13]. Both species roost in tree holes and man-made structures close to their foraging sites and form nursery colonies during the summer composed primarily of pregnant and lactating adult females. Nursery colonies form in May-June and split up once the once young are independent in August-September [13]. In this paper we define a 'colony' of bats as an aggregation of individuals at a single location. Both sexes of *M. nattereri* are highly philopatric, returning from hibernation to spend the summer at the site of their birth [14]. In *M. daubentonii*, males are likely to account for most dispersal whilst females are generally philopatric [15]. It has been proposed that summer bachelor colonies of *M. daubentonii* are excluded from areas of high quality foraging habitat by females [16–19]. *M. nattereri* also, though less frequently, form bachelor colonies of up to 28 individuals [20]. Like other *Myotis* bats, both species attend swarming sites, typically cave or mine entrances, from late summer to early autumn. These sites are thought to be important for mating, though mating may also occur at summer roosting sites [15] and hibernaculae [18].

Based on evidence that *M. daubentonii* and *M. nattereri* tend to form female dominated social groups, and that *M. daubentonii* males form separate bachelor roosts [15–18], we expected the species' social networks to reflect this structure. We set out to test the following:

i) Both species will exhibit long lasting intra-sex associations.

ii) The physical space within the wood occupied by roosting social groups will overlap, since tree dwelling bats change roost site frequently and potential roosts are in excess at this study site.

iii) *M. daubentonii* bachelor colonies will occupy roosts further from the highest quality foraging sites (in this case, The River Thames and Farmoor Reservoir) due to competitive exclusion by female maternity groups from roost sites closest to foraging areas [16–18].

Materials and Methods

Fieldwork

Bats were captured and ringed between May and mid-October annually, from 2006 to 2010, at Wytham Woods, Oxfordshire, UK (Latitude: 51.7743, Longitude: −1.3379). This 415 hectare site is composed of semi-natural ancient deciduous woodland and 18th–20th century plantations. Over 1150 woodcrete bird boxes of very similar design are dispersed through the woods, many of these are occupied by blue tits (*Parus caeruleus*) and great tits (*Parus major*) until chicks fledge in the second half of May. After this time the boxes are not used by birds but are frequently used by bats up until mid-October, after which the bats migrate to unknown hibernation sites. To minimise disturbance, boxes were not checked more than once within a two week period and females with attached young were not handled. Areas with higher occupancy rates (*pers. obs.*) were sampled more frequently to maximise data collection (Figure S1). Bats were ringed with 2.9 mm aluminium armbands bearing a unique identification number. The individuals were classed juvenile if the joints between the metacarpals and phalanx were not fully ossified [21,22].

Ethical considerations

All methods were approved by the University of Exeter Biosciences Ethical Review Committee and by the University of Oxford Ethics Committee and conducted in accordance with Oxford University's Local Ethical Review Procedures, overseen by the Zoology Department Local Ethical Review Committee. The work and was conducted under permit to conduct research within Wytham Woods. Rings were supplied by The Mammal Society, UK and were applied under Natural England licence no. 20113601 and previous licences.

Social network analysis

A social interaction, or 'association', was considered to exist between two individuals if they were found roosting together. Our analyses made no assumptions about the direction of association, as this would require identification of which individuals initiated and which received the behaviour. The link between a pair is therefore scored once in the data we present (ie. the link A-B is not considered separately from B-A). Since the sample size of this study was limited due to the practicality of fieldwork, associations were assumed to be binary and were not given weighting [9].

Structural analysis

Construction of the association matrix was undertaken in SocProg [23]. Visualisation of the networks was undertaken using Netdraw v.2 [24] - individual bats are represented by nodes and an association between two individuals is represented by a line connecting them. Individuals captured only once (Table 1) were excluded from the analysis, and individuals captured more than once but which had no associations (n = 10) were also removed.

Individuals were assigned to social groups using the Girvan-Newman method, which is particularly appropriate for populations with a strong social structure such as those studied here [25]. This top-down method, successively removes the association with the highest value of 'betweenness'. Betweenness is the number of shortest paths, connecting individuals in the network, which contain a given association. Associations with high values of betweenness are those that connect clusters with otherwise low interconnectivity and by removing them the network is broken down into an increasing number of unconnected components. Each time a new component is created the modularity of the network is calculated [26]. Modularity is derived from all associations from the original network and is the difference between the observed fraction of associations that are within components and the fraction expected if associations connected individuals at random. Modularity ranges from 0 to 1, with values over 0.3 regarded as evidence of social structure [26]. The division of individuals to components that produce the highest modularity value is selected as the best representation of social groups.

Evidence of assortment by sex within social networks was examined using join-count in UCINET [27] using 10,000 iterations. This test compares the number of male-male, female-female and intersex associations in the dataset with the number that would be expected by chance. Degree centrality was used to test the hypothesis that females were more central in the networks than males. Degree centrality is the simplest of the centrality measures and is calculated for each individual as the number of connections to other individuals in the network. Since individuals in a network are not independent, the significance of differences in degree centrality was calculated using permutation tests implemented in UCINET [27].

Spatial Analysis

Roost home ranges of social groups were estimated using 100% minimum convex polygons (MCPs) after the removal of roosts used by single bats (*M. daubentonii* = 42; *M. nattereri* = 27) and those isolated by over 1 km (*M. daubentonii* = 1; *M. nattereri* = 2) using ArcMap (ESRI v. 10.1, 2010) and Quantum GIS [28]. MCPs were created and cropped so that habitats such as grassland, which do not provide roosting opportunities, were removed.

Radio-tracking was undertaken in August 2009 and 2010 to compare roost home range estimates produced from the SNA to the roost use of individual bats. Three adult female *M. daubentonii*, known to have been present at the site for at least

Table 1. Frequency distribution of captured bats by species and sex.

Species	Sex	Number of times captured											% caught> once
		1	2	3	4	5	6	7	8	9	10	Total	
M. daubentonii	M	430	118	59	14	7	0	1	0	0	0	629	0.32
	F	204	55	33	27	13	11	4	0	2	0	349	0.42
	All	634	173	92	41	20	11	5	0	2	0	978	0.35
M nattereri	M	97	43	18	12	9	2	0	1	0	0	182	0.47
	F	101	71	42	40	25	14	8	7	4	3	315	0.68
	All	198	114	60	52	34	16	8	8	4	3	497	0.60

two consecutive summers (one parous but not breeding in the current season, and 2 post-lactation), and one juvenile female were fitted with radio transmitters weighing 0.35 g or 0.42 g (Holohil, Canada, type LB-2N). All tags weighed less than 5% of the body weight of the bat (4.1–4.7%) and were attached by a licensed bat worker using a previously described method [29]. Bats were located at their day roosts using an Australis receiver (Titley Electronics Ltd, Australia) and aYagi 3-element directional antennae (Biotrack Ltd, Wareham, UK). Tree roost locations were recorded by GPS and mapped using ArcMap (ESRI, USA).

Temporal analysis

The temporal structure of associations was examined using the lagged association rate [10,30]. This gives the probability that, after being found together, two individuals will be found together at a set time interval in the future. These trends were calculated for each of the four classes of association within each species (male-male, female-female, male-female and female-male) and compared to the expected trend if individuals were to associate randomly – the null association rate. Because individuals are included in the analysis only up until the point where they are last observed, emigration (or mortality) does not influence the values, except in the case of long-term migrations where an individual, having left the population subsequently returns to roost with the same companion. Standard errors were calculated for these trends by jack-knifing the data over a period of 30 days. We note that the error estimates produced using this method have previously been found to be too small, but the method allows for a more reliable interpretation of the data than other available techniques. We therefore recommend that the conclusions should be tested with more data [31].

Statistical analysis

All statistical analyses were undertaken in R version 2.11.0 [32]. The association between social group's roost home range size and the number of individuals in the social group, species and sampling effort was examined using multiple linear regression. Sampling effort was calculated as the average number of recaptures per individuals for each social group.

Results

Over 5 consecutive summers we performed 7578 box checks, finding bats on 627 occasions. Bats used numerous different boxes, but at any one time, only a minority were occupied, indicating an excess of potential roosting locations. For example, in 2010, bat droppings were found in 751 of 2279 box checks (33%), but only 146 (3%) had bats present. The two target bat species were never found in the same roost simultaneously, however, 27 roosts (of 293) were used by both species at different times (Figure S2). This is not significantly different from the number of boxes we would expect the species to share if they were randomly selecting empty roosts within the woods ($\chi2 = 0.48$, df = 1, p = 0.49).

A total of 490 *M. nattereri* and 978 *M. daubentonii* were ringed from 379 colonies. Of these, 643 bats were caught more than once, with the mean recapture frequency being 3.6 (range 2–10) for *M. nattereri* (n = 299) and 2.9 for *M. daubentonii* (range 2–9, n = 344)) (Table 1). *M. nattereri* colony size ranged from 2 to 35 individuals (median 7, n = 59), while *M. daubentonii* colonies ranged in size from 2 to 26 (median 10, n = 84). Due to limited opportunities for sampling during the nursery period, and the restrictions this placed on sample size, it was not possible to analyse the social structure separately for each year of the study. All data were therefore combined for SNA, and the nursery and post-nursery periods were considered together. While this approach means we are unable to examine the change in social structure between seasons and years it increases our confidence in results that show social isolation. If 2 social groups are found to have never associated when using 5 years data, we believe this is strong evidence that they do not socialise. The proportion of males captured in the adult population was 0.28 for *M. nattereri* and 0.62 for *M. daubentonii* (Table 1), whereas there was no sex ratio bias for juveniles (0.55 for *M. nattereri* and 0.54 for *M. daubentonii*). Given the relatively low sample size for juveniles (n = 77 *M. nattereri*; n = 98 *M. daubentonii*), we combined data for adults and juveniles in subsequent analyses.

Social structure of bat populations

For both species, female-female associations were significantly more frequent, and intersex associations significantly less frequent, than would be expected by chance (10,000 iterations, $p < 0.001$). Male-male associations were significantly more frequent in *M. daubentonii* (10,000 iterations, $p = 0.023$) and less frequent in *M. nattereri* (10,000 iterations, $p < 0.001$) than expected by chance. In both species, females had higher degree centrality than males (one-tailed t-test, 10,000 permutations, $p < 0.001$).

M. nattereri formed 11 social groups (Figure 1a) with 6 unconnected components. Despite evidence of assortment by sex, *M. nattereri* social groups were composed of a mix of males and females suggestive of a single social group with females at the core. Inter-group associations by either sex were rare, making up only 4.3% of all associations (n = 4258).

M. daubentonii also formed discrete social groups, with half of these containing more than 90% males (Figure 1b). This sexual segregation was apparent even when the analysis considered only males recaptured in two or three years, thereby removing 'transient males' who may only have been at the study site briefly. Consequently male and female *M. daubentonii* social networks were analysed separately. Individuals in the female network were assigned to 5 social groups (Figure 1c), with inter-group associations making up only 2.1% of all associations (n = 1091) (22 intergroup associations compared to 1069 intragroup associations). Males were assigned to 10 social groups (Figure 1d), however unlike the female *M. daubentonii* networks (and the *M. nattereri* network), there was a significant number of inter-group associations (15.4%, n = 1205, Figure 1d). This interconnectivity suggests that social group membership of *M. daubentonii* males is less specific than for the other networks. This, together with the relatively small sample size, precluded sensible assessment of the spatial organisation of male *M. daubentonii*.

Spatial distribution of social groups

Social groups showed roost site fidelity, each restricted to a sub-section of the woodland (Figure 2a and b). The four social groups for which 3 or fewer roosts were known (Figure 2a) were excluded from further consideration as accurate roost home range estimations were not possible. The mean minimum roost home range estimates were 0.16 km^2 (n = 4, range 0.09–0.30 km^2) for female *M. daubentonii* and 0.15 km^2 (n = 7, range 0.02–0.32 km^2) for *M. nattereri*. There was little spatial overlap between the estimated roost home ranges within species (female *M. daubentonii* = 5.9%, *M. nattereri* = 9.4%), and no area was shared by more than 2 social groups (Figure 2a and b). Between species however, there was significant overlap; 32% of the total area covered by both species was shared. Roost home range estimates were positively correlated to the number of individuals assigned to a social group (F = 6.62, df = 1, P = 0.03) but were not linked with sampling effort (F = 0.05, df = 1, P = 0.82) or species (F = 0.66,

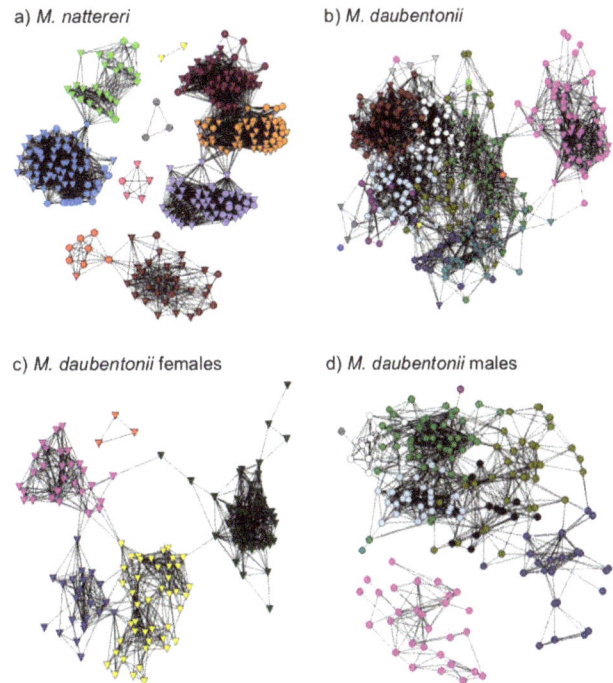

Figure 1. Social network visualisation a) male and female *M. nattereri*, b) male and female *M. daubentonii*, c) female *M. daubentonii*, and d) male *M. daubentonii*. a) *M. nattereri* male (n = 85) and female (n = 214), modularity = 0.74, b) *M. daubentonii* (n = 344), modularity = 0.66, c) female *M. daubentonii* (n = 145), modularity = 0.67, d) male *M. daubentonii* (n = 199), modularity = 0.64. Nodes represent individual bats (males, circles; females, triangles) and associations are represented by the lines that join them. Colours indicate the assignment of individuals to social groups using the Girvan-Newman algorithm. Colours do not correspond between panels. Colours in a) and c) are comparable to Figure 3. The position of individuals within these networks indicates their position in social space and is not an indication of an individual's geographical location.
doi:10.1371/journal.pone.0112225.g001

df = 1, P = 0.44). The spatial distribution of social groups did not reflect our sampling regime, and areas surveyed in a single day frequently contained more than one social group (an example of daily sampling is shown in Figure S1).

The roosting sites of four female *M. daubentonii*, two from each of two different social groups, were identified using daytime positioning for 51 tag-days (10–15 days per bat). These individuals were located in boxes on 29% of tag-days (range, 20–55%), and in natural tree roosts on all other occasions. The tracked bats changed roosts on average every 2 days (range, 1.1–3.5) and were located inside the roost home range of their group on 75% of occasions (range, 30–71%; Figure 2b). Of those roost locations that were outside the minimum roost home range, 28% were within 15 m and 42% were within 100 m of their range. On no occasion was a radio-tracked individual located in the known roost home range of another *M. daubentonii* social group, despite several other potential ranges lying within easy flight distance. *M. daubentonii* bachelor colonies observed during the nursery period were frequently found within the estimated roost home ranges of female social groups and of these, 5 bachelor colonies were identified in roost locations previously used by nursery colonies (Figure S3).

a) *M. nattereri*

Bird boxes

Woodland area

Boxes used by 2 or more bats

Boxes used by a single bat

Roost used by two social groups

Estimated female roost ranges

Radio-tracking fixes

N

0   250   500   750   1000 Metres

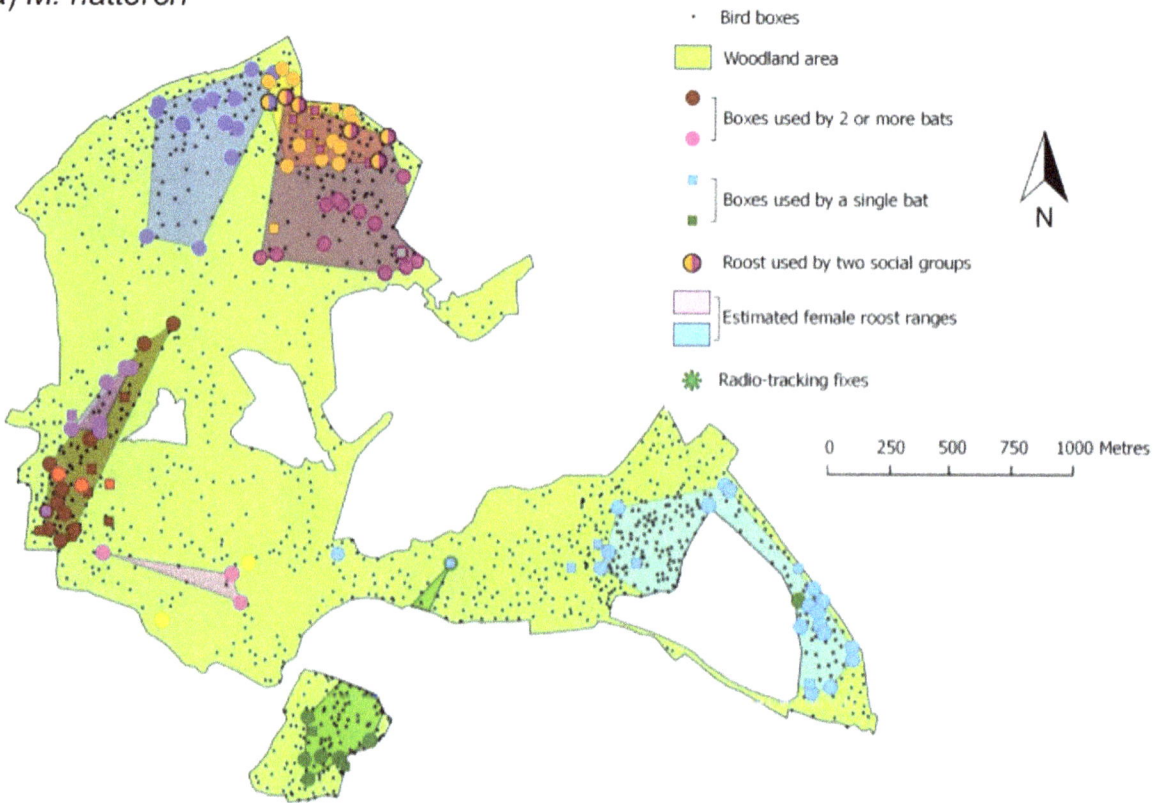

b) *M. daubentonii* females

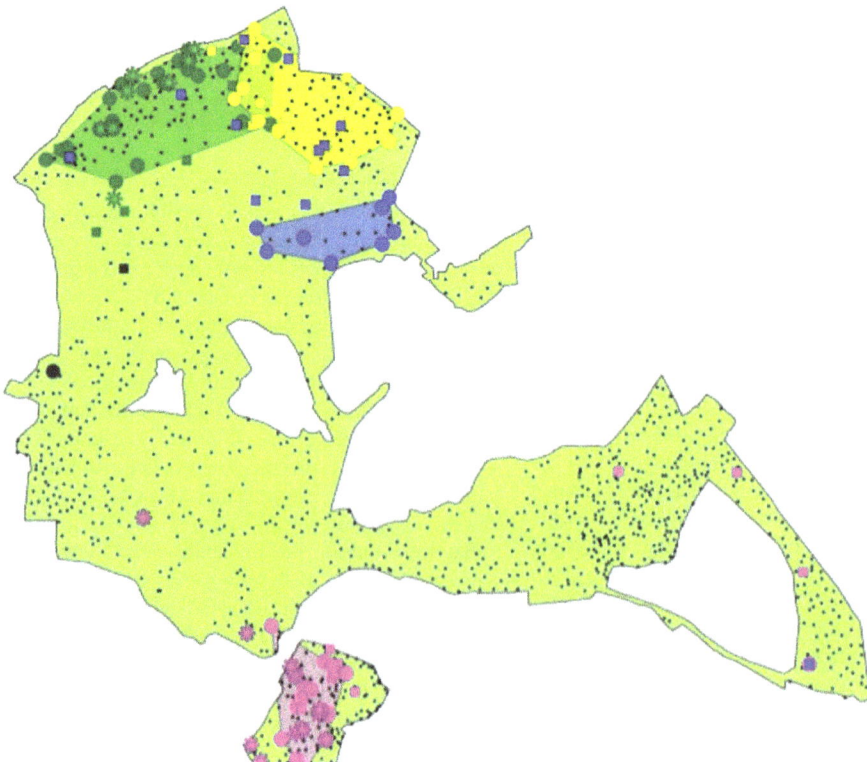

Figure 2. Distribution of a) *M. nattereri* **both sexes and b) female** *M. daubentonii* **social groups in Wytham Woods.** Roosts used by bats, and home range estimates are coloured according to social group - colours are comparable to Figure 2, panels a) and c) – symbols indicate colony size and roosts identified by radio-tracking. Roost home ranges are estimated using 100% minimum convex polygons (MCPs). MCPs exclude roosts occupied by a single individual (*M. nattereri*, n = 42; *M. daubentonii*, n = 44) or separated by over 1 km from a roost of the same social group (n = 1 for each species). Four adult female *M. daubentonii* were radio-tracked; two from each of two social groups. The daytime roosts (including trees) used by these individuals are indicated by asterisks and are coloured according to the social group to which they belonged.

Duration of association between individuals

Associations within and between sexes differed in their stability over time. This was true for both species (Figure 3). Up until approximately 400 days, all classes of *M. nattereri* association showed similar lagged association rates (Figure 3). Approximately half of associating pairs of *M. nattereri* were found associating after a few days, dropping by 100 days to 35–45% (range encompasses means, by sex, of the probability of a bat being found in future with the same individual i.e. M-M, M-F, F-M and F-F). There was then a gradual decline across all classes of association until about 400–500 days, suggestive of the breakdown of casual acquaintances. Beyond this point data were lacking for male-male and male-female associations; however female-male associations showed a continued decline suggestive of further breakdown of casual acquaintances, while female-female associations stabilised. These results suggest that *M. nattereri* have casual relationships lasting up to 400 days with some constant companionship between females beyond this. Overall there was some suggestion that the lagged association rates of same-sex associations were higher than those between sexes (Figure 3). Lagged association rates for all classes stayed above the null association rate for all time intervals, indicating the presence of preferred associations both within and between sexes.

Different trends are observed in the temporal structure of *M. daubentonii* associations (Figure 3): only a quarter of the associating pairs were found associating after a few days. After this point, same-sex associations approximated those seen for female-female *M. nattereri* after 500 days, indicating that stable long-term companionships exist. By contrast, between-sex associations showed a decline in lagged association rate following the first few days, plateauing at 100 days for male-female associations and 300 days for female-male associations (Figure 3). After these time points there was little difference between the observed level of association and that expected from a random network (null association rate) suggesting that between-sex associations amongst *M. daubentonii* represent casual acquaintances that last no longer than a year. Association rates for both species are below 50%, even at short time periods, indicating that most bats do not roost with the same individuals every day.

Discussion

This study identified multiple social groups in both *M. nattereri* and *M. daubentonii* populations within a continuous landscape in which roosts are not limiting. The social groups formed by *M. daubentonii* females and *M. nattereri* of both sexes show few inter-group interactions and little overlap between roost home ranges (Figure 1a, c and Figure 2a, b).

Social structure

As expected from work on other species [11], both *M. nattereri* and *M. daubentonii* formed multiple social groups centred on females. Almost all male *M. nattereri* also associated with only one social group, and male-male associations were less common than expected by chance.

Analysis of the temporal structure of associations support our prediction that intra-sex associations would be long lived. For both *M. nattereri* and *M. daubentonii* we observed enduring female to female and male to male associations. In each case, we found evidence of associations lasting more than one year, meaning that the individuals reformed their associations after prolonged absence from summer roosts during the hibernation period, as has previously been reported in *M. bechsteinii* [33]. Inter-sex associations amongst *M. daubentonii* were found to be short lived, but amongst *M. nattereri*, associations between sexes were seen to last more than a year. In both cases, this difference is likely to be the result of the dispersal behaviour of males, since male *M. nattereri* are thought to be philopatric [14] while a proportion of male *M. daubentonii* are thought to disperse [15].

Spatial structure

Wytham Woods contains an excess of roost sites, most of which are empty on any given day. We therefore predicted that intra-specific social group home ranges would overlap since competition for roosts is likely to be low. We found high levels of overlap in the roost home ranges of different species, but very little overlap in the roost home ranges of social groups within a species. One potential hypothesis to explain the lack of intra-specific overlap is that social groups are defending foraging resources. *M. nattereri* forage within woodland and it is possible that they are defending patches of woodland from other *M. nattereri* groups whilst *M. daubentonii*, which preferentially forage over water, might defend areas of woodland that give them easiest access to their prime foraging habitats. This could be tested by observing the foraging of individuals from known social groups using radio-tracking.

Previous studies suggest that *M. daubentonii* bachelor colonies are excluded from roosting in areas of high quality foraging habitat by females [15]. We therefore predicted that areas of the study site close to high quality foraging sites (The River Thames and Farmoor Reservoir) would host female colonies but not bachelor colonies. However, while female social groups were indeed found close to these foraging habitats, males were frequently found within the predicted roost home range of female social groups (Figure S3). The domination of territories by females may therefore be dependent on habitat quality, with males being tolerated where resources are abundant as may be the case at our study site. Alternatively there may be sexual segregation of foraging activity outside the woodland.

Broader implications

The results of this study have implications for bat conservation, disease dynamics, and the transfer of information through the population. Roost home range estimates were very small for both species (0.1–0.3 km^2 for *M. daubentonii* and 0.02–0.3 km^2 for *M. nattereri*). In addition, roosts identified by radio-tracking were close to, or within, the calculated roost home range. Thus, despite switching roosting locations frequently, woodland bat social groups rely on a network of roosts within a constrained geographical area. Small scale habitat changes, such as the felling of wood for timber, may therefore have a greater impact than previously suspected. Studies of *Chalinolobus tuberculatus*, a threatened New Zealand

M. daubentonii   M. nattereri

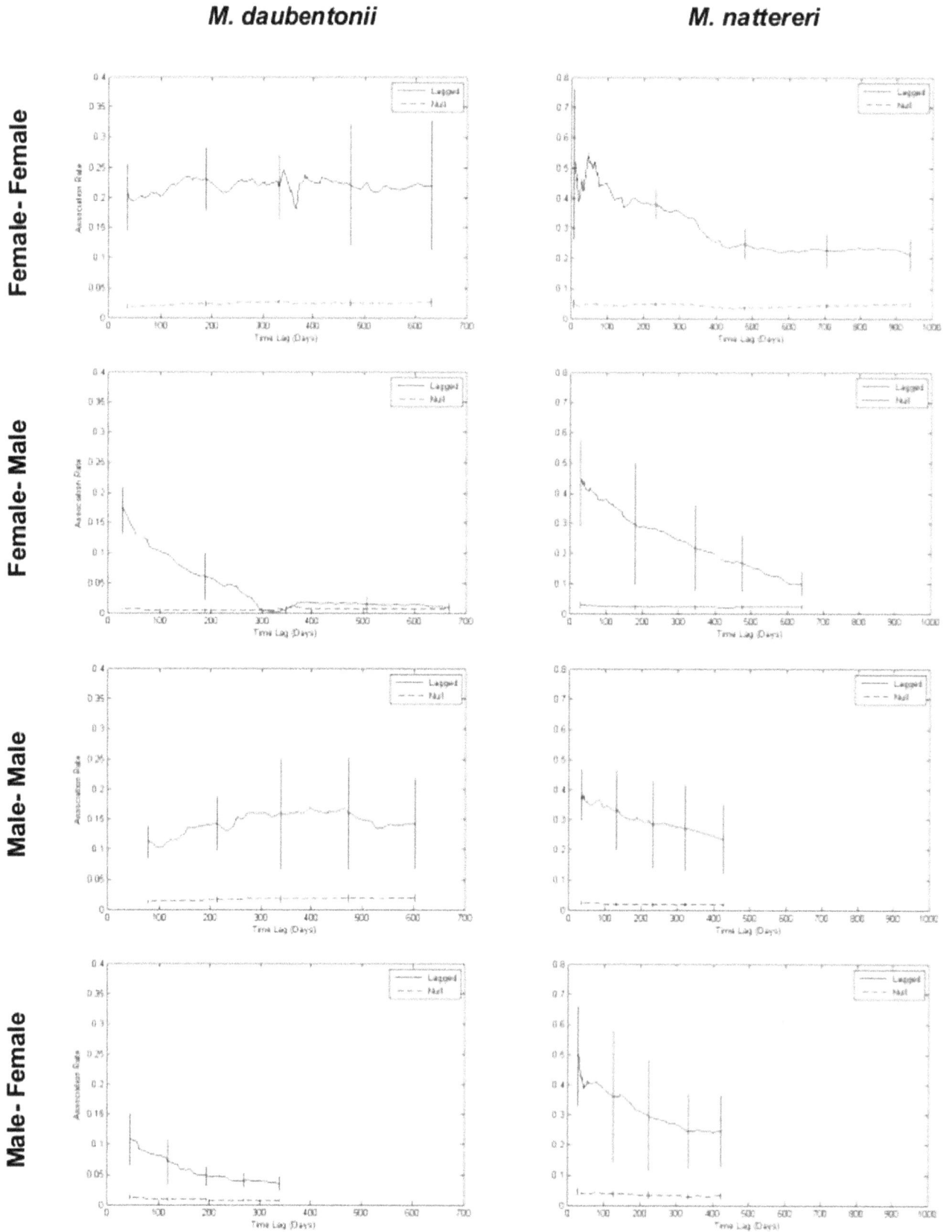

Figure 3. Lagged association rates within and between sexes of *M. daubentonii* **(left) and** *M. nattereri* **(right).** Standard error is calculated by jackknifing over a 30-day period.

bat species, have shown that their social groups have similarly restricted roost home ranges [3]. Within the year following tree felling, individuals in the area had smaller roosting home ranges and used fewer roosts than individuals in areas away from felling [34]. A substantial reduction in available roosting habitat within a social group's roost home range may also increase competition between social groups. It is therefore critical that the needs and locations of social groups are considered when undertaking alterations to woodlands with important bat populations.

The social structures we have identified suggest that pathogens are likely to spread rapidly within social groups of *M. nattereri* but slowly between them. For *M. daubentonii*, similar patterns would be expected for females, whilst in males, spread would also be rapid between groups (15.4% of all interactions were between-group). Such heterogeneity in transmission risk is commonly omitted from models of disease epidemiology, but the inadequacy of traditional random-mixing or frequency-dependent based models in describing many diseases is becoming increasingly apparent [35]. Bats are frequently the focus of infectious disease research: a number of recent outbreaks of highly infectious pathogens are thought to have their origins in wild bat populations [36–39], and bats are the ancestral host for some viruses that now infect a range of animals including humans [40]. Since males are primarily responsible for connectivity between female groups of *M. daubentonii* we hypothesise that they are likely to have a high probability of infection, and play an important role in disease transmission, as would be predicted by theoretical models [41]. However, this prediction needs to be tested empirically. In a well-characterised population of meerkats (*Suricata suricatta*), roving males had an increased risk of infection with TB (*Mycobacterium bovis*) but the groups visited were not found to be at increased risk of infection [42]. Not only is the social organisation of wild animals important to disease transmission, it is also likely to affect the transfer of information fundamental for individual and population

survival. We suggest that identifying the cryptic patterns of social structure and spacing in bats is an important step towards improved management and conservation.

Supporting Information

Figure S1   Distribution of sampling effort. Points show bird boxes (potential bat roosts). Three polygons show examples of the typical area of boxes checked in a day.

Figure S2   Spatial distribution of roosts. *M. nattereri* (red) and *M. daubentonii* (blue) and both species (white). Both species have been found in a large number of roosts though occupy few on any given day, suggesting that roosts are not limiting at this site.

Figure S3   Distribution of *M. daubentonii* bachelor colonies (defined as >90% male) observed during the nursery period compared to the MCPs of female social groups.

Acknowledgments

We thank B Sheldon and others at the Edward Grey Institute, Oxford University, for bird box location data. We also thank M Taylor for woodland boundary data, S Laurence and M Ryan for assistance with radio-tracking, and R Broughton and C Garroway for comments. The data on which this study is based are available on request from the authors and the Open Research Exeter repository (https://ore.exeter.ac.uk/repository/).

Author Contributions

Conceived and designed the experiments: FM TA MN. Performed the experiments: TA DL. Analyzed the data: TA AF. Contributed reagents/materials/analysis tools: TA FM. Wrote the paper: TA FM MN AF DL.

References

1. Altringham JD (1996) Bats Biology and Behaviour. Oxford: Oxford University Press.
2. Kunz TH, Fenton MB (2003) Bat Ecology. Chicago: The University of Chicago Press.
3. O'Donnell CFJ (2000) Cryptic local populations in a temperate rainforest bat *Chalinolobus tuberculatus* in New Zealand. Anim Conserv 3: 287–297.
4. Fortuna MA, Popa-Lisseanu AG, Ibáñez C, Bascompte J (2009) The roosting spatial network of a bird-predator bat. Ecology 90: 934–944.
5. Johnson JB, Mark Ford W, Edwards JW (2012) Roost networks of northern myotis (*Myotis septentrionalis*) in a managed landscape. For Ecol Manage 266: 223–231.
6. Garroway CJ, Broders HG (2007) Nonrandom association patterns at northern long-eared bat maternity roosts. Can J Zool 85: 956–964.
7. Patriquin KJ, Leonard ML, Broders HG, Garroway CJ (2010) Do social networks of female northern long-eared bats vary with reproductive period and age? Behav Ecol Sociobiol 64: 899–913.
8. Kerth G, Perony N, Schweitzer F (2011) Bats are able to maintain long-term social relationships despite the high fission-fusion dynamics of their groups. Proc Biol Sci 278: 2761–2767.
9. Chaverri G (2010) Comparative social network analysis in a leaf-roosting bat. Behav Ecol Sociobiol 64: 1619–1630.
10. Vonhof MJ, Whitehead H, Fenton MB (2004) Analysis of Spix's disc-winged bat association patterns and roosting home ranges reveal a novel social structure among bats. Anim Behav 68: 507–521.
11. Johnson JS, Kropczynski JN, Lacki MJ, Langlois GD (2012) Social networks of Rafinesque's big-eared bats (*Corynorhinus rafinesquii*) in bottomland hardwood forests. J Mammal 93: 1545–1558.
12. Park KJ, Masters E, Altringham JD (1998) Social structure of three sympatric bat species (Vespertilionidae). J Zool 244: 379–389.
13. Altringham JD (2003) British Bats. London: HarperCollins.
14. Rivers NM, Butlin RK, Altringham JD (2006) Autumn swarming behaviour of Natterer's bats in the UK: Population size, catchment area and dispersal. Biol Conserv 127: 215–226.
15. Senior P, Butlin RK, Altringham JD (2005) Sex and segregation in temperate bats. Proc Biol Sci 272: 2467–2473.
16. Encarnacao JA, Kierdorf U, Holweg D, Jasnoch U, Wolters V (2005) Sex-related differences in roost-site selection by Daubenton's bats *Myotis daubentonii* during the nursery period. Mamm Rev 35: 285–294.
17. Dietz M, Encarnação JA, Kalko EKV (2006) Small scale distribution patterns of female and male Daubenton's bats (*Myotis daubentonii*). Acta Chiropt 8: 403–415.
18. Angell RL, Butlin RK, Altringham JD (2013) Sexual segregation and flexible mating patterns in temperate bats. PLoS One 8: e54194.
19. Russo D (2002) Elevation affects the distribution of the two sexes in Daubenton's bats *Myotis daubentonii* (Chiroptera: *Vespertilionidae*) from Italy. Mammalia: 543–551.
20. Swift M (1997) Roosting and foraging behaviour of Natterer's bats (*Myotis nattereri*) close to the northern border of their distribution. J Zool: 375–384.
21. Racey PA (1974) Ageing and assessment of reproductive status of Pipistrelle bats, *Pipistrellus pipistrellus*. J Zool 173: 264–271.
22. Mitchell-Jones AJ, Mcleish AP (2004) Bat Worker's Manual. 3rd ed. Peterborough: Joint Nature Conservation Committee.
23. Whitehead H (2009) SOCPROG programs: analyzing animal social structures. Behav Ecol Sociobiol 63: 765–778.
24. Borgatti SP (2002) NetDraw: Graph Visualisation Software. Harvard Analytic Technologies.
25. Girvan M, Newman MEJ (2002) Community structure in social and biological networks. Proc Natl Acad Sci U S A 99: 7821–7826.
26. Newman M, Girvan M (2004) Finding and evaluating community structure in networks. Phys Rev E 69: 026113.
27. Borgatti SP, Everett MG, Freeman LC (2002) Ucinet 6 for Windows: Software for Social Network Analysis.
28. Quantum Geographic Development Team (2013) Quantum GIS Geographic Information System.
29. Kelly A, Goodwin S, Grogan A, Mathews F (2008) Post-release survival of hand-reared pipistrelle bats (*Pipistrellus spp*). Anim Welf 14: 375–382.
30. Whitehead H (2008) Analyzing animals societies. Chicago: The University of Chicago Press.
31. Whitehead H (2007) Selection of Models of Lagged Identification Rates and Lagged Association Rates Using AIC and QAIC. Commun Stat - Simul Comput 36: 1233–1246.

32. R Core Development Team (2011) R: A language and environment for statistical computing. R Foundation for Statistical Computing, Vienna, Austria. ISBN 3-900051-07-0. Available: http://www.R-project.org/.

33. Kerth G, Konig B (1999) Fission, fusion and nonrandom associations in female Bechstein's bats (*Myotis bechsteinii*). Behaviour 136: 1187–1202.

34. Borkin KM, O'Donnell C, Parsons S (2011) Bat colony size reduction coincides with clear-fell harvest operations and high rates of roost loss in plantation forest. Biodivers Conserv 20: 3537–3548.

35. Weber N, Carter SP, Dall SRX, Delahay RJ, McDonald JL, et al. (2013) Badger social networks correlate with tuberculosis infection. Curr Biol 23: R915-6.

36. Calisher CH, Childs JE, Field HE, Holmes KV, Schountz T (2006) Bats: important reservoir hosts of emerging viruses. Clin Microbiol Rev 19: 531–545.

37. Shi Z (2013) Emerging infectious diseases associated with bat viruses. Sci China Life Sci 56: 678–682.

38. Drexler JF, Corman VM, Wegner T, Tateno AF, Zerbinati RM, et al. (2011) Amplification of emerging viruses in a bat colony. Emerg Infect Dis 17: 449–456.

39. Kruse H, Kirkemo AM, Handeland K (2004) Wildlife as source of zoonotic infections. Emerg Infect Dis 10: 2067–2072.

40. Quan P, Firth C, Conte JM, Williams SH, Zambrana-torrelio CM (2013) Bats are a major natural reservoir for hepaciviruses and pegiviruses. Proc Natl Acad Sci USA 110: 8194–8199.

41. Miller MR, White A, Wilson K, Boots M (2007) The population dynamical implications of male-biased parasitism in different mating systems. PLoS One 2: e624.

42. Drewe JA (2010) Who infects whom? Social networks and tuberculosis transmission in wild meerkats. Proc Biol Sci 277: 633–642.

Permissions

List of Contributors

Tariq Halasa, Anette Boklund and Claes Enøe
Section of Epidemiology, The National Veterinary Institutes, Technical University of Denmark, Copenhagen, Denmark

Anders Stockmarr
Section of Epidemiology, The National Veterinary Institutes, Technical University of Denmark, Copenhagen, Denmark
Department of Applied Mathematics and Computer Science, Technical University of Denmark, Lyngby, Denmark

Lasse E. Christiansen
Department of Applied Mathematics and Computer Science, Technical University of Denmark, Lyngby, Denmark

Jean-Paul Chretien and Rohit A. Chitale
Division of Integrated Biosurveillance, Armed Forces Health Surveillance Center, Silver Spring, Maryland, United States of America

Dylan George
Division of Analytic Decision Support, Biomedical Advanced Research and Development Authority, Department of Health and Human Services, Washington, DC, United States of America

Jeffrey Shaman
Department of Environmental Health Sciences, Mailman School of Public Health, Columbia University, New York, New York, United States of America

F. Ellis McKenzie
Fogarty International Center, National Institutes of Health, Bethesda, Maryland, United States of America

Keren Cox-Witton, Rupert Woods and Victoria Grillo
Australian Wildlife Health Network, Mosman, New South Wales, Australia

Martin Phillips and Andrea Reiss
Zoo and Aquarium Association Australasia, Mosman, New South Wales, Australia

Rupert T. Baker
Healesville Sanctuary, Zoos Victoria, Healesville, Victoria, Australia

David J. Blyde
Sea World, Gold Coast, Queensland, Australia

Wayne Boardman and Ian Smith
Adelaide Zoo, Zoos South Australia, Adelaide, South Australia, Australia

Dion Wedd and Stephen Cutter
Territory Wildlife Park, Berry Springs, Northern Territory, Australia

Claude Lacasse
Australia Zoo Wildlife Hospital, Beerwah, Queensland, Australia

Helen McCracken
Melbourne Zoo, Zoos Victoria, Parkville, Victoria, Australia

Michael Pyne
Currumbin Wildlife Sanctuary, Currumbin, Queensland, Australia

Simone Vitali
Perth Zoo, South Perth, Western Australia, Australia

Larry Vogelnest
Taronga Zoo, Taronga Conservation Society Australia, Mosman, New South Wales, Australia

Chris Bunn and Lyndel Post
Australian Government Department of Agriculture, Canberra, Australian Capital Territory, Australia

M. Carolyn Gates and Mark E. J. Woolhouse
Epidemiology Group, Centre for Immunity, Infection and Evolution, School of Biological Sciences, University of Edinburgh, Ashworth Laboratories, Edinburgh, Scotland, United Kingdom

Shirley Abelman
School of Computational and Applied Mathematics, University of the Witwatersrand, Johannesburg, South Africa

Sansao A. Pedro
School of Computational and Applied Mathematics, University of the Witwatersrand, Johannesburg, South Africa
Modelling, International Center of Insect Physiology and Ecology, Nairobi, Kenya
Human Health, International Center of Insect Physiology and Ecology, Nairobi, Kenya
Departmento de Matemática e Informática, Universidade Eduardo Mondlane, Maputo, Mozambique

Henri E. Z. Tonnang
Modelling, International Center of Insect Physiology and Ecology, Nairobi, Kenya

Rosemary Sang
Human Health, International Center of Insect Physiology and Ecology, Nairobi, Kenya

Frank T. Ndjomatchoua
Modelling, International Center of Insect Physiology and Ecology, Nairobi, Kenya
Departement de Physique, Universite de Yaoundé I, Yaoundé , Cameroun

Shankar P. Mondal and Mat Yamage
Food and Agriculture Organization of the United Nations, Dhaka, Bangladesh

Christopher D. Hudson, Jonathan N. Huxley and Martin J. Green
School of Veterinary Medicine and Science, University of Nottingham, Sutton Bonington Campus, Sutton Bonington, Leicestershire, United Kingdom

Smaragda Tsairidou, John A. Woolliams, Mairead L. Bermingham, Ricardo Pong-Wong, Oswald Matika, Elizabeth J. Glass and Stephen C. Bishop
The Roslin Institute and RDVS, University of Edinburgh, Midlothian, United Kingdom

Adrian R. Allen, Robin A. Skuce, Stanley W. J. McDowell and Stewart H. McBride
Agri-Food and Biosciences Institute, Belfast, United Kingdom

David M. Wright
School of Biological Sciences, Queen's University of Belfast, Belfast, United Kingdom

Clement N. Mweya
National Institute for Medical Research, Tukuyu, Tanzania
Department of Veterinary Medicine and Public Health, Sokoine University of Agriculture, Morogoro, Tanzania

Niels Holst
Department of Agroecology, Aarhus University, Slagelse, Denmark

Leonard E. G. Mboera
National Institute for Medical Research, Dar es salaam, Tanzania

Sharadhuli I. Kimera
Department of Veterinary Medicine and Public Health, Sokoine University of Agriculture, Morogoro, Tanzania

Ryan A. Waters, Veronica L. Fowler, Bryony Armson, David J. Paton and Donald P. King
Livestock Viral Disease Program, The Pirbright Institute, Pirbright, Guildford, Surrey, United Kingdom

Noel Nelson and John Gloster
Atmospheric Dispersion and Air Quality, The Meteorological Office, Exeter, United Kingdom

Charlotte Carne, Stuart Semple and Julia Lehmann
Centre for Research in Evolutionary and Environmental Anthropology, University of Roehampton, London, United Kingdom

Helen Morrogh-Bernard
The Orang-utan Tropical Peatland Project, Centre for International Cooperation in Sustainable Management of Tropical Peatland, Universitas Palangka Raya, Palangka Raya, Central Kalimantan, Indonesia
Centre for Research in Animal Behaviour, College of Life and Environmental Sciences, University of Exeter, Exeter, United Kingdom

Klaus Zuberbühler
School of Psychology and Neuroscience, University of St Andrews, St Andrews, Fife, United Kingdom
Cognitive Science Centre, University of Neuchâtel, Neuchâtel, Switzerland
Cassidy Logan Rist, Carmen Sofia Arriola and Carol Rubin
Centers for Disease Control and Prevention, Atlanta, Georgia, United States of America

Juan Zhang
School of Mechatronic Engineering, North University of China, Taiyuan, Shan'xi, People's Republic of China
Complex Systems Research Center, Shanxi University, Taiyuan, Shańxi, People's Republic of China

Mingtao Li and Zhen Jin
Complex Systems Research Center, Shanxi University, Taiyuan, Shańxi, People's Republic of China

Gui-Quan Sun
Complex Systems Research Center, Shanxi University, Taiyuan, Shańxi, People's Republic of China
School of Mathematical Science, Fudan University, Shanghai, People's Republic of China

Baoxu Huang and Xiang-Dong Sun
The Laboratory of Animal Epidemiological Surveillance, China Animal Health & Epidemiology Center, Qingdao, Shandong, People's Republic of China

Qiang Hou
Department of Mathematics, North University of China, Taiyuan, Shańxi, People's Republic of China

Haiyan Wang
School of Mathematical & Natural Sciences, Arizona State University, Phoenix, AZ, United States of America

Mohammed El Amine Bekara, Aurélie Courcoul and Benoit Durand
University Paris Est, Anses, Laboratory of Animal Health, Epidemiology Unit, Maisons-Alfort, France

Jean-Jacques Bénet
University Paris Est, National Veterinary School of Alfort (ENVA), EpiMAI Unit, Maisons-Alfort, France

Sara Schärrer and Patrick Presi
Veterinary Public Health Institute/University of Berne, Berne, Switzerland

Jan Hattendorf and Jakob Zinsstag
Swiss Tropical and Public Health Institute/University of Basel, Basel, Switzerland

Nakul Chitnis
Swiss Tropical and Public Health Institute/University of Basel, Basel, Switzerland
Fogarty International Center, National Institutes of Health, Bethesda, Maryland, United States of America

Martin Reist
Federal Food Safety and Veterinary Office, Bern, Switzerland

Soo Jin Jeon, Manhwan Oh, Won-Sik Yeo and Kwang Cheol Jeong
Emerging Pathogens Institute, University of Florida, Gainesville, Florida, United States of America
Department of Animal Sciences, Institute of Food and Agricultural Sciences, University of Florida, Gainesville, Florida, United States of America

Klibs N. Galvão
Department of Large Animal Clinical Sciences, College of Veterinary Medicine, University of Florida, Gainesville, Florida, United States of America
D. H. Barron Reproductive and Perinatal Biology Research Program, University of Florida, Gainesville, Florida, United States of America

Sudarvili Shanthalingam, Subramaniam Srikumaran, William J. Foreyt and Kevin Lahmers
Department of Veterinary Microbiology and Pathology, Washington State University, Pullman, Washington, United States of America

Thomas E. Besser, Kathleen A. Potter and J. Lindsay Oaks
Department of Veterinary Microbiology and Pathology, Washington State University, Pullman, Washington, United States of America
Washington Animal Disease Diagnostic Laboratory, Washington State University, Pullman Washington, United States of America

E. Frances Cassirer
Idaho Department of Fish and Game, Lewiston, Idaho, United States of America

Gelin Xu, Zhizhong Zhang, Qiushi Lv, Yun Li, Ruidong Ye, Yunyun Xiong, Yongjun Jiang and Xinfeng Liu
Department of Neurology, Jinling Hospital, Nanjing University School of Medicine, Nanjing, Jiangsu Province, China

Mary M. Christopher
Department of Pathology, Immunology and Microbiology, University of California Davis, Davis, CA, 95616, United States of America

Michelle G. Hawkins
Department of Medicine and Epidemiology, University of California Davis, Davis, CA, 95616, United States of America

Andrew G. Burton
William R. Pritchard Veterinary Medical Teaching Hospital, University of California Davis, Davis, CA, 95616, United States of America

Mats Gunnar Andersson
Department of Chemistry, Environment and Feed Hygiene, The National Veterinary Institute, Uppsala, Sweden

Céline Faverjon
INRA UR346 Animal Epidemiology, VetagroSup, Marcy L'Etoile, France

Flavie Vial
Veterinary Public Health Institute, DCR-VPH, Vetsuisse Fakultät, Bern, Switzerland

Loïc Legrand
LABE´O - Frank Duncombe, Unité Risques Microbiens (U2RM), EA 4655, Normandie Universite, Caen, Normandy, France

Réseau d'EpidémioSurveillance en Pathologie Equine (RESPE), Caen, France

Agnès Leblond
Réseau d'EpidémioSurveillance en Pathologie Equine (RESPE), Caen, France
INRA UR346 Animal Epidemiologyet Département Hippique, VetAgroSup, Marcy L'Etoile, France

Miles A. Nunn
Centre for Ecology and Hydrology, Wallingford, Oxfordshire, United Kingdom

Tom A. August
Centre for Ecology and Hydrology, Wallingford, Oxfordshire, United Kingdom
University of Exeter, Exeter, Devon, United Kingdom

Amy G. Fensome
Biosciences, College of Life and Environmental Sciences, University of Exeter, Exeter, Devon, United Kingdom

Danielle M. Linton
Wildlife Conservation Research Unit, Oxford University, Oxford, Oxfordshire, United Kingdom

Fiona Mathews
Biosciences, University of Exeter, Exeter, Devon, United Kingdom

Index

www.ingramcontent.com/pod-product-compliance
Lightning Source LLC
Chambersburg PA
CBHW061247190326

41458CB00011B/3603